Immune Modulation Agents and Their Mechanisms

IMMUNOLOGY SERIES

NOEL R. ROSE

Professor and Chairman
Department of Immunology and
Infectious Diseases
The Johns Hopkins University
School of Hygiene and Public Health
Baltimore, Maryland

1. Mechanisms in Allergy: Reagin-Mediated Hypersensitivity
   Edited by Lawrence Goodfriend, Alec Sehon and Robert P. Orange
2. Immunopathology: Methods and Techniques
   Edited by Theodore P. Zacharia and Sidney S. Breese, Jr.
3. Immunity and Cancer in Man: An Introduction
   Edited by Arnold E. Reif
4. *Bordetella pertussis:* Immunological and Other Biological Activities
   J.J. Munoz and R.K. Bergman
5. The Lymphocyte: Structure and Function (in two parts)
   Edited by John J. Marchalonis
6. Immunology of Receptors
   Edited by B. Cinader
7. Immediate Hypersensitivity: Modern Concepts and Development
   Edited by Michael K. Bach
8. Theoretical Immunology
   Edited by George I. Bell, Alan S. Perelson, and George H. Pimbley, Jr.
9. Immunodiagnosis of Cancer (in two parts)
   Edited by Ronald B. Herberman and K. Robert McIntire
10. Immunologically Mediated Renal Diseases: Criteria for Diagnosis and Treatment
    Edited by Robert T. McCluskey and Giuseppe A. Andres
11. Clinical Immunotherapy
    Edited by Albert F. LoBuglio
12. Mechanisms of Immunity to Virus-Induced Tumors
    Edited by John W. Blasecki
13. Manual of Macrophage Methodology: Collection, Characterization, and Function
    Edited by Herbert B. Herscowitz, Howard T. Holden, Joseph A. Bellanti, and Abdul Ghaffar
14. Suppressor Cells in Human Disease
    Edited by James S. Goodwin

15. Immunological Aspects of Aging
    Edited by Diego Segre and Lester Smith

16. Cellular and Molecular Mechanisms of Immunologic Tolerance
    Edited by Tomáš Hraba and Milan Hašek

17. Immune Regulation: Evolution and Biological Significance
    Edited by Laurens N. Ruben and M. Eric Gershwin

18. Tumor Immunity in Prognosis: The Role of Mononuclear Cell Infiltration
    Edited by Stephen Haskill

19. Immunopharmacology and the Regulation of Leukocyte Function
    Edited by David R. Webb

20. Pathogenesis and Immunology of Treponemal Infection
    Edited by Ronald F. Schell and Daniel M. Musher

21. Macrophage-Mediated Antibody-Dependent Cellular Cytotoxicity
    Edited by Hillel S. Koren

22. Molecular Immunology: A Textbook
    Edited by M. Zouhair Atassi, Carel J. van Oss, and Darryl R. Absolom

23. Monoclonal Antibodies and Cancer
    Edited by George L. Wright, Jr.

24. Stress, Immunity, and Aging
    Edited by Edwin L. Cooper

25. Immune Modulation Agents and Their Mechanisms
    Edited by Richard L. Fenichel and Michael A. Chirigos

Other Volumes in Preparation

Immune Modulation Agents and Their Mechanisms

edited by

Richard L. Fenichel

Group Leader, Senior Research Scientist
Division of Experimental Therapeutics
Wyeth Laboratories, Inc.
Philadelphia, Pennsylvania

Michael A. Chirigos

Biological Response Modifiers Program
National Cancer Institute—Frederick
Cancer Research Facility
Frederick, Maryland

MARCEL DEKKER, INC. New York and Basel

Library of Congress Cataloging in Publication Data
Main entry under title:

Immune modulation agents and their mechanisms.

(Immunology series ; 25)
Includes index.
1. Immune response--Regulation. 2. Immunopharmacology. I. Fenichel, Richard L., [date].
II. Chirigos, Michael A. III. Series: Immunology series ; v. 25. [DNLM: 1. Adjuvants, Immunologic--pharmacodynamics. W1 IM53K v.25 / QW 800 I29]
QR186.I43 1984 616.99'40795 84-17468
ISBN 0-8247-7178-8

MARCEL DEKKER, INC.
270 Madison Avenue, New York, New York 10016

Current printing (last digit):
10 9 8 7 6 5 4 3 2 1

PRINTED IN THE UNITED STATES OF AMERICA

Preface

Over the past 20 years scientists studying the biological interactions between the tumor and the host, both in laboratory and clinical studies, have acknowledged that biological response modifiers (BRMs) will most likely have a role in cancer treatment. An appreciation of the clinical potential of BRMs has developed slowly. Like chemotherapy in the early 1940s, the usefulness of BRMs was met with skepticism. This was based on the initial clinical responses, with a limited number of BRMs, which resulted in a less significant response than was anticipated.

Biological response modifiers, which have also been referred to as immunomodulators, immunoaugmentors, immunostimulators, and immunorestoratives, are agents which can modify the relationship between the tumor and host by modifying a host's cellular immune response to tumor cells, with resultant therapeutic benefit. The modification can occur by one or several mechanisms: (a) by augmenting antitumor immunity by modulating cellular components of the immune system and inducing or restoring effector cells of immunity, including identifiable subsets of lymphocytes, cells of the monocyte-macrophage lineage, and natural killer cells; or (b) by protecting and/or reconstituting stem cell replication in bone marrow, which would also increase the ability of the host to tolerate damage by cytotoxic modalities of cancer treatment.

The possibility of augmenting the host response through selective modification of various components of the immune response has been demonstrated in animals with various chemicals, natural products, and physiological factors. Therapeutic benefits have been achieved by such an augmentation in tumor-bearing animals. Although similar beneficial effects in man will be necessarily far more difficult to achieve, some encouraging though tentative results have been reported in patients with certain types of cancer. The results with such agents suggest a prolongation of survival (with or without disease) and/or an increase in the remission duration induced by conventional therapy.

The purpose of this book is to provide a critical review of the studies dealing with biological response modifiers and their influence on immune functions and mechanisms through which effector cells are modulated. It will be informative and of interest to physicians, medical students, immunologists, immunopharmacologists, experimental and clinical oncologists, and other health professionals.

Michael A. Chirigos
Richard L. Fenichel

Contributors

Willem K. Amery Department of Clinical R & D, Janssen Pharmaceutica N. V. Research Laboratories, Beerse, Belgium

Tadao Aoki Research Division, Shinrakuen Hospital, Niigata, Japan

Anna Bartocci Immunopharmacology Section, Biological Therapy Branch, Biological Response Modifiers Program, National Cancer Institute-Frederick Cancer Research Facility, Frederick, Maryland

David Berd Thomas Jefferson University, Philadelphia, Pennsylvania

Uwe F. Bicker Product Development International, Boehringer Mannheim GmbH, Mannheim, Federal Republic of Germany

Nancy J. Bump Division of Protein Chemistry, Tufts University School of Medicine, Boston, Massachusetts

Nigel A. Byrom Immunology Unit, Department of Chemical Pathology, Westminster Medical School, London, England

Richard A. Carrano Department of Preclinical Research, Adria Laboratories Inc., Columbus, Ohio

Jan L. Ceuppens Laboratory of Clinical Immunology, Department of Medicine, University of Leuven School of Medicine, Leuven, Belgium

Joseph Chang Division of Experimental Therapeutics, Wyeth Laboratories, Inc., Philadelphia, Pennsylvania

Goro Chihara Bioactive Substances Research Laboratory, National Cancer Center Research Institute, Tokyo, Japan

Michael A. Chirigos Chief, Immunopharmacology Section, Biological Therapy Branch, Biological Response Modifiers Program, National Cancer Institute–Frederick Cancer Research Facility, Frederick, Maryland

Michel Colot Institute for Applied and Experimental Oncology, University of Vienna, Vienna, Austria

Cecil S. Cummins Department of Anaerobic Microbiology, Virginia Polytechnic Institute and State University, Blacksburg, Virginia

N. R. Di Luzio Department of Physiology, Tulane University School of Medicine, New Orleans, Louisiana

Julie Y. Djeu Center for Drugs and Biologics, Division of Virology, Food and Drug Administration, Bethesda, Maryland

Linda Eglin Department of Haematology, The University of Cape Town Medical School, Cape Town, South Africa

Gerald J. Elfenbein Division of Medical Oncology, Department of Medicine, The J. H. Miller Health Center, University of Florida, Gainesville, Florida

Judith A. Falk Department of Surgery, University of Toronto, Toronto, Ontario, Canada

Rudolf E. Falk Departments of Surgery and Pathology, University of Toronto, Toronto, Ontario, Canada

Isaiah J. Fidler* Cancer Metastasis and Treatment Laboratory, National Cancer Institute–Frederick Cancer Research Facility, Frederick, Maryland

Leo Filion Clinical Science Division, Department of Surgery, University of Toronto, Toronto, Ontario, Canada

William E. Fogler† Cancer Metastasis and Treatment Laboratory, National Cancer Institute–Frederick Cancer Research Facility, Frederick, Maryland

Bruce Freundlich Department of Medicine, Rheumatology Clinic, University of Pennsylvania, Philadelphia, Pennsylvania

H. Hugh Fudenberg Professor and Chairman, Department of Basic and Clinical Immunology and Microbiology, Medical University of South Carolina, Charleston, South Carolina

John P. Gibson Department of Pathology and Toxicology, Merrell Dow Pharmaceuticals, Inc., Cincinnati, Ohio

Theodore Ginsberg Newport Pharmaceuticals International, Inc., Newport Beach, California

Allan L. Goldstein Department of Biochemistry, The George Washington University School of Medicine and Health Sciences, Washington, D.C.

Current affiliations:

*Stribling Professor and Chairman, Department of Cell Biology, University of Texas. System Cancer Center, M.D. Anderson Hospital and Tumor Institute, Houston, Texas

†University of Texas System Cancer Center, M.D. Anderson Hospital and Tumor Institute, Houston, Texas.

James S. Goodwin Department of Medicine, University of New Mexico School of Medicine, Albuquerque, New Mexico

Francis J. Gregory Department of Microbiology, Wyeth Laboratories, Inc., Radnor, Pennsylvania

John W. Hadden Program of Immunopharmacology, Department of Internal Medicine, University of South Florida Medical Center, Tampa, Florida

Nicholas R. Hall Department of Biochemistry, The George Washington School of Medicine and Health Sciences, Washington, D.C.

Junji Hamuro Central Research Laboratories, Ajinomoto Co., Inc., Yokohama, Japan

Klaus Hartung* Division of Cancer Treatment, National Cancer Institute–Frederick Cancer Research Facility, Frederick, Maryland

John R. Hobbs Department of Chemical Pathology, Immunology Unit, Westminister Medical School, London, England

Fred K. Hoehler Newport Pharmaceuticals International, Inc., Newport Beach, California

William W. Hoffman Central Research Division, Pfizer Inc., Groton, Connecticut

Christian Hörig Janssen Pharmaceutica N. V. Research Laboratories, Beerse, Belgium

Anthony R. Imondi Department of Pharmacology, Adria Laboratories Inc., Columbus, Ohio

John D. Iuliucci Department of Safety Evaluation, Adria Laboratories Inc., Columbus, Ohio

Peter Jacobs Department of Haematology, The University of Cape Town Medical School, and Groote Schuur Hospital, Cape Town, South Africa

Ernest L. Jones Department of Physiology, Tulane University School of Medicine, New Orleans, Louisiana

Alan J. Lewis Division of Experimental Therapeutics, Wyeth Laboratories, Inc., Philadelphia, Pennsylvania

Teresa L. K. Low Department of Biochemistry, The George Washington University School of Medicine and Health Sciences, Washington, D.C.

James K. Luce Clinical Oncology Department, Adria Laboratories Inc., Columbus, Ohio

Henry C. Maguire, Jr. Division of Dermatology, Department of Medicine, Hahnemann University Medical School, and Thomas Jefferson University, Philadelphia, Pennsylvania

Leonard Makowka Departments of Surgery and Pathology, University of Toronto, Toronto, Ontario, Canada

Michael J. Mastrangelo Thomas Jefferson University, and Temple University School of Medicine, Philadelphia, Pennsylvania

---

*Current affiliation: Bundeswehrkrankenhaus, Klinische Medizin. Labor, Koblenz, Federal Republic of Germany.

Georges Mathé Service des Maladies Sanguines et Tumorales and Institute de Cancérologie et d'Immunogénétique, Villejuif, France

Rose B. McNamee Department of Physiology, Tulane University School of Medicine, New Orleans, Louisiana

Herbert Megel Department of Pathology and Toxicology, Merrell Dow Pharmaceuticals Inc., Cincinnati, Ohio

Michael Micksche Department of Immunodiagnosis and Immunotherapy, Institute for Applied and Experimental Oncology, University of Vienna, Vienna, Austria

Frederick L. Moffat Department of Surgery, Toronto General Hospital and University of Toronto, Toronto, Ontario, Canada

Victor A. Najjar Division of Protein Chemistry, Tufts University School of Medicine, Boston, Massachusetts

Bruce C. Nisula Development Endocrinology Branch, National Institute of Child Health and Human Development, National Institutes of Health, Bethesda, Maryland

James A. Page Medical Division, Adria Laboratories Inc., Columbus, Ohio

Vasilios Papademetriou Immunopharmacology Section, Biological Therapeutics Branch, Biological Response Modifiers Program, National Cancer Institute–Frederick Cancer Research Facility, Frederick, Maryland

Mario Piccoli* Immunopharmacology Section, Biological Therapeutics Branch, Biological Response Modifiers Program, National Cancer Institute–Frederick Cancer Research Facility, Frederick, Maryland

Keith M. Ramsey Center for Drugs and Biologics, Division of Virology, Food and Drug Administration, Bethesda, Maryland

P. Reizenstein Division of Hematology, Karolinska Hospital and Institute, Stockholm, Sweden and Visiting Professor, Institute de Cancérologie et d'Immunogénétique, Villejuif, France

Gerard Renoux Laboratoire d'Immunologie, Faculté de Médecine, Tours, France

Micheline Renoux Laboratoire d'Immunologie, Faculté de Médecine, Tours, France

Erich Schlick† Immunopharmacology Section, Division of Cancer Treatment, National Cancer Institute–Frederick Cancer Research Facility, Frederick, Maryland

Lionel N. Simon‡ Newport Pharmaceuticals International, Inc., Newport Beach, California

Julita A. Teodorczyk-Injeyan Department of Surgery, University of Toronto, Toronto, Ontario, Canada

Kwong Yok Tsang Department of Basic and Clinical Immunology and Microbiology, Medical University of South Carolina, Charleston, South Carolina

---

Current affiliations:
*Institute of General Pathology, State University of Rome, Rome, Italy.
†The Laboratory of Molecular Immunoregulation, National Cancer Institute, Frederick, Maryland.
‡International Pharmaceutical Products, Costa Mesa, California.

Atsushi Uchida* Institute for Applied and Experimental Oncology, University of Vienna, Vienna, Austria

Roy D. Welker Immunopharmacology Section, Division of Cancer Treatment, National Cancer Institute–Frederick Cancer Research Facility, Frederick, Maryland

David L. Williams Department of Physiology, Tulane University School of Medicine, New Orleans, Louisiana

Robert B. Zurier Rheumatology Section, Department of Medicine, University of Pennsylvania, Philadelphia, Pennsylvania

*Current affiliation: Christie Hospital and Holt Radium Institute, Manchester, England.

Contents

Immune Modulation Agents and Their Mechanisms

Part I

Biological Response Modifiers
Their Influence on Immune Function

Introduction

Richard L. Fenichel Wyeth Laboratories, Inc., Philadelphia, Pennsylvania

My interest in immunomodulating agents began in 1972 when I read the paper of Stjernsward and co-workers (1) showing the depletion of lymphocte populations in breast cancer patients after radiation treatment and indicating the long recovery time needed for these cells to regain their important functions. The pioneering work of Drs. Gerard and Micheline Renoux with levamisole (2) expressed the concept of immunomodulation of lymphocyte function by a chemical compound and demonstrated its antitumor and antimetastatic activity in murine tumor models. My own research was translated into the origination and initiation of a research program on immunomodulating agents (3,4). Wy-18,251, a thiazolobenzimidazole that emerged from this program, is now in clinical trial.

Part I of this book focuses our attention on defined organic agents—natural products and synthetic polymers that have undergone extensive laboratory investigation. Many of these agents are presently in various phases of clinical trials. The last two summarizing chapters of the section, one on tumors and metastases, the other on autoimmune disease, attempt to put in perspective the role of biological response modifiers in these diverse disease states.

Agents such as diethyldithiocarbamate, thiazolobenzimidazoles, cytoxan, lentinan, isoprinosine, NPT-15,396, tilorone, lipoidal amines, thymosin peptides, *Carynebacter parvum*, cyclosporine, tuftsin, and synthetic polymers MVE-2 and NED 137, are critically examined in this section. Emphasis is placed on the ways they influence the cellular immune system, the correlation of their in vitro with in vivo activities, and their effect on the interrelationship of the cellular immune with the humoral immune systems. The therapeutic implications and applications of these drugs are thoughtfully considered and, where possible, the results of clinical trials are insightfully examined.

ACKNOWLEDGMENT

I thank Dr. Maurits Dekker for encouraging me to undertake this project. The help of the staff of Marcel Dekker in solving the many problems faced during the preparation of these manuscripts is acknowledged with my thanks and appreciation. I thank Ms. Marsha Garsky and Ms. June Deitz for their help with the voluminous correspondence associated with this book. Special acknowledgment is made to Shirley Fenichel whose searching questions concerning resistance factors in cancer initiated my interest in immunomodulating agents. I particularly thank my daughter, Ms. Marilyn Fenichel, for her advice and guidance during the preparation of this book. Through her help, obstacles were overcome, crises were ameliorated, and continuity was maintained. Her assistance is gratefully acknowledged with my sincere appreciation.

REFERENCES

1. J. Stjernsward, M. Jondal, F. Vansky, and R. Sealy, *Lancet*, *2*:1352 (1972).
2. G. Renoux and M. Renoux, *Nature, New Biol.*, *240*:217 (1972).
3. R. L. Fenichel, F. J. Gregory, and H. E. Alburn, *Brit. J. Cancer*, *33*:329 (1976).
4. R. L. Fenichel, H. E. Alburn, P. A. Schreck, R. Bloom, and F. J. Gregory, *J. Immunopharmacology*, *2*:491 (1980).

Section A
Defined Organic Immunomodulating Agents

1

Diethyldithiocarbamate (DTC)

A Biological Augmenting Agent Specific for T Cells

Gerard Renoux and Micheline Renoux Laboratoire d'Immunologie, Faculté de Médecine, Tours, France

I. INTRODUCTION

When progress in clinical immunology revealed immune impairment or dysfunction associated with allergies, autoimmune diseases, infectious diseases, and cancers, it became tempting to develop agents that acted on the immune system, primarily for the treatment of cancer patients. The first clinical trials dealt with the systemic administration of bacille Calmette Guérin (BCG) to patients with acute lymphocytic leukemia (1), or the intralesional injection of BCG into metastases of malignant melanoma (2). The results generated exaggerated expectations of BCG therapy, and provided the impetus for the empirical utilization of a number of bacterial or biological products.

Almost simultaneously, our work on levamisole allowed us to express the concept that chemically defined compounds can modulate lymphocyte function in a way that could be better controlled than by the use of ill-defined biologicals.

Since the levamisole story has already been reviewed (3) and its present status is described in this volume (4), we will limit ourselves to a few introductory remarks we believe useful for the understanding of the pathways that led to our studies of sodium diethyldithiocarbamate (DTC).

We found the activities of levamisole on immune responses by using both a "prepared mind" and a 7% solution of an antihelminthic drug (Nemecide, Specia), the racemic isomer of 2,3,5,6-tetrahydro-6-phenylimidazo (2,1-b)thiazole hydrochloride, later known by us as tetramisole (Janssen). The first experiments, performed in 1969, were repeated

The name *Imuthiol* is now replacing the previous abbreviation DTC (for sodium diethyldithiocarbamate), as the latter could be confused with the chemotherapeutic agent DTIC, dimethyl-triazeno-imidazole-carboxamide.

and extended prior to communication (5-9), as we were well aware that they might introduce a new approach to immunostimulation.

Indeed, it marked the start of an extensive interdisciplinary research effort to investigate the effects of tetramisole and its optical isomers on the various host-defense mechanisms. However, conflicting data revealed an ambivalent influence of levamisole on T-cell responses. We therefore attempted to develop a synthetic sulfur compound devoid of the inhibitory effects of levamisole, which were likely associated with the cholinergic-like activity of the imidazole moiety (10, 11).

An overall appreciation of the reports on immunotherapeutic agents led us to conceptualize the following specifications and requisites for candidates to be suitable immunopharmacological agents for clinical trials. The agent should have defined influences on sets or subsets of immunocompetent cells as its essential activity. Known toxic levels and pharmacological effects should delineate the range of doses and predict most side effects. The absence of carcinogenicity, of tumor-promoting influence, and of antigenicity or sensitizing effect, is an essential prerequisite inasmuch as the agent will be administered for long periods of time to patients already at risk. Such requirements would reasonably eliminate most of the inconsistencies which have dampened confidence in most therapies used to modify the immune system. Immunomodulation remains a fascinating approach to the treatment, and even prevention, of the diseases where immunological disturbances have been demonstrated.

The present work reports immunopharmacological studies on sodium diethyldithiocarbamate (DTC), based along the aforementioned lines. DTC was selected from a large series of sulfur-containing drugs (12), seeking to obviate the ambivalent effect of levamisole and also to obtain an agent devoid of the sensitizing influence of thiazole or benzol ring structures (13). Available data show that DTC fulfills safety requirements and exerts a unique influence on the T-cell lineage. Furthermore, and interestingly, studies on the mode of action of DTC have provided new insights into the relationships between the immune system and other regulatory systems, the endocrine liver and the central nervous system.

II. PHARMACOLOGY IN ANIMAL AND MAN

The pharmacological characteristics of DTC have been extensively studied as it was known as a chelating agent employed in chemistry and agriculture and in the treatment of nickel poisoning. Taken from a recent review (14), the main features of interest for the immunopharmacologist follow.

A. Chemistry and Toxicology

Sodium diethyldithiocarbamate (DTC), mol wt 171, is obtained by reacting diethylamine with carbon disulphide in the presence of sodium hydroxide. Purified DTC (Institut Mérieux, Lyon, France) is a white, crystalline powder, readily soluble in water, buffers, and culture media; slightly alkaline buffers (pH 7.6-7.8) are preferable. Its acute toxicity for rodents and dogs is low ($LD_{50} > 2.5$ g/kg body weight). Chronic toxicity tests in rodents, dogs, or monkeys, evidence that DTC is devoid of side effects unless doses in excess of 200 mg/kg/day are employed for 3 months or more. DTC is not a sensitizing (haptenlike) agent for mice, guinea-pigs, and rabbits, and is devoid of pyrogenicity.

At doses ranging from 0.5 to 25 mg/kg, DTC has no effect on the weight of treated animals. However, administration of 2.5 mg/kg DTC prevents the wasting disease caused in mice by a phenol fraction of *Brucella melitensis*, and 25 days later induces a weight increase above that of normal, healthy controls.

In contrast with immunoadjuvants of bacterial origin, DTC does not lead to spleno-, adeno-, or hepatomegaly; indeed DTC, administered at the time of immunization, induces some splenocontraction, in comparison with animals immunized with sheep red blood cells. Treatment with DTC leaves unchanged the total number of nucleated spleen cells yet increases the percent of viable cells, in comparison with controls.

1. Absence of Carcinogenicity: Anticancer Effects

A recent study from The National Cancer Institute (15) reports a bioassay conducted by administering DTC in feed for 104-109 weeks to F 344 rats and (B6 C3)F_1 mice. Survival was not affected, and no clinical change could be related to administration of the drug. The high dose (about 140 mg/day) significantly prolonged the survival of female mice. The incidence of tumors in the experimental groups was not significantly higher than in the controls; furthermore, the incidence of certain spontaneous tumors, including lymphomas, was lower in the experimental groups than in the corresponding control groups.

As a free radical scavenger and through its effects on liver enzymes, DTC modifies the metabolic pathway of carcinogens, thereby protecting against a variety of chemically induced malignant tumors, such as those resulting from exposure to nitrosamines, polycyclic hydrocarbons, dimethylhydrazine, or azodyes. DTC inhibits in rats the nephrotoxicity of cis-platinum and reduces its gastrointestinal toxicity, without altering its antitumor efficacy (16-18). DTC was also found to regulate and potentiate bleomycin tumoricidal activity (19).

2. Detoxifying, Antibiotic, Radioprotective Effects

DTC is a nonmutagenic agent, which protects against the lethal effects of ionizing radiations better than cysteamine, dimethyldithiocarbamate, or tetraethylthiuram disulfide.

DTC has in vitro and in vivo antibiotic effects against a variety of bacteria, fungi, and parasites. It is of interest that DTC kills *Plasmodium falciparum* (20) or *Mycobacterium leprae* (21) by an antimetabolic mechanism, at doses inactive on mammalian cells.

DTC, through its action on monooxygenases, prevents and even cures the development of chemically induced diabetes and protects liver cells against the toxic effects of chemicals, such as chloroform, carbon tetrachloride, vinyl chloride, bromobenzene, benzopyrene, or paracetamol. It was also found to prevent excessive production of superoxydismutases.

These antibiotic and antitoxic activities should be of interest against the infections associated with immunodeficiencies and cancers, as well as in combined chemoimmunotherapy.

Most of these data on beneficial antitoxic or anticancer effects of DTC result from assays with doses higher than those that suffice for immunostimulant efficacy. Nevertheless, they attest to a safety factor for DTC use as a biological augmenting agent without fear of carcinogenicity or tumor-enhancing activity.

B. Clinical Pharmacology

Phase I-II studies were undertaken in informed-consent volunteers affected with chronic bronchitis or primary lung cancer. Chronic bronchitis patients were divided into three groups treated, respectively, with a single IV administration of either 2.5, 5, or 10 mg/kg DTC; a fourth group received two injections of 5 mg/kg at 1-days intervals, and a fifth groups was made up of a double-blind study of the effects of 5 mg/kg. Cancer patients were treated with 5 mg/kg.

The pharmacological and clinical follow-up paid particular attention to the following parameters. *Clinics*: mood changes, fatigability, or excitation; headache; dizziness or drowsiness; modification of recent or ancient memory; anorexia; stomach pain and vomiting; diarrhea or constipation; blood pressure, pulse, retinoscopy; Achilles and knee reflexes; venous irritation. *Hematology*: complete blood counts, including platelets, hemoglobin, coagulation tests. *Biochemistry*: (1) blood: glucose, urea, creatinine, uric acid, ionogram, cholesterol and triglycerides, liver tests; (2) urine: complete analysis, including ionogram

No untoward side effects were observed, and in a current double-blind study on weekly repeated treatment with 5 or 10 mg/kg DTC, no clinical differences have been noted among patients. However, when DTC was rapidly injected, at whatever dose, patients complained of a burning pain in the epigastric area and limbs, which vanished within minutes at the arrest of injection. The treatment was fully accepted without trouble if slowly administered, in 30 min at least, and the dose diluted in 125 ml of solvent. Alternatively, DTC can be given via the oral route or by aerosol (current studies) without incident.

Biochemical parameters were not modified by the treatments with DTC. However, we observed a slight but significant ($p = 0.03$) decrease in blood pressure in patients with high pressure at day 0, and a reduction in blood sugar levels (e.g., from 8.2 to 5.4 mEquiv.) in three patients.

DTC has a regulatory effect on leukocyte and platelet counts in chronic bronchitis patients. Table 1 summarizes the findings in 16 patients treated with 10 mg/kg at day 0. Highly significant correlation tests ($p = 0.001$) evidence that the effect to restore near normal values, either too high or too low figures, is not due to change. The tendency toward a return to normal values might be associated with the anti-inflammatory properties of DTC (current studies).

Thus, immunostimulant doses of DTC are devoid of toxicity, adverse effects on brain activity, and synergic activity with sedative and anesthetics. Weekly oral administration of 1-10 mg/kg for 1 month to children also shows no untoward effects (J. M. Lang, personal communication).

Table 1 Regulatory Influence on Blood Cell Counts

	Day 0	Day 7
Leukocytes (X 1000)		
$\bar{m}$ low counts	6.2	6.6
$\bar{m}$ low counts	17	12
Polymorphonuclears (%)		
$\bar{m}$ low counts	55.7	61.1
$\bar{m}$ high counts	80.2	70.6
Platelets (X 1000)		
$\bar{m}$ low counts	257	326
$\bar{m}$ high counts	741	593

III. EXPERIMENTAL IMMUNOSTIMULATION

As a biological response modified, DTC demonstrates a unique influence on the T-cell lineage, without affecting B cells.

A. Responses to Hetero- or Alloantigens and to Mitogens

DTC induces the production of immunoglobulin G (IgG) antisheep red blood cells (SRBC) circulating antibodies, a T-cell triggered event, as early as day 6 after immunization, whereas the level of specific IgM antibodies in serum is significantly reduced in comparison with untreated, immunized controls (22). A single administration in a range of doses between 0.5 and 25 mg/kg at various time intervals in relation to the antigenic stimulus (SRBC) in different mouse strains, elicits a marked increase in the number of IgM and of IgG plaque-forming spleen cells (PFC), whereas the nonspecific IgM-PFC response to horse red cells is abolished (22).

The kinetics of the DTC effect on functional activation was evaluated in C3H/He and BALB/c mice immunized with SRBC and simultaneously treated with 25 mg/kg DTC, and also by giving to C3H/He mice, at time intervals separated from SRBC immunization, various amounts of DTC suspended in drinking water. Table 2 shows that increased IgG-α SRBC responses were attained as early as day 2 and sustained for the 7 days of observation in treated mice of either strain, in comparison with controls. As indicated by Fig. 1, DTC

Table 2 The Influence of DTC on the Kinetics of the Primary Anti-SRBC Responses in Mice[a]

	Controls		Treated	
	C3H/He			
Day	IgM	IgG	IgM	IgG
1	362 ± 94	22 ± 8	346 ± 104	28 ± 10
2	537 ± 80	35 ± 8	1250 ± 148	121 ± 20
3	4895 ± 979	1383 ± 230	12,410 ± 1117	2927 ± 384
4	40,380 ± 8500	10,695 ± 2620	97,698 ± 10,170	27,390 ± 1660
5	20,450 ± 8250	25,130 ± 3610	20,785 ± 2370	35,435 ± 4650
6	3280 ± 710	10,390 ± 2840	2855 ± 1070	23,070 ± 3050
7	4159 ± 622	2502 ± 416	2515 ± 589	7383 ± 988
	BALB/c			
1	109 ± 34	11 ± 4	152 ± 28	17 ± 6
2	626 ± 72	70 ± 15	1890 ± 410	165 ± 40
3	15,020 ± 4020	1772 ± 210	21,950 ± 4600	7425 ± 1360
4	31,616 ± 2755	3987 ± 556	45,944 ± 2374	9586 ± 1075
5	10,909 ± 1328	5106 ± 1032	19,263 ± 3450	13,115 ± 967
6	6542 ± 1248	4875 ± 1250	8670 ± 1790	7966 ± 1175
7	2627 ± 935	1627 ± 315	4340 ± 360	2385 ± 275

[a]Female, 16-18 week old mice were immunized IV with 10^8 SRBC and simultaneously treated by SC injection of 25 mg/kg DTC or saline in controls. IgM- and IgG-antibody plaque-forming cells (PFC) were evaluated as PFC/10^6 splenocytes ± SE in five mice per group and day.

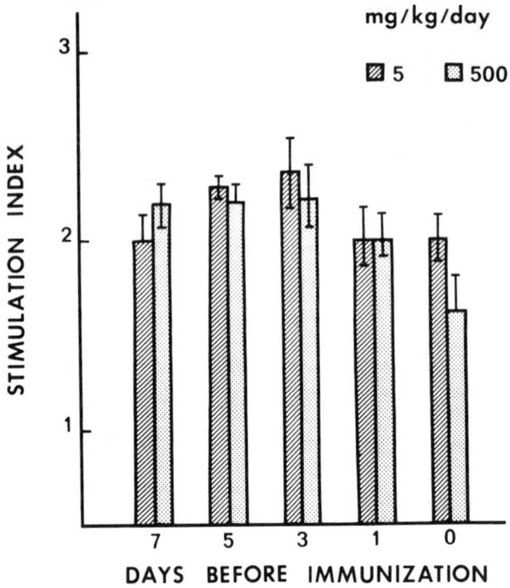

Figure 1 Effects of oral administration of DTC on the anti-SRBC response of female C3H/He mice. DTC was given in the drinking water during the time indicated and administered amounts were estimated on the basis of 2.2 ± 0.3 ml of water per mouse and per day (mean of 100 control mice and 100 treated mice). Counts of IgG plaque-forming spleen cells were performed 4 days after IV immunization with 10^8 SRBC.

was as active by the oral as via systemic administration, since as little as 5 mg/kg ingested induced increased functional activities at each time interval tested. The data show also that 1-week pretreatment with DTC caused augmented responses at a magnitude similar to administration concomitant with immunization. Moreover, DTC did not evidence time- or dose-dependent inhibitory influences.

A single injection of 2.5 or of 25 mg/kg DTC elicits in mice immunized with SRBC higher and more sustained levels of delayed-type hypersensitivity (DTH) than in controls (22). It is of interest for the planning of further studies and correlation with clinical assays to emphasize the finding that a high dose of DTC, 25 mg/kg, amplifies the feeble response induced by immunization with an excess of antigen (10^8 SRBC), whereas a low dose of the agent, 2.5 mg/kg, increases the already positive DTH response to a suboptimal dose (10^5 SRBC). It is also noteworthy that DTC impairs the immediate antibody-mediated hypersensitivity to dinitrophenol (DNP) and enhances the delayed hypersensitivity to bovine gammaglobulin (BGG) in guinea pigs immunized with BGG-DNP (23).

The kinetics of the DTC effect on mitogen-induced lymphoproliferation was evaluated in C3H/He, BALB/c, and C57B1/6 mice after a SC injection of 25 mg/kg DTC. As shown in Fig. 2, after an early decrease, lymphocytes of treated BALB/c mice show responses to stimulation by phytohemagglutinen (PHA) or concanavalin A (ConA) increased above controls at day 7 post-treatment, whereas C3H/He cells exhibit a double-peaked response curve to T-cell mitogens, the first peak appearing as early as 1 hr after treatment. In contrast, Fig. 2 evidences a striking dissociation of the influence of DTC on the responses of C57B1/6 cells to PHA or ConA. While ConA-induced lymphoproliferation is stimulated early after treatment with DTC, the response to PHA is symmetrically

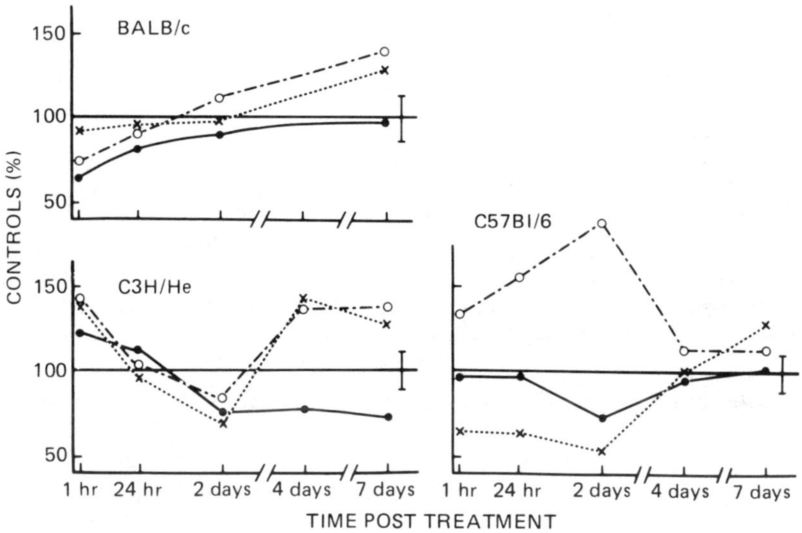

Figure 2 Kinetics of the influence of DTC on the proliferative responses to mitogens of female BALB/c, C3H/He, or C57B1/6 mice. DTC (25 mg/kg) was administered SC at time zero. Lymphoproliferative responses to PHA (X), ConA (○), or PWM (●) were assessed by [^{3}H] thymidine incorporation after 3 days in triplicate cultures at 37°C in a 5% CO_2 atmosphere following addition of 0.5 μC-labeled thymidine for the last 18 hr of incubation. n = five DTC-treated and five saline-treated mice per day.

inhibited, suggesting a preferential proliferation of the Lyt-1$^+$ subpopulation evoked by in vivo administration of DTC might be subjected to a genetic regulation. Responses to pokeweed mitogen (PWM), a B-cell mitogen in mice, are either unaffected or depressed. DTC alone is not a mitogen, as background counts in the absence of lectins are similar in DTC-treated and control mice (data not shown).

The delayed influence of DTC to increase PHA- or ConA-induced labeled thymidine incorporation was even more marked in guinea pigs, which augmented responses were attained not earlier than day 12 posttreatment (24). The data confirm that DTC should act indirectly to increase T cell-mediated responses.

DTC exerts a dose-dependent influence on the lymphoproliferative response to allogeneic antigens. C3H/He mice were treated either by 2.5 mg/kg or 25 mg/kg DTC, 4 days prior to sacrifice, and their spleen cells cocultured with mitomycin-treated C57B1/6 (H-2$\underline{b}$) spleen cells for 3-7 days. Results show that a 2.5-mg dose did not modify the mixed lymphocyte culture (MLC) response, whereas 25 mg/kg DTC markedly increased this response during the entire period of observation; they suggest that the agent could modify amounts of cell-surface antigens (manuscript in preparation).

B. Cytotoxic Responses

DTC could increase natural cytotoxic (NK) activity, depending on age of mice and on the dose, and at time periods differing from those where interferon and interferon inducers are active (25). These studies suggest complex relationships with features of the host and its ability to develop increased NK activity. The finding that a treatment with 25 mg/kg DTC significantly augmented NK activity of 26-week-old mice whose spontaneous response was lowered by age, might be of practical as well as basic interest, since NK-increased responses were obtained without involving augmentation of endogenous interferon levels (25).

C. Influence on Immunosuppression by Chemotherapeutic Agents

DTC was administered chronically (25 mg/kg three times a week for 4 weeks) to BALB/c mice treated for 4 weeks with cyclophosphamide (CY), azathioprine (AZA), or cortisone acetate, (HC) (26). DTC administered alone for 1 month stimulates the host to increased T cell-associated responses. Chronic treatment with the chemotherapeutic agents impairs or inhibits mitogen-induced lymphoproliferation and antibody response. DTC, administered simultaneously with AZA or HC, elevates these responses to levels comparable with those of mice treated with DTC alone, and partially restores the responses abrogated by CY. The results affirm the influence of DTC on T cells, the activities of which are suppressed by AZA.

Current studies have already shown that DTC has no direct influence on macrophages (27), nor does it modify antibody-dependent cell-mediated cytotoxicity for chicken red cells.

IV. INFLUENCE OF DTC ON IMMUNE PARAMETERS IN MAN

Low doses of DTC (0.5-2.2 mg/kg) administered prior to surgery prevent the immunodepression associated with surgical trauma, but also suffice to restore to normal values, and even more, the lymphocyte responses to T-cell mitogens that have been altered by cancer (28), without effects on PWM-induced response. A similar efficacy lasting for about 7 days is observed after treatment with 5 mg/kg for patients whose immune responsiveness was seriously impaired by chronic pulmonary infection (28, 29). The above data suggest that the restoring ability of DTC might depend on the PHA/ConA ratio observed before treatment more than on the magnitude of labeled thymidine incorporation. Either a defective PHA-responsive subset or a defective ConA subpopulation would result in DTC-increased responses, but not fully restored at day 7, whereas a similar impairment of both T-cell subsets would allow for a full restoration, as shown in Table 3. Since the net [^{3}H] thymidine incorporation response of a total, mixed-cell population exposed to ConA or PHA reflects not only the activity of mitogen-reactive cells, but also positive and negative interactions among subclasses of lymphocytes, more studies would be essential to understand the finding. If confirmed by further assays with other doses of the agent and in various conditions, the appraisal of PHA/ConA ratio prior to treatment will help to tailor the dose of DTC to fit the patient's needs. The background responses, in the absence of mitogens, were 638 ± 504 at day 0 (prior to treatment), 737 ± 541 at day 1, 482 ± 343 at day 2 and 554 ± 400 at day 7 in the treated groups, and very similar to those of untreated controls.

DTC has no significant influence on the immunoglobulin and complement levels, apart from those cases where an excess of IgA or of complement could be associated with an acute inflammatory process.

These studies have also shown a regulatory influence of DTC on the number of peripheral blood T cells. Counts of E rosettes were performed at day 0 (before treatment), than at days 1, 2, and 7 after administration of either 5 mg/kg (20 patients) or 10 mg/kg (16 patients). Table 4 summarizes the data on day 0 and day 7, as day 1 or day 2 results did not significantly differ from those of day 0, providing additional evidence that DTC

Table 3 Influence of the PHA/ConA Ratio on DTC-Induced Stimulation

PHA/ConA Ratio	Patients (N)		Day of Test 0	1	2	7
≃1	1	PHA[a]	9574	48,479	42,946	ND
		ConA	11,310	29,694	49,720	ND
	16	PHA	29,579	57,226	63,613	32,291
		ConA	28,109	21,742	32,231	47,340
	10	PHA	40,199	36,888	34,958	59,337
		ConA	42,014	32,588	22,876	54,327
<0,5	6	PHA	831	3454	8734	14,265
		ConA	6039	ND	13,259	15,733
	8	PHA	5282	24,112	14,586	24,700
		ConA	10,508	7859	7170	26,459
>2	5	PHA	14,804	39,242	ND	13,253
		ConA	4777	5047	18,596	24,652
	9	PHA	30,290	32,970	56,649	ND
		ConA	4600	40,541	45,745	ND
	13	PHA	11,714	14,260	10,794	36,599
		ConA	5855	2951	4415	18,266

[a]Mean cpm of triplicate assays. In 149 healthy controls, 25-35 years of age, corresponding values were: PHA, 38,635 ± 8488; ConA 41,415 ± 8935 (28).

has an indirect mode of action. In a study nearing completion, endogenous interferon levels are evaluated before and 2, 6, and 24 hr and days 2 to 7 after an intravenous administration of either 5 or 10 mg/kg DTC. In 27 patients, no variation in interferon levels is observed that differed from minor spontaneous changes in control untreated patients. The DTC-induced changes in immune responsiveness are obtained in man without intervention of interferon.

In a current study (manuscript in preparation), a single treatment with 10 mg/kg, or repeated administration of either 2 mg/kg or 5 mg/kg DTC in chronic pulmonary infections or bronchogenic cancers (a double-blind study), restored to control values the responses to T-cell mitogens and did not affect the response to PWM and seems to regulate to normal values the relative percentages of T-cell subsets, evaluated by monoclonal antibody assays.

Table 4 The Regulatory Effect of DTC on E Rosettes

Treatment[a]	Day of Sampling[b] 0	+7	Significance
5 mg/kg			
11 patients	54.1	60.1	$p = 0.01$
9 patients	73.6	63.2	$p < 0.01$
10 mg/kg			
8 patients	62.2	66.9	$p = 0.07$
8 patients	76.7	69.3	$p < 0.06$

[a]Chronic bronchitis patients.
[b]Tests performed on fasting individuals and between 8:30 and 9:30 a.m. to minimize bioperiodicity.

The data confirm that in man as in animals, DTC is neither a mitogen, a polyclonal activator, nor an interferon inducer. DTC regulates the activities of the T-cell lineage, and without apparent direct effects on B cells.

V. MECHANISMS OF ACTION

The increase in T-cell associated events which follows systemic administration of DTC is accompanied by an augmentation in the numbers of splenic Thy–1$^+$ cells (30), of Qa–1^a cells (31), and of the amount of Lyt–1 antigen (current studies). Administered to congenitally athymic mice, DTC induces the in vivo acquisition of specific T-cell markers by precommitted and undifferentiated percursor spleen cells and concomitant functional immune activation, without modifying the percent of B (CR$^+$) cells (14, 29, 30, 32, 33).

A. DTC as a Trigger of Hormonal Production

The finding that DTC replaces a signal missing in nu/nu mice allowing futther differentiation steps in the T-cell lineage and increasing the number of T cells and their functional activation in athymic mice, suggested to us that DTC was able to trigger, or augment, the production of a hormone specific for T cells and inactive on B cells.

The serum of DTC-treated nu/nu mice, like the serum of treated thymus-bearing mice, allows precursor spleen cells of nu/nu mice to differentiate in vitro into Thy–1$^+$ cells in a 3.5-hr induction assay, whereas even 18-hr incubation did not increase the percentage of B (CR$^+$) cells (32 - 34).

As little as 0.01 ml of serum of a DTC-treated mouse suffices to convert 7-12% HTLA$^-$ human lymphocytes into T (HTLA$^+$) cells, and to increase ConA-induced proliferation, without appreciable modification in the percentage of B cells. Moreover, the serum of DTC-treated mouse induces blast cells that are suppressive in mixed lymphocyte culture (MLC) tests (35).

DTC promotes or stimulates the in vivo synthesis of a potent inducer of prothymocyte maturation and acquisition of functional activities, an inducer active across the species barrier.

B. The Liver as a Site for the Synthesis of a Specific T-Cell Inducer

As DTC is able to trigger in athymic mice the production of a specific inducer of T-cell maturation, it seems obvious that the thymus is not required for such synthesis. Accordingly, spleen, kidney, lymph node, and liver were tested for their ability to produce the inducer in vitro, spontaneously or in the presence of DTC. The heat-stable fractions from either unconditioned or DTC (10^{-3}-10^{-10} mM/ml)-conditioned spleen, lymph nodes, or kidney cultures were unable to modify the spontaneous percentage (4 ± 3) of nu/nu spleen Thy–1$^+$ cells in induction assays.

In contrast, we found a heat-stable active T-cell differentiating and maturation factor (mol wt between 2 and 5 kD) in liver cultures (36). The product from unconditioned cultures induced appreciable T-cell differentiation in a range of doses between 10 pg and 500 ng/ml. The product from DTC-conditioned cultures was called hepatosin, to recall its origin. Between 1 pg and 1μg of hepatosin per ml induced prothymocytes to maximally express Thy–1, while as little as 100 fentograms also evoked appreciable induction. Throughout the entire range of tested concentrations, hepatosin generates only thymocytes and did not modify the percentage of B (CR$^+$) cells. Propanolol, a β-adrenergic blocking agent which ablates induction by ubiquitin (37), does not prevent induction of thymocytes by hepatosin. One can thus infer that hepatosin is not biologically related to ubiquitin.

The in vivo effects of hepatosin were determined in congenitally athymic nu/nu mice. The percent of Thy-1$^+$ or B (CR$^+$) spleen cells induced in vivo was evaluated 4 days after a subcutaneous dose of either 0.1, 0.01, or 0.001 μg per mouse, with four mice per group. As little as 1 ng/mouse of hepatosin induced appreciable T-cell differentiation, and the increase in the number of thymocytes induced in nu/nu mice by hepatosin appeared to be dose dependent (36). In vivo and in vitro hepatosin did not modify the percentage of spleenic B cells.

The activity of hepatosin cannot be ascribed to the remote presence of nonspecific, varied, or unrelated agents because the pharmacological agents already tested induce in vitro both T and B cells (37), whereas hepatosin induces only T cells in vivo and in vitro. A latent viral infection, either of cultured cells or of recipient nu/nu mice, cannot account for the findings since spleen, lymph node, or kidney supernatants from the same donor mice were ineffective, and control of in vitro or in vivo induction assays have few or no Thy-1$^+$ cells. Products of tissue breakdown remaining in supernatants do not explain the results, as control supernatants were devoid of influence. Finally, that ubiquitin (38) is not the active factor can be inferred from the inefficacy of hepatosin on the B-cell lineage, the lack of effect of propanolol on induction by hepatosin, and the ability of hepatosin to induce T cells after a single administration.

The evidence provided indicates that liver of normal mice synthetize a hormone specific for cells of the T-cell lineage and that DTC increases this production.

C. The Brain Neocortex Control the T-Cell Lineage and the Efficacy of DTC

The influence of DTC on the immune system and its efficacy against endotoxin-induced wasting disease suggested the operation of a central control (14,22). That neurological centers could influence normal host immune competence can be deduced from studies showing that destructive lesions of the hypothalamus, or of the pituitary, as well as chemical destruction of sympathetic nerve ending, decreases immune responsiveness, mostly in terms of antibody responses.

As the hypothalamus and the pituitary receive signals which modulate their activities, we postulated that other regions of the central nervous system could be involved in the modulation of immune responsiveness. Ablation of a part of the left cerebral neocortex indeed inhibited T-cell mediated responses and NK activities, as well as the serum levels of the T-cell specific inducer, while a similar lesion of the right neocortex had no other effects than a mere but reproducible increase in these activities. The number of activities of B cells were unchanged (14, 30, 39-45). The results demonstrate that the influence of the brain on the T-cell lineage is unequally represented between the two hemispheres in a population of laboratory rodents.

Experiments to determine the influence of the brain neocortex on the T-cell recruiting activity of DTC are nearing completion and will be published in detail elsewhere. In brief, administration of DTC to mice that underwent surgery 10 weeks earlier reconstitutes all the impaired responses in left decorticated animals, whereas treatment of right decorticated mice does not modify these responses, although they are not significantly different from those of the controls.

Taken together the data show that the cerebral neocortex controls a most elaborate arm of the immune system, the T-cell lineage. The impact of the cerebral neocortex on T cells is all the more interesting since the ablation involved approximately only one-third of the total left or right neocortex, and since the responses were measured 10 weeks afterwards at a time when a possibility exists for readaptation of cortical activities.

Present findings reveal hemispheric lateralization for the modulation of T-cell associated activities. The left brain neocortex maintains body integrity in response to environment through the control of the T-cell lineage, and an intact right neocortex is needed for the in vivo efficacy of DTC.

VI. DISCUSSION

The data obtained in these investigations show a unique influence of DTC on the immune system. From a practical point of view, DTC has no influence on B cells, on unspecific polyclonal activities of in vitro enhancing effects, but it does recruit T cells from precommitted precursors and induces T cells to generate enhanced levels of cytotoxic activities and responses to mitogens and alloantigens. Resting T cells are induced by DTC to develop suppressive activities, B cells to secrete antibodies of the IgG class, and monocytes and macrophages to participate in delayed-type hypersensitivities.

These actions are evoked in the absence of events initiated by other triggering influences, and contrast with those of other immunostimulants known to act as promoters to increase an already developing immune event, or as adjuvants to augment the responses to an antigen. It is noteworthy that DTC does not evince time- or dose-dependent characteristics to enhance or inhibit immune responses, a feature which clearly distinguishes DTC from other adjuvants or immunomodulators. DTC does not give rise to granulomatous disease, such as is induced by adjuvants of bacterial origin. DTC has no sensitizing or pyrogenic effects, and is not a carcinogenic agent.

That DTC is not an interferon inducer, although promoting increased NK activity, could be of practical interest, as J. Chany (personal communication) has found a synergistic effect of DTC and interferon against encephalomyocarditis virus infection.

Aware of the difficulties and pitfalls that could arise during the development of a biological augmenting agent, we deliberately adopted a slow pace for clinical testing. Now, more than 100 patients treated with 0.5-10 mg/kg DTC allow us to emphasize the absence of clinical toxicity and stress the T-cell restoring capacity of the agent. These preliminary assays will now safely permit clinical studies in those ailments where T-cell defects are involved. In addition, these studies provided a new glimpse of the complex relationships among the immune system, the endocrines, and the brain.

Since DTC and DTC-induced factors are neither active on B cells nor mitogenic or tumor promoting, their mechanism of action does not involve the mediation of a general lymphocyte activator such as produced by 2-mercaptoethanol and related thiols, including levamisole (reviewed in 46).

DTC, however, does not act directly to differentiate T cells but, through stimulation of the central nervous network, influences the endocrinological network to synthesize a hormone specific for the T-cell lineage.

The finding that DTC increases the liver synthesis of hepatosin, a specific T-cell inducer, indicated a new role for this organ already known as a main detoxifying site. Taken together, available results are consonant with the notion of a feedback regulation between hepatosin and thymic hormones; in this situation hepatosin would trigger the thymic release of active hormones, and the activated thymus would control the synthesis of hepatosin. Thymic activities are not a prerequisite for the elaboration of the inducer; the finding that extrathymic agents can lead to the production of T cells explains the preservation of T-lymphocyte functions in the elderly (47, 48).

The indirect effectiveness of DTC led to the discovery of a role displayed by the brain neocortex in the control of T-cell function and production of the specific hormone. The influence of the thymus, likely functioning as a relay, is under current study: in experiments on the distribution and fate of [^{35}S] DTC we found that radiolabeled DTC settles within minutes in brain neocortex, liver, and thymus and not in other organs or brain areas (manuscript in preparation). Importantly, these three organs are those involved in the regulation of T-cell function. Since an athymic animal treated with DTC can generate T cells, but an animal deprived of the right neocortex and then treated with DTC cannot increase the number and activitiy of its T cells, it is concluded that the primary site of action of DTC involves the brain neocortex and is controlled by it, and that DTC might replace a signal from the thymus.

More generally, the data suggest that brain lateralization for cognitive processes should be extended to immune recognition. The brain may control the immune mechanisms aimed at maintaining body integrity in response to environmental agression just as it controls behavioral and psychic mechanisms to maintain individual personality. Indeed, the central nervous system may well be the great organizer of diversity (GOD) which programs each segment of the immune system to adequately play its role, through the modulation of hormonal and pharmacological mediator synthesis.

DTC satisfies the criteria of an agent devoid of untoward side effects, carcinogenicity, and antigenicity, and with recruiting and regulating abilities on a set of immunocompetent cells. The data suggest it would be an effective agent for the treatment of syndromes and disease states where the underlying defect is a T-cell deficiency or dysfunction. It has already been of value as a tool for study of the relationships and mutual controls within the central nervous system, the endocrine liver, and the immune system.

ACKNOWLEDGMENTS

The work was supported by grants-in-aid from Institut Mérieux and in parts by the University of Tours, INSERM, Ligue Nationale contre le Cancer, Fondation Langlois, and New York Cancer Research Institute.

REFERENCES

1. G. Mathé, J. L. Amiel, L. Schwartzenberg, M. Schneider, A. Cattan, J. R. Schlumberger, M. Hayat, and F. de Vassal, *Lancet*, *1*:697 (1969).
2. D. L. Morton, R. R. Eilber, R. A. Malmgren, and W. C. Woods, *Surgery*, *68*:158 (1970).
3. G. Renoux, *Pharmacol. Ther. A.*, *2*:397 (1978).
4. J. Symoens, this volume.
5. G. Renoux and M. Renoux, *C. R. Acad. Sci. (Paris)*, *272 D*:349 (1971).
6. G. Renoux and M. Renoux, *C. R. Acad. Sci. (Paris)*, *274 D*:756 (1972).
7. G. Renoux and M. Renoux, *Nature* (New Biol.), *240*:217 (1972).
8. G. Renoux and M. Renoux, *Infect. Immunity*, *8*:554 (1973).
9. G. Renoux and M. Renoux, *J. Immunol.*, *113*:779 (1974).
10. J. W. Hadden, R. G. Coffey, E. M. Hadden, E. Lopez-Corrales, and G. H. Sunshine, *Cell. Immunol.*, *20*:98 (1975).
11. G. Renoux and M. Renoux, in *Control of Neoplasia by Modulation of the Immune System* (M.A. Chirigos, ed.), Raven Press, New York, 1977, p. 67.
12. G. Renoux and M. Renoux, *C. R. Acad. Sci. (Paris)*, *278 D*:1139 (1974).

13. N. W. Blacow (ed.), *Martindale The Extra Pharmacopoeia*, 26th ed., The Pharmaceutical Press, London, 1972, *passim*.
14. G. Renoux, *J. Pharmacol. (Paris)*, *13*:95 (1982).
15. National Cancer Institute, *Tech. Rep. Series* n° 172 (1979).
16. R. F. Borch and M. E. Pleasant, *Proc. Natl. Acad. Sci. USA*, *76*:6611 (1979).
17. R. F. Borch, J. C. Katz, P. H. Lieder, and M. E. Pleasant, *Proc. Natl. Acad. Sci. USA*, *77*:5441 (1980).
18. G. R. Gale and L. M. Atkins, *J. Clin. Hematol. Oncol.*, *11*:41 (1981).
19. P. S. Lin, L. Kwock, and N. T. Goodchild, *Cancer*, *46*:2360 (1980).
20. L. W. Scheibel, A. Adler, W. Trager, *Proc. Natl. Acad. Sci. USA*, *76*:5303 (1979).
21. K. Prabhakaran, E. B. Harris, and W. F. Kirchheimer, in *Pigment Cell* (V. Riley, ed.), Karger, Basel, 1976, p. 152.
22. G. Renoux and M. Renoux, *J. Immunopharmacol.*, *1*:247 (1979).
23. P. J. Neveu, *Clin. Exp. Immunol.*, *32*:419 (1978).
24. P. J. Neveu, D. Perdoux, and L. Lafleur, *Int. J. Immunopharmacol.*, *4*:9 (1982).
25. G. Renoux, P. Bardos, D. Degenne, and M. Musset, in *Natural Cell-Mediated Immunity* (R. B. Herberman, ed.), Academic Press, New York, 1982, p. 443
26. G. Renoux and M. Renoux, *Clin. Immunol. Immunopath.*, *15*:21 (1980).
27. P. J. Neveu, P. H. Lagrange, D. Thierry, and D. Perdoux, *Nouv. Rev. Franç. Hematol.*, *22*:139 (1980).
28. G. Renoux, M. Renoux, J. Greco, J. Baudoin, M. Lavandier, and E. Lemarié, in *Trends in Human Immunology and Cancer Immunotherapy* (B. Serrou and C. Rosenfield, eds.), Doin, Paris, 1980, p. 974.
29. G. Renoux and M. Renoux, in *Augmenting Agents in Cancer Therapy* (E. M. Hersh, M.A. Chirigos, and M. J. Mastrangelo, eds.), Raven Press, New York, 1981, p. 427.
30. G. Renoux, in *Trends in Human Immunology and Cancer Immunotherapy* (B. Serrou and C. Rosenfeld, eds.), Doin, Paris, 1980, p. 986.
31. G. Renoux and M. Renoux, *Abst. 4th Int. Congr. Immunol., Paris*, 1980, 3.3.21.
32. G. Renoux and M. Renoux, *J. Exp. Med.*, *145*:466, (1977).
33. G. Renoux, M. Renoux, L. Gyenes, and J. M. Guillaumin, *Int. J. Immunopharmacol.*, *2*:167 (1980).
34. G. Renoux, M. Renoux, J. M. Guillaumin, and C. Gouzien, *J. Immunopharmacol.*, *1*: 415 (1979).
35. G. Renoux, J. L. Touraine, and M. Renoux, *J. Immunopharmacol.*, *2*:49 (1980).
36. G. Renoux and M. Renoux, *Abst. 8th Int. Cong. Pharmacol. Tokyo*, 1981, p. 437.
37. M. P. Scheid, G. Goldstein, and E. A. Boyse, *J. Exp. Med.*, *147*:1727 (1978).
38. G. Goldstein, *Nature*, *147*:11 (1974).
39. G. Renoux, K. Biziere, M. Renoux, and J. M. Guillaumin, *C. R. Acad. Sci. (Paris)*, *290 D*:719 (1980).
40. G. Renoux, K. Bizière, M. Renoux, L. Gyenes, D. Degenne, J. M. Guillaumin, P. Bardox, and Y. Lebranchu, *Int. J. Immunopharmacol.*, *2*:156 (1980).
41. P. Bardos, D. Degenne, Y. Lebranchu, K. Bizière, and G. Renoux, *Scand. J. Immunol.*, *13*:609 (1981).
42. G. Renoux, K. Bizière, and M. Renoux, *Bull. Acad. Med. (Paris)*, *166*:88 (1982).
43. K. Bizière, M. Renoux and G. Renoux, *Neuroscience (suppl. to vol. 7)*:528 (1982).
44. G. Renoux, K. Bizière, P. Bardos, D. Degenne, and M. Renoux, in *Natural Cell-Mediated Immunity* (R. B. Herberman, ed.), Academic Press, New York, 1982, p. 639.
45. G. Renoux, K. Bizière, M. Renoux, and J. M. Guillaumin, *Scand. J. Immunol.* (1982), accepted for publication.
46. G. Hewlett, H -G. Opitz, and H. D. Schlumberger, in *Lymphokines*, vol. 4 (E. Pick and M. Landy, eds.), Academic Press, New York, 1981.
47. M. E. Weksler and T. H. Hutteroth, *J. Clin. Invest.*, *53*:99 (1974).
48. S. Gupta and R. A. Good, *J. Immunol.*, *122*:1214 (1979).

2

Thiazolobenzimidazole and Thiazolobenzothiazole Compounds as Biological Response Modifiers

Francis J. Gregory Wyeth Laboratories, Inc., Radnor, Pennsylvania

I. INTRODUCTION

For the past ten years we have been engaged in a search for chemical agents that are capable of modifying the immune response. Among many promising types of synthetic materials we studied, the most encouraging have been the thiazolobenzimidazoles and the thiazolobenzothiazoles. Many members of these two familes of compounds have effected rapid and reproducible changes in the immune response, resulting in suppression of metastatic disease in tumor-bearing animals; potentiation of cell-mediate immunity as measured by delayed hypersensitivity reactions in the guinea pig; increased numbers of T cells in the peripheral blood of rats on a dose-response basis; potentiation of lymphocyte proliferation of concanavalin A (ConA) activated lymphocytes; depression of circulating immunoglobulins in mice bearing genetic autoimmune disease; extension of the median survival time of animals suffering from systemic lupus erythematosis; stimulation of interleukin production; and stimulation of blastogenesis in cultures of phytohemagglutinin (PHA) sensitized lymphocytes from patients with bone marrow transplant.

Although hundreds of compounds have been synthesized in each family, extensive studies have been carried out with one representative of each of these two groups; their structures are shown in Fig. 1.

These two compounds were selected because Wy-18,251 showed the best stimulation of rosette formation of rat lymphocytes (1) and Wy-40,453 demonstrated the greatest ability to inhibit the production of immunoglobulin G (IgG) and IgM in the Cunningham modification of the Jerne plaque assay.

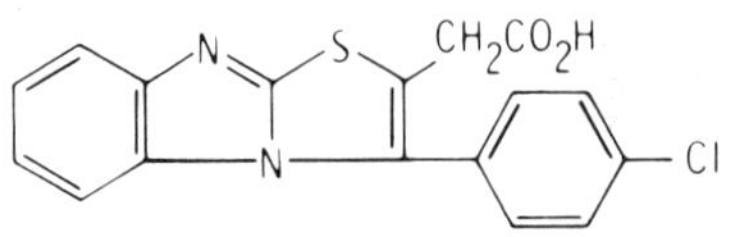

Wy-18,251

3-(p-chlorophenyl) thiazolo (3,2-a) benzimidazole-2-acetic acid

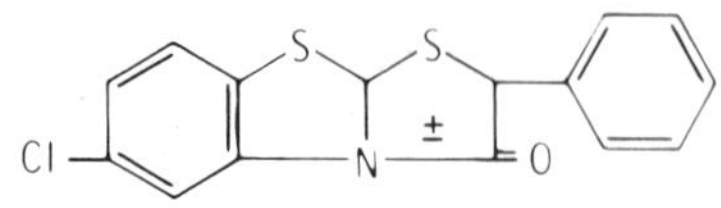

Wy-40,453

6-chloro-2-phenylthiazolo (2,3-b) benzothiazol-3 (2H)-one, mesoionic didehydro derivative

Figure 1 Thiazolobenzothiazole compounds.

II. THIAZOLOBENZIMIDAZOLES

An analog of Wy-18,251, 3-(p-chlorophenyl)-2, 3-dihydro-3-hydroxythiazolo [3,2-a] benzimidazole-2-acetic acid) (Wy-13,876), showed marked capacity to inhibit metastatic disease in Lewis lung-tumor-bearing mice (1), but was not cytotoxic as shown by its ED_{50} of 198 μg/ml against HEP-2 (human epidermal tumor) in vitro and a chronic LD_{50} (10 daily doses) of 263 mg/kg in mice. Wy-18,251 was selected to overcome the toxicity of the other compound for thyroid tissue. The following discussion summarizes the results obtained with Wy-18,251.

A. Effect on Maturation and Proliferation of T Lymphocytes

The incubation system for rosette formation was a modified form of the procedure of Siegel and Sherman (3) in which a 4:1 ratio of 2-aminoethylisothiouronium-bromide-treated guinea pig red blood cells, obtained by the method of Kaplan and Clark (4), was mixed with separated rat lymphocytes and the rosettes per 100 cells determined. The results (Table 1) indicate that Wy-18,251 increased the relative number of circulating T lymphocytes in the normal rat by over three-fold in some instances.

Elfenbein et al. (5) observed that transplant patients have cells which can be induced by Wy-18,251 in vitro to express the receptor for sheep erythrocytes as detected by rosette formation. The interpretation (based on studies with thymosin and levamisole) is that Wy-18,251 is driving the maturation of immature T cells. In a study on the effect of thymosin on rosetting of lymphocytes from patients with bone marrow transplants (5), Elfenbein et al. found that those showing normal rosetting behavior, for example patient B in Table 2, do not respond, but patients with impaired rosetting such as patient A, respond dramatically. He believes that Wy-18,251 is behaving in the same manner as thymosin in his detailed study.

Wy-18,251 was administered orally to normal rats and its effect on T-cell surface antigens was measured by the formation of a tertiary complex (antigen-antibody-complement) that injures the surface membrane, permitting entry of an indicator dye, trypan blue. The theta index, determined by counting the marked cells under a microscope, rose significantly with a single oral dose of 25 mg/kg or after three doses (one per day) of 7.5 or 10 mg/kg (Table 3).

Using mouse splenocyte cultures, Wy-18,251 could either stimulate or inhibit T-cell blastogenesis, although studies using peripheral lymphocytes from immunodepressed humans showed solely stimulation. Fenichel et al. (6) have shown that with enriched

Table 1 Effect of Wy-18,251 on T-Cell Marker Expression by Normal Rat[a] Lymphocytes

Dose[b] (mg/kg)	No. Doses	Rosettes/100 Cells[c] (Mean + SD)
0	1	1.6 ± 0.3
150	1	5.3 ± 0.7
0	1	3.0 ± 0.6
150	1	4.3 ± 0.9
0	1	5.0 ± 0.6
150	1	6.6 ± 0.3
0	2	1.7 ± 0.6
150	2	4.0 ± 0
100	2	3.0 ± 1
50	2	2.3 ± 1.2

[a]CD rats from Charles River Farms, Wilmington, Mass.
[b]Compound suspended in water and dosed by gavage once daily.
[c]For three groups of cells from three incubation tubes.

T-lymphocyte splenocyte cultures obtained from CBA/J mice (Charles River, Minnesota), in the presence of a suboptimal concentration of ConA (0.025 μg/culture), Wy-18,251 effectively increased lymphocyte proliferation at concentrations of 0.05, 0.1, 0.25, and 1 μg/culture (Table 4). A significant increase was not seem at 0.5 μg/culture. When Wy-18, 251 was cultured with enriched T lymphocytes in the absence of ConA, no significant proliferation was observed. In a further study by Fenichel et al. (7), they show that enriched T cells from tumor-injected mice treated with 5 mg/kg of Wy-18,251 display augmented mitogenic activity which correlates with increased T-cell function. Further, macrophages harvested from the peritoneal cavity of Lewis lung-tumor-bearing mice display significantly increased phagocytic activity against opsonized chicken red blood cell targets. However, in carbon clearance studies with non-tumor-bearing animals, phagocytosis was not stimulated (7). The fact that Wy-18,251-stimulated macrophages from tumor-bearing mice attack opsonized targets appears to indicate some degree of specificity.

Table 2 Effect of Wy-18,251 on Rosetting by Lymphocytes from Bone Marrow Transplant Patients

Wy-18,251 (μg/ml)	Rosettes/100 Cells: Patient A 1 hr	Patient A 18 hr	Patient B 1 hr	Patient B 18 hr
0	19	24	44	33.5
0.025	50	44.5	39	48.5
0.25	50.5	27	47	37.5
2.5	39	31.5	46.5	41.0

Table 3 Effect of Wy-18,2551 on T Surface Antigens of Rat Lymphocytes

Dose[a] (mg/kg)	No. of Rats	No. Doses	T-Lymphocyte Count (Theta Index) (Mean + SEm)
0	5	1	2.3 ± 0.7
15	5	1	3.3 ± 0.6
0	4	1	4.1 ± 0.8
20	4	1	5.7 ± 0.9
0	5	1	3.4 ± 0.7
25	5	1	7.7 ± 0.9[b]
0	4	1	2.6 ± 0.7
25	4	1	2.0 ± 0.4
0	5	3	3.3 ± 0.8
10	5	3	8.2 ± 1.4[b]
0	5	3	3.1 ± 0.6
7.5	5	3	7.7 ± 2.0[c]
0	4	3	1.9 ± 0.6
5	4	3	2.0 ± 0.5

[a]Suspended in PEG 400 and dosed PO by gavage once per day; blood samples obtained by cardiac puncture 18 hr postprandially.
[b]$p < 0.01$.
[c]$p < 0.05$.

When B lymphocytes were measured using fluorescence-conjugated rabbit-antirat IgG antiserum (Cappel Labs.) with cell suspensions from the control and treated groups (6), Wy-18,251 did not have any effect at doses of 50, 100, and 150 mg/kg PO given daily for 2 consecutive days.

B. Effect of Wy-18,251 on Interleukin 2

Interleukin 2 (IL2) is a soluble substance secreted by lymphoid cells which stimulates T-cell proliferation and has been reported to augment natural killer cell activity (8). Wy-18,251 has been shown to stimulate IL2 production in vitro at concentrations of 10-50 $\mu g/10^6$ cells (8). When an optimal dose of Wy-18,251 (50 $\mu g/10^6$ cells) was compared with an optimal dose of indomethacin (1 $\mu g/10^6$ cells), the level of stimulation caused by Wy-18,251 either exceeded or equaled that of indomethacin (Table 5). Cultures not responding to Wy-18,251 did not respond to indomethacin; these cultures often produced high levels of IL2 when stimulated by PHA alone (10).

C. Effect of Wy-18,251 on Delayed Hypersensitivity

Probably one of the most reliable indicators of drugs that affect the cell-mediated immune system is alterations in the delayed hypersensitivity (DH) reaction. Guinea pigs from Buckshire Breeders (Perkasie, Pennsylvania), weighing 200-300 g, were used with a de novo

Table 4 Effect of Wy-18,251 on $[^3H]$ Thymidine Uptake by Enriched Mouse T Splenocytes Cultured with Suboptimal Concentration of Concanavalin A

Agent	μg/Culture	μg/Culture	N	$[^3H]$ Thymidine CPM (Means ± SE)	Stimulation Index
Blank			4	1872 ± 159	
ConA		0.025	5	4703 ± 224[b]	
ConA + Wy-18,251		1.0	5	7088 ± 486[a]	1.5
		0.5	5	6677 ± 860	1.4
		0.25	4	7351 ± 540[a]	1.6
		0.1	5	10,822 ± 592[b]	2.3
		0.05	5	10,766 ± 1387[a]	2.3

[a]$p < 0.01$.
[b]$p < 0.001$.

antigen dinitrochlorobenzene (DNCB) following the procedure of Campbell et al. (11). The diameter of the hyperemic area of the skin surface was measured with Vernier calipers. The largest dimension was designated length, the dimension at right angles to it width, and the Student's t-test was employed to determine the significance of the difference in area from that of the control site. In order to increase the sensitivity of the animals to DNCB, they were previously immunosuppressed with a 200-mg/kg IP dose of cyclophosphamide (Cytoxan, Mead-Johnson). Wy-18,251 was administered orally by gavage. The results (Table 6) show that Wy-18,251 significantly potentiated the DH reaction at 50, 100, and 150 mg/kg; it was not effective at 25 mg/kg.

In another model designed to measure specificity of the augmentation of the subliminal delayed hypersensitive response, Lewis et al. (12) used mice injected in the hand paw with carrageenan to produce edema. Footpad swelling is measured after 3 and 24 hr

Table 5 Effects of Wy-18,251 and Indomethacin on In Vitro Production of Interleukin2 by Human Lymphocytes

Donor	Stimulation Index[b] Wy-18,251 (50 μg/10^6 cells)	Indomethacin (1 μg/10^6 cells)
CM[a] 136	1.7[c]	–
CM 140	2.5[c]	–
CM 146	7.3[c]	3.6[b]
CM 157	2.6[c]	1.3[b]
CM 158	2.0[c]	1.6[b]
CM 164	1.4[c]	1.8[b]
CM 150	–	2.6[b]
CM 155	0.74[c]	0.99
CM 156	0.83	0.99

[a]Conditioned medium prepared from lymphocytes of different donors according to the methods in Ref. 8.

$$^{b}SI = \frac{\text{Mean CPM of compound - stimulated culture}}{\text{Mean CPM of culture control}}$$

[c]$p < 0.05$.

Table 6 Effect of Wy-18,251 on the Delayed Hypersensitivity Reaction in Immunosuppressed Guinea Pigs

Dose (mg/kg)	No. Guinea Pigs	Area of Erythema (mm^2 = SEm)
0	20	444 ± 5
50	10	610[a] ± 48
25	10	508 ± 35
0	16	671[b] ± 40
150	7	913[b] ± 41
100	10	888[b] b 42
50	10	860[b] ± 46

[a] $p < 0.05$.
[b] $p < 0.01$.

using a mercury plethysmograph. The results (Table 7) indicate that Wy-18,251 is able to produce a reduction in the hindpaw edema over that of the control.

D. Wy-18,251 as an Adjuvant in Vaccine Prophylaxis

The adjuvant effect of Wy-18,251 was tested by Moore (13) with a vaccine designed for veterinary use, inactivated equine herpesvirus type I (EHV-1) vaccine, and by Hjorth (13) with one designed for human use, inactivated subunit A/Bangkok influenza virus vaccine. An antigen extinction type of hamster protection test is used for EHV-1 vaccine, and the ability of drugs to augment the protective effect of the vaccine is measured by survival time. All of the unvaccinated hamsters died from the infection as expected (Table 8), while vaccine in diluent along protected the animals at low dilutions with a PD_{50} of 22.4. The PD_{50} of 64.8 for Wy-18,251 at 5 mg/kg and 132 for the positive control, aluminum phosphate, both show enhancement or adjuvant activity.

Table 7 Effect of Levamisole and Wy-18,251 on Carrageenan Hindpaw Edema in Mice[a]

		3 hr		24 hr	
Treatment	Oral Dose (mg/kg)	Edema Volume (μl)	Change from Control (5)	Edema Volume (μl)	Change from Control (%)
Control	–	36 ± 4	–	15 = 4	–
Levamisole	3	39 ± 9	±9	15 = 3	0
	10	17 ± 5	-52	13 = 4	-13
	30	17 ± 5	-52	7 = 3	-53
Wy-18,251	0.1	41 ± 8	+14	16 = 4	+1
	1	35 ± 5	-3	5 = 6	-66
	10	27 ± 11	-25	8 = 4	-47

[a]Mice were treated with drug or vehicle 1 hr prior to carrageenan administration (0.1 ml of 0.01% solution). Each point represents the mean ± SE of six animals.

Table 8 Adjuvant Effects of Wy-18,251 and $ALPO_4$ in Hamster Protection Tests with Equine Herpesvirus Type I Vaccine

Antigen Dilution	Diluent Control	Dead/Total Wy-18,251 (5 mg/kg)	$AlPO_4$ (10 mg/kg)
12.5	1/5	0/5	0/5
25	3/5	2/5	1/5
50	4/5	2/5	1/5
100	5/5	2/5 1	1/5
200		5/5	3/5
400			5/5
PD_{50}[a]	22.4	64.8	132

[a]PD_{50} = The dilution of antigen which protects 50% of the hamsters; Reed-Meunch Analysis (12).

In measuring the adjuvant effect of Wy-18,251 on influenza virus vaccine, the elicitation of antibody in mice as determined by hemagglutination inhibition titers was employed (Table 9).

By either the Probit Analysis or the Spearman-Karber Analysis, it is evident that Wy-18,251, tested at 25 mg/kg, enhanced vaccine protection in a manner superior to that of the $AlPO_4$ control.

E. Effect of Wy-18,251 on Metastatic Disease

Six- to eight-week-old $B_6D_2F_1$ male mice weighing 19-21 g were used for the tumor studies. The tumor employed was mainly the Lewis lung (obtained from Fiddler), using a modification of a system described by James and Salsbury (15) for axillary implant studies, or modifications of the techniques described by Post and Fidler and colleagues (16-18) for footpad implants with or without surgical amputation. The stock tumor line was carried in the $C57BL_6$ mouse. Either trochar implants of 2-4 mm fragments of LL tumor or brei inocula of 2×10^6 viable cells were employed as inocula for the axillary region, while a brei inoculum of 1×10^5 cells in 0.05 ml of phosphate buffered saline (PBS) was always used for the footpad. The extent of metastatic disease after axillary implant was determined in the animals sacrificed after 13-16 days. The lungs were injected with 10% buffered formalin, removed, and immersed in this fixative. All lobes were sectioned and stained with hematoxylin eosin. The slides were coded and examined microscopically by a pathologist (J. Steinberg, Burlington Memorial Hospital, Burlington,

Table 9 Effects of Wy-18,251, Freund's Complete Adjuvant, and $AlPO_4$ in Antigen Extinction Tests with Influenza Vaccine

Treatment Group	Antigenic $Dose_{50}$: Probit Analysis	Antigenic $Dose_{50}$: Spearman-Karber Analysis
Diluent Control	1	19
Wy-18,251 (25 mg/kg)	2529	1398
Freund's complete adjuvant	22	33
$AlPO_4$ (5 mg/kg)	1918	1069

New Jersey) who recorded numbers and sizes of metastatic foci on all lung areas. The results obtained on two such assays may be found in Table 10 (6). In both assays trochar implants of tumor tissue in the right axilla were the inoculum, and drugs were administered once daily, intraperitoneally, for the duration of the assay (14 days for the first experiment and 13 days for the second).

Doses of 100 mg/kg or greater produced a significant reduction in metastatic disease; a dose of Wy-18,251 of 150 mg/kg reduced metastatic spread by 60% when compared with the vehicle-treated control animals. The low score achieved with cyclophosphamide is due to its excellent activity against the primary tumor.

In an additional study (6) three dose levels of Wy-18,251 were employed using four different dose regimens in an effort to establish the best combination. The inocula, 2×10^6 viable LL tumor cells, were implanted in the right axilla. Treatment was initiated 24 hr after challenge. The results, shown in Table 11, indicate that mice which received only one dose of Wy-18,251, and at the lowest dose level, had the best reduction in the number of metastases and in metastases per section.

Clearly, the best results were achieved by dosing 1 day/week which gave reductions in metastases per section of 57, 46, and 31% at doses of 50, 100, and 150 mg/kg, respectively. In addition, the overall best score of 57% reduction (metastases per section) or 58% reduction (mean number metastatic foci) was achieved by the lowest dose.

Following these observations, Wy-18,251 was evaluated in two subsequent assays using one IP dose per week with doses ranging from 5 to 50 mg/kg in one trial and 1 to 5 mg/kg in the second (6). The results, shown in Table 12, once again indicate that the greatest reduction in metastatic disease was achieved by the lowest dose levels of 5 mg/kg (59%) and 1 mg/kg (47%). Levamisole at 3 mg/kg also had a very respectable score of 70%.

When Wy-18,251 was evaluated in an assay in which the Lewis lung tumor is implanted in the $B_6D_2F_1$ mouse footpad (220,000 viable cells in 0.02 ml) and the tumor-bearing foot amputated on day 12, with dosing initiated on day 13, the mean and median survival times of treated and control mice evaluated, a minimal extension of survival time is often seen (Table 13). An analysis of variance using Dunnett's comparison was used to determine significant difference from the controls (19).

Table 10 Effect of High Doses of Wy-18,251 on Lewis Lung Metastases[a]

Drug	Dose (mg/kg)	N	Metastases Section (Mean)	Reduction (%)	Mice with Large Metastases (%)
Wy-18,251	25	15	1.50	6	33.3
Wy-18,251	100	12	1.17	25	16.6
Levamisole	25	14	1.21	24	28.5
Cytoxan	15	7	0.24	85	0
Vehicle control	–	16	1.58	–	43.8
Wy-18,251	150	11	0.33[b]	60	–
Wy-13,876[d]	150	10	0.51[b]	38	–
Vehicle control	–	9	0.82[c]	–	–

[a]Drugs administered intraperitoneally once daily for duration of assay.
[b]$p < 0.0005$.
[c]$p < 0.05$.
[d]3-(p-chlorophenyl)-2,3dihydro-3-hydroxythiazolo [3,2–a] benzimidazole-2-acetic acid.

Table 11 Effect of Varying Doses and Regimes upon the Antimetastatic Effect of Wy-18,251 Against the Lewis Lung Tumor

Dose Regime[a]	Dose (mg/kg)	N	No. Metas. (Mean + SE)	Metas./Sect. (Mean + SE)	Reduction (%)
MWF	50	10	23.3 ± 6.8	1.9 ± 0.44	+19
WThF	50	9	18.4 ± 2.6	1.14 ± 0.16	8
W	50	10	9.0 ± 2.3[b]	0.54 ± 0.14[b]	57
Daily	50	9	18.3 ± 4.9	1.14 ± 0.31	8
MWF	100	9	22.3 ± 3.8	1.43 ± 0.24	+16
WThF	100	8	12.0 ± 2.8	1.02 ± 0.16	18
W	100	10	11.4 ± 2.7	0.72 ± 0.17	46
Daily	100	10	22.3 ± 4.0	1.42 ± 0.27	+19
MWF	150	8	16.8 ± 4.4	1.00 ± 0.26	19
WThF	150	9	19.2 ± 2.6	1.13 ± 0.15	8
W	150	10	14.9 ± 3.8	0.85 ± 0.20	31
Daily	150	9	32.4 ± 5.6	1.76 ± 0.30	+43
Cytoxan MWF	25	10	2.00 ± 0.7[c]	0.13 ± 0.40[c]	95
Vehicle cont. daily	–	31	21.3 ± 3.2	1.23 ± 0.18	–

[a]All dosing intraperitoneal 24-hr after challenge.
[b]$p < 0.05$.
[c]$p < 0.0015$.

Table 12 Effect of Intraperitoneal Administration on One Dose Per Week of Wy-18,251 or Levamisole on Lewis Lung Metastases

Treatment[a]	Dose (mg/kg)	N	Metastases (Mean + SE)	Metas./Sect. (Mean + SE)	Reduction (%)
18,251	5	8	10.6 ± 2.5	0.76 ± 0.18[c]	59
18,251	10	7	22.3 ± 7.0	1.57 ± 0.50	15
18,251	25	6	30.8 ± 11.3	1.82 ± 0.62	2
18,251	50	10	20.0 ± 6.8	1.21 ± 0.41	35
Levamisole	3	6	9.3 ± 4.2[c]	0.56 ± 0.25[b]	70
Levamisole	25	7	15.1 ± 3.3	0.80 ± 0.18	57
Cytoxan	25	9	6.6 ± 1.1[d]	0.48 ± 0.08[d]	73
Control	–	17	28.8 ± 6.0	1.84 ± 0.36	–
18,251	1	18	13.9 ± 3.0[b]	0.96 ± 0.21[b]	43
18,251	3	18	19.7 ± 4.3	1.39 ± 0.31	24
18,251	5	20	16.6 ± 2.6	1.18 ± 0.18	35
18,251	50	17	15.5 ± 2.2	1.04 ± 0.16	43
CMC control	–	20	26.4 ± 5.2	1.81 ± 0.36	–

[a]Brei inoculation of 2.0×10^6 viable cells in axillary region. Intraperitoneal injection of agent started 24 hr after tumor cell implantation. Mice sacrificed on day 15.
[b]$p < 0.05$.
[c]$p < 0.03$.
[d]Dosed Monday, Wednesday, and Friday of each week.

Table 13 Effect of Wy-18,251 on Survival Time of Mice Dying from Metastatic Lewis Lung Tumor (Primary Tumor Removed Surgically)

Drug	Dose (mg/kg)	Regime	N	Survival Time Mean	Survival Time Median	p Value (Mantel-Haenszel)
Wy-18,251	5	1 time week	20	14.4	14.0	0.4433
Wy-18,251	5	2 times week	20	16.1	16.0	0.0309[a]
Wy-18,251	1	5 times week	20	15.6	15.0	0.1178[b]
Vehicle control	–	–	19	13.5	14.0	–

[a] $p < 0.05$.
[b] $p < 0.01$ day 13; < 0.02 day 14.

This is a severe test of a drug's antimetastatic activity since the highly virulent LL tumor begins metastasizing on days 5-7, and lung foci are probably well established by day 13 when dosing is initiated. Earlier treatment might show more dramatic results.

F. Effect of Wy-18,251 on Primary Tumor Growth

In all cases of tumor experimentation with Wy-18,251, primary tumor size was determined on day 12 or at sacrifice by measuring two dimensions and applying the formula mg = $L \times W^2/2$ or by excising and weighing the tumor. Significance of inhibition was determined according to the protocols of the National Cancer Institute (20). No significant reduction in primary tumor size by Wy-18,251 was observed in any of the experiments.

G. Summary of Studies on Wy-18,251

Wy-18,251, a noncytoxtoxic agent, is significantly active in reducing the spread of metastasis of the highly virulent Lewis Lung tumor in mice, even when severe tumor loads of 2×10^6 viable cells are used as inocula for primary tumor growth, and these evaluations based on histopathological examination of 1-μm sections of the entire lung. These studies indicate that maximum dose levels for this drug should generally be 1-5 mg/kg on a once weekly basis. The drug appears to have a biphasic response, so that excessive dose loads may be inactive or slightly stimulating to metastatic growth.

In other studies (1) it has been demonstrated that injection of antilymphocyte serum or antitheta serum can reduce the effectiveness of a close analog of Wy-18,251 (Wy-13,876) in preventing the establishment of metastatic foci. This drug increases the relative numbers of T cells in the peripheral blood of rats as shown by rosetting and by the more sensitive antigen-antibody assay, clearly demonstrating that T-lymphocyte stimulation is involved in the activity of this compound. Wy-18,251, therefore, should play a role in delayed hypersensitivity (DH) reactions. Accordingly, when evaluated in immunosuppressed guinea pigs sensitized against the de novo antigen dinitrochlorobenzene, Wy-18,251 markedly increased the DH reaction at oral doses ranging from 50 to 150 mg/kg. The accumulated evidence of the activities of Wy-18,251 described above points to its potential use as an antimetastatic agent, and also as a possible enhancer of immunomodifying activity in immunosuppressed patients with life-threatening infections in combination with anti-infective therapy. Its possible role in autoimmune disease requires clarification.

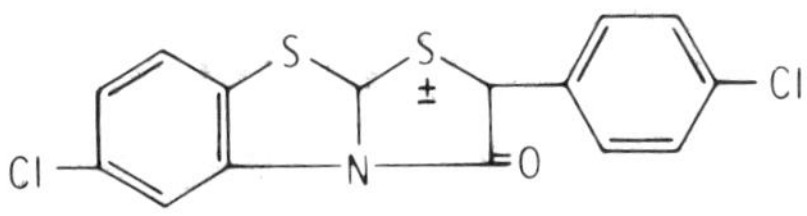

Wy-43,502

6-chloro-2 (4-chlorophenyl) thiazolo (2,3-b) benzothiazol-3(2H)-one, mesoionic didehydro derivative

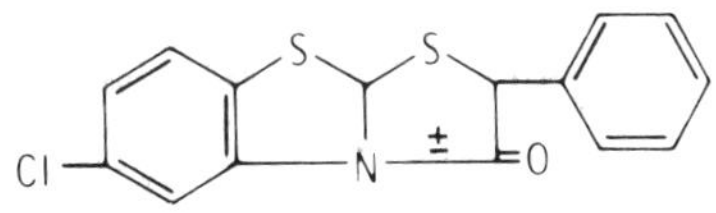

Wy-40,453

6-chloro-2 phenylthiazolo (2,3b) benzothiazole-3(2H)-one, mesoionic didehydro derivative

Figure 2 Thiazolobenzothiazole compounds.

III. THIAZOLOBENZOTHIAZOLES

The above two tricyclic thiazolobenzothiazole mesoionic compounds were the most active of a large number studied. These mesoionic compounds markedly inhibit immunoglobulin synthesis (20).

A. Antimetastatic Activity

When originally evaluated against metastatic disease using the Lewis lung tumor, it was noted that daily doses of 200 and 100 mg/kg of Wy-40,453 had a prometastatic effect as shown in Table 14. It was felt that once again this was a biphasic response and that antimetastatic results might be obtained with a minimal treatment of one dose, 1 day/week. The results of such an experiment are shown in Table 15.

The initial two assays were based on the histopathological examination of lung tissues as described previously. When the Wexler technique (21), employing India ink plus a bleaching fixative was employed, a similar result was obtained and the results, given in Table 16, show 85% inhibition of metastases with an intraperitoneal dose of 100 mg/kg on day 1 only, and 67% inhibition with a single intramuscular dose of 200 mg/kg. In

Table 14 Effect of Wy-40,453 on Lewis Lung Metastases[a]

Drug	Dose (mg)[b]	D/T	Primary Tumor (mg)[b]	Primary Tumor (T/C%)	Metastatic Tumor Total Metas.	Metastatic Tumor Metas./Sect.	Change Tumor Metas./Sect. (%)
Wy-40,453	200	0/10	810	58	411	2.22	+753
Wy-40,453	100	0/10	1070	77	127	0.45	+265
Wy-40,453	50	0/10	1140	82	24	0.12	-54
Wy-40,453	25	0/10	1530	110	54	0.27	+3
Wy-40,453	12.5	0/10	920	66	25	0.16	−39
Vehicle Cont.	–	0/13	1390	–	50	0.26	

[a]Implant = 1.2×10^6 cells in 0.1 ml right axilla.

[b] $M = \frac{L \times W}{2}$

Table 15 Effect of Intraperitoneal Administration of One Dose Per Week of Wy-40,453 on Lewis Lung Metastases[a]

Drug	Dose (mg/kg)	N	Metastatases (Mean + SE)	Metastases Section (Mean + SE)	Reduction (Metas./Sect.) %
Wy-40,453	50	9	12.6 ± 5.0[b]	0.87 ± 0.36[c]	54
Vehicle	–	17	28.8 ± 6.0	1.84 ± 0.36	–

[a]Brei inoculum of 2.0 $\times 10^6$ cells right axilla.
[b]$p < 0.052$, Kruskil-Wallis test.
[c]$p < 0.059$, Kruskil-Wallis test.

addition, there was activity when 5 mg/kg was given twice per week by either the intraperitoneal or intramuscular route.

An additional method we have employed to study the effect of drugs on metastatic disease is an assay in which the tumor is implanted in the footpad which is later amputated and the activity of the drug is measured by survival time. The technique is as follows.

Lewis lung tumor grown for 12-day days in $C57BL_6$ female mice is made into a brei by mixing one part tumor with three parts of minimum essential medium (MEM) media containing all of the additive described by Fidler (17) for maintenance of the B-16 melanoma cell line. Two-tenths of the finely divided brei is injected into the right hind footpad toward the front of the foot near the toes. On day 12 postinoculum (this date may be varied) all mice without at least a 10-mm tumor are discarded. The remainder (> 95%) are randomized into test groups and anesthetized with 20 mg/kg of sodium nembutal in 5% ethyl alcohol. The tumor-bearing foot is surgically removed, cauterized, and the wound treated with an antiseptic dressing, New Skin (New Skin Co., Cody, Wyoming). Dose regimens are usually initiated on day 1 postsurgery. Animals dying during the course of treatment are examined to confirm metastatic lung disease. Usually tumor tissue has replaced almost all of the normal lung tissue. Mean survival time (MST) calculations are computed beginning with the day prior to the first metastatic death in the controls. Treated-to-control-survival-time (T/C) ratios expressed as a percentage are computed as follows:

$$\frac{\text{MST treated}}{\text{MST control}} \times 100 = \text{T/C\%}$$

Table 16 Effect of Wy-40,453 on Metastatic Spread of the Lewis Lung Carcinoma as Evaluated by the Wexler Technique

Drug	Dose (mg/kg)	Regimen	Route	Primary Tumor T/C (%)	Avg. No. Metas. Fici	Reduction (%)
Wy-40,453	200	Day 1 only	IP	81	4.4	63
Wy-40,453	200	Day 1 only	IM	70	4.4	67
Wy-40,453	100	Day 1 only	IP	78	2.0	85
Wy-40,453	5	2 times/week	IP	84	6.4	52
Wy-40,453	5	2 times/week	IM	97	6.8	49
Levamisole	5	2 times/week	IP	101	12.1	10
Vehicle Control	–	2 times/week	IP	–	12.9	–

Table 17 Effect of Mesoionic Derivatives on Median Survival Time (MST) from Metastatic Disease

Drug	N	Dose (mg/kg)	Route	Regimen	MST (Days)	T/C (%)	Activity
Wy-40,453	24	100	IP	Day 1 only	14.3	124	Active
Wy-40,453	23	100	PO	Day 1 only	13.9	125	Active
Wy-40,453	23	100	IP	Every 14 days	15.3	138	Active
Wy-40,453	23	100	PO	Every 14 days	12.2	110	NS
Vehicle Control	24	–	IP	Every 14 days	11.1	–	–
Wy-40,453	10	50	IP	Day 1 only	19.0	170	Active
Wy-40,453	10	12.5	IP	Day 1 only	12.5	112	NS
Wy-40,453	10	5.0	IP	Day 1 only	11.8	105	NS
Wy-40,453	10	50	IP	1 time/week	13.4	120	NS
Wy-40,453	10	12.5	IP	1 time/week	13.7	122	NS
Wy-40,453	10	5.0	IP	1 time/week	18.4	164	Active
Wy-40,453	9	50	IP	2 times/week	16.0	143	Active
Wy-40,453	10	12.5	IP	2 times/week	14.4	129	Active
Wy-40,453	10	5.0	IP	2 times/week	17.3	154	Active
Wy-40,453	8	50	IP	Day 5 only	12.0	152	Active
Wy-40,453	8	12.5	IP	Day 5 only	10.4	93	NS
Vehicle Control	20	–	IP	2 times/week	11.2	–	–
Wy-40,453	10	25	PO	2 times/week	14.6	124	Active
Wy-40,453	10	50	PO	2 times/week	15.4	131	Active
Wy-40,453	9	25	IP	2 times/week	16.7	142	Active
Wy-40,453	10	25	IP	1 time/week	16.4	139	Active
Vehicle Control	20	–	IP	2 times/week	11.8	–	–

A drug giving a score of ⩾125% is considered active. The results obtained with Wy-40,453 and Wy-43,502 in a number of such assays may be found in Table 17.

It may be seen that both Wy-40,453 and Wy-43,502, given parenterally or orally, significantly extended the survival time of mice dying solely from metastatic disease. Again, smaller and less frequent doses seemed to yield the best results, indicating an agent with a biphasic response.

B. Effect on Antibody Production

The Cunningham modification (22) of the Jerne plaque assay (23) was employed to determine the effect of these drugs on antibody-secreting cells (ASCs). In these preliminary studies the only antigen employed was sheep red blood cells (SRBC). The results obtained with Wy-40,453 are shown in Table 18. Doses of 25-200 mg/kg significantly decrease the number of ASCs. Spleens appeared grossly normal, and spleen mass was unchanged.

In a series of additional assays in which only IgM plaques were measured, both Wy-40,453 and Wy-43,502 markedly inhibited antibody production as shown in Table 19.

C. Effect on Thymus Gland

In an attempt to define the mode of attack of Wy-40,453, animals were dosed with varying amounts of drug intraperitoneally for 9 consecutive days, sacrificed by cervical separation,

Table 18 Effect of Wy-40,453 upon Antibody Secreting Cells: Jerne Plaque Assay[a, b]

Control No.	Drug	(mg/kg)	IgM Plaques	IgG	p Values
16	Wy-40,453	200	110.643	22,875	<0.01
	Wy-43,502	200	74,025	0656	<0.01
	Vehicle	–	295,785	168,210	
17	Wy-40,453	200	55,518	117,337	$<0.001/0.01$
	Wy-43,502	200	50,250	49,218	<0.001
	Vehicle	–	142,143	242,570	<0.001
20	Wy-40,453	25	78,300	–	<0.01
	Vehicle	–	141,500	–	
21	Wy-40,453	25	66,600	–	<0.01
	Vehicle	–	135,300	–	

[a]CDF_1 mice immunized with 25% SRBC on day 0.
[b]Dosed on day 1, IgM read on day 4, and IgG read day 6.

and spleen, liver, lymph nodes, heart, thymus, and adrenals removed, weighed, and processed for histopathology. The only organ showing any abnormality was the thymus which was atrophied with a large weight loss (Table 20) and showed almost complete depletion of lymphocytes, with an otherwise normal structure on histological examination. Other groups of mice treated in a similar manner for 9 days and then allowed to rest for 2 weeks, showed on sacrifice a normal thymus both by weight and histopathological examination. The thymic effect was completely reversible.

D. Effect on Autoimmune Disease

Because of the profound activity of Wy-40,453 and Wy-43,502 in reducing serum antibody levels, it was decided to evaluate these compounds against an experimental model of autoimmune disease. Female NZB/W F_1 or MRL/1pr mice obtained from Jackson Memorial Laboratories, Bar Harbor, Maine, were employed in these studies. Mice were bled bimonthly from the retro-orbital sinus and the serum tested for IgG and IgM levels using quantitative immunodiffusion plates (25). Samples were pooled by cage, and standards and unknowns were assayed in duplicate. Antinuclear antibody (ANA) levels were also determined using an indirect immunofluorescent assay (26). In calculating these

Table 19 Effect of Two Mesoionic Derivatives upon IgM Plaque Formation

Assay No.	Drug	Dose (mg/kg)	PFC[a]	P Value[b]	Control PFC	Direction
68-79	Wy-40,453	100	63,992	0.001	209,012	↑
723-79	Wy-40,453	25	78,300	0.01	141,500	↑
729-79	Wy-40,453	25	66,600	0.01	135,300	↑
813-79	Wy-40,453	25	126,666	0.001	220,000	↑
614-79	Wy-43,502	200	74,025	0.01	295,285	↑
619-79	Wy-43,502	200	50,250	0.001	142,143	↑

[a]Plaque-forming cells.
[b]Student's T-test.

Table 20 Effect of Graded Doses of Wy-40,453 on Thymus Gland Weight

Compound	Dose (mg/kg)	D/T	Avg. Thymus Wt (mg)	Reduction (%)
Wy-40,453	400	1/15	6.7	86
Wy-40,453	200	4/15	13.3	73
Wy-40,453	100	1/15	21.0	56
Wy-40,453	50	0/15	34.2	29
Wy-40,453	25	1/15	40.3	16
Wy-40,453	12.5	0/15	42.3	12
Wy-40,453	6.25	0/15	38.1	21
Wy-40,453	3.125	2/15	40.2	16
Vehicle control	–	0/15	48	–

values an accuracy of ± 10% of the diffusion zone diameter reading was assumed. Time of death is recorded and median survival times computed and statistically evaluated according to the technique of Mantel-Haenszel (27). Survival curves for Wy-40,453, Wy-43,502, and levamisole may be seen in Figs. 3-5. Survival data are also expressed numerically in Table 21.

Histophathological examination of long-term survivors reveals renal changes consistent with long-term systemic lupus erythematosis. There have been no cures with this therapy to date. When IgG or IgM levels are plotted over an extended period of time, no useful pattern emerges that would be indicative of a favorable response (Fig. 6).

IV. SUMMARY

The immunomodifying effect of a thiazolobenzimidazole (Wy-18,251) has been described. The compound elevates circulating levels of T lymphocytes as indicated by increased

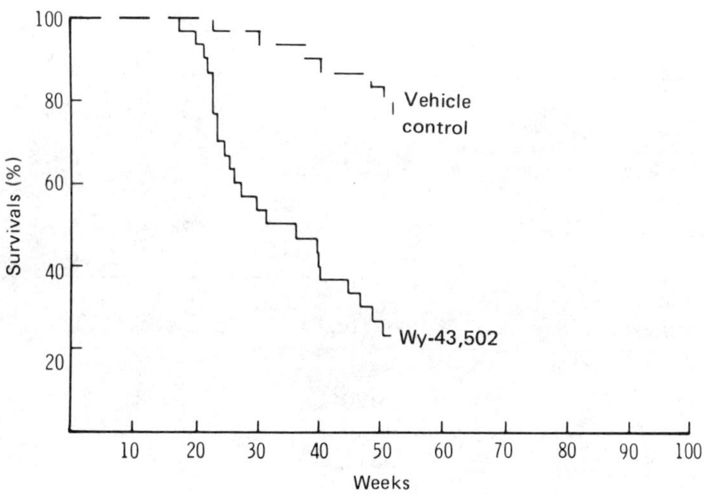

Figure 3 Effect of Wy-43,502 on survival of NZB/W mice.

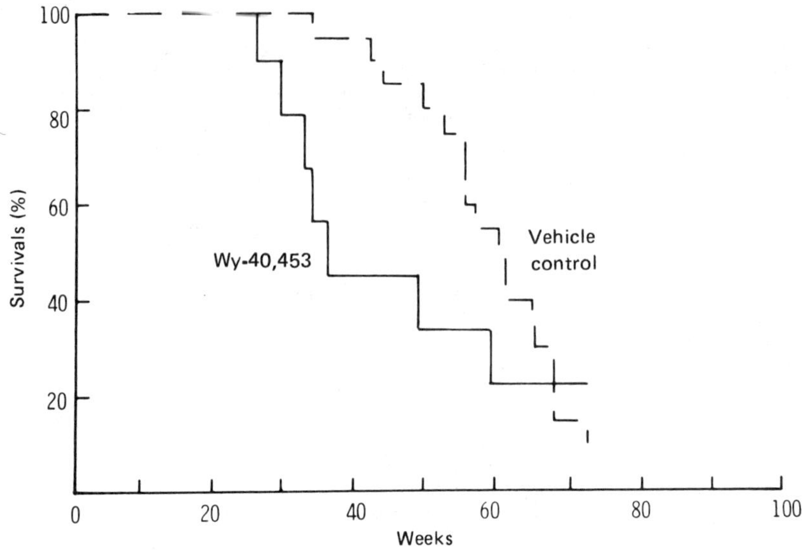

Figure 4 Effect of Wy-40,453 on survival time of NZB/W mice.

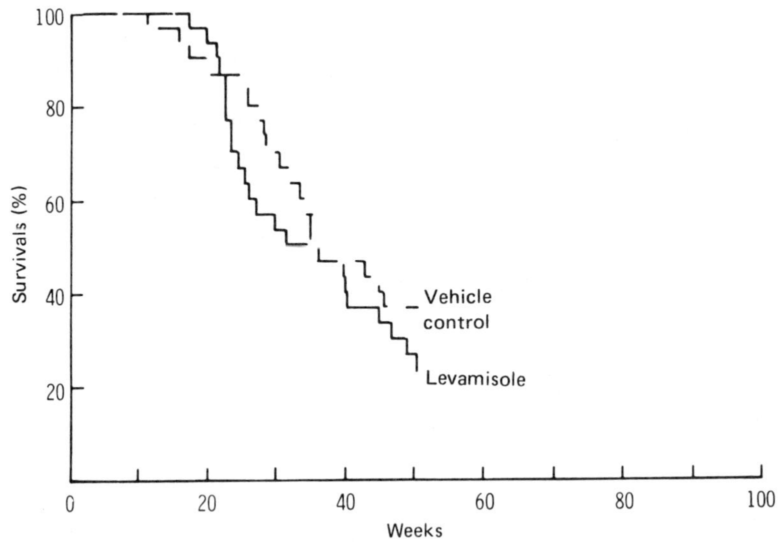

Figure 5 Effect of levamisole on survival time of NZB/W mice.

Table 21 Survival Rates of NZB/W F_1 Mice Treated with Mesoionic Derivatives and Levamisole

Drug	Dose (mg/kg)	ANA (58 weeks)	Alive/Total	Survival (72nd week) (%)
Wy-40,453	100	1:20	6/20	30
Wy-40,453	50	1:30	13/20	65
Wy-43,502	5	1:30	16/20	80
Saline	1 ml	1:120	2/18	11
Wy-43,502	5	1:120	19/20	64
Levamisole	5	1:150	10/30	30
Saline	1 ml	1:160	6/30	20

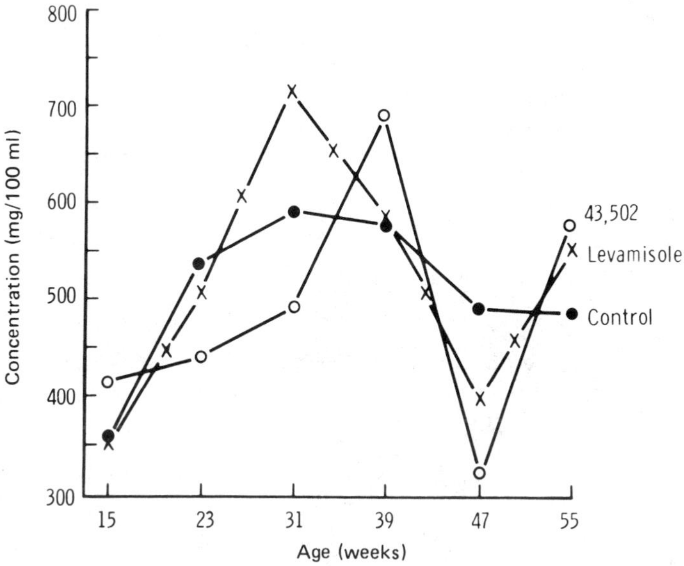

Figure 6 Effect of Wy-43,502 and levamisole on IgG levels.

rosette formation and stimulates humoral immunity as measured by an antigen-antibody reaction. The drug significantly increases the delayed hypersensitivity reaction in immunocompromised guinea pigs at oral doses ranging from 50 to 150 mg/kg. At the low doses of 1 and 5 mg/kg, once per week, Wy-18,251 prevented the metastatic spread of the highly virulent Lewis lung tumor as determined by histopathological evaluation of the entire lung area by a consulting pathologist as a blind study.

The mesoionic compounds, Wy-40,453 and Wy-43,502, are highly effective in inhibiting the production of antibody at doses ranging from 25 to 100 mg/kg. Both drugs are capable of causing a reversible depletion of lymphocytes from both the medulla and cortex of the thymus gland. Use of these drugs in the NZB/W F_1 autoimmune disease model extends the survival time over the vehicle-treated controls and prevents the development of antinuclear antibody, although no cures were effected. When tested in the Lewis lung tumor system at high-dose levels, the drugs have a prometastatic effect, but at dose levels of 50- to 5-mg/kg per week there is a marked reduction in lung metastasis.

REFERENCES

1. R. L. Fenichel, F. J. Gregory, and H. E. Alburn, *Brit. J. Cancer*, *33*:329 (1976).
2. F. J. Gregory, H. E. Alburn, and P. H. L. Wei, *Augmenting Agents in Cancer Chemotherapy*, (E. M. Horisch, ed.), Raven Press, New York, 1981.
3. I. Siegel and W. B. Sherman, *J. Allergy Clin. Immunol.*, *50*:65 (1972).
4. M. E. Kaplan and C. Clark, *J. Immunol. Meth.*, *5*:131 (1974).
5. G. C. Elfenbein, A. D. Goldstein, S. J. Adams, and H. M. Ravlin, *Transplantation*, *29*:113 (1980).
6. R. L. Fenichel, H. E. Alburn, P. A. Schreck, R. L. Bloom, and F. J. Gregory, *J. Immunopharmacol.*, *2*(4):491 (1980).
7. R. L. Fenichel, S. K. Dheer, N. H. Grant, D. P. Scott, R. L. Bloom, and F. J. Gregory, *J. Immunopharmacol.*, *5*(4):333 (1983).

8. C. S. Henney, K. Kuribashi, D. E. Kern, and S. Gillis, *Nature*, *291*:335 (1981).
9. R. Rappaport and G. R. Dodge, *Int. J. Immunopharmacol.*, *4*:377 (1982).
10. R. Rappaport, personal communication.
11. D. H. Campbell, J. S. Garvey, N. E. Cremer, and D. H. Sussdorf, in *Methods in Immunology*, 2nd ed., W. A. Benjamin, Inc., Reading, Mass., 1970.
12. A. J. Lewis, J. Parker, J. DiLuigi, L. J. Datko, and R. P. Carlson, *J. Immunopharmacol.*, *3*:344 (1981-2).
13. B. G. Moore, personal communication.
14. R. Hjorth, personal communication.
15. S. E. James and A. J. Salsbury, *Cancer Res.*, *34*:839 (1974).
16. G. Poste and I. J. Fidler, *Nature*, *283*:139 (1980).
17. I. J. Fidler, *Science* (*Wash, D.C.*), *208*:1469 (1980).
18. I. J. Fidler, Z. Barnes, W. E. Fogler, R. Korish, P. Bugelski, and G. Poste, *Cancer Res.*, *42*:496 (1982).
19. J. L. Gill, *Design and Analysis of Experiments in the Animal and Medical Sciences*, vol. 1, Iowa State University Press, Ames, Iowa, 1978.
20. R. L. Geran, N. H. Greenberg, M. M. MacDonald, A. M. Schumaides, and B. J. Abbott, *Cancer Chemother. Rep.*, *3*:1 (1972).
21. H. Wexler, *J. Natl. Cancer Inst.*, *36*:4;641 (1966).
22. A. J. Cunningham, *Nature*, *207*:1106 (1965).
23. N. K. Jerne and A. A. Nordin, *Science*, *140*:405 (1963).
24. J. L. Fahey and E. M. McKelvely, *J. Immunol.*, *94*:84 (1965).
25. A. S. Lubiniechi and C. A. Dorsch, *Am. J. Clin. Pathol.*, *66*:982
26. D. J. Finney, in *Statistical Methods in Biological Assay*, Macmillan, New York, 1978.
27. N. Mantel, *J. Am. Statistical Assoc.*, *58*:690 (1963).

3

Immunopotentiation by Cyclophosphamide and Other Cytotoxic Agents

David Berd Thomas Jefferson University, Philadelphia, Pennsylvania

Henry C. Maguire, Jr. Hahnemann University Medical School, and Thomas Jefferson University, Philadelphia, Pennsylvania

Michael J. Mastrangelo Thomas Jefferson University, and Temple University School of Medicine, Philadelphia, Pennsylvania

I. INTRODUCTION

Until recently, to characterize a cytotoxic drug as an immunopotentiating agent would have been considered self-contradictory. It was thought that if killing or damage of lymphocytes had any functional consequence, it would have to be suppression of immune responsiveness. Indeed, a major impetus to the development of cytotoxic drugs was the need to achieve sufficient immunosuppression for successful allogeneic organ transplatation.

We now realize that although the interaction of a lymphocyte with a cytotoxic drug often does lead to immunosuppression, it can also result in quite remarkable augmentation of an immune response. The cytotoxic drug whose immunopotentiating effects have been most extensively studied is cyclophosphamide (CY). Therefore, the bulk of this chapter will be devoted to a summary and analysis of studies with that drug. Other cytotoxic drugs that seem to be capable of acting as immunopotentiators will be briefly discussed at the end of the chapter. We have placed the major emphasis on clinical studies, but animal data are included to provide information not yet obtained in humans and to give historical perspective.

II. BIOCHEMISTRY AND PHARMACOLOGY

CY was developed as an oncostatic agent by Brock and Wilmanns (1). The structure is shown in Fig. 1. CY consists of a nitrogen mustard group (bis-chloroethylamine) attached to an oxazophosphorine ring. This compound is nontoxic to tumor cells and lymphocytes in vitro. CY was designed with the expectation that it would be selectively activated by enzymes within tumor cells which would result in toxicity for tumor cells with relative sparing of normal cells. However, cytotoxic metabolites appear in the serum shortly after

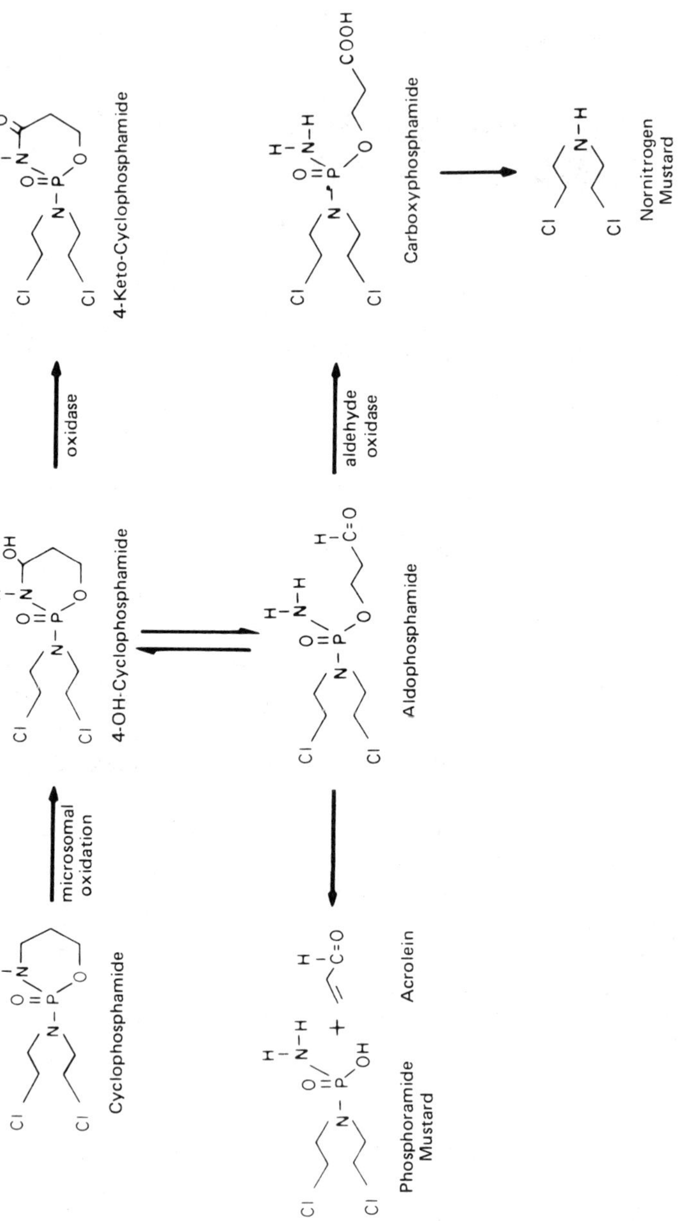

Figure 1 Metabolism of CY. (From Ref. 3.)

administration of CY, and it has been shown that activation occurs in the liver (2). CY can be activated in vitro by incubation with liver homogenates or with isolated liver microsomes (2).

There is still considerable debate over the role played by the various metabolites in producing cytotoxic effects. Figure 1 is a summary of what is currently known of the metabolism of CY (3, 4). CY is converted by liver mixed-function oxidases to 4-hydroxy-cyclophosphamide, which is highly cytotoxic; this compound is in equilibrium with aldo-phosphamide. Hydroxycyclophosphamide is released from liver, enters cells, and decomposes to phosphoramide mustard and acrolein, both of which are cytotoxic and may have biologically significant cytotoxic effects. The noncytotoxic compounds, carboxyphosphamide and 4-ketocyclophosphamide, are formed mainly in the liver, and constitute the major urinary metabolites. Nornitrogen mustard is actively cytotoxic at acid pH and may be important in the development of the bladder toxicity characteristically produced by CY (5). Hydroxycyclophosphamide and phosphoramide mustard are considered to be the compounds most important in producing antitumor effects, and the former might be a transport form of the latter. A synthetic compound, 4-hydroperoxy-cyclophosphamide (4-HP-CY), spontaneously converts to 4-hydroxycyclophosphamide in aqueous solutions, but is more stable than the natural metabolite (6). 4-HP-CY has been useful for in vitro studies, and these will be discussed later in this chapter.

The clinical pharmacology of CY has been studied by measuring plasma alkylating activity and by direct assay of CY and its metabolites (3,4,7-9). After IV administration, the half-life of unchanged CY is about 6 hr. Active metabolites appear within 30 min and reach peak levels at 2-3 hr. The half-life of disappearance of the active metabolites is about 8 hr with little activity detected at 24 hr. After administration of radiolabeled CY, most of the radioactivity is excreted in the urine, and only a small fraction of this is unchanged CY. CY is well absorbed orally. Although the pharmacokinetics of orally administered CY has not been extensively studied, it seems to be similar to that of an intravenously administered drug. Bagley et al. (7) have shown that repeated administration of CY over 5 days alters the pharmacokinetics. By the third day of CY administration, there was a 31% decrease in the half-life of unchanged CY and a 73% increase in maximum plasma levels of active metabolites. There are few data on the effect of the administration of CY on the pharmacokinetics of a dose given 3-4 weeks later. Since CY is commonly given as a bolus every 3-4 weeks, this is worthy of study.

The active metabolites of CY are potent alkylating agents, and damage cells mainly by alkylating DNA bases (10). Since they are bifunctional, each molecule can alkylate two different purine or pyrimidine bases, resulting in cross-linking. This can cause cellular damage by producing direct breakdown of the DNA, or the alkyl group can remain bound to the DNA and interfere with replication. Most cells have enzymes with the capacity to repair the damage done by alkylating agents, and the repair capabilities vary among different normal and malignant cell types. Cells are most sensitive to CY in the phases of the cell cycle in which they are producing DNA (i.e., in G1 and S phases). However, susceptible cells, such as some tumor cells and lymphocytes, are susceptible to damage by alkylating agents even in the resting phases of the cell cycle.

CY has been used for the treatment of human tumors since 1960 (11-13). Although sometimes used as a single agent, CY is usually given in combination with other cytotoxic drugs. CY alone or CY combinations have been shown to be effective for the treatment of acute leukemia, lymphomas, myeloma, breast carcinoma, and oat cell carcinoma of the lung. It has proven less useful in the other common human cancers, such as gastrointestinal, squamous cell of the lung, and melanoma. CY is given as an intravenous bolus of 1000-2000 mg/M^2 every 3-4 weeks, or orally as 40-80 mg/M^2 daily. Currently, the intravenous bolus is preferred by most cancer chemotherapists. The most important toxicity of CY is granulocytopenia which is most severe 7-14 days after a bolus dose. Thrombocytopenia and anemia occur much less frequently. Hemorrhagic cystitis is a characteristic toxicity, and as noted above, may be due to the metabolite nornitrogen mustard, which is found in urine and is an active alkylating agent at acid pH. In addition, a yet unidentified urinary metabolite can directly damage the renal tubules producing transient, but sometimes clinically significant, water retention (10). Other short-term toxicities of CY include nausea and vomiting and reversible alopecia. CY, like most alkylating agents, is a weak carcinogen, and second malignancies have been observed in cancer patients who have received CY for long duration (14). Other toxicities observed with long-term administrations are sterility and, rarely, pulmonary fibrosis (15).

III. IMMUNOSUPPRESSION: HUMAN STUDIES

CY came into clinical usage at a time when there was a great deal of interest in immunosuppressive drugs. Not only was this the beginning of the era of human allogeneic transplantation, but also investigators were becoming interested in the possibility of controlling autoimmune diseases with drugs. Consequently, there have been a number of studies on the effect of CY on the human immune system (Tables 1-3). Because these vary greatly in their experimental design, they are difficult to compare with one another. In some studies, the subjects were patients with a variety of autoimmune diseases and in others the subjects had metastatic cancer. Controls were often nonexistent or inappropriate (e.g., normal subjects without CY compared with autoimmune disease patients with CY). Finally, the dose and/or duration of administration of CY differed from study to study.

Despite these difficulties, several conclusions can be drawn from the data. The administration of CY to patients with autoimmune diseases is followed by a fall in the number of circulating lymphocytes (Table 1). Daily oral administration of CY 1-2 mg/kg/day (40-80 mg/M^2/day) causes the lymphocyte count to decrease by 40-80%. The nadir is reached within 3 weeks (18), and the count does not appear to decline further even if CY is continued for a year or more. Although some authors have suggested that CY preferentially depletes B cells (18), the data indicate that T cells are equally depleted. After an IV bolus of CY 40 mg/kg (1600 mg/M^2) was given to patients with metastatic cancer, the lymphocyte count fell by more than 50% by 1 week and was just beginning to recover at 3 weeks, without selectivity for B or T cells (21). Finally, Mullins et al. (20) administered an extraordinarily large dose of CY 120 mg/kg (4800 mg/M^2) to cancer patients and observed a profound (>80%) fall in circulating lymphocytes, although there was partial recovery by 2.5 weeks.

The effect of CY on in vitro lymphoproliferative responses is not so clear, as shown by the variability of the data in Table 2. The studies of Alepa et al. (16) and Winkelstein et al. (17, 23) indicated that chronic oral administration of CY 1-2 mg/kg (40-80 mg/M^2) resulted in marked reduction of the proliferative response of blood lymphocytes to phytohemagglutinin (PHA) and pokeweed mitogen (PWM). This was true whether the responses of CY-treated patients were compared with those of control subjects or with their own pre-CY responses. On the other hand, neither Horwitz (18) nor Cupps et al. (22) observed a significant change in PHA or PWM proliferative responses, although the latter authors reported a decrease in concanavalin A-induced proliferation. These conflicting results

Table 1 Published Studies on the Effect of CY on Human Circulating Lymphocytes[a]

Reference	Year	Study Subjects: No.	Study Subjects: Disease	Study Subjects: Concomitant Steroids	Controls	Dose of CY	Duration of CY	Result
Alepa et al. (16)	1970	9	RA	+	Same, pre-CY	100-150 mg/day	4-15 months	Ly ↓ 42%
Winkelstein et al. (17)	1972	47	RA	+	RA, no CY	50-100 mg/day	9 months	Ly ↓ 55%
		9	RA	+	Same, pre-CY	50-100 mg/day	4 months	Ly ↓ 46%
Horwitz (18)	1974	11	RA, SLE	+	Same, pre-CY	1.5-2 mg/kg/day	3 weeks	Ig + Ly and Ig − Ly ↓ 50%
Hurd and Giuliano (19)	1975	8	SLE	+	SLE, no CY	2 mg/kg/day	41 weeks	T Ly ↓ 51% B Ly ↓ 83%
		7	A	+	A, no CY	2 mg/kg/day	21 weeks	T Ly ↓ 78% B Ly ↓ 76%
Mullins et al. (20)	1975	12	C	−	Same, pre-CY	60 mg/kg, two doses	8 days	Ly ↓ 82%
Smit et al. (21)	1979	10	C	−	Same, pre-CY	40 mg/kg, one dose	1 week	Ly ↓ 58%, no change in % T Ly or B Ly
Cupps et al (22)	1982	16	A	+	Normals	2 mg/kg/day	14 months	Ly ↓ 45% T Ly ↓ 27% B Ly ↓ 33%

[a]Abbreviations: RA, rheumatoid arthritis; SLE, systemic lupus erythematosus; A, various autoimmune diseases; C, cancer; Ly, peripheral blood lymphocytes; T Ly, T lymphocytes; B Ly, B lymphocytes.

Table 2 Published Studies on the Effect of CY on Human Lymphoproliferative Responses[a]

Reference	Year	Study Subjects: No.	Study Subjects: Disease	Study Subjects: Concomitant Steroids	Controls	Dose of CY	Duration of CY (Months)	Results
Alepa et al. (16)	1970	9	RA	+	Same, pre-CY	100-150 mg/day	4-15	PHA ↓ 60% PWM ↓ 55%
Winkelstein et al. (17)	1972	47	RA	+	RA, no CY	50-100 mg/day	9	PHA ↓ 75%
		9	RA	+	Same, pre-CY	50-100 mg/day	4	PHA ↓ 54%
Winkelstein et al. (23)	1974	12	RA	+	RA, no CY	1 mg/kg/day	3	PHA ↓ 53% PWM ↓ 61%
Horwitz (18)	1974	11	A	+	Same, pre-CY	1.5-2 mg/kg/da6	2-6	PHA ↓ in 3/11, ↑ in 4/11
Cupps et al. (22)	1982	16	A	+	Normals, and unspecified other	2 mg/kg/day	14	PHA, no change PWM, no change ConA ↓ 34%

[a]Abbreviations: RA, rheumatoid arthritis; A, various autoimmune diseases; PHA, proliferative response to phytohemagglutinin; PWM, proliferative response to pokeweed mitogen; ConA, proliferative response to concanavalin A.

Table 3 Published Studies on the Effect of CY on Human Primary Immune Responses[a]

Reference	Study Subjects: Year	No.	Disease	Concomitant Steroids	Controls	Dose of CY	Duration of CY	Results
Santos et al. (24)	1964	4	MC	–	None	7 mg/kg/day for 7 days IV	1 day	0/4 made antibody to Vi
Fauci et al. (25)	1971	9	WG	+	Normals	50-125 mg/day PO	3-12 months	2/9 had antibody and DTH response to KLH vs. 8/10 controls
Mullins et al. (20)	1975	12	MC	–	None	60 mg/kg/day for 2 days IV	1 day	3/12 made antibody to Vi
Mackay et al. (26)	1973	6	A	+	(1) A, receiving azathioprine (2) unrelated diseases	2.6 mg/kg/day PO	3-12 months	Impaired antibody response to flagellin
Curtis et al. (27)	1973	11	RA	–	RA, prospectively randomized group receiving placebo	1 mg/kg/day PO	2 weeks	Antibody and DTH to KLH, no difference; antibody to GLAT, no difference; DTH to GLAT, increased in CY group

[a]Abbreviations: MC, metastatic cancer; WG, Wegener's granulomatosis; A, various autoimmune diseases; RA, rheumatoid arthritis; Vi, *E. coli* Vi antigen; DTH, delayed-type hypersensitivity; KLH, keyhole limpet hemocyanin; GLAT, see text.

could be explained by variations among the studies in regard to control subjects and the amount of concomitant corticosteroid administration. It is also possible that changes in the status of a patient's autoimmune disease over a period of several months could produce alterations in lymphoproliferative responses independent of CY or could mask alterations produced by CY.

It is noteworthy that Cupps et al. (22) observed a marked impairment of the PWM-driven immunoglobulin production of lymphocytes from patients chronically receiving CY. This finding appeared to be due to functional impairment of the B cells, since the helper function of T cells from CY-treated patients was normal. Whether this change was truly induced by CY can only be determined by a confirmatory study performed with appropriate controls and without the confounding effect of corticosteroids.

Table 3 summarizes the studies of the effect of CY on the development of antibody and delayed-type hypersensitivity (DTH) responses to primary antigens. Santos et al. (24), Fauci et al. (25), and Mullins et al. (20) demonstrated that patients with advanced cancer or Wegener's granulomatosis receiving CY had marked impairment of primary antibody and DTH responses. However, since none of these studies included appropriate controls, it is uncertain whether these authors observed the immunosuppressive effects of CY or of the underlying diseases. Mackay et al. (26) compared the antibody response to flagellin of patients with immunopathic disease treated with CY versus a similar but not prospectively randomized group treated with azathioprine and a third group of patients with unrelated diseases who were receiving neither drug. They found that the increase in antibody titer of the CY group was less than that of the azathioprine and control groups. Although their data suggest an immunosuppressive effect of CY, they are also consistent with an immunostimulating effect of azathioprine (28). The most rigorously controlled study of the effect of CY on human immune responses is that of Curtis et al. (27). They randomly assigned patients with rheumatoid arthritis to receive either CY or placebo, and after 2 weeks tested the ability of the patients to make primary antibody and DTH responses to keyhole limpet hemocyanin (KLH) and to a copolymer of glutamic acid, lysine, alanine, and tyrosine (GLAT). CY had no significant effect on the antibody or DTH response to KLH or to the antibody response to GLAT. However, patients receiving CY had significantly increased DTH responses to GLAT. The mean DTH responses (diameter of skin reaction) were 12.7 mm in the CY group versus 1.8 mm in the control group. This finding, which must have seemed peculiar to the authors, was not discussed in the publication and does not appear to have been the subject of follow-up investigations.

In summary, the administration of CY to humans causes a marked decrease in the number of circulating lymphocytes and probably some impairment of in vitro lymphoproliferative responses. However, the net effect of these changes on the development of antibody and DTH responses has not been clearly defined. The few studies performed over the past 20 years are compatible with the concept of CY as an immunomodulating rather than simply as an immunosuppressive agent.

IV. IMMUNOSUPPRESSION: EXPERIMENTAL ANIMALS

The reputation of CY as a potent immunosuppressant has a firmer basis in the studies in experimental animals. The first paper to demonstrate an immunological effect of CY in experimental animals was that of Stender et al. (29). These investigators showed that the antibody response of rats to killed *Brucella melitensis* organisms was suppressed when CY was given at the time of antigen administration. Soon afterward, our laboratory (30, 31) demonstrated the inhibition by CY of primary antibody formation in guinea pigs; primary antibody formation was markedly inhibited when CY was given at the time of antigen administration. We further observed that specific immunological tolerance could be induced by treating guinea pigs with CY at the time that they were being immunized (32). Thus, most guinea pigs given CY and the antigen ovalbumin not only failed to make antibody against ovalbumin, but, when reimmunized with ovalbumin 3 months later (no further CY), again did not make antibody to ovalbumin, although they did make antibody against an unrelated foreign protein, namely, horse serum. Control groups of guinea pigs that were immunized in parallel responded readily both to ovalbumin and to horse sera.

Many subsequent studies in a variety of experimental animals have had the common theme that CY suppresses antibody formation and that it can be used to induce specific immunological tolerance (33). The suppression of B-cell immunity has been demonstrated with a wide array of immunogens including both soluble and particulate materials (34-36). In studies where a comparison has been made of the degree of immunosuppression induced by several cancer chemotherapeutic drugs, CY is generally one of the most active, if not the most active drug. In the avian species, severe damage to the bursa of Fabricius results from the administration of CY to newly hatched chickens (37). Such chemically bursectomized chickens fail to make significant levels of antibody to all antigens and provide an experimental model for human agammaglobulinemia.

The ability of CY to inhibit antibody synthesis has been applied to diverse animal models of human disease. For instance, with aging, NZB/W F1 mice develop an immune complex disease that resembles lupus erythematosis; their disorder is secondary to the production of antibody directed against DNA. Chronic treatment with CY reduces the synthesis of anti-DNA antibodies and thereby retards development of the disease (38). A variety of infections, whose resistance depends upon the development of specific antibodies, have been shown to be accelerated in animals treated with CY (39, 40).

Early work has also revealed that CY can suppress reactions of delayed-type hypersensitivity (DTH). Maguire and Maibach (41), studying the effect of CY and other drugs (6-mercaptopurine, vincaleukoblastine, and actinomycin D) on the acquisition of allergic contact dermatitis in guinea pigs, observed that CY, but not the other drugs, were immunosuppressive when given during the induction of the contact hypersensitivity; in contrast, already established allergic contact dermatitis was resistant to CY immunosuppression. Turk and Stone (42) studies the histological changes in the lymph nodes regional to the sensitization site during the incubation of the allergic contact dermatitis. Normally, several days following the application of a strong contact allergen, an abundance of pyroninophilic cells is observed in the paracortical areas of the regional lymph nodes. In animals treated with CY shortly after application of sensitizer, the number of pyroninophilic cells in the regional lymph node cells is markedly reduced, and of those cells that can be found, many are abnormal in appearance. Immunosuppression by CY of microbial hypersensitivity and of transplantation immunity in experimental animals has been reported by many investigators (43, 44).

V. IMMUNOPOTENTIATION: EXPERIMENTAL ANIMALS

In the course of our studies of the modulation by CY of the induction and expression of allergic dermatitis, we (45) discovered that guinea pigs treated with CY and then contact-sensitized developed much more intense and prolonged allergic contact dermatitis reactions than did control guinea pigs that had received sensitizer alone. This phenomenon was not due to the induction by CY of a nonspecific increase in skin reactivity, since the reactions to croton oil, a primary irritant, were not effected by the CY. A digest of data taken from the original report of that work is shown in Figure 2; the finding was soon confirmed (46). In addition, CY was observed to immunopotentiate the acquisition of DTH to a variety of microbial products as well as to immunopotentiate the acquisition of DTH in the guinea pig to a soluble protein (ovalbumin) incorporated in Freund's incomplete adjuvant (47-49). Indeed, CY has been used to facilitate the induction of DTH to syngeneic testicular tissue (50).

Not only does CY, under appropriate circumstances, immunopotentiate cellular immune responses, but the antibody response can also be heightened (51). This is particularly evident in the instance of immunoglobulin E (IgE) (52). In addition, in several systems, genetically low-antibody responders are rendered high responders when CY is given prior to stimulation with antigen (53).

The critical factor determining whether CY depressed or potentiated an immune response in these experimental systems was the timing of administration of CY and antigen. The importance of timing has been particularly well illustrated in the studies of Turk and Parker (51). They observed that administration of CY to guinea pigs 2 days *before* sensitization to 2,4-dinitrofluorobenzene *increased* the contact hypersensitivity response three- to fourfold, whereas administration of CY 2 days *after* sensitization completely *suppressed* it. In the studies cited above, the interval between administration of CY and antigen varied from 1 to 4 days.

The dose of CY, although the object of much attention (54) seems to be much less important. The immunopotentiating dose of CY most commonly reported in the literature is 100 mg/kg in mice, equivalent to 300 mg/M^2. [Expressing doses on the basis of body surface area instead of weight allows comparison of doses among different species (55).]

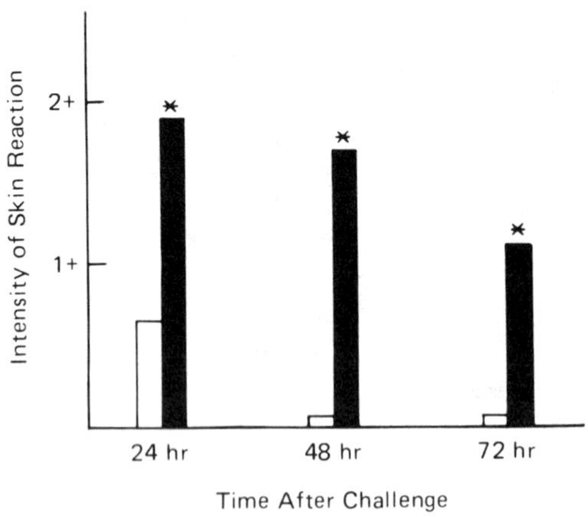

Figure 2 Enhancement of DNCB contact sensitization by CY in the guinea pig. A group of 12 Hartley albino guinea pigs was treated with CY 10 mg (approximately 25 mg/kg or 175 mg/M^2) IP daily for 5 days. On day 5, these guinea pigs as well as a control group of equal number were putatively sensitized by the application of 0.5 mg DNCB (1-chloro,2, 4-dinitrobenzene) to the skin. Ten days later both groups were challenged by topical application of 0.1% DNCB. The mean intensity of the challenge reaction of each group is shown (open bars = controls, solid bars = CY pretreatment). *, solid vs. open bars, $p < 0.0001$.

However, it has varied from 20 mg/kg in mice (54), equivalent to 60 mg/M^2, to 300 mg/kg in guinea pigs (51), equivalent to 2100 mg/M^2. Most investigators have pretreated animals with a single injection of CY. Administration of a dose of CY over a 5-day period was also effective (45), but immunopotentiation was not observed when CY was given daily over a 2-week period (56).

VI. IMMUNOPOTENTIATION: HUMAN STUDIES

These animal studies on CY-induced immunopotentiation stimulated our interest in the question of whether CY could augment human immune responses (57). We studied 22 patients with far advanced cancer, 12 with malignant melanoma, and 10 with colorectal carcinoma. All patients had metastatic disease that was beyond surgical cure and had failed to respond to standard chemotherapy. Most of the patients had visceral metastases with a low clinical performance status (median Karnovsky score = 70) and had been treated previously with two or three chemotherapeutic agents. The blood lymphocyte count was markedly depressed compared with 30 age-matched control subjects.

Because of the demonstrated importance of timing in the animal systems, we designed the study so that CY was administered 3 days before antigen. The dose of CY, 1000 mg/M^2 given as a single IV injection, was chosen because it is commonly used to achieve oncostatic effects in cancer patients. Although that is higher than the dose of 300 mg/M^2 most commonly used in experimental animals, it is within the reported immunopotentiating range (see discussion above).

The immune response to two primary antigens, keyhole limpet hemocyanin (KLH) and 1-chloro-2,4-dinitrobenzene (DNCB), was measured before or after the administration of CY, according to the protocol outlined in Fig. 3. Patients were alternatively assigned to one of two groups: Group I patients were pretested with KLH and posttested with DNCB; group II patients were pretested with DNCB and posttested with KLH. For each antigen, the responses of group I patients were compared with those of group II patients. Patients were given a sensitizing dose of the first antigen and a challenge dose 14 days later. After 48 hr the DTH response was measured, and CY was administered. Three days

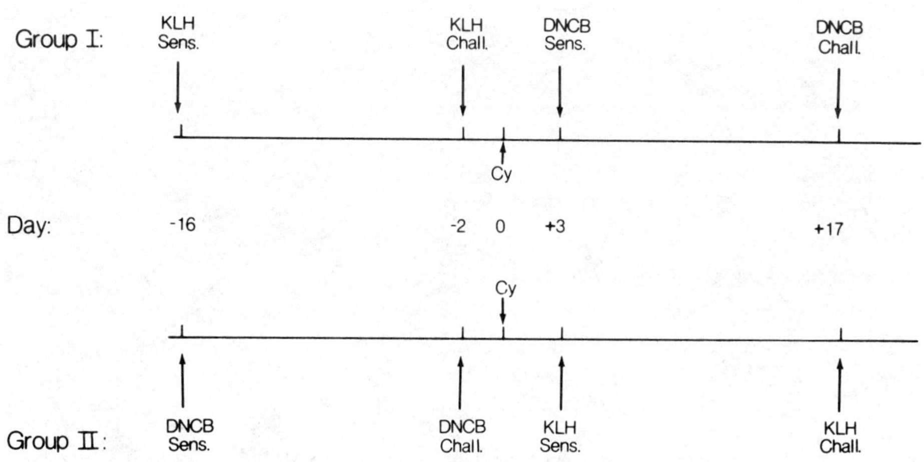

Figure 3 Schema of study of CY-induced immunopotentiation in humans. Abbreviations: Sens. = sensitization dose; Chall. = challenge dose. (From Ref. 57.)

after CY, patients were given a sensitizing dose of the second antigen. Fourteen days later they were given a challenge dose. After 48 hr the DTH response was measured. Serum for antibody determination was collected before and 14 days after the initial injection of KLH.

The most striking finding of this study was that pretreatment of patients with CY significantly augmented the development of DTH to KLH (Fig. 4). The DTH reactions of patients given KLH 3 days after CY (group II) were significantly greater than those of patients given KLH without prior CY (group I) (medians: KLH alone, 0; KLH after CY, 19 mm; $p < 0.025$, Mann-Whitney U test). With CY pretreatment, 11 of 11 patients developed a DTH response of greater than 5 mm compared with 4 of 11 without CY ($p < 0.002$, Student's t-test for proportions).

Of 10 patients given DNCB without CY, none developed DTH. Of 11 patients given DNCB 3 days after CY, 3 developed a positive DTH response. The difference (0 of 10 versus 3 of 11) was of borderline significance ($p = 0.082$, Student's t-test for proportions).

Pretreatment with CY neither augmented nor suppressed the agglutinating antibody response to KLH. There was no correlation, either positive or negative, between DTH and antibody responses.

Of the 22 patients, 3 (13.6%) demonstrated a partial regression of tumor following CY administration. Two of these were melanoma patients who had a greater than 50%

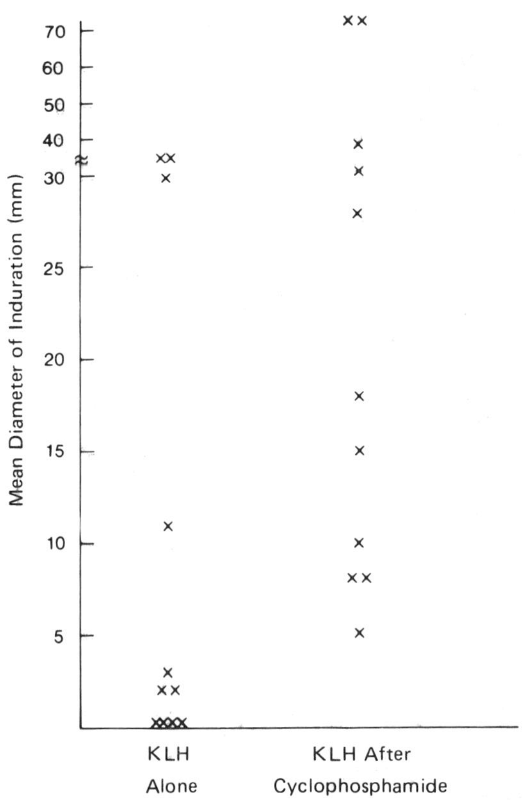

Figure 4 DTH responses to KLH. Patients were sensitized with KLH without CY or 3 days after CY 1000 mg/M^2. All patients were challenged with ID KLH 14 days after sensitization, and DTH was measured after 48 hr. X = size of the DTH reaction of one patient. (From Ref. 57.)

shrinkage of cancerous lymph nodes. The other was a patient with colon carcinoma who had a 50% decrease in the size of the liver. One of these patients was in group I and the other was in group II; all developed DTH to DNCB or KLH when sensitized 3 days after CY. Of the 22 patients on the study, 17 have died with a median survival time from CY administration of 5 months (identical for groups I and II).

This study demonstrated that pretreatment with CY could augment a human cell-mediated immune response, even in subjects with far advanced cancer, some of whom were terminally ill. We did not attempt to define the optimal conditions for immunopotentiation, and it is possible that other doses or times of administration of CY would be even more effective.

VII. MECHANISM OF IMMUNOPOTENTIATION

A. Animal Studies

The first hypothesis proposed to explain CY-induced augmentation of T cell-mediated immunity was inhibition by suppressor B cells (58) or their products (59). This explanation seemed reasonable in view of the fact that a number of manipulations in addition to CY administration can produce reciprocal effects on antibody formation and DTH (60). However, the hypothesis was questioned by Askenase et al. (54) who showed that a small dose of CY (20 mg/kg) would augment murine DTH reactions to sheep erythrocytes without impairing the antibody response. Subsequently, Burrows et al. (61) and Maguire et al. (62) showed that mice lacking detectable B cells and B-cell products could be immunopotentiated with CY as effectively as normal mice. Thus, the B-cell depletion hypothesis has not withstood experimental testing and no longer appears to be valid.

Currently, the leading hypothesis is that CY augments immunity by selectively depleting suppressor T cells, and the data generated so far from experimental systems support this hypothesis. Several investigators (63, 64) have shown that adoptive transfer of normal T cells abrogates immunopotentiation by CY. Diamantstein et al. (65) demonstrated that spleen cells from mice treated with CY showed an increased (fourfold) mitogenic response to dextran sulfate and that this could be reversed by the addition of normal thymocytes, but not by thymocytes treated with 4-hydroperoxycyclophosphamide (4-HP-CY), a synthetic compound that spontaneously hydrolyzes to the active metabolite, 4-hydroxycyclophosphamide. The response to dextran sulfate could also be augmented by treatment of spleen cells with 4-HP-CY in vitro, but not if the spleen cells had first been depleted of T cells.

Kaufmann et al. (66) compared the sensitivity to 4-HP-CY of two populations of splenic T cells: (a) those capable of adoptively transferring specific DTH (T_{DH} cells), and (b) those capable of specifically suppressing DTH (T_s cells). The former were resistant to concentrations of 4-HP-CY of 3 μg/ml, while the latter were inactivated by 1 μg/ml. Moreover, spleen cells from mice injected with supraoptimal doses of antigen were incapable of adoptively transferring DTH, but regained that capability after exposure to 3 μg/ml of 4/HP-CY. Finally, these investigators showed that pretreatment with CY enabled mice to make a DTH response after a supraoptimal dose of antigen. This could be reversed by adoptively transferring normal spleen cells but not by spleen cells that had been exposed to 4-HP–CY, even to concentrations of 4-HP-CY as low as 0.3 μg/ml. These results suggested that antigen-primed suppressor T cells were more sensitive to activated CY than antigen-primed T_{DH} cells, and that precursors of these antigen-primed suppressor cells were the most sensitive of all. B cells, as measured by the mitogenic response to lipopolysaccharide, were about as sensitive to 4-HP-CY as T suppressor cells.

Although these data support the hypothesis that CY augments immunity because of selective toxicity for suppressor T cells or their precursors, Schwartz et al. (67) have suggested that the explanation might be more complicated. They reported that CY augmented the DTH response of mice to sheep erythrocytes when the dose of antigen was supraoptimal, but could depress the response when the dose of antigen was optimal. To explain their data, they postulated that CY depleted a population of ***amplifier*** T cells (i.e,, capable of amplifying DTH and capable of amplifying suppression of DTH). This hypothesis predicts that CY would suppress responses that are "destined" to be strong and augment responses that are "destined" to be weak.

B. Human Studies In Vitro

Most of the investigation on the mechanism of augmentation of human immunity by CY has involved attempts at showing that CY is selectively cytotoxic for suppressor T cells in vitro. Such studies require the use of active CY metabolites, since CY itself is inactive in vitro. Stevenson and Fauci (68) obtained activated CY from the serum of a CY-treated monkey and tested its effect on human lymphocyte function in vitro. They observed that activated CY suppressed PWM responses, even at a concentration that had only a slight effect on lymphocyte viability. However, if only T lymphocytes were exposed to activated CY and then added to untreated B cells, the PWM response was augmented compared with that of untreated B and T cells. This work suggests that activated CY killed or inhibited a subset of T cells that normally modulated the PWM response.

Ozer et al. (69) tested the effect on human lymphocytes of 4-HP-CY. These investigators found that a 1-hour treatment with 4-HP-CY did not kill lymphocytes, but did result in marked inhibition of their response to lectins when the concentration exceeded 30 nmol/ml. However, when purified T cells were treated with 4-HP-CY and then mixed with untreated B cells, the production of immunoglobulin after stimulation with PWM was increased. This occurred when the concentration of 4-HP-CY was 20 nmol/ml or less, and even when it was as low as 10^{-3} nmol/ml. Thus, similar to the study of Stevenson and Fauci cited above, these authors had circumstantial evidence that activated CY was selectively toxic to suppressor T cells or their precursors.

Ozer et al. also studied the effect of in vitro treatment with 4-HP-CY on concanavalin A (ConA) inducible suppressor T cells. A 1-hr incubation with 4-HP-CY in concentrations ranging from 20 nmol/ml to 10^{-2} nmol/ml completely prevented the development of T cells that could suppress pokeweed mitogen-driven immunoglobulin production. On the other hand, treatment of T cells with 4-HP-CY after they had been activated by ConA to become suppressors had no effect on their ability to suppress immunoglobulin production. Thus, 4-HP-CY appeared to be working by preventing the development of mature suppressor cells, possibly by selective toxicity for a "presuppressor" cell. Ozer et al. and others have presented evidence that the presuppressor might have a helper-inducer phenotype (Leu-3 or OKT-4+), rather than the expected suppressor-cytotoxic phenotype (Leu-2 or OKT-8+).

Although these data are interesting and provocative, they must be interpreted with caution, because in vitro conditions may be quite different from the in vivo environment. In the experiments of Ozer et al., lymphocytes were exposed to a single active metabolite of CY, 4-hydroxycyclophosphamide, to which 4-HP-CY is spontaneously converted. Yet the plasma of animals and humans who have received a dose of CY contains not only 4-hydroxycyclophosphamide, but also phosphoramide mustard, acrolein, and possibly other as yet unidentified cytotoxic compounds. Moreover, in the in vitro experiments cells were exposed to the metabolite for an arbitrary length of time, generally 1 hr.

However, cytotoxic compounds are found in the plasma of CY-treated patients for up to 24 hr after administration and may persist even longer in some tissues.

C. Human Studies In Vivo

These concerns led us to conduct a study of the effect of exposure to CY in vivo on human lymphocyte composition and function. We administered CY 1000 mg/M^2 to 19 patients with advanced cancer. Before and at various times after CY, we collected blood samples and separated peripheral blood mononuclear cells by density gradient centrifugation on Ficoll-metrizoate. Cells were frozen in a controlled-rate freezer and cryopreserved in liquid nitrogen until needed for testing, so that all the cells serially collected from a patient could be tested simultaneously.

If CY is selectively toxic for suppressor T cells, than one would expect to observe a decrease in the number of circulating suppressor T cells and/or an impairment of their function. We first studied the composition of blood lymphocytes by staining with fluoresceinated monoclonal antibodies and analyzing with the fluorescence-activated cell sorter. As shown in Fig. 5, the administration of CY resulted in a fall in the number of circulating

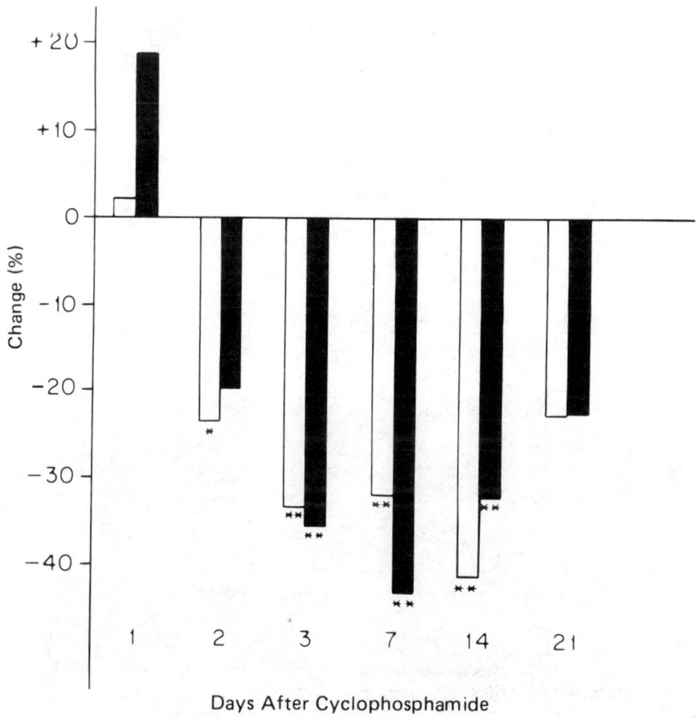

Figure 5 Change in number of circulating T lymphocytes (open bars) and B lymphocytes (solid bars) after CY administration to cancer patients. Nineteen patients with advanced cancer were given CY 1000 mg/M^2 IV. Blood lymphocytes were serially collected and tested for binding to fluoresceinated antihuman immunoglobulin to detect B lymphocytes and to the monoclonal antibody anti-Leu-4 (Becton Dickinson) to detect T lymphocytes. At each time point the percent change from the pre-CY number was calculated for each patient. Then the significance of the group of changes at each time point was determined by the Student's t-test for nonindependent samples. $^*p < 0.05$; $^{**}, p < 0.01$; others, not significant.

lymphocytes by day 2, which continued through day 14 with recovery beginning by day 21. There was no selective depletion of T cells (Leu-4+) or B cells (Ig+). Figure 6 shows the effect of CY on two subsets of T cells—Leu 2+ cells, which mediate suppression and cytotoxicity, and Leu-3+ cells, which provide help for antibody responses. The number of cells in the two subsets was decreased to the same degree at every time point. Thus, CY did not selectively kill suppressor T cells, at least not those defined by the Leu-2 phenotype. This apparent lack of selectivity could be explain by some recent studies which suggest that some types of suppressor T cells bear the Leu-3 phenotype (69). The CY-sensitive target cell could be a subset of Leu-3+ cells, the idenitification of which awaits the development of new monoclonal antibody reagents.

Next, we sought to determine whether suppressor function was selectively impaired. As shown in Fig. 7, ConA-inducible suppressor T-cell activity was significantly impaired at 1, 2, and 3 days after CY. Although it seemed to recover partially on day 7, it was again significantly diminished on days 14 and 21. In contrast was the effect of CY

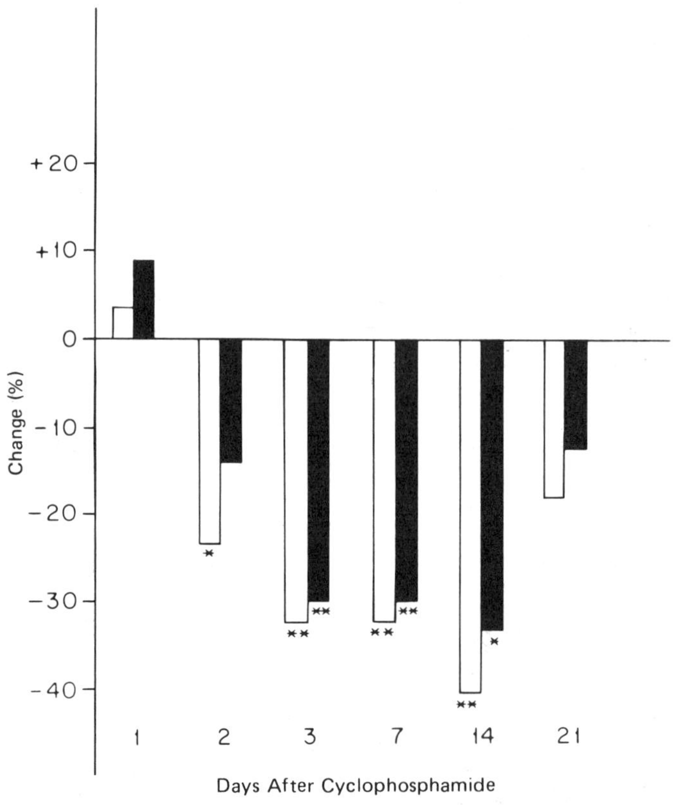

Figure 6 Change in number of circulating T suppressor cells (solid bars) and T helper cells (open bars) after CY administration to cancer patients. Nineteen patients with advanced cancer were given CY 1000 mg/M^2 IV. Blood lymphocytes were serially collected and tested for binding to the fluoresceinated monoclonal antibodies anti-Leu-2 to detect suppressor-cytotoxic T cells and anti-Leu-3 to detect helper-inducer T cells (Becton Dickinson). At each time point the percent change from the pre-CY number was calculated for each patient. Then, the significance of the group of changes at each time point was determined by the Student's t-test of nonindependent samples. *,$p<0.05$; **, $p<0.01$; others, not significant.

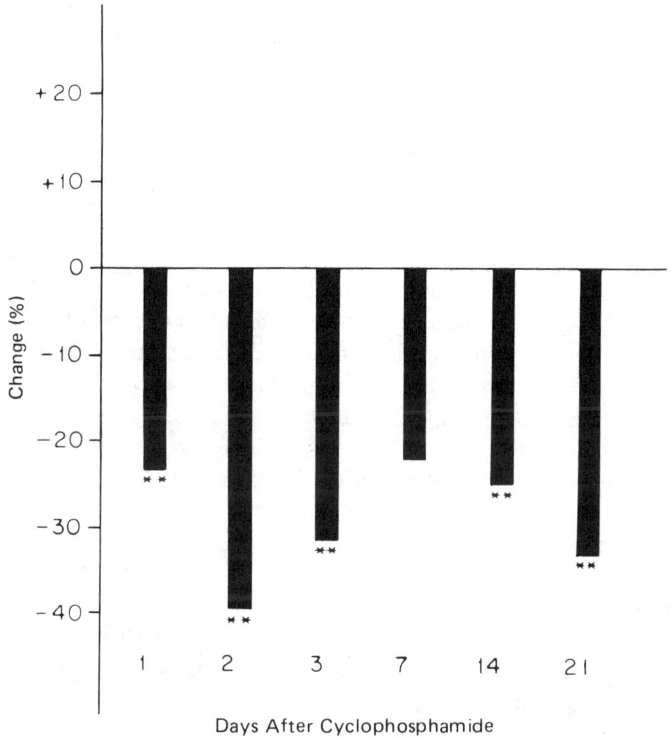

Figure 7 Change in ConA-inducible suppressor activity after CY administration to cancer patients. Nineteen patients with advanced cancer were given CY 1000 mg/M^2 IV. Blood lymphocytes were serially collected and tested for ConA-inducible suppressor activity. Lymphocytes were incubated with or without ConA 25 μg/ml for 3 days, treated with mitomycin C, and repeatedly washed. They were then added to allogeneic lymphocytes (indicator cells) from a single donor at a suppressor/indicator ratio of 0.5:1. Suppression was defined as the percent decrease in the response of indicator cells to a suboptimal concentration of PHA in the presence of ConA-stimulated patient's cells versus nonstimulated patient's cells. At each time point the percent change from the pre-CY value in the amount of ConA inducible suppression was calculated for each patients. Then, the significance of the group of changes at each time point was determined by the Student's t-test for non-independent samples. **, $p < 0.01$; others, not significant.

administration on lymphoproliferative responses. The response to a suboptimal concentration (0.1 μg/ml) of PHA was decreased by a mean of 12.6% ($p < 0.01$) on day 1. However, it recovered to pretreatment levels by day 2 and was slightly, but not significantly, above baseline levels on day 7. A similar pattern was noted for proliferative responses to an optimal concentration (1.0 μg/ml) of PHA and for proliferative responses to PWM, ConA, and pooled allogeneic lymphocytes (mixed lymphocyte response).

Thus 2-3 days after administration of CY 1000 mg/M^2, we found an impairment of ConA-inducible suppressor T-cell activity that seemed to be selective (i.e., not associated with a generalized impairment of lymphocyte function). This observation fits well with our original observation that the administration of a primary antigen on day 3 results in augmentation of DTH. However, it is premature to conclude that the impairment of this type of T-suppressor activity consitutes the explanation for the agumentation of DTH.

There could be other varieties of T suppressor cells (e.g., those inducible by tolerogenic concentrations of antigens, that are even more CY sensitive). Also, we have not excluded the possibility that CY diminishes monocyte-mediated suppression (70).

VIII. IMMUNOPOTENTIATION BY OTHER CYTOTOXIC DRUGS

Since there is nothing highly unique about the pharmacology or biochemistry of CY, it would be surprising if it were the only cytotoxic drug capable of augmenting immune responses. Indeed, Goto et al. (56) showed that in mice not only CY but also Thio-TEPA, mitomycin, adriamycin, fluorouracil, vincristine, and methotrexate could augment the development of DTH to an antigen given 4 days later. These authors also observed that augmentation was observed if antigen was given after a single dose of drug, but not after the same dose of drug had been given by daily administration over a 2-week period.

There have been no studies showing that the administration of cytotoxic drugs other than CY can augment human immune responses. Hersh et al. (71) observed that patients challenged with Vi antigen or tularemia vaccine 3 days after the completion of a course of chemotherapy with methotrexate or 6-mercaptopurine developed antibody responses that were the same as those of untreated patients, just as we have shown with anti-KLH antibody responses after CY. Those authors did not measure the development of DTH.

Several investigators have studied the effect of administration of various combinations of cytotoxic drugs to cancer patients on in vitro lymphocyte function. In general, lymphoproliferative responses to lectins, soluble antigens, and allogeneic lymphocytes are markedly depressed during the period of administration of drugs, but recover to pretreatment levels by 3-4 days after drug administration is stopped (72-74). Thus, the kinetics of recovery of lymphoproliferative responses after combinations of drugs is similar to what we have observed after CY alone. Frequently, an increase in proliferative responses 9-14 days after combination chemotherapy has been observed, a phenomenon that has been referred to as "rebound overshoot" (74). Although it is tempting to attribute rebound overshoot to selective elimination of suppressor cells, there are not sufficient data to warrant such a conclusion. Overshoot could just as likely be due to regeneration of functionally efficient lymphocytes from precursor pools, in the same manner as circulating neutrophils recover and rebound after initial depression. Moreover, rebound overshoot of lymphoproliferation has been observed mostly in patients in whom chemotherapy causes tumor regression (74, 75) and, therefore, could be a consequence of the decreased tumor burden, rather than a result of the drugs themselves. Braun and Harris (70) reported that 14 of 20 cancer patients developed rebound overshoot of PHA proliferation at at least one point between 7 and 28 days after chemotherapy. In each case, rebound overshoot was temporally associated with a decrease in the augmentation of proliferation obtained by adding indomethacin or depleting adherent cells. The authors concluded that rebound overshoot was caused by drug-induced elimination or reduced function of suppressor monocytes. However, they did not directly demonstrate suppression by showing that proliferation could be "resuppressed" by the addition of the putative suppressor monocytes. Thus, the significance of rebound overshoot remains uncertain.

The work of Dimitriu and Fauci (28) suggests that the antimetabolite, azathioprine, may be selectively toxic for human suppressor T cells. They found that normal human T cell-enriched mononuclear cells that had been treated in vitro with azathioprine augmented the polyclonal antibody response of untreated mononuclear cells. Moreover, azathioprine pretreatment prevented the development of ConA-inducible suppressor cells and even abolished the effect of suppressor cells that had already been induced by ConA.

It seems highly likely that properly controlled studied would demonstrate that a number of cytotoxic drugs can augment human immune responses given theproper dose and timing in regard to administration of antigen. As with CY, selective toxicity for some type of suppressor mechanism is likely to be the basis of the immunopotentiation.

IX. TUMOR-ASSOCIATED IMMUNITY

Although it has not been shown that human cancer cells have tumor-specific antigens, serological data (76) and work using monoclonal antibodies (77) suggest that there are antigens on tumor cells that cannot be detected on most normal cells or most tumors of a histologically different type, and these surface antigens could provide functional specificity. Unfortunately, great difficulty has been encountered by investigators attempting to demonstrate that patients develop an immune response against these antigens (76, 78). One obvious explanation for the difficulty is that tumor antigens are not recognized by the autologous host as foreign and that an immune response is never initiated. However, an alternative explanation is that tumor cells are immunogenic but that the host in which they arise becomes tolerant to them.

Although the mechanisms of immunological tolerance are incompletely understood, evidence from many experimental systems (79) suggests that antigen-specific suppressor T lymphocytes play a major role. Tumor-associated antigens may induce immunological tolerance, and the failure of the host to make an effective immune response could be due to activity of specific suppressor cells.

The reasons for considering such a hypothesis have been reviewed (80). There are several experimental systems in which tumor-specific suppressor cells appear shortly after the transplantation of syngeneic tumors: (a) the methylcholanthrene-induced sarcoma system of Fujimoto et al. (81); (b) the P815Y mastocytoma system of Takei et al. (82); (c) the UV-induced tumor system of Fisher and Kripke (83); and (d) the methylcholanthrene-induced sarcoma system of Berendt and North (84). In these systems, it appears that in the initial stages of growth, tumors stimulate a specific, measurable immune response, but that this response is transient because of the development of T cells that suppress it.

Patients with primary cancers, even those detected early, probably correspond to mice with large, transplanted tumors, and it is reasonable to hypothesize that the tumor-directed immune response of these patients has already passed through the initial phase and is in a suppressor phase at the time of diagnosis. This hypothesis would account for the difficulty in measuring tumor-directed immunity and also for the failure of conventional forms of immunotherapy.

The suppressor hypothesis predicts that a reduction in tumor-specific T-suppressor activity would facilitate the successful use of immunotherapy. This question has been addressed in the experiments of Berendt and North (84) and North (85). They have shown that adoptive transfer of tumor-immune spleen cells to tumor-bearing mice had no effect on tumor growth. However, if mice had been depleted of T cells by thymectomy, lethal irradiation, and bone marrow reconstitution, or pretreated with CY, then adoptive transfer of immune spleen cells resulted in complete and permanent regression of established tumors. The tumor regression could be prevented by administration of splenic T cells from mice with established tumors, but not by spleen cells from normal mice. Thus, depletion or impairment of CY-sensitive suppressor T cells allowed the expression of immunity to tumor-associated antigens.

There are a number of other studies in rodent models suggesting that the principle of CY immunopotentiation might be applied to heighten the immune response to tumor antigens (64, 86-93). CY pretreatment followed by tumor cells increased the number of cytotoxic T cells, as judged by in vitro cytotoxicity or by Winn testing (64, 88). CY given 3 days prior to tumor cells decreased the growth rate of an implant of that tumor in syngeneic mice (87). Properly timed low-dose CY treatment of the MOPC-315 myeloma in syngeneic mice decreased tumor growth by immunological means (90). CY treatment of mice bearing a MCA fibrosarcoma resulted in the maintenance or restoration of tumor immunity as judged by the activity of spleen cells in a Winn assay (86). Terishimna et al. (91) found enhanced immunogenicity of xenogenized tumor cells in syngeneic rats pretreated with CY. Similarly, Baldwin et al. (92), again in rats, found that CY pretreatment rendered effective an otherwise ineffective 3M KCl extract of a hepatoma when that extract was used as a vaccine to protect against subsequent transplantation of the tumor. In histocompatible mice, Nicolin et al. (93) obtained immunopotentiation by CY pretreatment of an immunizing inoculum of viable L1210/DTIC cells, once more using an immunoprotection assay.

Curiously, the particularly pertinent issue of using CY to immunopotentiate a tumor vaccine so as to cause rejecton of an established syngeneic tumor has not been investigated in an animal model. The ability of CY immunopotentiation to facilitate the immunological rejection of autologous tissue and its ability to break natural and acquired specific immunological tolerance *when used with antigen* (50, 94, 95) provides precedent and encouragement that a similar immunologically based rejection of autologous (syngeneic) tumor tissue can be obtained. Our initial studies in man of the immunopotentiation by CY of an autologous tumor vaccine have been encouraging (96). Systematic investigations to optimize parameters of immunization with tumor antigen plus CY alone, and with CY combined with other immunopotentiators, in animals bearing syngeneic or autologous tumors could be of great practical importance and are urgently needed.

X. SUMMARY AND CONCLUSIONS

CY is a potent cytotoxic drug, and among the cells that are very sensitive to its cytotoxic effect is the lymphocyte. This chapter has attempted to show that killing of, or damage to, lymphocytes does not necessarily lead to immunosuppression, but can just as readily result in immunopotentiation. Although this concept is widely accepted, and even considered mundane, by experimental immunologists, it is not yet fully appreciated by clinical immunologists and clinicians who study cytotoxic agents.

The data accumulated so far suggest that the most important variable determining whether CY is immunosuppressive or immunopotentiating is the timing of the administration of CY and antigen. In animal systems, immunopotentiation is produced by administering CY 1-4 days before antigen, while administration of CY after antigen generally results in no effect or in immunosuppression. Although we achieved immunopotentiation in patients by giving CY 3 days before antigen, we did not determine whether this interval was optimal, and further clinical study of this variable is needed.

The dose of CY is probably less important than the timing. Doses that have been reported to produce immunopotentiation in experimental animals have varied from 60 mg/M^2 to 2100 mg/M^2. In the one clinical study reported, augmentation of immunity was observed with a dose of 1000 mg/M^2. It is possible that lower doses would be more effective in humans, especially in patients with advanced cancer whose immune system is often severely damaged by the combined effects of the disease and therapies.

We believe it important that immunopotentiation by CY be evaluated by measuring its effect on actual immune responses (i.e., cell-mediated or humoral immunity to specific antigens, rather than on nonspecific parameters of lymphocyte functions). Although parameters such as lymphoproliferative responses to lectins could be useful in working out the mechanisms of immunopotentiation, they are not per se measures of immunity and could even be misleading. For example, since both suppressor and helper T cells respond to commonly used lectins (97), CY-induced depletion of suppressor T cells could result in augmentation of DTH in the face of impaired lymphoproliferative responses.

Finally, it is premature to speculate on the potential usefulness of CY in augmenting immunity to clinically important antigens in patients with cancer or other disease states associated with immunosuppression. However, it is clear that the realization that cytotoxic drugs can be immunopotentiating has given us a new perspective on immunoregulation. At the very least, these drugs will be valuable tools in the study of human immune responsiveness and the factors that modulate it.

REFERENCES

1. N. Brock and H. Wilmanns, *Dtsch. Med. Wochenschr.*, *83*:453 (1958).
2. N. Brock and H. J. Hohorst, *Arzneim Forsch.*, *13*:1021 (1963).
3. M. Colvin and J. Hilton, *Cancer Treatment Rep.*, *65*, (Suppl. 3):89 (1981).
4. L. B. Grochow and M. Colvin, *Clin. Pharmacokinetics*, *4*:380 (1979).
5. M. Colvin, R. B. Brundrett, M. -N. N. Kan, I. Jardine, and C. Fenselau, *Cancer Res.*, *36*:1121 (1976).
6. A. Takamizawa, S. Matsumoto, T. Iwata, K. Katagiri, Y. Tochino, K. Yamaguchi, *J. Am. Chem. Soc.*, *95*:3 (1973).
7. C. M. Bagley, Jr., F. W. Bostick, and V. T. DeVita, Jr., *Cancer Res.*, *33*:226 (1973).
8. F. D. Juma, H. J. Rogers, and J. R. Trounce, *Brit. J. Clin. Pharm.*, *8*:209 (1979).
9. S. C. Sarpel and R. B. Epstein, *Exp. Hematol.*, *9*:223 (1981).
10. B. A. Chabner and C. W. Myers, *Cancer, Principles and Practice of Oncology*, Lippincott, Philadelphia, 1982, pp. 172-175.
11. H. Haar, J. Marshall, H. Bierman, et al., *Cancer Chemother. Rep.*, *6*:41 (1960).
12. R. Papac, N. Petrakis, F. Amini, et al., *JAMA*, *172*:1387 (1960).
13. P. Coggins, R. Ravdin, and S. Eisman, *Cancer*, *13*:1254 (1960).
14. C. C. Harris, *J. Natl. Cancer Inst.*, *63*:275 (1979).
15. C. S. Alvarado, T. F. Boat, and A. J. Newman, *J. Pediatr.*, *92*:443 (1978).
16. F. P. Alepa, N. J. Zvaifler, and A. J. Sliwinski, *Arthritis Rheum.*, *13*:754 (1970).
17. A. Winkelstein, J. M. Mikulla, N. R. Nankin, B. H. Pollock, and B. L. Stolzer, *J. Lab. Clin. Med.*, *80*:506 (1972).
18. D. A. Horwitz, *Arthritis Rheum.*, *17*:363 (1974).
19. E. R. Hurd and V. J. Giuliano, *Arthritis Rheum.*, *18*:67 (1975).
20. G. M. Mullins, P. N. Anderson, and G. W. Santos, *Cancer*, *36*:1950 (1975).
21. B. Smit, J. Stjernsward, E. Dowdle, G. R. Sealy, E. Wilson, D. Beatty, P. Jacobs, and M. B. Bennett, *Int. J. Radiation Oncol. Biol. Phys.*, *5*:1841 (1979).
22. T. R. Cupps, L. C. Edgar, and A. S. Fauci, *J. Immunol.*, *128*:2453 (1982).
23. A. Winkelstein, F. L. Ruben, S. F. Tolchin, and B. M. Pollock, *J. Lab. Clin. Med.*, *83*:504 (1974).
24. G. W. Santos, A. H. Owens, and L. L. Sensenbrenner, *Ann. N.Y. Acad. Sci.*, *114*:404 (1964).
25. A. S. Fauci, S. M. Wolff, and J. S. Johnson, *N. Engl. J. Med.*, *285*:1493 (1971).
26. I. R. Mackay, J. M. Dwyer, and M. J. Rowley, *Arthritis Rheum.*, *16*:455 (1973).
27. J. E. Curtis, J. T. Sharp, M. D. Lidsky, and E. M. Hersh, *Arthritis Rheum.*, *16*:34 (1973).

28. A. Dimitriu and A. S. Fauci, *Trans. Proc.*, *11*:878 (1979).
29. H. S. Stender, D. Ringlieb, D. Stranch, and H. Winter, *Strahlentherapie*, *43*:392 (1959).
30. H. C. Maguire, Jr., H. I. Mailbach, and L. W. Minisce, Jr., *J. Invest. Derm.*, *36*:235 (1961).
31. H. C. Maguire, Jr. and E. Steers, *Experientia*, *19*:591 (1963).
32. H. C. Maguire, Jr. and H. I. Mailbach, *J. Allergy*, *32*:406 (1961).
33. P. Dukor and F. M. Dietrick, *J. Immunol.*, *105*:118 (1970).
34. A. W. Frische and G. Davis, *Cancer Res.*, *25*, 745 (1965).
35. M. C. Berenbaum and I. N. Brown, *Immunology*, *7*:65 (1964).
36. G. Santos, *Fed. Proc.*, *26*:907 (1967).
37. S. P. Lerman and W. P. Weidanz, *J. Immunol.*, *105*:614 (1970).
38. J. Zulman, J. Michalski, C. McCombs, J. Greenspan, and N. Tabal, *Clin. Exp., Immunol.*, *31*:321 (1978).
39. S. Faine and B. Adler, *Infect. Immunity*, *14*:703 (1976).
40. J. Pacha, M. Metzger, W. Smogor, E. Michalska, J. Podwinska, and J. Ruczkowska, *Arch. Immun. Ther. Exp.*, *27*:45 (1979).
41. H. C. Maguire, Jr. and H. I. Mailbach, *J. Invest. Derm.*, *37*:427 (1961).
42. J. Turk and S. Stone, *Cell Bound Antibodies*, Wistar, Philadelphia, 1963, p. 15.
43. A. Hafizi and P. Z. Modabber, *Clin. Exp. Immunol.*, *33*:389 (1978).
44. M. C. Berenbaum, *Nature*, *200*:84 (1963).
45. H. C. Maguire, Jr. and V. L. Ettore, *J. Invest. Derm.*, *48*:39 (1967).
46. N. Hunziger, *Dermatologica*, *136*:187 (1968).
47. S. I. Katz, D. Parker, G. Sommer, and J. L. Turk, *Nature*, *248*:612 (1974).
48. J. F. Finerty and E. P. Kresh, *Infect. Immunity*, *14*:1103 (1976).
49. F. Y. Liew, S. M. Russell, and I. M. Brand, *Eur. J. Immunol.*, *9*:783 (1979).
50. S. Yoshida, K. Nomoto, K. Himeno, and K. Takeya, *Clin. Exp. Immunol.*, *38*:211 (1979).
51. J. L. Turk and D. Parker, *Immunol. Rev.*, *65*:99 (1982).
52. N. Chiorazzi, D. A. Fox, and D. H. Katz, *J. Immunol.*, *117*:1629 (1976).
53. P. Debre, C. Waltenbaugh, M. E. Dorf, and B. Benacerraf, *J. Exp. Med.*, *114*:277 (1976).
54. P. W. Askenase, B. J. Hayden, and R. K. Gershon, *J. Exp. Med.*, *141*:697 (1975).
55. E. J. Freireich, E. A. Gehan, D. P. Rall, L. N. Schmidt, and H. E. Skipper, *Cancer Chemother. Rep.*, *50*:219 (1966).
56. M. Goto, A. Mitsuoka, M. Sugiyama, and M. Kitano, *J. Exp. Med.*, *154*:204 (1981).
57. D. Berd, M. J. Mastrangelo, P. F. Engstrom, A. Paul, and H. Maguire, *Cancer Res.*, *42*:4862 (1982).
58. S. I. Katz, D. Parker, and J. L. Turk, *Nature*, *251*:550 (1974).
59. P. H. LaGrange, G. B. Mackaness, and T. E. Miller, *J. Exp. Med.*, *139*:528 (1974).
60. C. R. Parish, *Eur. J. Immunol.*, *2*:143 (1972).
61. P. D. Burrows, R. K. Gershon, A. R. Lawton, and R. W. Mowry, *Fed. Proc.*, *35*:861 (1976).
62. H. C. Maguire, Jr., L. Faris, and W. Weidany, *Immunology*, *37*:367 (1979).
63. M. Rollinghoff, A. Starzinski-Powitz, K. Pfizenmaier, and H. Wagner, *J. Exp. Med.*, *145*:455 (1977).
64. M. Glaser, *Cell. Immunol.*, *48*:339 (1979).
65. R. Diamantstein, E. Willinger, and J. Reiman, *J. Exp. Med.*, *150*:1571 (1979).
66. S. H. E. Kaufmann, H. Hahn, and T. Diamantstein, *J. Immunol.*, *125*:1104 (1980).
67. A. Schwartz, P. W. Askenase, and R. K. Gershon, *J. Immunol.*, *121*:1573 (1978).
68. H. C. Stevenson and A. S. Fauci, *Immunology*, *39*:391 (1980).
69. H. Ozer, J. W. Cowens, M. Colvin, A. Nussbaum-Blumenson, and D. Sheedy, *J. Exp. Med.*, *155*:276 (1982).
70. D. P. Braun and J. E. Harris, *Clin. Immunol. Immunopathol.*, *20*:193 (1981).

71. E. M. Hersh, P. P. Carbone, and E. J. Freireich, *J. Lab. Clin. Med.*, *67*:566 (1966).
72. E. M. Hersh and J. J. Oppenheim, *Cancer Res.*, *27*:98 (1967).
73. J. E. Harris, R. C. Bagai, and T. H. M. Stewart, *Proc. 7th Leukocyte Culture Conf.*, Academic Press, New York, 1973, pp. 443-457.
74. J. E. Harris, and T. H. M. Stewart, *Proc. 6th Leukocyte Culture Conf.*, Academic Press, New York, 1972, pp. 555-579.
75. A. R. Cheema and E. M. Hersh, *Cancer*, *28*:851 (1971).
76. L. J. Old, *Cancer Res.*, *41*:361 (1981).
77. M. Herlyn, W. H. Clark, M. J. Mastrangelo, D. Guerry, D. Elder, D. LaRossa, R. Hamilton, E. Bondi, R. Tuthill, Z. Steplewski, and H. Koprowski, *Cancer Res.*, *40*:3602 (1980).
78. W. H. Clark, M. J. Mastrangelo, A. M. Ainsworth, D. Berd, R. E. Bellet, and E. A. Bernardino, *Adv. Cancer Res.*, *24*:267 (1977).
79. R. K. Gershon, *Contemp. Top. Mol. Immunol.*, *3*:1 (1974).
80. S. Broder and T. A. Waldmann, *N. Engl. J. Med.*, *299*:1335 (1978).
81. S. Fujimoto, M. I. Green, and A. H. Sehon, *J. Immunol.*, *116*:791 (1976).
82. F. Takei, J. G. Levy, and D. G. Kilburn, *J. Immunol.*, *116*:288 (1976).
83. M. S. Fisher and M. L. Kripke, *Proc. Natl. Acad. Sci. USA*, *74*:1688 (1977).
84. M. J. Berendt and R. J. North, *J. Exp. Med.*, *151*:69 (1980).
85. R. J. North, *J. Exp. Med.*, *149*:774 (1979).
86. G. Steele, Jr., H. O. Sjogren, and T. Ankers, *Int. J. Cancer*, *14*:743 (1974).
87. M. C. Maguire, Jr., *Proc. Am. Assoc. Cancer Res.*, *18*:185 (1977).
88. M. Glaser, *J. Exp. Med.*, *149*:774 (1979).
89. S. Yu, D. R. Lannin, A. L. Tsui-Collins, and C. F. McKhann, *Cancer Res.*, *40*:2756 (1980).
90. J. C. D. Hengst, M. B. Mokyr, and S. Dray, *Cancer Res.*, *40*:2135 (1980).
91. M. Terishimma, N. Takeichi, K. Suzaki, T. Itaya, E. Gotohoda, and H. Kobayashi, *Tohoku J. Exp. Med.*, *132*:355 (1980).
92. R. W. Baldwin, V. S. Byers, D. Hannant, J. A. Jones, M. V. Pimm, and M. R. Price, *Recent Results Cancer Res.*, *80*:338 (1982).
93. A. Nicolin, F. Veronese, O. Marelli, and A. Goldin, *Cancer Immunol. Immunther.*, *9*:43 (1980).
94. L. Polak, H. Geleick, and J. L. Turk, *Immunology*, *28*:939 (1975).
95. A. M. Mowat, S. Strobel, H. E. Drummond, and A. Ferguson, *Immunology*, *45*:105 (1982).
96. D. Berd, H. Maguire, and M. J. Mastrangelo, *Proc. Am. Soc. Clin. Oncol.*, *2*:56 (1983).
97. E. G. Engleman, C. J. Benike, F. C. Grumet, and R. L. Evans, *J. Immunol.*, *127*:2124 (1981).

4
Lentinan

Tadao Aoki Shinrakuen Hospital, Niigata, Japan

I. INTRODUCTION

Numerous immunomodulating agents have been derived from plants, including mushroom, fungi, and bacteria. Since the discovery by Chihara and his colleagues (1,2), one of these agents, *Lentinan*, because of its significant antitumor activity and unique characteristics, has attracted the attention of clinical and preclinical investigators as a potent cancer immunotherapeutic agent.

When the antitumor effect of Lentinan was studied in 1969, using transplanted mouse tumors, no significant results were obtained (unpublished observations) because of compound overdosage as defined by our current findings (see below). Recently, the acting mechanisms as well as the clinical efficacy of Lentinan have been clarified to such an extent that the optimal dosage can be determined and its applicability utilized for the treatment of infectious diseases. Moreover, better understanding of its mechanisms of action has improved tremendously the clinical effectiveness of Lentinan. Thus, Lentinan, specifically its application in the treatment of infectious diseases caused by bacteria, viruses, and parasites, has been and is being studied in experimental animals and human systems.

This chapter will review the biological activity and mechanisms of action of Lentinan in humans from an immunological point of view. The data in experimental animal systems will be presented as supplementary information to the results obtained in the human systems. The general properties of Lentinan will also be described.

II. PHYSICOCHEMICAL PROPERTIES

Lentinan is a completely purified neutral polysaccharide extracted from the fruit bodies or myelium of basidiomycetes, ***Lentinus edodes*** (Berk.) Sing., an edible mushroom prevalent in Japan. Its physicochemical characteristics are as follows: (a) Molecular formula $(C_6H_{10}O_5)n$, a β (1,3)-D-glucan as the main chain with two β (1,6)-D-glucopyranoside branchings for every five β (1,3)-glucopyranoside linear linkages (Fig. 1) (3); (b) average molecular weight 5×10^5, ranging from 3 to 7×10^5 daltons as determined by gel chromatography (G. Chihara, personal communications); (c) glucose sugar components; (d) a right-handed triple-helix structure according to x-ray analysis (4); (e) water-soluble (5); (f) heat-stable (T. Hirata, personal communications); and (g) acid-stable but alkali-labile (T. Hirata, personal communications).

In terms of a correlation between the chemical structure of polysaccharides and their antitumor effects, the higher-order structure or micelle formation seems to play a more important role than the primary structure (6,7). In other words, among glucans with the same β (1,3)-glucopyranoside as the main chain, some compounds, such as Lentinan or pachymaran, possess strong antitumor activity (5,8), but others are devoid of this activity. For instance, it is well known that pachyman has no antitumor effects. However, when this compound is converted to U-Pachyman by treatment with urea, without conversion of its primary structure, U-Pachyman becomes a strong antitumor agent (5,9). This fact suggests the presence of a specific mechanism in the biological system which identifies the essential conformation of polysaccharides. Thus, both a formulized Lentinan with low molecular weight of about 6250 daltons (10) and a debranched Lentinan (11) showed significant antitumor activity.

III. DOSAGE

A. Optimal Dosage

When the antitumor activity of Lentinan was examined experimentally in the cradle of Lentinan development, the rule, "the larger the dose, the better the results," was automatically applied. Consequently, the experimental results were often negative on the basis of our current knowledge, due to overdosage (9,12-14); that is, subcutaneous administration of Lentinan caused the complete regression of Sarcoma-180 transplanted into ICR mice at a dose of 1 mg/kg for 10 days, while a larger dose of 80 mg/kg of Lentinan for 5 days showed no antitumor activity in comparison with the untreated control mice. By focusing our attention on this critical problem, the method of administration of Lentinan was improved in the clinic rather than in the experimental system.

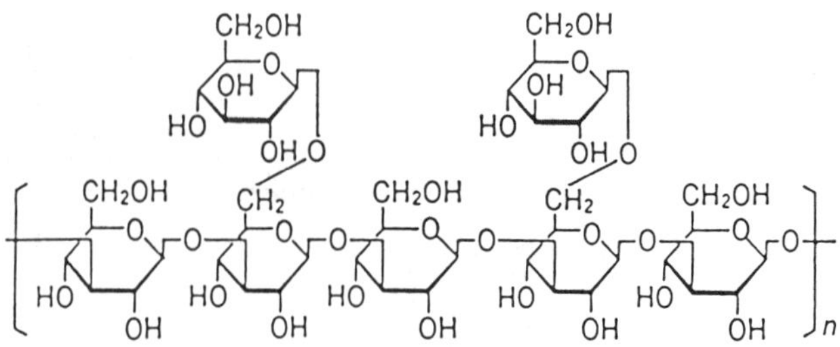

Figure 1 The main part of chemical structure of Lentinan.

In the clinic, 1 mg per person of Lentinan twice a week has been found to be the optimal dosage for intravenous (IV) or intramuscular (IM) injection (15,16). Of course, this amount is flexible within a certain permissible range. When overdoses (e.g., 10 mg per person) of Lentinan were injected daily IV or IM into cancer patients, the host immune response was markedly depressed as indicated by several measurements (see below). However, when an effective method of oral administration of Lentinan, though not available yet, becomes available dosages considered excessive for injections may be found to be optimal for oral usage (under investigation). For now, the optimal dosage of almost all immunomodulators including Lentinan can be individually determined for the corresponding route of administration.

B. Toxicology

Acute and subacute toxicological studies of Lentinan were determined by IV injection into mice, rats, dogs, and monkeys. In all species tested, the LD_{50} was more than 100 mg/kg (15). Chronic toxicity of Lentinan was also examined by injecting it IV daily for 25 weeks in various amounts (0.5, 2, 8, and 30 mg/kg) into four groups (two males and two females each) of rhesus monkeys. Although the group injected with the lowest dosage showed no side effects or histological changes, the other groups demonstrated both clinical and histological changes such as skin rashes, bleeding, foam cells in the liver, spleen, and lymph nodes, renal granuloma and vasculitis, and subepithelial hemorrhage and vasculitis in the urinary bladder. In anaphylaxis tests, all guinea pigs preinjected with Lentinan, regardless of the presence or absence of accompanying adjuvant, were not hypersensitized by the IV or intracutaneous injection of Lentinan.

Therefore, the regular dosage of Lentinan, 1 mg IV injection for humans, is quite safe and is given in the clinic for the reasons described above.

IV. BIOLOGICAL ACTIVITY

Several immune parameters have been employed in order to enquire into the host immune responses, including natural killer (NK) activity, killer T cell-mediated cytotoxicity, DNA synthesis and proliferative responses of peripheral mononuclear cells (PMNC) to mitogens, interferon (IFN) titer, opsonin titer, phagocytic activity of neutrophils, etc. First, the results obtained in the human system will be described, and second, the data reported in an experimental animal system will be supplementarily summarized (Table 1).

A. NK Activity and Interferon (IFN) Titers

The ^{51}Cr-release of human myeloid K-562 cells was measured as NK activity by incubation at 37°C for 6 hr at ratios to effector cells of 1:20 and/or 1:40. International units of IFN were determined by measuring the protection capacity of cytopathic effects of vesicular stomatitis virus (VSV) on human FL cells.

When IFN titers in plasma and NK activity of PMNC from patients with various types of cancer were sequentially measured before and after the initiation of Lentinan administration, the peak of IFN titer preceded that of NK activity (17), e.g., the former appeared 12 hr after Lentinan administration and the latter after 24 hr. Since IFN directly activates NK cells in vitro and in vivo very quickly (within 1 or 2 hr) (18-20), the 12 hr interval between the appearance of the peaks of IFN titer and NK activity seems to be too long to interpret by the in vitro findings. A possible explanation is that IFN-activated

Table 1 Comparison Between Biological Activities of Lentinan in Experimental Animals and Human Systems

Items	Experimental Animal System		Human System	
	In Vitro	In Vivo	In Vitro	In Vivo
Humoral factors				
Inhibition of immunosuppressive substance production	ND[a]	++	ND	++
Immunopotentiative substance production	ND	++	ND	++
C3 splitting activity	ND	+	ND	ND
Antibody production	ND	+	ND	+
Opsonin production	ND	ND	ND	+
Production of CSF[b]	+	ND	ND	ND
Production of LAF (IL1)[c]	+	+	+	ND
Inhibition of prostraglandin release	−	+	ND	ND
IFN[d] production	−(?)	+(γ type?)	− ~ ±	+(γ type)
Cellular factors				
NK[e] activation	−	+	± ~ +	++
Activation of helper T cells	ND	+	+	ND
Activation of killer T cells	+	+	+	ND
Activation of cytotoxic macrophages	−	+	ND	+
DTHR[f]		+		+ ~ ++
Mitogenicity	ND	ND	± ~ +[g]	++

[a]ND: not done.
[b]CSF: colony-stimulating factor.
[c]LAF (IL1): lymphocyte-activating factor (interleukin 1).
[d]IFN: interferon.
[e]NK: natural killer.
[f]DTHR: delayed-type hypersensitivity reaction.
[g]Coexistence of T cells, B cells, and monocytes is essential for stimulating mitogenicity by Lentinan.

effector cells for cytotoxicity may penetrate into malignant tissues, causing their disappearance from the peripheral blood circulation soon after the administration of Lentinan. Afterwards, when the surplus of effector cells has been boosted with IFN produced by the host, augmentation of NK activity of PMNC can be recognized. Thus, intervals of 12-24 hr may be necessary. To substantiate this explanation, a case of paraganglioma is described here.

Metastatic paraganglioma of a 42-year-old male was diagnosed by clinical and histological examinations. Its onset began in the spring of 1979. The SC metastases were found and biopsied in June 1981. Mononuclear cells were collected from either the metastatic tumor tissues or the peripheral blood. In the autochthonous system—namely, using fresh paraganglioma cells from the patient as target cells, mononuclear cells from the patient as attacker cells, and the patient's own plasma—the mononuclear cells from the malignant tissues showed a certain cytotoxicity, but the cells from peripheral blood did not. On the other hand, NK activity against K-562 cells was quite positive with the latter, but almost completely negative with the former. According to cytological examination with May-Giemsa, the mononuclear cells from the malignant tissues look most like NK cells, large granular lymphocytes (LGL) (21), suggesting the presence of at least two different subpopulations of LGL.

In the context of the findings in this patient and the general kinetics of both IFN production and cell-mediated cytotoxicity induced by Lentinan administration, the above explanation seems most likely. Further, Lentinan may activate NK cells directly and/or through IFN induction; the former suggests the presence of an alternative pathway for NK cell activation (22).

When Lentinan was administered continuously for a long period of time, the IFN titer in peripheral blood was high as indicated by periodically performed tests. Of course, the IFN titers fluctuated with each individual Lentinan administration as described above. Therefore, unless Lentinan was used properly, the IFN titers in the body fluid could not have been constantly maintained at a high level. In vitro, however, IFN induction did not take place in the experimental animal system (J. Hamuro, personal communications), despite the in vivo induction of IFN and NK cell activation (23,24). Whether IFN induction occurred in vitro in humans remains undetermined, although weak IFN production was observed in vitro.

Based on the physicochemical characteristics of IFN induced by Lentinan administration (i.e., heat-labile and acid-labile), this IFN can be considered to be human IFN-γ (25). The final determination of the IFN type will be determined with antisera against human IFN-α, -β, and -γ.

One way mixed lymphocyte culture (MLC) reaction-induced killer T-cell activity was measured by ^{51}Cr-release using blastoid stimulating cells, incubated with phytohemagglutinin (PHA), as target cells (25,26). This MLC-induced killer T-cell activity was augmented by adding Lentinan in vitro only when suboptimal numbers of stimulator cells were added to responder cells. By contrast, no stimulatory effect of Lentinan was observed when it was added with optimum numbers of stimulator cells. These findings suggest the presence of a certain stimulus that induces effective cell-to-cell reaction.

B. PMNC-Proliferative Responses

In general, the ^{3}H-TdR (tritiated methyl thymidine) incorporation of PMNC from cancer patients significantly declined with the progression of the disease in contrast with that of PMNC from healthy donors (15,27,28). This trend was also observed after in vitro stimulation with well-known mitogens such as PHA, staphage lysate (SPL), pokeweed mitogen (PWM), and concanavalin A (ConA). However, the suppressed PMNCs from cancer patients were activated in vitro by various dosages of Lentinan, ranging from 10^{-5} to 10^3 μg/ml, and in vivo by Lentinan administration of 1 mg/day twice weekly. It is of great interest that PMNCs from healthy donors were similarly activated in vitro and in vivo with Lentinan, whereas PMNCs from patients who had already been given Lentinan did not respond in vitro to Lentinan. These findings indicate that, since they had been maximally activated in vivo by Lentinan, PMNCs were not able to respond further to Lentinan. Of course, the level of ^{3}H-TdR incorporation by PMNCs was much higher after the Lentinan treatment than before. After the termination of Lentinan administration, the PMNCs from the cancer patients again showed lowered spontaneous and proliferative responses to mitogens and became reactive to Lentinan in vitro after several weeks (27,28).

Before a couple of years ago, Lentinan had been considered to be an immunorestorative agent (i.e., Lentinan restored the suppressed host immune response to the normal level but not above it). In light of the above results Lentinan, at various concentrations, can clearly augment in vitro the proliferative reaction of PMNC from healthy donors. Consequently, Lentinan, more properly, should be categorized as an immunopotentiator. This theoretical modification has been substantiated by in vivo animal experiments as mentioned below.

Concerning the in vitro activation of PMNC subpopulations with Lentinan, neither human T cell-rich PMNCs, B cell-rich PMNCs, nor adherent PMNC alone responded at all to ^{3}H-TdR incorporation, although the whole PMNCs or the reconstructed mixture of T-cell-rich PMNCs, adherent PMNCs, and non-T cell-rich PMNCs were clearly activated by Lentinan. Because of the absence of in vitro stimulation of any two subpopulation combinations among those three PMNC subpopulations, it may be concluded that the coexistence of all three PMNC subpopulations—B cells, T cells, and adherent cells—are essential for the in vitro Lentinan activation of PMNCs (15,27,28). This action of Lentinan differs clearly from that of other known mitogens, such as PHA, PWM, SPL, and ConA, which can stimulate in vitro the interaction between two individual subpopulations of PMNCs (29).

When a B cell-activating mitogen, PWM or SPL, was added in vitro with Lentinan to PMNCs, the PWM-induced IgG and IgM syntheses of PMNCs were elevated by adding a certain amount of Lentinan (15,27,28). However, the SPL-induced IgG synthesis of PMNC was decreased by adding Lentinan while no significant changes in the SPL-induced IgM synthesis occurred. These findings may be interpreted by the following three possible explanations: (a) suppresser T cells were relatively inactivated by Lentinan; (b) helper T cells were activated by Lentinan; and (c) the above two possibilities occurred simultaneously and canceled each other's actions.

The PWM-induced IgG and IgM syntheses of PMNCs decreased to one-half or one-third by adding PMNCs preincubated with ConA. This suppressive effect of PMNCs on the immunoglobulin synthesis was reduced by preculturing with both Lentinan and ConA (15,27,28). Therefore, Lentinan itself seems to augment the immunoglobulin synthesis of PMNCs, although the IgG synthesis of PMNCs was only somewhat diminished by adding PMNCs preincubated with Lentinan alone. These results suggest that Lentinan affects two subpopulations, suppressor and helper T cells. This suggestion has been substantiated by a report that Lentinan recovered and sometimes heightened the depressed activity of helper T cells in cancer patients as well as in tumor-bearing mice (14,30,31), thus qualifying Lentinan as a T-cell adjuvant (32-34). Particularly since the immunosuppressed status of cancer patients has been considered to be caused predominantly by the elevation of suppressor T-cell activity (35-37), these biological characteristics of Lentinan, as an immunopharmacological agent, may allow it to be considered increasingly as an effective defense against the lowered immune status of cancer patients.

C. Humoral Immune Factors

Knowledge of the effects of Lentinan on specific humoral antibody formation is still very poor. Only a specific opsonin against *Mycobacterium tuberculosis* has been investigated. Lentinan was administered to three patients who excreted, for more than 10 years, bacilli resistant to antituberculosis drugs (38). After Lentinan administration (IM injection, 1 mg/day, twice a week), the titer of specific opsonin toward the bacilli which the patients excreted was elevated so appreciably that the bacillus excretion in one of these patients ceased.

Treatment of ICR mice injected with Sarcoma-180 10 days earlier with 1 mg/kg/day of Lentinan for 10 days caused complete regression of the tumors. At the same time, the amount of three serum proteins, LA, LB, and LC, increased markedly 4-7 days after the initiation of Lentinan administration (39). LA is an α-globuline while LB and LC are β-globulins. These glycoproteins, LA, LB, and LC, may be identified as ceruloplasmin, hemopexin, and complement C3, respectively (40-42). In contrast, overdosages of

Lentinan (10 mg/kg/day) induced progressive tumor growth, without a significant increase of these three serum proteins. Thus, these proteins are assumed to play a necessary role in influencing the host immune response. A similar specific serum protein fraction has been demonstrated in cancer patients (43-45). This human serum protein is also an α-globulin, which is an immunosuppressive factor as indicated by its effects on MLC reaction, proliferative responses of PMNCs to mitogens, and NK activity. Interestingly, Lentinan administration to cancer patients not only abolished this immunosuppressive serum fraction but also produced a new protein fraction, a β-globulin which stimulates MLC, PMNC-proliferative responses, and NK activity (43-45). These special changes in serum proteins were detected in 4 of 12 patients with either stomach or lung cancer, and among these 4, 3 showed noticeable improvement with Lentinan treatment. These serum fractions differ from tumor necrosis factor, ceruloplasmin, and haptoglobin. The immunosuppressive factor was found in sera from lung cancer patients and, when these sera were injected into mice, the plaque-forming cell (PFC) response to sheep red blood cells (SRBC) was suppressed (45). This suppression was also significantly inhibited by Lentinan (47).

One of the most important biological activities of Lentinan is its capacity to function as a prostaglandin inhibitor; prostaglandin release from peritoneal macrophages is remarkable suppressed in Lentinan-administered mice (48). Since prostaglandin depresses T-cell differentiation, Lentinan may potentiate cell-mediated immunity. This may also be true in the human system.

D. Supplementary Data in the Experimental Animal System

So far, the mechanism of action of Lentinan has been described mainly by using the data obtained in the human system. When attention was shifted to the experimental animal system, almost the same findings were observed as in the human system, indicating that Lentinan may activate essentially the host immune response through the stimulation of immune effector cell interaction as indicated:

1. Lentinan selectively activated the cytotoxicity of murine peritoneal macrophages against malignant cells when systematically used in vivo but not when cocultured in vitro with macrophages (49,50). This in vivo activation of peritoneal macrophages may be attributed to the restoration of tumor-specific antigen-directed delayed-type hypersensitivity reaction (DTHR) due to Lentinan, or to the activation of an alternative pathway of the complement system (51).
2. Less antitumor action of Lentinan was observed in athymic nude mice (30,52). Antitumor activity of Lentinan was completely abolished by neonatal thymectomy plus administration of antilymphocyte serum in the mouse (15,30,53).
3. Lentinan could induce IFN in vivo but, although this should be examined further, not in vitro. Lentinan did not induce any types of IFN in vitro in the mouse system (J. Hamuro, personal communication), but IFN-production was detected in the culture supernatants of spleen cells from CBA/J mice injected IP, IV, SC, or IM with 1 mg/kg/day of Lentinan for 3 days. Furthermore, the ddI mouse produced IFN 240 IU/ml in serum in response to one injection of a high dose of Lentinan (200 mg/kg, IP injection) (N. Ishida, personal communication). The type of mouse IFN has not been identified as either α or β but may be classified in the future as γ-type using antimouse IFN-γ serum.
4. Prostaglandin release from macrophages was markedly depressed by Lentinan administration, suggesting the potentiation of cell-mediated immunity (48).

5. Lentinan augments the production of lymphocyte-activating factor, Interleukin 1 (IL1), from immune response-regulated macrophages directly and/or via the colony stimulating factor production with Lentinan-stimulated T cells (34). Since IL1 is able to transform premature T cells into immunopotent mature T cells (54), the augmented IL1 production may enhance the maturation of premature T cells into mature T cells which, in turn, become effector cells in the presence of lymphokines as a second signal.
6. The characteristics of Lentinan as a macrophage activator were accompanied by its enhancement of the cytotoxic and cytostatic activities of mouse peritoneal cells against different tumor cells in vivo (49,50). Lentinan, however, did not augment either in vivo phagocytic activity as measured by conventional carbon clearance or in vitro phagocytic and cytotoxic activities of macrophages (49).
7. In the murine system Lentinan activated markedly the alternative pathway of the complement system (51) as well as the classical pathway (K. Nishioka, personal communications). Lentinan was also able to split C_3 into C_{3a} and C_{3b}. This ability appears to enhance macrophage activation (55). These findings are among the first effects of Lentinan in the host, undergoing nonspecific activation of macrophages. Moreover, Lentinan increases absolute value of C_3 and stimulates C_4 (A. Davies, personal communications), which may help cancer-bearing hosts with lowered complement levels.
8. Lentinan augments both PFC induction against SRBC in vivo and in vitro and DTHR to SRBC. After SC injection of the SRBC antigen into mice of several strains on day 0 in various inoculum sizes, Lentinan was injected IP three times, on days 0, 1, and 2 over a wide range of doses from 0.02 to 100 mg/kg. Although augmenting and inhibiting effects of Lentinan on PFC induction varied depending upon the amount of inoculated SRBC, the smaller the amount of SRBC, the larger the dose of Lentinan required to show optimal augmentation (34). By measuring footpad swelling as DTHR to SRBC, injection of 5 mg/kg of Lentinan clearly revealed significant elevation of DTHR in all of the strains of mice tested (34). This DTHR indicated again the dose response to SRBC, exhibiting lower DTHR at 10^4 and 10^8 of SRBC than that at 10^6, and additionally, the augmentation of DTHR by Lentinan reflected the dose response (47).

These findings again indicate clearly that Lentinan is not only an immunorestorative agent, but also an immunopotentiating agent.

E. Others

Lentinan possesses some characteristics different from those of other known immunomodulating agents:

1. Lentinan strengthens mouse sensitivity to histamine or serotonin in the same way that pertussis vaccine, in contrast to the suppressive activity of Lentinan, strengthens mouse sensitivity to the histamine shock of pertussis-treated mice (56). This characteristic seems relevant to the fact that Lentinan can prevent what appears to be toxic death caused by the administration of cyclocytidine or vincristine (57) because of the following findings. Administration of 500 mg/kg cyclocytidine for 20 days resulted in death, but this toxication like action appeared to be depressed by the use of Lentinan in combination with cyclocytidine for the same reason that no death occurred during the corresponding period. This might be induced by the action of physiologically active amines, such as vascular permeability, which effect the mechanisms of action of Lentinan.

2. The difference within the wide range of the antitumor effect of Lentinan on LOU immunocytoma in rats according to the timing of its administration may be due to the action of serotonin or catecholamines (58).
3. The antitumor activity of Lentinan was greatly inhibited by thyroxin, its activity dropping from 96 to 22% (59). As thyroxin serves to enhance tumor growth, it still remains possible that this inhibition may result from an antagonism between the actions of Lentinan and thyroxin. In any case, it is an interesting and important problem for future studies of host defense mechanisms against cancer, that the thyroid gland plays some role in tumor growth, because cancer incidence is high in myxedema but low in hyperthyroidism.
4. The antitumor activity of Lentinan was also inhibited by hydrocortisone (59). Since the action of cortisol to attack specifically thymus-derived lymphocytes was synergistic with that of antilymphocyte serum (60), it should be reasonable to consider that the antitumor effect of Lentinan may be inhibited by hydrocortisone acetate. Therefore, endocrinological homeostasis could be affected by Lentinan.

V. APPLICATIONS

A. Possible Use for the Treatment of Bacterial Infection

Although Lentinan was originally developed as a candidate for an antitumor agent, it has gradually become evident that Lentinan can be also applied to the treatment of infectious diseases on the basis of the above findings. For example, three patients with pulmonary tuberculosis who had excreted drug-resistant *M. tuberculosis* for at least 10 years were treated with Lentinan and the excretion of *M. tuberculosis* ceased (38). In these patients the opsonin effect on or the phagocytic activity of neutrophils to the *M. tuberculosis* excreted by these same patients was augmented in addition to the improvement of general conditions. These findings have been supported by examining the immunopotentiating effects of Lentinan on experimental mouse tuberculosis, especially on postchemotherapy relapse (61). Infected mice were first treated by intensive chemotherapy with a three-drug combination (streptomycin + isoniazid + rifampicin or ethambutol + isoniazid + rifampicin) for 5 months. After termination of chemotherapy, the mice of one group were treated with Lentinan for 4 weeks and then for another 4 weeks after a 1-month pause, reducing this persistent bacilli to undetectable levels (determined by examining the growth of latent tubercle bacilli in the lungs and spleen by cultivation of tissue homogenates). Thus, the application of Lentinan was highly effective in limiting the relapse rate in the lungs.

Lentinan also potentiated host resistance to infection with *Listeria monocytogenes*, therefore, prolonging the survival time through the macrophage route (62).

B. Initial Trials of Lentinan Administration for Virus Infection

Due to induction of IFN production, Lentinan had potential value against virus infection. Actually, mouse encephalitis caused by VSV was markedly improved by postinfection treatment with Lentinan (63). Significant protection against VSV infection was more effectively achieved by pretreatment with Lentinan, even though the effectiveness of Lentinan treatment depended upon the mouse strains used. At present, clinical trials of Lentinan administration to aged patients with chronic infectious diseases such as chronic bronchitis are being conducted by us. We can at least state so far that some significant results have been obtained.

The original application of Lentinan in the clinic should be for the treatment of cancer. In general, however, this kind of immunomodulator is always open to utilization for the prevention as well as the treatment of malignancy, whatever the oncogenesis. What mechanisms of action of Lentinan as an immunomodulator are important, or essential, for cancer prevention are still unclear. However, it has been known that Lentinan possesses some prophylactic activity to virus induction of malignancy [e.g., adenovirus-12 (64) and Abelson's tumor virus (63)]. Recent discovery of a novel type-C retrovirus in T-cell leukemia patients (65,66) has raised a new implication for the immunotherapy and immunoprophylaxis of T-cell leukemias or malignant lymphomas. Some animal experiments are under investigation for treatment of chemical carcinogen-induced tumors or spontaneous tumors. Since this kind of work is of great interest from both practical and theoretical points of view, we should remain attentive to this project.

C. Preliminary Trials for Experimental Parasitism

In experimental mouse parasitism, it has been reported (67) that Lentinan potentiated granuloma formation against the eggs of *Shistosoma mansoni* and *Shistosoma japonicum* up to an eight-fold increase above that of controls in the lung, and in addition it caused necrosis in the center of granulomas. However, that this did not occur in nude mice suggests again an important role for T cells in these phenomena.

Possible mechanisms of action of Lentinan, based on the above findings, are schematically illustrated in Fig. 2.

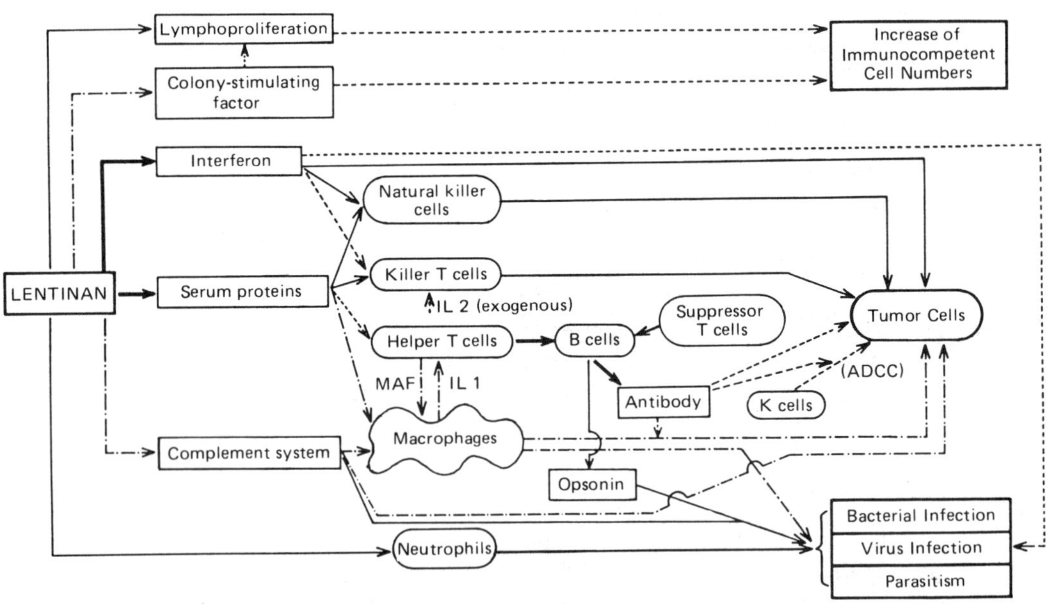

Figure 2 A schema of possible acting mechanisms of Lentinan. ——→, Known in both the human and experimental animal systems; ——→, known only in the human system; —·—·→, known only in the experimental animal system; – – – –→, unknown yet.

D. Usage for the Treatment of Cancer Patients

The antitumor activity of Lentinan was originally found against the Sarcoma-180 transplanted SC tumor in ICR mice. It was then observed that Lentinan exhibited no direct cytotoxicity to tumor cells but showed this activity through host-mediated immunity (52); and furthermore that there is some optimal dosage of Lentinan for inducing the above phenomena (9). In addition a most important finding was that methylcholanthrene-induced primary tumors in C3H/HeN mice regressed after Lentinan administration even when it was used in combination with cyclophosphamide injection (68), since there was neither interference with transplantation immunity, nor the presence of a precancerous stage before these treatments. Nonetheless, these positive results in this experimental tumor system encouraged clinical investigators to pursue the application of Lentinan administration in the treatment of human neoplasias.

Lentinan was also able to prevent chemical carcinogenesis: 1 mg/kg of Lentinan was administered daily for 10 days after methylcholanthrene injection into SWM/Ms mice, resulting in a 30% tumor incidence in the treated mice 30 weeks after the treatment with the chemical carcinogen and an 83% tumor incidence in the controls (69). This suggests the possible prophylactic use of Lentinan for chemical carcinogenesis.

By phase I and II clinical trials using a total of 235 patients with various types of cancer, the optimal dosage– 1 or 2 mg per person once or twice a week in combination with chemotherapy–was used to obtain favorable clinical antitumor efficacy with improved host immune responses as mentioned above (16). Guided by these results, a phase III (70) randomized controlled trial was conducted on patients with advanced or recurrent gastric cancer by administering the optimal dosage of Lentinan in combination with the following two kinds of basic chemotherapy: one was the combination treatment of mitomycin C with 5-fluorouracil (5-FU) (MF); the other was the single administration of tegafur (FT). In the MF treatment, mitomycin C (IV) and 5-FU (IV or oral, PO) were administered at the dosages of 4 and 500 mg per person per day, respectively, twice a week for the first 2 weeks and once weekly thereafter; FT (PO, IV, or suppository) treatment was at the dosage of 1 mg per person everyday. Lentinan was prepared as a lyophilized vial containing mannitol and dextran-40 as the excipients.

Of the patients examined in the trial, 60 were eligible for MF, 76 for the combination treatment of MF with Lentinan, 72 in FT, and 77 for the combination treatment of FT with Lentinan. Evaluations of clinical efficacy of Lentinan were judged on (a) the basis of the prolongation of life measured by using survival curves according to the Kaplan-Meier method; (b) the antitumor effect against measurable and/or evaluable lesions of solid tumors; (c) improvement of host immune responses, measured by PPD skin tests and peripheral blood lymphocyte counts; and (d) side effects. The statistical significance of life span prolongation was estimated by the generalized Wilcoxon's test.

The first three criteria consistently showed that the combination treatment of Lentinan with MF or FT was statistically more effective than the chemotherapy alone. Furthermore, since greater statistical significance was observed in patients both with primary lesion and without prior chemotherapy, it should be emphasized that the initiation of Lentinan administration prior to chemotherapy was essential in order to maximize the therapeutic efficacy of Lentinan. The following symptoms in 15 cases (10 patients) were suspected of being caused by side effects of Lentinan administration: 2 cases of nausea and vomiting, 4 cases of heaviness felt in the chest, 2 cases each of heat sensation, skin rash, and sweating, and 1 case each of face flush, blood pressure rise, and heaviness felt in the head. All side effects were transitional and not particularly serious.

Theoretically, the "regional" use of antitumor agents would be reasonable either to reduce harmful side effects or to augment the clinical effect of these agents. On the other hand, immunotherapy with nonspecific immunomodulators must be achieved "systematically" to induce the greatest host immune response. For these reasons, the following protocols of immunochemotherapy have been proposed and examined for inoperable gastric cancer patients (71). Intraaortic infusion of anticancer agents for carcinomatous peritonitis or hepatic arterial infusion for hepatic metastases were selected as examples of regional chemotherapy, and IM injection of Lentinan and/or picibanil (a preparation of attenuated *Streptococcus hemolyticus*) (72,73) was chosen for systemic nonspecific immunotherapy.

More than half of the 30 patients observed showed much better results than those obtained in cancer patients who were treated with "systemic immunochemotherapy" alone; that is, (a) survival time was prolonged, (b) the absolute number of peripheral leukocytes, lymphocytes, and erythrocytes did not fall permanently, and (c) the host immune response increased or at least did not decrease.

Moreover, intravenous hyperalimentation and blood transfusion may also help these patients by providing some materials favorable for the host defense mechanisms such as essential amino acids and complement. Another way to improve immunochemotherapy might be to use several different immunomodulating agents together to take advantage of their specific mechanisms of action. These possibilities should be investigated by further studies.

VI. CONCLUSION

Lentinan helps to create conditions favorable for the host defense mainly through the augmentation of humoral as well as cell-mediated immunity against exogenous invadors (e.g., bacteria, viruses, parasites, and endogenous non-self, neoplasias). Thus, Lentinan is a strong candidate as an immunomodulating agent for various therapeutic and prophylactic purposes, and additionally because of the absence of serious side effects.

Besides these utilities, Lentinan may be used to strengthen the biological activities of aged persons, regardless of health status, and to prevent the exhaustion of the activities in healthy persons from overwork. Especially, since it is evident that oral administration of Lentinan induces the same effective activity as that found for other routes of administration, the application of Lentinan treatment should expand to such additional fields as hypoglobulinemia, hypoimmune disorders, etc.; and furthermore it will be easier to treat outpatients. Endocrinological homeostasis could be maintained by Lentinan administration, which is an activity that is different from other immunomodulating agents.

On the other hand, it should be kept in mind that Lentinan administration cannot definitely cure malignant diseases at this time, although its administrations still remains to be improved by further studies. Since "specific" immunotherapy of cancer seems to be critical, and since "nonspecific" immunotherapy with immunomodulating agents has as its objective enhancement of specific immunity, development of specific immunotherapy is not only crucial but is also an ultimate goal of cancer immunotherapy (74,75). Accordingly, researchers must keep their eyes open to other, possibly more fruitful ways to conquer malignancy.

ADDENDUM

Since this chapter was written, an important report has been written [J. P. Fruehauf, G. D. Bonnard, and R. B. Herberman, *Immunopharmacology* (in press).] that indicates that the IL1 production by human monocytes is augmented in vitro by Lentinan. The importance of Lentinan's effect on the interaction between monocytes and T cells thus becomes more evident.

ACKNOWLEDGMENTS

The author is indebted to Mr. H. Miyakoshi for his valuable discussion and to Miss K. Igarashi for her excellent aid in preparation of this manuscript.

REFERENCES

1. G. Chihara, Y. Y. Maeda, J. Hamuro, T. Sasaki, and F. Fukuoka, *Nature*, *222*:687 (1969).
2. G. Chihara, Y. Y. Maeda, J. Hamuro, T. Sasaki, and F. Fukuoka, *Cancer Res.*, *30*:2776 (1970).
3. T. Sasaki and N. Takasuka, *Carbohyd. Res.*, *47*:99 (1976).
4. T. H. Bluhm and A. Sarko, *Can. J. Chem.*, *55*:293 (1977).
5. J. Hamuro, Y. Yamashita, Y. Ohsaka, Y. Y. Maeda, and G. Chihara, *Nature*, *233*:486 (1971).
6. J. Hamuro, Y. Y. Maeda, F. Fukuoka, and G. Chihara, *Chem. Biol. Interac.*, *3*:69 (1971).
7. J. Hamuro and G. Chihara, *Nature*, *245*:40 (1973).
8. G. Chihara, J. Hamuro, Y. Y. Maeda, Y. Arai, and F. Fukuoka, *Nature*, *225*:943 (1970).
9. Y. Y. Maeda and G. Chihara, in *Immunopotentiation* (G. E. W. Wolstenholme and J. Knight, eds.), Ciba Found. Symposium, new series 18, Elsevier, Excerpta Medica, Amsterdam, 1973, p. 251.
10. T. Sasaki, N. Takasuka, G. Chihara, and Y. Y. Maeda, *Gann* (*Jap. J. Cancer Res.*), *67*: 191 (1976).
11. J. Hamuro, in *Chemico-Biological Studies on Antitumour Polysaccharides*, Ph. D. dissertation, Kyoto University, 1973.
12. J. Hamuro, H. Wagner, and M. Röllinghoff, *Cell. Immunol.*, *38*:328 (1978).
13. J. Hamuro, M. Röllinghoff, and H. Wagner, *Cancer Res.*, *38*:3080 (1978).
14. G. Chihara, in *Manipulation of Host Defence Mechanisms* (T. Aoki, I. Urushizaki, and E. Tsubura, eds.), Excerpta Medica, Amsterdam, 1981, p. 1.
15. T. Aoki, H. Miyakoshi, Y. Horikawa, and Y. Usuda, in *Augmenting Agents in Cancer Therapy* (E. M. Hersh, M. A. Chirigos, and M. Mastrangelo, eds.), Raven Press, New York, 1981, p. 101.
16. T. Taguchi, T. Aoki, H. Furue, and H. Mazima, in *Manipulation of Host Defence Mechanisms* (T. Aoki, I. Urushizaki, and E. Tsubura, eds.), Excerpta Medica, Amsterdam, 1981, p. 259.
17. T. Aoki, H. Miyakoshi, Y. Horikawa, A. Shibata, Y. Aoyagi, and M. Mizukoshi, in *NK Cells and Other Effector Cells* (R. B. Herberman, ed.), Academic Press, New York, 1982, p. 1297.
18. J. Y. Djeu, J. A. Heinbaugh, H. T. Holden, and R. B. Herberman, *J. Immunol.*, *122*: 175 (1979).
19. R. B. Herberman, J. R. Ortaldo, and G. D. Bonnard, *Nature*, *277*:221 (1979).

20. N. Minato, L. Reid, H. Cantor, P. Lengyel, and B. R. Bloom, *J. Exp. Med., 152*:124 (1980).
21. T. Timonen, J. R. Ortaldo, and R. B. Herberman, *J. Exp. Med., 153*:569 (1981).
22. M. J. Brunda, R. B. Herberman, and H. T. Holden, in *Natural Cell-Mediated Immunity Against Tumors* (R. B. Herberman, ed.), Academic Press, New York, 1980, p. 525.
23. R. B. Herberman and M. E. Nunn-Hargrove, in *Manipulation of Host Defence Mechanisms* (T. Aoki, I. Urushizaki, and E. Tsubura, eds.), Excerpta Medica, Amsterdam, 1981, p. 188.
24. F. Sendo, K. Seiji, S. Fuyama, S. Watabe, and S. Arai, in *Manipulation of Host Defence Mechanisms* (T. Aoki, I. Urushizaki, and E. Tsubura, eds.), Excerpta Medica, Amsterdam, 1981, p. 178.
25. H. Miyakoshi, T. Aoki, and M. Mizukoshi, *Int. J. Immunopharmacology* (in press).
26. H. Miyakoshi, T. Shimizu, Y. Usuda, M. Mizukoshi, S. Abe, and T. Aoki, in *Immunomodulation by Microbial Products and Related Synthetic Compounds* (S. Kotani, ed.), Excerpta Medica, Amsterdam, 1981, p. 472.
27. H. Miyakoshi and T. Aoki, *Int. J. Immunopharmacology* (in press).
28. H. Miyakoshi, T. Aoki, and Y. Usuda, in *Manipulation of Host Defence Mechanisms* (T. Aoki, I. Urushizaki, and E. Tsubura, eds.), Excerpta Medica, Amsterdam, 1981, p. 118.
29. H. Miyakoshi, T. Aoki, and M. Mizukoshi, *Biomed. Res., 2*:629 (1981).
30. Y. Y. Maeda and G. Chihara, *Nature, 229*:634 (1971).
31. S. Haba, T. Hamaoka, K. Takatsu, and M. Kitagawa, *Int. J. Cancer, 18*:93 (1976).
32. G. Dennert and D. Tucker, *J. Natl. Cancer Inst., 51*:1727 (1973).
33. D. W. Dresser and J. M. Phillips, *Immunology, 27*:895 (1974).
34. Y. Akiyama, S. Kashima, T. Hayami, M. Izawa, K. Mitsugi, and J. Hamuro, in *Manipulation of Host Defence Mechanisms* (T. Aoki, I. Urushizaki, and E. Tsubura, eds.), Excerpta Medica, Amsterdam, 1981, p. 227.
35. S. Fukimoto, M. I. Greene, and A. H. Sehon, *J. Immunol., 116*:791 (1976).
36. S. Fukimoto, M. I. Greene, and A. H. Sehon, *J. Immunol., 116*:800 (1976).
37. M. A. Bean, M. Akiyama, Y. Kodera, B. Dupont, and J. A. Hansen, *J. Immunol., 123*:1610 (1979).
38. Y. Usuda, K. Imai, S. Takahashi, S. Abe, H. Miyakoshi, K. Watanbe, and T. Aoki, in *Manipulation of Host Defence Mechanisms* (T. Aoki, I. Urushizaki, and E. Tsubura, eds.), Excerpta Medica, Amsterdam, 1981, p. 50.
39. Y. Y. Maeda, G. Chihara, and K. Ishimura, *Nature, 252*:250 (1974).
40. T. Torikai, O. Itoh, S. Toyoshima, and T. Osawa, *Gann (Jap. J. Cancer Res.), 69*:657 (1978)
41. O. Itoh, T. Torikai, M. Satoh, and T. Osawa, *Gann (Jap. J. Cancer Res.), 71*:644 (1980).
42. T. Torikai, O. Itho, M. Satoh, O. Okumura, and T. Osawa, *Gann (Jap. J. Cancer Res.), 72*:92 (1981).
43. I. Urushizaki, K. Ishitani, T. Nagai, Y. Gocho, and R. Koyama, *Gann (Jap. J. Cancer Res.), 68*:413 (1977).
44. T. Aoki, I. Urushizaki, H. Miyakoshi, and K. Ishitani, in *Cancer Immunology and Parasite Immunology* (L. Israël, P. Lagrange, and J. C. Salomon, eds.), Les Colloques de l'INSERM, Paris, 1980, p. 85.
45. I. Urushizaki and K. Ishitani, in *Manipulation of Host Defence Mechanisms* (T. Aoki, I. Urushizaki, and E. Tsubura, eds.), Excerpta Medica, Amsterdam, 1981, p. 127.
46. T. Izumi, S. Nagai, and T. Suginoshita, *Cancer Res., 40*:444 (1980).
47. T. Izumi, in *Manipulation of Host Defence Mechanisms* (T. Aoki, I. Urushizaki, and E. Tsubura, eds.), Excerpta Medica, Amsterdam, 1981, p. 45.
48. J. Hamuro, M. Röllinghoff, H. Wagner, M. Seitz, W. Grimm, and D. Gemsa, *Z. Immun-Forsch., 155*:248 (1979).

49. Y. Y. Maeda and G. Chihara, *Gann (Jap. J. Cancer Res.)*, *64*:351 (1973).
50. J. Hamuro, M. Röllinghoff, and H. Wagner, *Immunology*, *39*:551 (1980).
51. J. Hamuro, U. Hadding, and D. Bitter-Seuermann, *Immunology*, *14*:695 (1978).
52. Y. Y. Maeda and G. Chihara, *Int. J. Cancer*, *11*:53 (1973).
53. Y. Y. Maeda, J. Hamuro, and G. Chihara, *Int. J. Cancer*, *8*:41 (1971).
54. In *Immunological Reviews*, vol. 51 (G. Möller, ed.), Munksgaad, Copenhagen, 1980.
55. T. Okuda, Y. Yoshida, T. Ikekawa, G. Chihara, and K. Nishioka, *Nature (New Biol.)*, *238*:59 (1972).
56. R. Homma and K. Kuratsuka, *Experientia*, *29*:290 (1973).
57. R. Tokuzen, M. Okabe, and W. Nakahara, *Gann (Jap. J. Cancer Res.)*, *67*:327 (1976).
58. G. Chihara, F. Garandente, and F. Halberg, *Proc. Am. Soc. Cancer Res.*, *20*:111 (1979).
59. K. Ishimura, Y. Y. Maeda, and G. Chihara, in *Corynebacterium Parvum in Experimental and Clinical Oncology* (B. Halpern, ed.), Plenum Press, New York, London, 1975, p. 300.
60. E. M. Lance and S. Cooper, in *Hormones and Immune Response* (G. E. W. Wolstenholme and J. Knight, eds.), Ciba Found. Study Group, No. 36, Churchill, London, 1970, p. 73.
61. K. Kanai and E. Kondo, in *Manipulation of Host Defence Mechanisms* (T. Aoki, I. Urushizaki, and E. Tsubura, eds.), Excerpta Medica, Amsterdam, 1981, p. 65.
62. T. Kawamura and Y. Numasaki, *Proc. Jap. Cancer Assoc.*, *39*:134 (1980).
63. K. S. S. Chang, in *Manipulation of Host Defence Mechanisms* (T. Aoki, I. Urushizaki, and E. Tsubura, eds.), Excerpta Medica, Amsterdam, 1981.
64. C. Hamada, in *Manipulation of Host Defence Mechanisms* (T. Aoki, I. Urushizaki, and E. Tsubura, eds.), Excerpta Medica, Amsterdam, 1981, p. 76.
65. B. J. Poiesz, F. W. Ruscetti, A. F. Gazdar, P. A. Bunn, J. D. Minna, and R. C. Gallo, *Proc. Natl. Acad. Sci. USA*, *77*:7415 (1980).
66. M. S. Reitz, B. J. Poiesz, F. W. Ruscetti, and R. C. Gallo, *Proc. Natl. Acad. Sci. USA*, *78*:1887 (1981).
67. J. E. Byrum, A. Sher, J. Dipietro, and F. von Lichtenberg, *Am. J. Pathol.*, *94*:201 (1979).
68. T. Shiio, T. Yoshihama, and Y. Yugari, *Proc. Int. Congr. Cancer*, *12*:39 (1978).
69. T. Shiio and Y. Yugari, *Int. J. Immunopharmacol.*, *2*:172 (1980).
70. T. Taguchi, H. Furue, T. Hattori, T. Kondo, T. Kimura, I. Itoh, and N. Ogawa, in *Immunomodulation by Microbial Products and Related Synthetic Compounds* (S. Kotani, ed.), Excerpta Medica, Amsterdam, 1981, p. 467.
71. T. Shimizu, T. Aoki, and H. Miyakoshi, in *Manipulation of Host Defence Mechanisms* (T. Aoki, I. Urushizaki, and E. Tsubura, eds.), Excerpta Medica, Amsterdam, 1981, p. 199.
72. H. Okamoto, S. Shoin, and S. Koshimura, *β-Hemolytic Streptococcus as a Cancer Controller*, Chugai Pharmaceutical Co., Ltd., Tokyo, 1972.
73. T. Aoki, J. P. Kvedar, V. W. Hollis, Jr., and G. S. Bushar, *J. Natl. Cancer Inst.*, *56*:687 (1976).
74. T. Aoki and L. R. Sibal, *Cancer Res.*, *36*:591 (1976).
75. E. M. Hersh, G. M. Mavligit, J. U. Gutterman, and S. P. Richman, in *Cancer: A Comprehensive Treatise* (F. F. Becker, ed.), Plenum Press, New York, 1977, p. 425.

5

Immunostimulating Compounds
Isoprinosine and NPT 15396

Kwong Yok Tsang and H. Hugh Fudenberg Medical University of South Carolina, Charleston, South Carolina

Fred K. Hoehler Newport Pharmaceuticals International, Inc., Newport Beach, California

John W. Hadden University of South Florida Medical Center, Tampa, Florida

I. INTRODUCTION

Several developments have served to focus the interest of immunologists on purine metabolism of lymphocytes. The discovery that adenosine deaminase defects are associated with severe combined immunodeficiency has prompted a number of studies on how this defect is preferentially destructive of lymphocytes. While a number of metabolic explanations have been put forth (see Ref. 1 for review), a general consensus has not been reached. One possibility is that lymphocytes, or subsets thereof, produce an inosine-containing essential substance not synthesized by other cell types. The recent demonstration that transfer factor contains inosine supports such a possibility. A focus on inosine-containing drugs with immunomodulating activity is suggested by these observations on transfer factor. Two novel compounds of this type are Isoprinosine, an inosine-containing complex, and 9-erythro(2-hydroxy, 3-nonyl) hypoxanthine (NPT 15392), a synthetic molecule similar to inosine in structure. Both of these compounds have potent immunomodulating activity, particularly for T lymphocytes. This review will summarize recent studies with these compounds and discuss important features of their immunopharmacologies. The reader is referred to other reviews for more complete information (2-4).

II. ISOPRINOSINE

A. Formula and Description

Isoprinosine is a compound formed by inosine and N-N-dimethylamino-2-propanol p-acetoamidobenzoate (DIP PAcBA) in a 1:3 molar ratio (Fig. 1). Isoprinosine is a water-soluble white crystalline powder, with maximal ultraviolet absorption at 260 nm in aqueous solution. It has also been shown to have antiviral activity in several experimental

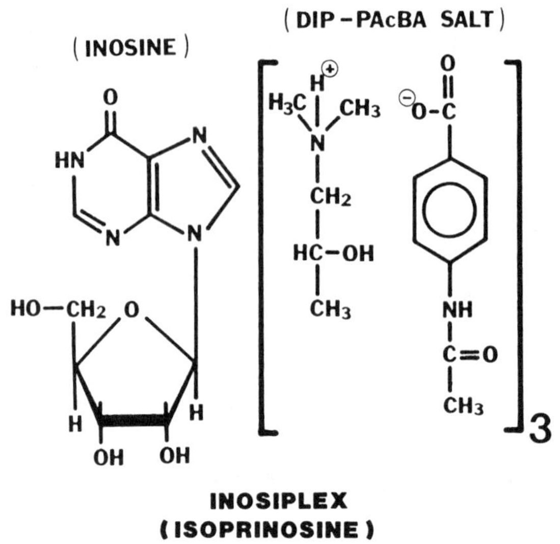

Figure 1 Structure of Isoprinosine.

systems (5-7) and to be effective in clinical viral infections (8-10). Isoprinosine is also an immunopotentiator in that it enhances the differentiation, proliferation, and function of lymphocytes (2,11).

B. Immunopharmacology

The current interpretations of Isoprinosine's clinical efficacy involves both antiviral activity and "prohost" enhancement of immune responses in varying degrees (12,13). For example, in subacute sclerosing panencephalitis (SSPE), treatment with Isoprinosine significantly increases survival (14) in the absence of any demonstable capacity to inhibit the replication of the measles virus (15). On the other hand, in influenza infection, Isoprinosine treatment improves symptoms in humans (16) and increases survival in mice (17) in association with the inhibition of influenza virus replication (16,17). In mice infected with influenza, lymphoproliferative and antibody responses are impaired and treatment with Isoprinosine restores both responses (15,18). This effect is due to the restoration of T-lymphocyte function as is demonstrated by lymphocyte transfer experiments (18). The mechanism appears to involve an augmentation of total ribonucleic acid and messenger ribonucleic acid (mRNA) synthesis of lymphocytes (which is ordinarily depressed during influenza infection), and a specific suppression of viral mRNA (18). Aspects of interferon action may be involved since Isoprinosine augments the production of immune interferon both in vitro (15) and in vivo (19). In immunosuppressive disorders, unassociated with virus infection, as occur in cancer patients, Isoprinosine has been found to increase various immune responses both in vitro (20) and in vivo (21). Thus, in a variety of disorders, Isoprinosine can be used to improve host resistance. Other examples include influenza infection (15,18) and autoimmune disease in mice (22) and herpes (23), and rhinovirus infection in humans (24).

The immunopharmacological effects of Isoprinosine provide the basis for extending the use of this drug to immunodeficiency states associated with cancer and aging. Hadden et al. first reported that Isoprinosine augments lymphocyte responses to mitogens (11).

These observations have been extensively confirmed with a variety of mitogenic agents (see Ref. 2 for review). This augmentation appears to involve principally an effect on T cells, since B-cell responses to lipopolysaccharide (LPS) are variably affected by Isoprinosine (25,26). Direct effects of Isoprinosine on B lymphocytes are possible since induction of Complement Receptor Markers (CR) (2) and enhancement of pokeweed-induced immunoglobulin production (3) have also been observed. A role for lymphokines and monokines is implied since, in several experimental systems, Isoprinosine has been observed to promote the production of a helper or mitogenic factor, lymphotoxin, and interferon, and to promote the actions of lymphokines and interferon (see Ref. 2 for review).

An important aspect of Isoprinosine's action involves its thymic hormonelike properties. This feature has been demonstrated in vitro by the induction of differentiation of both human and murine prothymocytes (2,22,26) and the promotion of the receptor display of T cells as manifested by active and autologous rosetting (27). These observations have been confirmed in vivo (28,29) but should be extended to bring out more fully this thymic-hormonelike action. In addition to its effects on both T- and B-lymphocyte function, Isoprinosine modulates macrophage receptors, increases phagocytosis, and potentiates lymphokine-induced proliferation and activation for microbicidal function. Variable effects on granulocytes and natural killer (NK) cells have been described (see Ref. 2 for review).

In vivo treatment with Isoprinosine is associated with augmentation of both cellular and humoral immunity in animals (2,18). The effects on humoral immunity involve both the primary immunoglobulim M (IgM) and secondary IgG responses and can be attributed in part to effects on T helper cells (18). Effects of Isoprinosine on T suppressor cells have been described in vitro (2,3,30); in vivo the activation of suppressor cells has been observed in autoimmune mice but not in normal mice (22). In general, the more potent effects of Isoprinosine, in vitro and in vivo, have been on cell-mediated immune responses rather than humoral responses.

The collected immunopharmacological data on Isoprinosine indicate its potential usefulness in treating immunodeficiency in general. This is supported by a number of recent observations. For example, Isoprinosine augments responses that have been depressed by chemotherapeutic agents in mice (15). It has also been reported that Isoprinosine alone (31) or in combination with interferon (32) augments the survival of mice following tumor challenge. Lesourd et al. (33) studied Isoprinosine prognosis and therapy in 42 acute encephalitides of various causes and found that Isoprinosine can restore depressed cell-mediated immunity in these patients as assayed by the lymphocyte nuclear refringency test. Isoprinosine treatment significantly accelerated the restoration of immune function depressed by radiotherapy in patients with cancer of the breast, mouth, neck, and uterus (34). It has also been found to restore the graft versus host reactivity of patients with cancer (35).

C. Animal Models of Human Osteosarcoma and Aging

While the ability of Isoprinosine to restore immune responses of human patients with cancer and nonviral diseases has not yet been evaluated with respect to increased survival or reduced morbidity, more than adequate rationale exists for investigating its use in a variety of immunodeficiency disorders. Since both aging and cancer involve immunodeficiency, the immunopotentiating capacity of Isoprinosine has been investigated in both an animal (hamster) model of human osteosarcoma (36) and in aging hamsters (37).

Table 1 Effect of Isoprinosine (ISO) on ConA-Induced Proliferation of Lymphocytes from Normal Hamsters[a]

Concentration of ISO ($\mu g/ml^{-1}$)	[^{3}H] Thymidine-Uptake (Mean cpm per 105 lymphocytes ± SD) Control	ConA only	ConA and ISO	Increase (%), ISO vs. ConA Only
10	275 ± 16.2	6781 ± 261.4	10,102 ± 406.4	48.9 $p < 0.01$[b]
20	306 ± 18.7	7182 ± 249.6	8867 ± 396.4	23.4 $p < 0.01$
50	242 ± 15.8	7504 ± 210.8	10,981 ± 398.1	46.3 $p < 0.01$
100	307 ± 21.9	8686 ± 209.7	12,204 ± 382.1	40.5 $p < 0.01$

[a]ConA was added at 5 $\mu g/ml^{-1}$ (final concentration). Control, no ISO and no ConA added.
[b]Statistical significance as determined by Student's t-test.

Human osteosarcoma (OS) was induced in inbred hamsters (LSH/SsLAK) by the following procedure (36). A laparotomy was performed on pregnant hamsters at approximately 12 days of gestation. A homogenate of 2 × 10^6 OS cells (TE-85) (38) in 0.1 ml of medium 199 was injected into each fetus through the intact uterine wall. After birth, 2 × 10^6 TE-85-M-MSV cells (TE-85 cell productively infected with MSV-RD-114 pseudo-type virus) (39) suspended in 0.25 ml of medium 199, were injected adjacent to the midshaft of the femur of the 4-day-old newborn hamsters. Tumors were palpable 10-15 days later.

The in vitro effects of Isoprinosine on concanavalin A (ConA) induced lymphocyte proliferation by cells from normal and OS-bearing hamsters were studied. ConA responses of OS-bearing hamsters were depressed compared with normal controls. Isoprinosine increased ConA-induced lymphocyte proliferation over control levels at all cell concentrations tested in both the normal and OS-bearing hamsters (Tables 1 and 2). The effects of Isprinosine on the response of lymphocytes from OS-bearing hamsters were greater than the effects of Isoprinosine on lymphocytes from normal hamsters. The effects of in vivo Isoprinosine administration on ConA-induced lymphocyte stimulation, monocyte chemotactic responsiveness, and NK cell cytotoxicity were also investigated (Table 3).

Table 2 Effect of Isoprinosine (ISO) on ConA-Induced Proliferation of Lymphocytes from Tumor-Bearing Hamsters[a]

Concentration of ISO ($\mu g/ml^{-1}$)	[^{3}H] Thymidine Uptake (Mean cpm per 105 lymphocytes ± SD) Control	ConA only	ConA and ISO	Increase (%), ISO vs. ConA Only
10	307 ± 7.6	3,264 ± 176.4	5,162 ± 367.1	58.1 $p < 0.01$[b]
20	298 ± 9.4	3,492 ± 113.6	6,077 ± 319.2	74.0 $p < 0.01$
50	267 ± 6.5	3,062 ± 189.7	5,984 ± 291.4	82.3 $p < 0.01$
100	312 ± 8.9	2,896 ± 133.8	6,008 ± 365.6	107.4 $p < 0.01$

[a]ConA was added at 5 $\mu g/ml^{-1}$ (final concentration). Control, no ISO and no ConA added.
[b]Statistical significance as determined by Student's t-test.

Table 3 Effect of Isoprinosine (ISO) on Monocyte Chemotactic Responsiveness (MCR) in Tumor-Bearing Hamsters[a]

Day Post-injection of ISO	Functional Chemotactic Index (Mean ± SD) Control	ISO	Increase (%)
1	49 ± 5.4	80 ± 4.7	63.2 $p < 0.001$[b]
3	49 ± 4.3	78 ± 8.7	59.1 $p < 0.001$
5	49 ± 4.2	77 ± 5.1	97.4 $p < 0.001$
7	51 ± 4.8	50 ± 6.2	–

[a]ISO (2 mg/kg^{-1} body weight) was injected IP on day 0. Control, saline injected IP on day 0.
[b]Statistical significance as determined by Student's t-test (36).

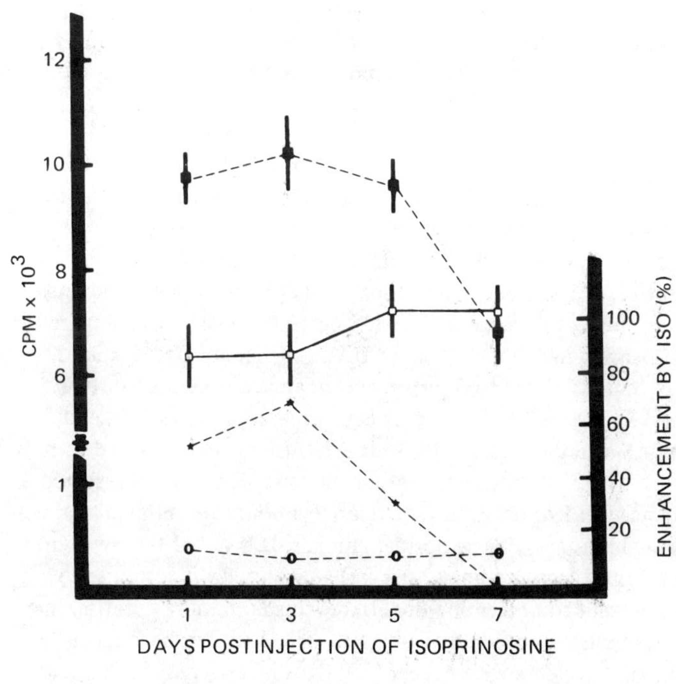

Figure 2 Effects of Isoprinosine (ISO) administered in vivo on ConA-induced proliferation by lymphocytes from normal hamsters in vitro. ■ - - - ■, with ISO, and ConA; □ - - - □, with ConA only; o - - - o, control (no ISO and no ConA); * - - - *, percent enhancement. (From Ref. 36.)

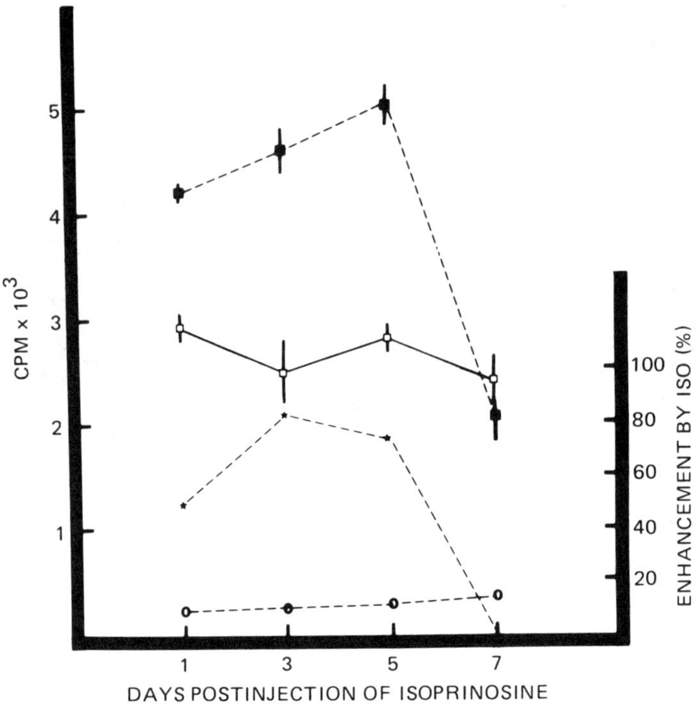

Figure 3 Effects of Iosprinosine (ISO) administered in vivo on ConA-induced proliferation by lymphocytes from OS-bearing hamsters in vitro. ■ - - - ■, with ISO and ConA; □ - - - □, with ConA only; o - - - o, control (no ISO and no ConA); * - - - *, percent enhancement.

ConA-induced lymphocyte stimulation was increased in both normal and OS-bearing hamsters treated in vivo with Isoprinosine. Lymphocyte responsiveness was increased on days 1, 3, and 5 postinjection and returned to control levels on day 7 in both the normal and OS-bearing hamsters (Figs. 2 and 3). The macrophage chemotactic response was significantly enhanced in the Isoprinosine-treated OS-bearing hamsters as compared with the control group (OS-bearing hamsters injected with phosphate-buffered saline). The response was enhanced on days 1, 4, and 5 postinjection and returned to control levels on day 7 (Tables 4 and 5). NK cell activity was also increased on days 1, 3, and 5 after Isoprinosine injection in both normal and OS-bearing hamsters, and returned to normal levels on day 7 (Table 6). These studies indicate that they are significantly restored in vitro and in vivo by treatment with Isoprinosine. The relative amount of immune augmentation is greater in OS-bearing hamsters than in normal animals. It is noted that with in vivo treatment a single injection of Isoprinosine (2 mg/kg) augmented the responses over a 5-day period. It will be important to determine the effects this immunorestoration may have on survival in conjunction with cytoreductive therapy. These studies have recently been extended to cells of human patients with cancer (20). It was observed that patients with melanoma, lung cancer, and breast cancer show uniform reductions of ConA response, NK cell activity, and monocyte chemotaxis. A short in vitro incubation with Isoprinosine (50 μg/ml) generally and markedly restored these responses. This restoration

Table 4 Effect of Isoprinosine (ISO) on Natural Killer (NK) Cytotoxicity in Normal Hamsters[a]

Day Post-Injection of ISO	(%) Cytotoxicity (Mean ± SD) Control	ISO	Increase (%)	
1	28.7 ± 4.6	37.8 ± 2.5	31.7	$p < 0.01$[b]
3	26.9 ± 2.3	49.4 ± 1.8	83.6	$p < 0.01$
5	20.8 ± 1.6	34.6 ± 3.6	66.3	$p < 0.01$
7	27.1 ± 4.1	26.5 ± 1.7	0	–

[a]ISO (2 mg/kg^{-1}) was injected IP on day 0. Control, saline injected IP on day 0.
[b]Statistical significance as determined by Student's t-test (36).

may result from the elaboration of a helper function(s) (20) similar to that observed by Wybran (29,40).

The effects of Isorpinosine on the immune responses of aging hamsters were also investigated. The strain used in this study was the Lak:LvG(Syr) outbred hamster. Immune competence declines with advancing age in hamsters. Beginning at approximately 14 months of age, we found significant alterations in the functions of natural killer cells, T cell, monocytes, and suppressor cells. NK cytotoxicity, phytohemagglutinin (PHS) induced lymphocyte stimulation, and monocyte chemotaxis were significantly decreased, while the suppressor cell activity for the lymphocyte response to PHA was increased in aging hamsters.

The effects of Isoprinosine treatment on the lymphocyte stimulation response to PHA, NK cytotoxicity, and monocyte chemotaxis were studied in three age groups of hamsters (14, 18, and 24 months old). Increases in lymphocyte stimulation, NK activity, and monocyte chemotaxis were seen on days 1, 3, and 5 after Isoprinosine injection. These immune responses returned to control levels by day 7 in all three age groups

Table 5 Effect of Isoprinosine (ISO) on Natural Killer (NK) Cytotoxicity in Tumor-Bearing Hamsters[a]

Day Post-injection of ISO	(%) Cytotoxicity (Mean ± SD) Control	ISO	Increase (%)	
1	13.9 ± 1.6	21.5 ± 3.6	54.6	$p < 0.01$[b]
3	6.9 ± 0.8	19.6 ± 3.7	184.0	$p < 0.01$
5	10.6 ± 2.4	17.9 ± 2.5	68.8	$p < 0.01$
7	11.5 ± 1.9	11.8 ± 3.4	2.6	–

[a]ISO (2 mg/kg^{-1}) was injected on day 0. Control, saline injected IP on day 0.
[b]Statistical significance as determined by Student's t-test (36).

Table 6 Effects of Isorpinosine (ISO) Treatment on Suppressor Cell Activity in Aging Hamsters

	Before ISO Treatment		After ISO Treatment	
Culture[a]	cpm[b]	Suppression (%)[c]	cpm[b]	Suppression (%)
Y_1	6349 ± 593	–	7996 ± 449	–
$Y_1 + 0_1$	1097 ± 69	82.8	7814 ± 560	3.0
$Y_1 + 0_2$	1541 ± 87	75.8	8062 ± 671	0
$Y_1 + 0_3$	1112 ± 98	82.5	7094 ± 698	1.2
$Y_1 + 0_4$	987 ± 56	84.5	7126 ± 709	11.0
$Y_1 + 0_5$	1610 ± 107	74.7	7012 ± 604	12.4
$Y_1 + 0_6$	1812 ± 124	71.5	6984 ± 587	12.7
$Y_1 + 0_7$	1937 ± 94	69.5	5837 ± 439	27.1
$Y_1 + 0_8$	1406 ± 119	77.9	6019 ± 672	24.8
$Y_1 + 0_9$	2013± 143	68.3	7504 ± 714	6.2
$Y_1 + 0_{10}$	2436 ± 109	61.7	8126 ± 568	0
Y_2	9817 ± 746	–	8964 ± 765	–
$Y_2 + 0_1$	1916 ± 114	80.6	8166 ± 643	9.0
$Y_2 + 0_2$	1314 ± 134	86.7	8431 ± 747	6.0
$Y_2 + 0_3$	1659 ± 156	83.2	7561 ± 564	16.0
$Y_2 + 0_4$	1927 ± 148	80.5	7844 ± 766	13.0
$Y_2 + 0_5$	1762 ± 114	82.2	7124 ± 567	20.6
$Y_2 + 0_6$	1845 ± 125	81.6	7344 ± 671	18.1
$Y_2 + 0_7$	1978 ± 116	80.0	8126 ± 562	9.4
$Y_2 + 0_8$	2042 ± 187	79.4	6021 ± 413	32.9
$Y_2 + 0_9$	2137 ± 104	78.4	6124 ± 409	31.7
$Y_2 + 0_{10}$	1534 ± 109	84.5	6849 ± 514	23.6

[a]Lymphocytes from 18-month-old hamsters (0_1–0_{10}) were cocultures with lymphocytes from the pooled blood of two different groups of three 4-month-old hamsters (Y_1 and Y_2).
[b]Mean ± SE for three determinations.
[c]Percent suppression = [1 0 (cpm Y + 0)/(cpm Y)] × 100 (37).

Fig. 4a-c). Eighteen-month-old hamsters were employed for the investigation of possible effects of Isorprinosine on suppressor cell activity. Suppressor cell assays were conducted prior to and 4 days after injection of Isoprinosine. The suppressor cell activity for PHA-induced lymphocyte proliferation was significantly reduced in all of the 18-month-old hamsters treated with Isorpinosine (Table 6). Continuous weekly intraperitoneal injections of Isoprinosine, beginning at the fourteenth month, resulted in restoration of each of the responses studied to normal or near-normal levels (Figs. 5 and 6). These studies indicate that Isoprinosine significantly restored depressed immune responses in aging hamsters after both single and multiple weekly injections. In separate studies, weekly administration of Isoprinosine produced a significant prolongation of life span in hamsters (37).

We conclude that Isoprinosine is a safe and effective immune-response modifier with immunopharmacological characteristics suggesting usefulness in a variety of immunodeficiency disorders.

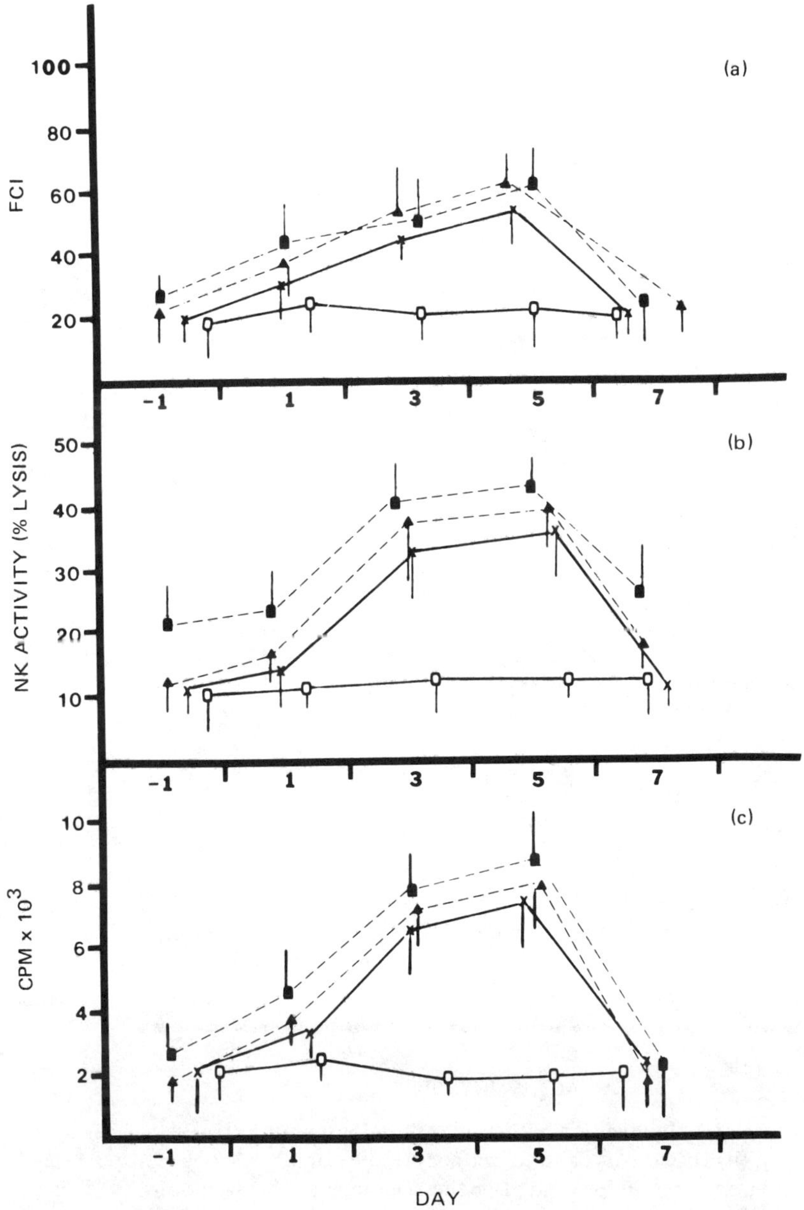

Figure 4 Effects of single injection of Isoprinosine (ISO) on (a) PHA-induced lymphocyte proliferation, (b) NK activity, and (c) monocyte chemotaxis in aging hamsters: (■) 14 months, (▲) 18 months, (x) 24 months, (□) control (14 months old).

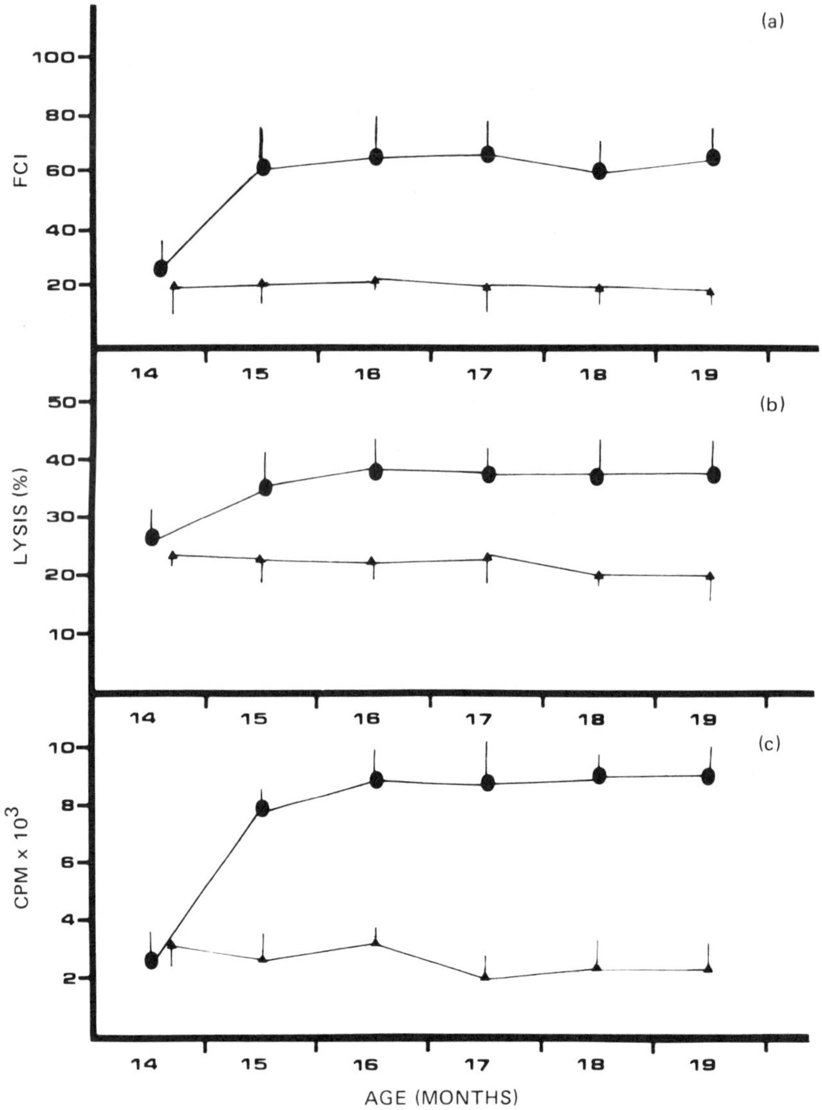

Figure 5 Effects of weekly injections of Isorpinosine (ISO) on (a) PHA-induced lymphocyte proliferation, (b) NK activity, and (c) monocyte chemotaxis in aging hamsters. Immune assays were performed before and after the beginning of ISO injections. (●) ISO-treated hamsters, 14 months old at the beginning of treatment; (▲) age-matched controls.

III. NPT 15392

A. Formula and Description

Inosine was shown by Hadden (41) to be active in promoting lymphocyte proliferation in vitro. The dose-response function was similar to that of Isoprinosine, although the magnitude of the effect was less. While the components of Isoprinosine (inosine and the DIP PAcBA salt) are not individually effective in vivo (15), it was surmised that inosine-

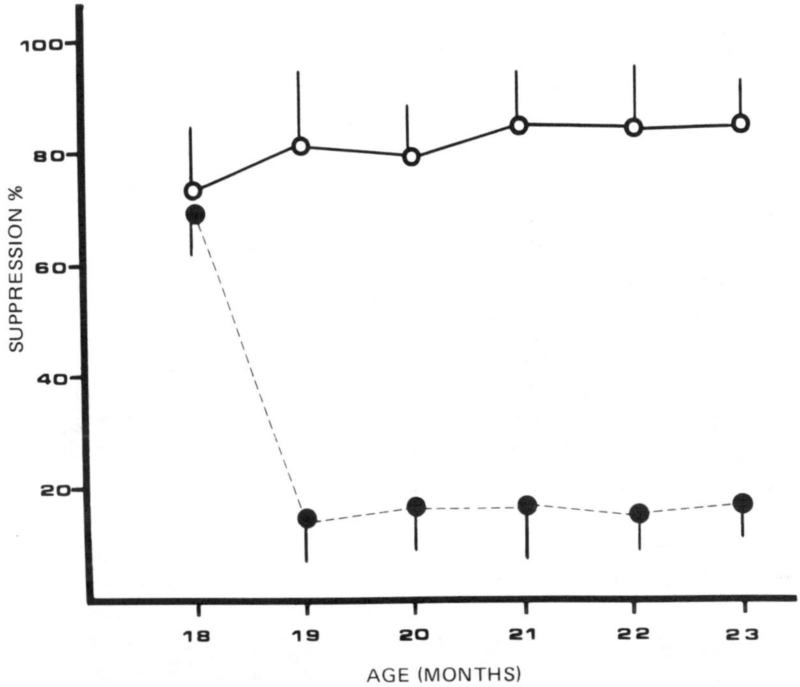

Figure 6 Effects of weekly injections of Isoprinosine (ISO) on suppressor cell activity in aging hamsters. SC assays were performed before and after the beginning of ISO injections. (●) ISO-treated hamsters, 18 months old at the beginning of treatment; (o) age-matched controls.

NPT-15392

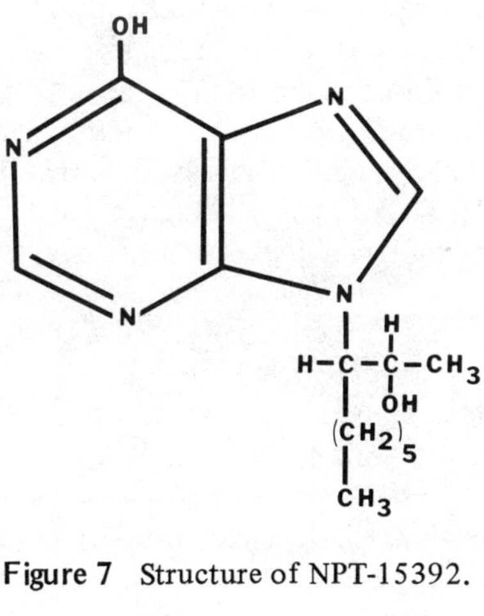

Figure 7 Structure of NPT-15392.

related compounds might also be active. Under a joint development program sponsored by Newport Pharmaceuticals International, Inc. and Sloan-Kettering Institute for Cancer Research, NPT 15392 (9-erythro (2-hydroxy, 3-nonyl hypoxanthine) was synthesized. NPT 15392 (Fig. 7) is a white crystalline powder having a melting point of 198-200°C and slight solubility in water (42). Saturated aqueous solutions of 0.75 mg/ml were prepared and tested for physical and chemical stability following storage at room temperature for 6 months. No degradation was observed. NPT 15392 is soluble in a variety of organic solvents. Toxicity tests indicate an oral LD_{50} in excess of 3 g/kg in mice and no significant side effects in mice, rats, rabbits, and humans at immunopharmacologically active doses.

B. Immunopharmacology

NPT 15392 has many immunopharmacological properties similar to Isoprinosine, yet its effects are observed at 1/10=1/1000 the concentration. In general, its effects are more modulating in nature, and suppressive effects are apparent at concentrations above 10 μg/ml in vitro or 1 mg/kg in vivo. NPT 15392 augments mitogen and antigen responses of human lymphocytes in vitro in some but not all individuals (43,44). The effects, when observed, are generally small (10-40%) and occur at concentrations as low as 0.01 μg/ml. NPT 15392 induces suppressor cell activity in vitro and promotes the suppressor cell induction of ConA (43). However, the variability of mitogen and antigen responses of human lymphocytes in vitro has not yet been shown to result from this effect. The mitogen responses of mice are more consistently augmented by in vitro incubation with low doses of NPT 15392 (26,42).

Like the thymic hormones and Isoprinosine, NPT 15392 induces murine and human T-cell differentiation (26,30) and augments active rosetting by human T cells (43, 45). Variable effects of NPT 15392 have been observed on B lymphocytes. LPS responses of spleen cells from C57B1/6 mice have been reported to be augmented (26) while those from BALB/c mice are unchanged (46). Induction of plasmablasts and plasma cells from human B lymphocytes is promoted by NPT 15392, particularly in combination with pokeweed mitogen or phorbol myristic acetate (47).

The functions of macrophages and granulocytes are both augmented by NPT 15392 (42,45). NK cells are not stimulated in vitro by NPT 15392, either directly or in the presence of optimal interferon (43). However, at low doses of interferon, NPT 15392 potentiates NK cell activity (48). It has not been demonstrated that this effect is the result of interferon induction. Tsang and Fudenberg (49) found that NPT 15392 may induce interferon in vitro while Hadden et al. (43) reported that it does not.

The mechanism of action of NPT 15392 is not known. However, nuclear refringence data implicate RNA metabolism (50), and unpublished observations indicate that higher concentrations of NPT 15392 inhibit cyclic GMP (cGMP) phosphodiesterase and adenosine deaminase while lower concentrations may mildly inhibit purine nucleoside phosphorylase. The latter action is variable but may act as an inosine-sparing mechanism to provide the basis for the variable potentiation of Isoprinosine effects observed with NPT 15392 (22). NPT 15392 does not appear to possess direct antiviral activity.

In vivo studies with NPT 15392 have demonstrated optimal effects at 0.01=0.3 mg/kg. In mice, augmentation of T cell-dependent and T cell-independent antibody and mitogen responses have been observed (42,51,52). These effects were observed consistently in BALB/c mice but inconsistently in C57B1/6 mice. In the latter strain, depressions of both plaque-forming cells (PFC) and the mitogen response have been observed (53). Jones et al. (46) examined mitogen responses in normal and thymectomized adult BALB/c mice which had received either multiple intraperitoneal injections or oral doses of NPT 15392 (0.1-0.3 mg/kg) or saline. In instances where the thymidine incorporation in spleen cells from saline-control animals was suppressed, NPT 15392 enhanced the mitogenic response. Conversely, maximal control-group responses were always accompanied by slightly depressed responses of cells from NPT 15392-treated animals. ConA responses were enhanced by NPT 15392 in BALB/c mice thymectomized at 9 weeks of age assessed for immunocompetence at 12 and 14 weeks. Thymectomy resulted in a diminished ConA response that was normalized by NPT 15392.

Florentin et al. (51) observed a variable increase in the ConA response in BALB/c mice which received a single injection of NPT 15392. PHA responses in these animals were more consistent, the overall effect of NPT 15392 being one of suppression. Over a 14-day period following a single intraperitoneal injection of NPT 15392, PHA-induced mitogenic responses were diminished an average of 40%. Florentin et al. (51) also found that NPT 15392 augments the mitogenic response of BALB/c mice to the B-cell mitogen, dextran sulfate. A single intraperitoneal injection of NPT 15392 on day 0 was followed by a 14-day period during which the response was enhanced by at least 60%. Almost complete abrogation of the dextran sulfate response and its augmentation by NPT 15392 were observed if adherent cells were eliminated from the cell cultures. These results, in conjunction with the understanding that many B-cell mitogens actually act on macrophages, present the possibility that macrophages may be a target of NPT 15392. Hadden and colleagues (2,43) have obtained results which indicate that NPT 15392 promotes lymphokine-induced macrophage proliferation and the production of interleukin 1, a soluble mediator which is produced by macrophages and interacts with T and B cells.

While the effects of NPT 15392 on ConA and PFC responses have been variable in normal mice, the drug more consistently increases both responses in mice immunosuppressed by virus, chemotherapy, or tumor (1,46,54). Delayed-type hypersensitivity reactions were increased in both normal and tumor-bearing mice treated with NPT 15392 (51,54). NPT 15392 modulates a variety of cytocidal functions. Florentin et al. (51) measured NK activity present in spleen or peritoneal cells harvested from BALB/c mice which received a single IP or IV injection of NPT 15392 (0.1 mg/kg) 1-14 days prior to cytotoxicity testing. In both cell populations the ability to lyse the YAC-1 tumor target cells was increased at least threefold by NPT 15392. The response was maximal 3-7 days after drug administration. The degree of augmentation was related to the route of administration. As expected, more NK activity was exhibited by peritoneal cells following an intraperitoneal injection of NPT 15392. Likewise, spleen cells expressed a higher level of NK activity after an IV administration of NPT 15392. The magnitude of the increase was comparable with that noted for interferon. Florentin et al. (53) also showed that combinations of interferon and NPT 15392 in vivo appear to produce a synergistic effect in augmenting NK cell activity. Micksche et al. (55) have also reported that NPT 15392 can augment NK cell activity in patients with malignant melanoma or gastrointestinal tract cancer. The consistent effects of NPT 15392 on NK activity in vivo contrast with the absence of any demonstrable augmentation of NK cell acitivy in vitro (43).

The level of T lymphocyte-mediated cytotoxicity expressed by spleen cells immunized in vitro with allogeneic tumor cells is increased by NPT 15392 (51,52). Spleen cells taken from mice which received a single or multiple doses of NPT 15392 possess higher lytic activity against tumor cell lines than matched controls. At an effector-target ratio of 100:1, spleen cells from animals which received multiple doses of NPT 15392 (0.1 mg/kg) exhibited 2.6-fold higher cytotoxic activity against the P815 mastocytoma than controls (52). Against another tumor line, the EL-4 lymphoma, increases in the maximum lytic activity of 2.7-fold were noted in mice which received a single IP injection of NPT 15392 (0.2 mg/kg) (52).

Tsang et al. (56) investigated the effects of NPT 15392 on the immune responses of hamsters in different age groups and showed that enhancement of both PHA-induced lymphocyte proliferation and NK cell cytotoxicity were observed on days 1 and 3 after injection of NPT 15392 (100 μg/kg), with the maximum augmentation observed on day 3. A greater percentage of augmentation was seen in the young (2 month) and old-age groups (14 month old), as compared with the mature age group (4-6 months).

C. Activity in Cancer and Autoimmune Disease

Sato and Tsurufuji (54) have measured NPT 15392-mediated restoration of immune function in tumor-bearing mice. In all experiments mice were administered NPT 15392 IP, either prior to tumor inoculation or both before and after exposure to the tumor. As a result of drug treatment, the suppressed DTH response in the Ehrlich ascitic tumor, Ehrlich lung tumor, sarcoma-180, and L1210 leukemia models was partially reversed. An otherwise depressed mitogenic response, in Ehrlich ascitic tumor or the L1210 leukemia model, was normalized by treatment with NPT 15392. In mice with Ehrlich lung metastatic tumor, the number of PFCs was increased from 27 to 97% (relative to nontreated controls) by NPT 15392. PFC levels in NPT 15392-treated Ehrlich ascitic carcinoma-bearing animals were elevated two- to threefold over nontreated tumor-bearing controls. The degree of improvement in PFC depended on the drug dose and administration regimen. In general, the most effective dose of NPT 15392 was 0.1 mg/kg.

Sato (57) has also utilized the AH series of hepatomas as a model system for evaluating NPT 15392 action in vivo. Survival was followed in groups of six control or drug-treated (IP, 0.5 mg/kg or PO, 5 mg/kg) animals for a period of 60 days. The drug was judged to have positive efficacy if the increased life span (ILS) was greater than 200% relative to the untreated control, and mixed efficacy if the improvement was between 50 and 150%. All untreated animals, regardless of AH tumor type received, died within 20 days. NPT 15392, administered PO, was found to be a positive treatment against AH-44. More than 50% of these animals survived to the 60-day test limit. Animals with AH-66 and AH-130 hepatoma types also responded positively to the drug treatment, although the magnitude of improvement was only sufficient to classify drug efficacy as mixed. Nevertheless, two animals from the AH-66 group were still alive when the test terminated. In rats with chemically induced bladder carcinoma (BC-47), a significant increase in survival was reproducibly obtained in animals treated with NPT 15392 compared with saline-treated controls. In addition, 10-20% of the animals in the drug-treated group appeared to exhibit cures (survival greater than 51 days). Enhancement by NPT 15392 of a depressed cytotoxic T-cell response of spleen cells isolated from tumor-bearing animals was also noted. Florentin et al. (53) have reported that treatment with NPT 15392 decreases lung metastases in the Lewis lung carcinoma model without significant effect on the primary tumor.

Wybran (45,58) and Mickshe et al. (55) have reported studies of NPT 15392 in human patients with a variety of cancers. They found statistically significant increases in the number of T cells, percentage of E rosette-forming cells, autologous rosette-forming cells, active rosette-forminc cells, and NK cell activity. In general, significant effects were observed in patients with depressed immune responses but not those who were normal.

Jones et al. (59) have reported that daily injections of 0.1 mg/kg NPT 15392 retarded the development of antierythrocyte antibody in young (11 week old) New Zealand Black (NAB) mice, while 0.4 mg/kg NPT 15392 reduced the levels of that antibody in older (38 week old) NZB mice. This apparent therapeutic efficacy in an animal model of autoimmune disease indicates that the normalizing properties of NPT 15392 may be useful in the treatment of human autoimmune disorders.

The accumulating immunopharmacological data on NPT 15392 indicate that it has immunomodulating activity on a variety of immunological responses and promotes both T-cell differentiation and NK cell activation. Its stimulating effects are most clearly observed in individuals immunodepressed by chemotherapy, aging, or cancer. It remains to be determined whether the immunomodulating properties of NPT 15392 will prove to be useful in the treatment of patients with immune system disorders.

IV. CONCLUSION

The demonstrated clinical utility of Isoprinosine and the potential for such manifested by NPT 15392 indicate that, by whatever mechanism, inosinelike compounds show remarkable immunopharmacological activity. For the therapeutically oriented scientist this observation should warrant continued synthetic development in this area, and for the basic scientist, it should encourage studies to further unravel the mysteries of the purine "salvage" pathway in lymphocytes.

REFERENCES

1. J. Hadden, E. Hadden, and R. Coffey, *Transplant. Clin. Immunol., 10*:143 (1978).
2. J. Hadden and A. Giner-Sorolla, in *Augmenting Agents in Cancer Therapy* (E. M. Hersh, ed.), Raven Press, New York, 1981.
3. A. Morin, J. Touraine, G. Renoux, and J. Hadden, in *Current Concepts in Human Immunology and Cancer Immunomodulation* (B. Serrou, C. Rosenfeld, and J. Daniels, eds.), Elsevier, Amsterdam, 1982.
4. T. Ginsberg and J. Hadden, *Int. Symp. Rec. Adv. Immunomodulators,* Viarregio, Italy, May, 1982.
5. T. Chang and L. Weinstein, *Am. J. Med. Sci., 265*:143 (1973).
6. P. Gordon, B. Ronsen, and E. Brown, *Antimicrob. Agents Chemother., 5*:153 (1974).
7. R. Muldoon, L. Menzy, and G. Jackson, *Antimicrob. Agents Chemother., 2*:224 (1972).
8. L. N. Simon, K. Maxwell, T. Ginsberg, and A. J. Glasky, in *Advances in Immunopharmacology* (J. Hadden, L. Chedid, P. Mullen, and F. Spreafico, eds.), Pergamon Press, Oxford, 1981.
9. R. Khakoo, G. Watson, R. Waldman, and R. Ganguly, *J. Antimicrob. Chemother., 7*: 389 (1981).
10. P. Dyken, A. Swift, and A. DuRant, *Ann. Neurol., 11*:359 (1982).
11. J. Hadden, E. Hadden, and R. Coffey, *Infect. Immunol. 13*:382 (1976).
12. L. N. Simon and A. J. Glasky, *Cancer Treat. Rep., 62*:1963 (1978).
13. G. H. Werner, *Pharmacol. Ther., 6*:235 (1979).
14. C. Jones, P. Dyken, P. Huttenlocher, J. Jabbour, and K. Maxwell, *Lancet, 1*:1034 (1982).
15. H. Shinkai, H. Kosuzume, H. Inaba, and H. Ohnishi, *1st Int. Conf. Immunopharmacol.,* Brighton, U.K., July 1980.

16. R. Betts, R. Douglas, Jr., S. George, and C. Rinehart, *78th Ann. Meeting Soc. Microbiol.*, Las Vegas, Nevada, May 1978.
17. P. Gordon and E. Brown, in *Advances in Antimicrobial and Antineoplastic Therapy* (M. Hejzler, M. Semonski, and S. Masak, eds.), University Park Press, Baltimore, 1972.
18. H. Ohnishi, H. Kosuzume, H. Inaba, M. Okura, Y. Morita, H. Mochiyuki, and Y. Suzuki, *Infect. Immunol., 38*:243 (1982).
19. E. Kott, N. Gadoth, S. Levin, T. Hahn, V. Bergman, R. Avidor, and C. Braun, *13th Symp. Israeli Immunol. Soc.*, 1981.
20. K. Y. Tsang, M. J. Gnagy, C. B. Phillips, and H. H. Fudenberg, *Int. J. Immunopharm.*, in press.
21. H. Fridman, R. Calle, and A. Morin, *Int. J. Immunopharm., 2*:194 (1980).
22. J. Touraine, G. Gay-Ferret, K. Sanadji, O. Othmane, G. Fournie, and F. Touraine, in *Current Concepts in Human Immunology and Cancer Immunomodulation* (B. Serrou, C. Rosenfeld and J. Daniels, eds.), Elsevier, Amsterdam, 1982.
23. L. Bradshaw and H. Sumner, *Ann. N.Y. Acad. Sci., 284*:190 (1977).
24. R. Waldman and R. Ganguly, *Ann. N.Y. Acad. Sci., 284*:153 (1977).
25. H. Inaba, H. Kosuzume, M. Okura, H. Ohnishi, and Y. Suzuki, *8th Int. Congr. Pharmacol.*, Tokyo, Japan, July 1981.
26. S. Ikehara, J. Hadden, R. Good, D. Lunzer, and R. Pahwa, *Thymus, 3*:87 (1981).
27. J. Wybran, *J. Immunol., 121*:1184 (1978).
28. G. Renoux, M. Renoux, J. Guillaumin, and C. Gouzien, *J. Immunopharm., 1*:415 (1979).
29. J. Wybran, in *Current Concepts in Human Immunology and Cancer Immunodulation* (B. Serrou, C. Rosenfeld, and J. Daniels, eds.), Elsevier, Amsterdam, 1982.
30. J. L. Touraine, B. Serrou, J. W. Hadden, A. Morin, and F. Touraine, in *International Symposium on New Trends in Human Immunology and Cancer Immunotherapy* (B. Serrou and C. Rosenfeld, eds.), Doin-Editeurs, Paris, 1981.
31. C. Fellous, A. Carbone, and L. Bradshaw, *4th Int. Congr. Immunol.*, Paris, France, July 1980.
32. I. Cerutti, C. Chany, and J. Schlumberger, *Int. J. Immunopharm., 1*:59 (1979).
33. B. Lesourd, G. Rancurel, J. Huraux, A. Pompidou, C. Jacque, D. Denvil, A. Buge, and R. Moulias, *Int. J. Immunopharm., 2*:195 (1980).
34. H. Fridman, R. Calle, and A. Morin, *Int. J. Immunopharm., 2*:194 (1980).
35. M. Talpaz and G. Mavligit, *2nd Int. Conf. Immunopharmacol.*, Washington, D.C., July 1982.
36. K. Y. Tsang and H. H. Fudenberg, *Int. J. Immunopharm., 13*:383 (1981).
37. K. Y. Tsang and H. H. Fudenberg, *J. Clin. Invest.*, in press.
38. R. M. McAllister, M. B. Gardner, A. E. Green, C. Bradt, W. W. Nichols, and B. H. Landing, *Cancer, 27*:397 (1971).
39. P. A. Jones, J. S. Rhim, H. Isaacs, and R. M. McAllister, *Int. J. Cancer, 16*:616 (1975).
40. Wybran, J., *8th Int. Pharmacol. Congr.*, Tokyo, Japan, July 1981.
41. J. Hadden, in *The Pharmacology of Immunoregulation,* (G. H. Werner and F. Floc'h, eds.), Academic Press, New York, 1978.
42. L. Simon, R. Settineri, E. Pfadenhauer, C. Jones, K. Maxwell, and A. Glasky, *Int. J. Immunopharm., 2*:200 (1980).
43. J. Hadden, E. Hadden, T. Spira, R. Settineri, L. Simon, and A. Giner-Sorolla, *Int. J. Immunopharm., 4*:235 (1982).
44. A. Vecchi, M. Sironi, N. Serraglia, A. Mantovani, and F. Spreafico, *Int. J. Immunopharm., 2*:204 (1980).
45. J. Wybran, *Int. J. Immunopharm., 2*:201 (1980).

46. C. Jones, B. Binko, R. Settineri, and K. Maxwell, unpublished data.
47. A. Pompidou, in *Advances in Immunopharmacology* (J. Hadden, L. Chedid, P. Mullen, and F. Spreafico, eds.), Pergamon Press, Oxford, 1981.
48. A. Goutner, *Int. J. Immunopharm., 2*:197 (1980).
49. K. Y. Tsang and H. H. Fudenberg, *Clin. Res., 30*:564A, 1982.
50. A. Pompidou, B. Mace, N. Duchet, J. Leymeyer, and M. Cooper, *Int. J. Immunopharm., 4*:286 (1982).
51. I. Florentin, E. Taylor, M. Davigny, G. Mathe, and J. Hadden, *Int. J. Immunopharm., 4*:225 (1982).
52. V. Merluzzi, M. Walker, N. Williams, B. Susskind, and J. Hadden, *Int. J. Immunopharm., 4*:219 (1982).
53. I. Florentin, L. Krause, G. Mathe, and J. Hadden, in *Current Concepts in Human Immunology and Cancer Immunomodulation* (B. Serrou, C. Rosenfeld, and J. Daniels, eds.), Elsevier, Amsterdam, 1982.
54. S. Sato and M. Tsurufuji, *Int. J. Immunopharm., 2*:200 (1980).
55. M. Micksche, E. Kokuschka, H. Rainer, and A. Uchida, *Int. J. Immunopharm., 4*: 283 (1982).
56. K. Y. Tsang, C. B. Phillips, M. J. Gangy, and H. H. Fudenberg, *Fed. Proc., 41*:812 (1982).
57. S. Sato, unpublished data.
58. J. Wybran, in *Current Concepts in Human Immunology and Cancer Immunomodulation* (B. Serrou, C. Rosenfeld, and J. Daniels, eds.), Elsevier, Amsterdam, 1982, pp. 1014-1020.
59. C. Jones, C. Lee, F. Hoehler, P. Koyama, W. Skinner, and J. Lamott, *Int. J. Immunopharm., 5*:85 (1983).

6

Tilorone and Related Analogs

Herbert Megel and John P. Gibson Merrell Dow Pharmaceuticals Inc., Cincinnati, Ohio

I. INTRODUCTION

Tilorone hydrochloride [2,7-bis (2-diethylaminoethoxy) fluoren-9-one hydrochloride] was first discovered by Krueger and Mayer in the late 1960s as an orally active, small molecular weight, chemical entity with antiviral activity resulting primarily from the induction of interferon (1,2). Shortly, thereafter, it was found that tilorone was capable of modulating the immune system in that it had opposing influences on the immune system. It enhanced humoral immunity while it suppressed cell-mediated immune responses in several animal model systems (3,4). It was also found to possess anti-inflammatory activity (5). The oral antiviral and interferon-inducing actions of tilorone and many of its congeners have been amply confirmed and are the subject of several comprehensive reviews (6-10). Our objectives are to describe the immunomodulatory aspects of tilorone in more detail, to briefly refers to its analogs and point out where their actions differ from those of the parent compound, and to summarize the chemistry, antiviral, and anticancer activities for completeness of this review. We will also give our opinions as to its possible modes of action and attempt to discuss tilorone's activity in light of current immunological concepts.

II. CHEMISTRY

Over a ten-year period, more than 800 compounds were synthesized in the tilorone series in search of orally active antiviral and immunoregulatory compounds. The chemistry and results of biological testing of 350 such compounds have been reviewed (11,12) with 24 literature citations to the syntheses and biological activities. In addition, 39 of these compounds were evaluated morphologically for their capacity to deplete lymphocytes from the T-cell areas of spleen and lymph nodes, since a correlation appears to exist between lymphocyte depletion from these areas and the ability to suppress cell-mediated immune responses such as experimental allergic encephalomyelitis (13,14). Structures and biological activities of tilorone and eight active analogs most often referred to in the literature are shown in Fig. 1 and Table 1, respectively. The generic structure can be represented as R_2N-aliphatic group-X-nucleus-X-aliphatic group-NR_2.

The several hundred compounds that were synthesized consisted primarily of those in which the nucleus was one of 22 classes (Fig. 2) of polycyclic or aromatic compounds with permutations of the terminal amine groups (-NR_2), aliphatic group, and X in the side chain. Since a large number of these compounds were tested in models of humoral and cell-mediated immunity, a structure-activity relationship (SAR) can be described for compounds with immunological activity. Active compounds, many of which had parenteral activity only, generally had the following characteristics.

1. The compounds required a basic side chain since any substitution for the terminal nitrogen atom (e.g., sulfur, oxygen) resulted in reduced or no immunological activity.
2. The alkyl chain could vary from one to five carbon atoms and still retain biological activity.
3. The structure had to be symmetrical since monobasic or asymmetrical compounds had reduced or no biological activity.
4. Substitutions of the tertiary terminal amine (-NR_2) had little effect on immunological activity.
5. The X function on the side chain could be a ketone, ester, or ether. Any substitution for the oxygen atom or any direct linkage of the aliphatic group to the nucleus resulted in reduced biological activity.

Table 1 Biological Activity of Tilorone and Selected Analogs[a]

Compound	Oral activity	EMC[b]	Antibody[c] IgG	IgM	Cell-mediated[d] EAE	Lymphoid Depletion	Inflammation[e] Carr. Paw.	Arthus.	Adj. Arthr.
Tilorone	A	A	A	A	A	A	A	A	A
RMI 9563	I	A	A	A	A	A	A	A	A
RMI 10024	A	A	A	I	I	A	I	I	I
RMI 10874	A	A	A	A	A	0	A	0	0
RMI 11002	A	A	A	A	A	A	I	I	A
RMI 11513	A	A	A	I	I	0	I	I	0
RMI 11567	A	A	A	A	A	A	A	0	A
RMI 11877	A	A	A	I	A	A	I	0	A
RMI 12358	A	A	A	A	A	0	A	I	0

[a]A = active; I = inactive; 0 = not tested.
[b]Antiviral activity as measured by a lethal challenge of encephalomyocarditis (EMC) virus in mice as described in Ref. 9.
[c]Antibody production was measured by the methods described in Ref. 4.
[d]Cell-mediated immune responses were evaluated by noting the effect on inhibiting paralysis in the experimental allergic encephalomyelitis (EAE) model as described in Ref. 4 and on lymphoid depletion in spleen and lymph nodes as in Ref. 14.
[e]Effects on inflammation were assessed using carrageenan paw edema as in Ref. 4, direct passive Arthus reaction as in Ref. 5, and adjuvant arthritis models as in Ref. 4.

Tilorone (RMI 10,008)

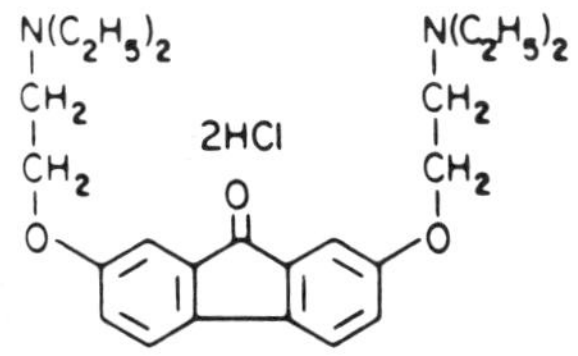

2, 7-Bis (2-diethylaminoethoxy) fluoren-9-one dihydrochloride

RMI 9563

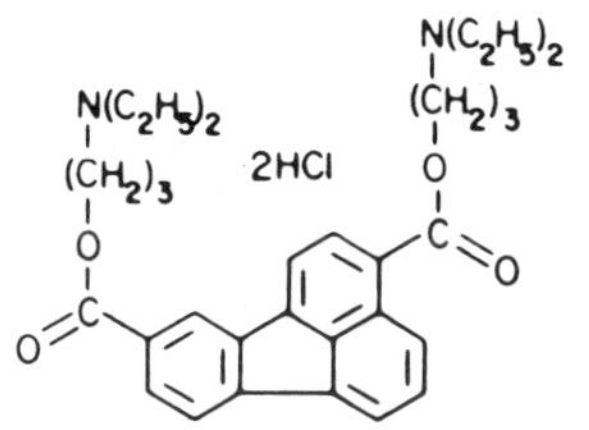

Bis (3-diethylaminopropyl) fluoranthene-3, 9 dicarboxylate dihydrochloride

RMI 10,024

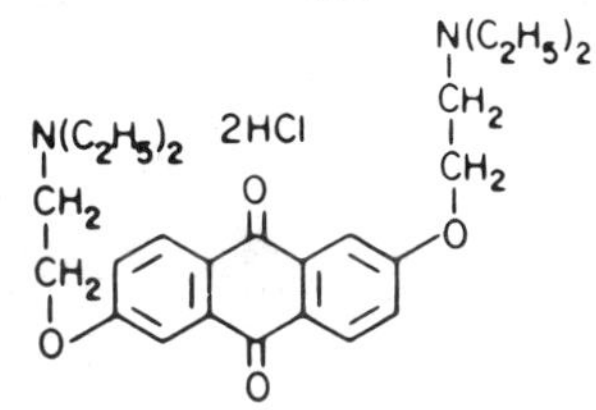

2, 6-Bis (2-diethylaminoethoxy) anthraquinone dihydrochloride

RMI 10,874

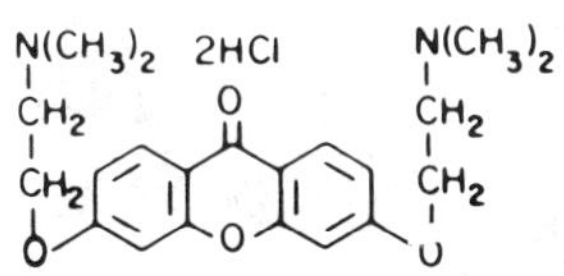

3, 6-Bis [2-(dimethylamino) ethyoxy]-9-xanthone dihydrochloride

RMI 11,002

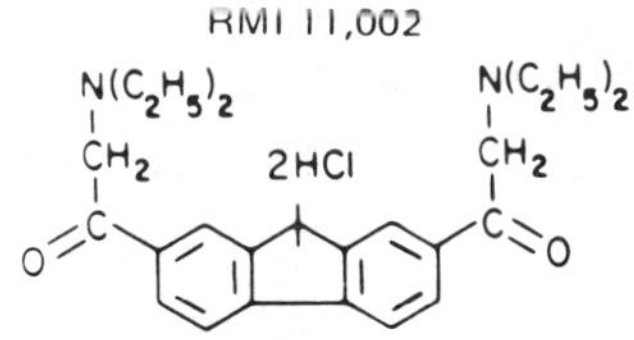

2, 7-Bis [2-(diethylamino) acetyl] fluorene dihydrochloride

RMI 11,513

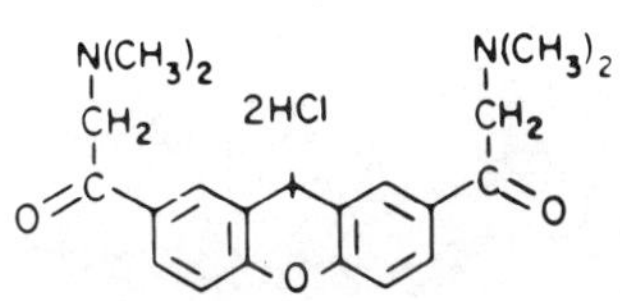

2, 7-Bis [2-(dimethylamino) acetyl] xanthene dihydrochloride

RMI 11,567

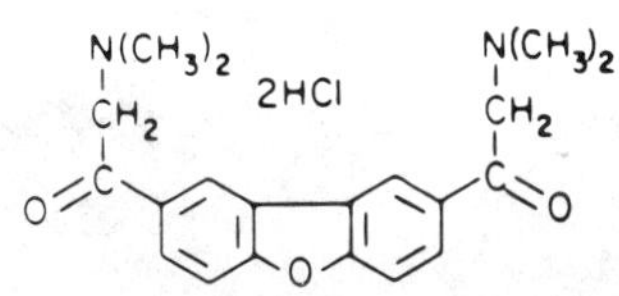

2, 8-Bis [2-(dimethylamino) acetyl] dibenzofuran dihydrochloride

RMI 11,877

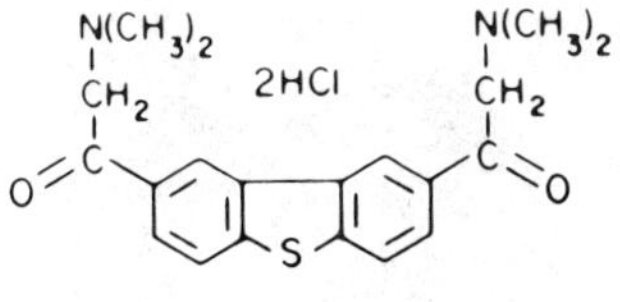

2, 8- [Bis(2-dimethylamino) acetyl] dibenzothiophene dihydrochloride

RMI 12,358

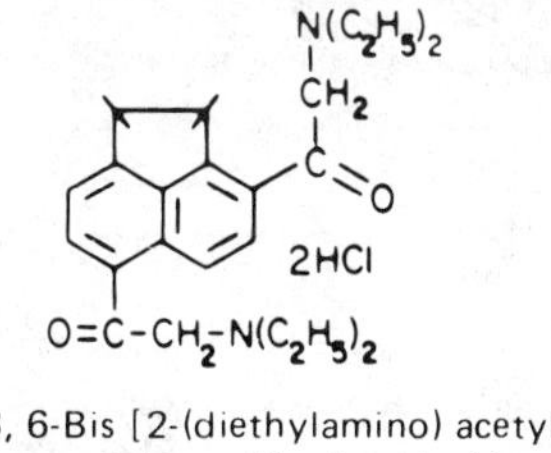

3, 6-Bis [2-(diethylamino) acetyl] acenaphthene dihydrochloride

Figure 1 Analogs of tilorone hydrochloride referred to in text.

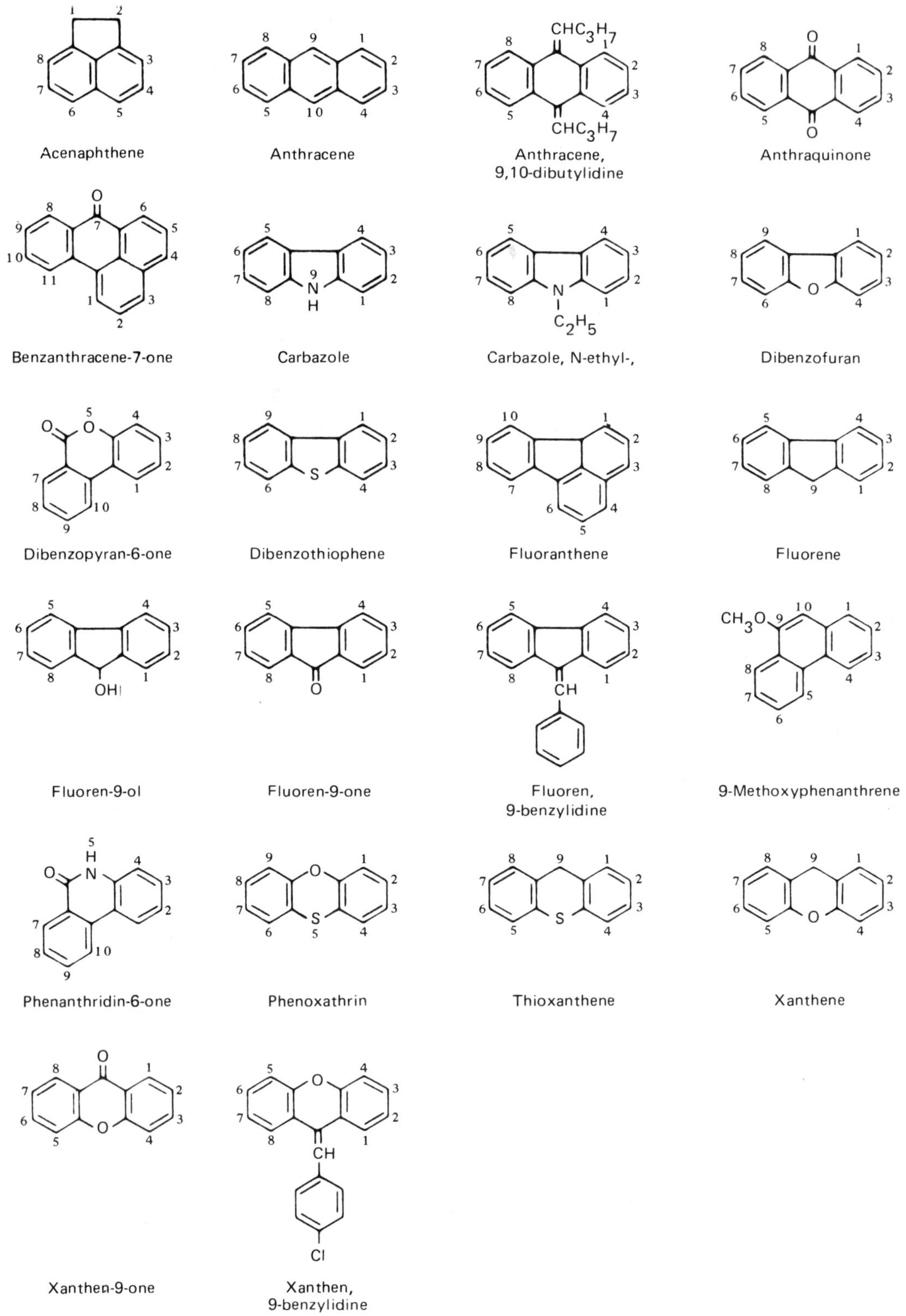

Figure 2 Aromatic and polycyclic nuclei used in the synthesis of tilorone analogs. (From Ref. 12.)

Since a large number of compounds were also tested for antiviral activity, an SAR for antiviral activity has been described (8). Examples of inactive antiviral compounds included fluorenones with a single side chain (monobasic), fluorenes or fluorenols with no free functional groups. In general, a good correlation exists between active antiviral compounds and active immunomodulatory compounds (Table 1).

III. HOST DEFENSE

A. Antiviral Activity

Anitiviral activity manifested by increased survival incidence, increase survival time, and/or prevention of viremia following a live virus challenge has been reported for mice, rats, and monkeys for a number of DNA and RNA viruses (Table 2) (9). Tilorone and analogs were active after oral, topical, intraperitoneal, and subcutaneous routes of administration and generally most active when given prophylactically about 12-24 hr prior to a virus challenge (at the time of peak serum interferon levels), depending on virus and route of infection.

Antiviral activity in mice has been ascribed to interferon induction (2). Serum from mice was shown to have antiviral activity against a broad spectrum of viruses in tissue culture (vesicular stomatitis virus, encephalomyocarditis virus, yellow fever virus); the active component in serum was nondialyzable, resistant to ribonuclease but not to trypsin, and stable at pH 2 (2).

Interferon was induced in mice after oral and subcutaneous administration of tilorone but not after intravenous administration (9). It induced less interferon in rats than in mice, had questionable activity in monkeys (9), and no interferon was detected in sera of hamsters, ferrets, cats, and dogs. Tilorone and analogs, as well as other interferon inducers, produced a state of hyporesponsiveness in mice and rats in that a second dose elicited less of an interferon response than the first dose (15-18). Maximum hyporesponsiveness occurred when the doses were given 72 hr apart, and full responsiveness returned after a 6-day separation.

Table 2 In Vivo Antiviral Spectrum of Tilorone Analogs[a]

Compound	EMC[b]	SFV[c]	VEE[d]	Influenza A	Influenza PR	TBE[e]	Vaccinia	HVR[f]
Tilorone	A	A	A	A	A	A	A	A
RMI 10024	A	A	0	I	I	0	A	0
RMI 10874	A	A	A	I	0	0	A	0
RMI 11002	A	A	A	I	I	A	I	A
RMI 11513	A	A	0	A	0	0	I	0
RMI 11567	A	A	A	I	I	A	A	A
RMI 11877	A	A	A	A	I	A	A	A
RMI 12358	A	A	0	A	0	0	A	0

[a]A = active; I = inactive; 0 = not tested.
[b]Encephalomyocarditis virus.
[c]Semliki forest virus.
[d]Venezuelan equine virus.
[e]Tick-borne encephalitis.
[f]Herpes virus.
Source: Adapted from Ref. 9.

The nature of the interferon protein(s) induced by tilorone and analogs has yet to be defined. One molecular species was found in mice (34,800 mol wt) and two in rats (27,000 and 80,000 mol wt) after oral tilorone administration; however, two molecular species were found in mice after the administration of other tilorone analogs (RMI 11,877, RMI 11645, RMI 11,513, and RMI 11,567) (9). Two peaks of interferon activity have been detected by affinity chromatography in mice after oral tilorone administration (19, 20). The major peak (85%) was similar to that produced by viruses and mitogenic stimulation of B lymphocytes [similar to type I interferon of Youngner and Salvin (21)]. The smaller peak (15%) was similar to that produced by the in vitro PHA stimulation of T lymphocytes that have characteristics of type II interferon or "immune interferon" of Falcoff (22) and Volle et al. (23). These results are in agreement with previous findings that interferon could be induced in athymic (nu/nu) mice (24) and in mice treated with antilymphocytic serum (ALS) (6) which lack T lymphocytes—possibly type I. The increased quantity of interferon induced by tilorone in the phenotypically normal nude mice (nu/+) which have T lymphocytes may have resulted from the induction of both types of interferon as mentioned above (24).

Mechanisms other than interferon induction may also contribute to the antiviral activity of tilorone. Tilorone and analogs intercalate with DNA (7,25-27) and inhibit DNA polymerases from RNA viruses (28,29). Direct incubation of herpes simplex virus type 1 and vaccinia virus, but not RNA viruses, with tilorone inhibited growth of these viruses in tissue culture (155). Infectivity of these viruses, however, was not altered (155). Direct photoinactivation of vesicular stomatitis virus in vitro by RMI 9563, a tilorone analog, has also been reported (30). Giron et al. reported protection against MM virus in mice in vivo with low doses of tilorone that did not induce serum interferon (31).

B. Antitumor Activity

Antitumor effectiveness of tilorone and several analogs has been tested in rodents against spontaneous, chemically induced, and viral-induced tumors as measured by survival time, tumor growth, and numbers of metastases. The data have been summarized by Mayer and Krueger (9) and are shown in Table 3. By way of summary, tilorone was more active after oral administration than when given parenterally; the compound was more active when given before or at the time of tumor challenge than after; and multiple dosing, even at weekly intervals, was more effective than a single dose, which was reported to exacerbate the oncogenesis of a transplantable virus-induced sarcoma in mice when given 24 hr prior to tumor challenge (43,44). Tilorone also was reported to potentiate the antitumor activity of cyclophosphamide against a murine mammary tumor even though tilorone was ineffective against the tumor when used by itself (45). Of interest was that analog RMI 11,002 was more active against Friend's leukemia, Lewis lung carcinoma, and B16 melanoma than the parent compound (32,34).

Antitumor properties of tilorone did not appear to result from the direct cytotoxicity of the compound itself. Tilorone, which was cytotoxic against several tumor cell lines in vitro, was ineffective against these same cell lines in vivo (40,46). However, in vivo effectiveness may have been mitigated by tumor challenge and/or drug blood-tissue levels which may not have reached the required cytotoxic concentrations due to tissue and protein binding. With regard to viral-induced tumors, inhibition of RNA-directed DNA polymerase (reverse transcriptase) could block the viral transformation of normal cells into malignant cells (28,47,48). Tilorone activation of natural killer (NK) cells by means of interferon induction could also play a role in the surveillance and cytotoxicity against tumor cells (49-54).

Table 3 Antitumor Responses to Tilorone

Response	Tumor	References
Active	Reticulum cell sarcoma A-RCS	147
	Walker carcinosarcoma 256	147, 148
	Morris hepatoma 3942A	148
	Morris hepatoma 7777	147
	Morris hepatoma 7794	148
	Lewis lung carcinoma (oral treatment)	32
	B_{16} melanoma	33
	Friend leukemia	34-36
	Leukemia K 1964	37
	Leukemia YLL	37
	Leukemia YALL	38
	Spontaneous lymphoma, development in immunosuppressed mice	39
Equivocal	B_{16} melanoma	40
	Murine sarcoma	41
Inactive	Ehrlich adenocarcinoma	34
	Prostatic adenocarcinoma	42
	Mast cell tumor P815	147
	Plasma cell tumor YPC-1	147
	Lewis lung carcinoma (parenteral treatment)	40
	L1210 leukemia	32, 147
	P388 leukemia	32, 147

Source: Adapted from Ref. 9.

C. Antimicrobial Activity

For the most part, tilorone has either had no effect or has exacerbated microbial infections. When administered to mice in the diet, it inhibited the multiplication of slow-growing *Mycobacterium leprae* in the footpad, but exacerbated the swelling of footpads inoculated with faster-growing *M. marinum* and *M. leprae murium* (55). Tilorone had little or no effect on mortality in mice infected with *Pasteurella tularensis* (56), *Diplococcus pneumoniae* (56), *Staphylococcus aureus* (57), and the protozoan *Trypanosoma equiperdum* (58). Tilorone exacerbated infections in mice inoculated with *Listeria monocytogenes* (57,59,60), *M. bovis* (59,60), *M. tuberculosis* (60), and *Salmonella enteritidis* (60). The effectiveness of tilorone as an antimicrobial agent may reside in the nature of the host's defense against those organisms. For those infections in which resistance is primarily mediated by antibody, prior exposure to antigen is required to mount such a response. Tilorone appeared to exacerbate those bacterial infections where resistance is primarily mediated by cellular immunity (T lymphocytes and/or macrophage) (60).

IV. HUMORAL IMMUNITY

Enhanced antibody production as originally observed by Hoffman et al. (61, 62), in which increased serum hemolytic titers and increased numbers of plaque-forming cells (PFC) were found in the spleens of mice sensitized to sheep red blood cells (SRBC), has been amply confirmed (3,4,34,63-66). These observations were further extended to show that both the primary and secondary immune responses to SRBC, a thymus-dependent antigen, involving antibodies of the IgG and IgM classes, were also enhanced as well as antibody to *Escherichia coli* lipopolysaccharide, a thymus-independent antigen (Table 4) (3,4). Tilorone was most effective as a single dose when given 24 hr prior, to 2 hr after, antigen but not at other times (61,67). In another system, Chang and colleagues reported that intraperitoneal inoculation of mice with EL_4 lymphoma cells enhanced complement-dependent cytotoxic antibody in a dose-dependent fashion following daily oral doses of tilorone starting 24 hr before tumor challenge (68,69).

A natural extension of enhanced antibody production by tilorone and analogs was its potential as a vaccine adjuvant. Tilorone-treated mice vaccinated with inactivated influenza A_2 virus and later challenged with live virus were protected to a greater extent than nonvaccinated mice or mice treated with tilorone alone (9,70). Hemagglutination inhibition titers (HAI) to influenza A_2 vaccine were enhanced four-fold (equivalent to the effectiveness of complete Freund adjuvant) in guinea pigs given tilorone and vaccine intramuscularly (71). Adjuvanticity was observed when the vaccine and tilorone were administered either in combination or were injected separately at different sites. Tilorone analog RMI 11,567, in addition to protecting mice against a live virus challenge of Venezuelan equine encephalomyelitis (VEE), was shown to potentiate a formalin-inactivated VEE vaccine by enhancing survival and elevating serum antibody titers over control levels (72). RMI 11,567 also enhanced primary (four-fold) and secondary (12-fold) antibody titers to VEE in monkeys, equivalent to that produced by Freund complete adjuvant (72). In the

Table 4 Effects of Tilorone (50 mg/kg subcutaneously) on the Primary and Secondary Immune Response in Mice

Antigen	No. of days after immunization	Immune response	Treatment	Type of antibodies	PFC/10^6 spleen cells Mean ± SD	P
SRBC[a]	3	Primary	Control (10)[b]	(19S)	160 ± 16[e]	< 0.01[f]
	3	Primary	Tilorone (10)	(19S)	390 ± 38	
SRBC	4	Primary	Control (9)	(19S)	640 ± 55	< 0.01
	4	Primary	Tilorone (10)	(19S)	890 ± 55	
SRBC	10	Primary	Control (10)	(19S)	50 ± 8	< 0.01
	10	Primary	Tilorone (10)	(19S)	75 ± 4	
	10	Primary	Control (10)	(7S)	420 ± 35	< 0.01
	10	Primary	Tilorone (10)	(7S)	910 ± 84	
E. coli[c]	3	Primary	Control (10)	(19S)	80 ± 9	< 0.01
	3	Primary	Tilorone (10)	(19S)	190 ± 19	
E. coli	4	Primary	Control (10)	(19S)	210 ± 12	< 0.01
	4	Primary	Tilorone (10)	(19S)	460 ± 36	
SRBC	24[d]	Secondary	Control (10)	(19S)	200 ± 12	< 0.01
	24	Secondary	Tilorone (10)	(19S)	380 ± 30	
SRBC	24	Secondary	Control (15)	(7S)	710 ± 58	< 0.01
	24	Secondary	Tilorone (14)	(7S)	1300 ± 98	

[a]Adult female CF1 mice immunized with 0.1 ml of 20% SRBC intravenously.
[b]Number of mice per group.
[c]Adult female CF1 mice immunized with 10 μg *E. coli* endotoxin intravenously.
[d]A second immunization with SRBC was given on day 21.
[e]Mean = SD.
[f]Level of confidence as determined by the Student's t-test.
Source: Ref. 4.

monkey, however, low doses of RMI 11,567 (10 mg/kg) enhanced, whereas high doses (100 mg/kg) had little effect on antibody production.

An increase in IgE serum levels to ovalbumin was demonstrated in rats given seven doses of tilorone orally in an every-other-day (EOD) regimen (4). Under similar conditions, hydrocortisone (subcutaneous) and 6-mercaptopurine (oral) totally suppressed IgE. In vitro, an IgE-secreting rat myeloma was stimulated by tilorone (73).

As to possible mechanisms of antibody enhancement with tilorone, Kettman (65) demonstrated that enhanced antibody production occurred when both drug and antigen (SRBC) were given to mice in vivo. Spleen cells taken from tilorone-treated mice and stimulated in vitro with SRBC did not produce any more PFC than untreated control mice. Kettman concluded that the action of tilorone was to remove suppressor T lymphocytes rather than alter B-lymphocyte function. This concept was further advanced by the increased synthesis of IgE noted in rats following tilorone administration, since IgE production, more so than other immunoglobulins, is regulated by suppressor T lymphocytes (74).

V. CELL-MEDIATED IMMUNITY

A. Delayed Hypersensitivity

Delayed-type hypersensitivity (DTH) reactions, as manifested by the classic tuberculin skin reaction in guinea pigs, can also be induced in rats following subplantar injection of *M. tuberculosis* in light mineral oil (75). Subsequent intradermal skin challenge with purified protein derivative (PPD) of tuberculin resulted in erythema and induration 24-48 hr after antigen challenge due to lymphokine release, attraction of mononuclear cells, and macrophage activation. Tilorone and analog RMI 9563 inhibited the tuberculin skin reaction in rats 14 days later when the drugs were given at the time of initial sensitization and continued on an EOD regimen (4,76,77). A similar effect with tilorone was noted in guinea pigs (78). Tilorone was also effective therapeutically in rats after the tuberculin skin reaction had already been established (76).

A corollary of DTH can be induced in mice and guinea pigs by the intraperitoneal or intravenous sensitization with antigen, followed by subplantar challenge. The difference in the thickness of footpads 24 hr later between that challenged with antigen and the contralateral footpad challenged with vehicle is an indicator of DTH. Tilorone given orally inhibited the DTH response to SRBC in mice (59,79), and to *M. tuberculosis* in mice (80) and guinea pigs (81). Tilorone also inhibited the tuberculin skin reaction in sensitized chickens as measured by wattle size (82).

The effectiveness of tilorone in suppressing DTH reactions is temporally related to sensitization, drug administration, and subsequent challenge. Kettman demonstrated that tilorone given subcutaneously to mice as a single dose on the day of challenge (4 days after sensitization) reduced footpad swelling 24 hr later (79). He further showed that DTH could be adoptively transferred with spleen cells of sensitized mice and that tilorone treatment of donor mice 24 hr (but not 4 hr) prior to cell transfer inhibited the DTH response in the recipient. Drug treatment of recipient mice 24 hr prior to cell transfer also inhibited the DTH reaction. Kettman concluded that tilorone did not block the generation of DTH effector cells but altered their responsiveness (79). An alternative explanation is that the leukopenia that occurred 24 hr after tilorone administration (13,24,83), also observed by Kettman (79), reduced or destroyed T lymphocytes at the time of sensitization or at the time primed T lymphocytes were required for DTH expression.

B. Allograft Survival

Tilorone prolonged survival time of skin grafts in mice and rats (84-86), heterotopic heart transplants in rats (85,86), and renal grafts in dogs (87). In rats, tilorone prolonged allograft survival across both major and minor histocompatability barriers and to a greater extent when given in combination with methylprednisone. In dogs given tilorone subcutaneously (35 mg/kg), starting on the day prior to renal transplant and continued on the day of surgery and EOD thereafter, lymphopenia occurred 24 hr after the first dose. Lymphopenia was no longer present 48 hr after surgery, even though tilorone was still continued.

C. Graft Versus Host (GVH)

The GVH reaction is that produced when competent lymphoid cells from a donor (parent), which cannot be rejected by a recipient (offspring), recognize the antigens of the recipient as foreign and mount an immunological attack against the recipient. The systemic introduction of donor lymphoid cells in the host causes splenomegaly, runting, wasting away, and finally death. If the lymphoid cells are injected locally in a footpad, the popliteal lymph node on the ipsilateral side becomes enlarged and increases in weight (local or regional GVH response). GVH responses are mediated by T lymphocytes.

Single doses of tilorone given to recipient (CBA × C57BL/6J) F_1 hybrid mice on the day of or 2 days after the transfer of splenic cells markedly suppressed the local GVH responses, whereas prior drug treatment (48 hr) of the donor C56BL/6J mice enhanced the GVH response slightly (88,89). In rats in which donor spleen cells from Lewis rats were injected into the footpad of Lewis × Brown Norway recipients, tilorone given orally to the donors suppressed the local GVH response if three daily doses of 100 mg/kg or a single dose of 250 mg/kg were given 24 hr prior to cell transfer (90). A single dose of 100 mg/kg was ineffective (90). In chickens, tilorone given orally during the sixth week of life had no effect on systemic GVH as measured by spleen weight after the intravenous introduction of peripheral white blood cells (82); however, tilorone itself has been shown to increase spleen weight and may have interfered with the interpretation of the results (71,91,92). Zschiesche and colleagues (89) found no difference in numbers of T and B lymphocytes in spleen cell suspensions taken from donor mice treated 24 hr before with tilorone compared with controls not receiving the drug; these results are in agreement with those of Raychaudhuri and Megel (93) where the percentage of B and T cells in the spleens of mice did not change after a single oral dose of tilorone, but marked changes in the B and T lymphocyte distribution occurred on repeated oral dosing (93).

D. Experimental Allergic Encephalomyelitis (EAE)

EAE is a useful experimental model of an autoimmune disease for evaluating drugs in which cell-mediated immunity plays a primary role. EAE is generally induced in inbred Lewis rats by the subplantar injection of an encephalitogenic emulsion consisting of nervous tissue in complete Freund adjuvant (CFA). The disease is manifested by hind limb weakness and paralysis, flaccid tail, incontinence, rapid loss of weight, leading generally to complete recovery. Deaths have occurred on occasion. Histologically, perivascular inflammation is noted in the spinal cord and brain (94). Onset of these clinical symptoms occurs 8-12 days after sensitization. The disease can only be transferred by T lymphocytes and not by antibody (94-97). EAE can be exacerbated and onset of clinical signs accelerated (hyperacute form of EAE) by using the more antigenic neural tissue or basic protein isolated from guinea pig and given in conjunction with a subcutaneous injection of *Bordetella pertussis* (98).

Tilorone and analogs suppressed completely or delayed the onset of paralysis significantly when the disease was produced by active sensitization or by adoptive transfer of spleen cells (4,71,77,99-102). The effectiveness of tilorone was dependent upon the severity of the induced disease, dose and dosing regimen, and the time of drug administration with relation to injection of the encephalitogenic emulsion. Tilorone completely suppressed clinical signs and prevented histological change when the disease was mild, and delayed the onset of symptoms significantly in the hyperacute form. Tilorone appeared to alter the inductive phase of the disease rather than the effector cells since two doses given to rats orally the day before and on the day of sensitization completely suppressed paralysis, whereas two doses given on the sixth and seventh days failed to alter the course of EAE (Table 5). The action of tilorone and analogs in suppressing EAE was clarified to some degree when it was shown that these compounds selectively depleted lymphocytes from the T-cell areas of spleen, lymph nodes, and Peyer's patches (13,14,99,103). The effect was rapid, occurring within 24 hr after tilorone administration. Suppression of EAE could simply result from the unavailability of T lymphocytes at the time of antigen presentation.

Tolerance to EAE could be induced by two daily doses of tilorone when given up to 28 days prior to encephalitogenic challenge (Table 6). Tolerance to EAE could also be produced by injection of CFA up to several weeks before sensitization with basic protein in CFA (104). Of further interest is the observation that lymph node cells taken from rats made tolerant by prior CFA injection and transferred to rats actively sensitized with an encephalitogenic emulsion could suppress EAE in the recipient rats (104). The passive transfer of suppressor T lymphocytes was postulated.

E. Cytotoxicity

Cytotoxic lymphocytes and activated macrophages have been implicated in the defense against tumors. In a unique model described by Chang and Hoffman (68), EL_4 cells, a tumor cell line passaged in syngeneic C57BL/6 mice, were injected intraperitoneally into

Table 5 Effect of Tilorone on EAE in Lewis Rats

Treatment	Dosage[a]			Paralysis	
	No. doses	mg/kg	Route	Day 15	Day 18
Control	—	—	—	17/20	17/20
Tilorone	8 on alternate days	100	PO	0/10[b]	3/10[b]
	2 at 24 hr and day 0	100	PO	0/10[b]	0/10[b]
	2 on days 3 and 4	100	PO	3/10[b]	3/10[b]
	2 on days 6 and 7	100	PO	7/10	8/10
Hydrocortisone	8 on alternate days	25	SC	2/10[b]	4/10[c]

[a]Administration of compounds was started on the day of sensitization with emcephalitogen.
[b]$p < 0.01$ by chi-square test.
[c]$p < 0.05$ by chi-square test.
Source: Ref. 4.

Table 6 Tolerogenic Effect of Tilorone on Experimental Allergic Encephalomyelitis in Lewis Rats

Treatment[a]	Time intervals (days) last dose to immunization	Paralysis	
		Days 13-17	Day 28
Control	–	26/28	26/28
Tilorone	0	1/17[b]	3/17[b]
(100 mg/kg, PO) × 2	7	4/18[b]	13/18
	14	7/18[c]	12/18
	28	8/10	8/10
Tilorone	0	0/18[b]	1/18[b]
(250 mg/kg, PO) × 2	7	0/18[b]	4/18[b]
	14	0/17[b]	6/17[c]
	28	3/10[c]	5/10[c]

[a]Two daily doses of tilorone were given.
[b]$p < 0.01$ by chi-square test.
[c]$p < 0.05$ by chi-square test.
Source: Ref. 91.

mice. Cytotoxicity of spleen cell suspensions was measured 16 days later by the release of ^{51}Cr from labeled EL_4 cells in the absence of complement. Under these conditions, the oral administration of tilorone starting at the time of tumor cell inoculation and continuing throughout the 16-day period depressed the cytotoxic response in a dose-related fashion.

Under a different set of conditions, tilorone was shown to elicit a population of killer cells independent of prior sensitization. The cytotoxicity of spleen cells from CD-1 mice against P815Y mastocytoma target cells was significantly increased following oral or intraperitoneal tilorone given 24 hr prior to sacrifice (49,105). More recently a natural killer (NK) lymphocyte population has been identified in spleen and other lymphoid tissues of mice that do not have surface markers of B or T lymphocytes (51,53). Tilorone given orally to mice 24 hr prior to spleen removal stimulated the cytotoxicity of these NK cells to target YAC-1 cells; activation of the NK cells was attributed to interferon induction (50-54,106).

Tilorone and analogs have been reported to regulate phagocytosis implicated in tumor surveillance and antimicrobial activity. Phagocytosis was enhanced 24 hr after the administration of tilorone and other analogs as shown by the increased vascular clearance of colloidal carbon (34,107). In contrast, macrophage activity was impaired in mice infected with *Salmonella* and treated with tilorone for longer periods of time (60). Macrophage mobilization into the pleural cavity of rats following the injection of carrageenan into the pleural space was impaired following tilorone (108). Additionally, tilorone administered orally to mice as a single dose elicited a serum macrophage migration-inhibitory factor (MIF_t) apparently RES in origin, which resembled the MIF of lymphocyte origin; the appearance, peak activity, and decay of this serum MIF_t paralleled that of serum interferon (151-154). The role of tilorone in the activation, mobilization, and regulation of phagocytic cells still remains to be more completely explored.

VI. ANTI-INFLAMMATORY EFFECTS

A. Carrageenan Paw Edema

The carrageenan paw edema model in rats as originally described by Winter et al. (109) detects nonsteroidal anti-inflammatory drugs (NSAID), such as indomethacin, aspirin, phenylbutazone, and many of the newer proprionic acid (profen) derivatives. The anti-inflammatory nature of these compounds is generally attributed to the inhibition of prostaglandin synthesis (110). Tilorone and several congeners inhibited carrageenan-induced paw edema, provided the compounds were given 24 hr prior to challenge (5,77,111,112). Tilorone was inactive when given 1 hr before challenge–a marked difference from NSAIDs that are usually effective when given shortly before the carrageenan insult.

The anti-inflammatory action of tilorone did not result from inhibition of prostaglandin synthesis (113), nor did it rely on the induction of interferon (114). Rather, tilorone may have interfered with the mobilization of inflammatory cells to the site of the insult (60,108,113). The phlogistic action of carrageenan may result from its ability to activate complement with the formation of chemotactic factors (115). Tilorone has been shown to interfere with cellular infiltration into the pleural space, following the instillation of carrageenan (108), or into implanted polyvinyl sponges (113). Continued oral tilorone administration to rats markedly elevated total serum complement levels but failed to inhibit its activation in vitro with carrageenan, inulin, cobra venom factor, and aggregated gamma globulin (76). From this standpoint, tilorone's anti-inflammatory action may depend on its ability to interfere with chemotactic action rather than its formation from complement. In contrast, RMI 9563 administered subcutaneously to rats also elevated total serum complement levels (77,149,150) and was found to inhibit C1 esterase in vitro (77). Elevated serum complement levels following RMI 9563 could have resulted from its ability to inhibit activation of complement, but it is Doherty's opinion that the elevated serum complement levels were a result of irritation caused by the subcutaneous administration of the drug (149,150). The causative factors in serum complement elevation following oral tilorone and subcutaneous RMI 9563 still remain to be elucidated.

B. Adjuvant Arthritis

Adjuvant arthritis in rats is considered to be a model of inflammation that is immunologically induced (116,117) although a viral etiology has been more recently proposed (69,118). It is induced by a subplantar injection of *M. tuberculosis* in light mineral oil. An initial swelling occurs in the injected paw after 3-4 days (nonspecific response), subsides slightly, and is followed by a secondary inflammation in both paws (immunological response). Tilorone (and other analogs) started at the time of paw injection and continued on an EOD or daily regimen inhibited both the primary and secondary responses (4,68,71,111,114). Tilorone was also effective when the drug was started on day 14 in established adjuvant arthritis (71). Chang and colleagues demonstrated that a single oral dose given on day -3, day 0, or day 3, but not on day 10, relative to challenge, was capable of suppressing adjuvant arthritis (111). They further demonstrated that rat interferon, obtained from fibroblasts in vitro or produced in serum in vivo by live virus challenge, suppressed paw swelling when given intraperitoneally over a 16-day period–thereby implicating a viral etiology in rat adjuvant arthritis and tilorone's effectiveness as an interferon inducer.

C. Arthus Response

The Arthus response is considered an immunologically mediated model of inflammation in which complement activation plays a predominant role. In the direct passive Arthus reaction (DPAR) in rats, antibody is given intravenously 1 hr prior to the injection of antigen into the paw. Paw edema 3 hr later is taken as the inflammatory response. The intravenous administration of cobra venom factor or carrageenan, agents that activate complement in vivo when given 30 min before antigen challenge, abrogated the inflammatory response. Tilorone and other analogs given 24 hr prior to DPAR inhibited paw edema in a dose-dependent fashion (5,77). Similar results were obtained in rats and guinea pigs in the reverse passive Arthus reaction where antigen is given intravenously and the animals are challenged with an intradermal injection of antibody (119). The role of tilorone on complement and its activation has already been discussed (see Sec. VI. A).

VII. MORPHOLOGICAL CHANGES

Many of the functional immunological effects described can be explained, in part, by the changes noted in peripheral blood and in lymphoid tissues.

A. Hematological and Histological Effects

Following a single dose of tilorone or its analogs, a distinct lymphopenia occurred in mice and rats that reached its nadir in 24 hr and returned to normal levels within 48-72 hr (13,24,83,93). A similar finding was observed in dogs given tilorone subcutaneously (87). The lymphopenia was accompanied by a mild to moderate granulocytosis about 8 hr after dosing which returned to normal levels within 24 hr (24). At the time the lymphopenia was most priminent, a depletion of lymphocytes was observed in the thymus-dependent areas of spleen, lymph nodes, and Peyer's patches, although the thymus itself remained normal (13,14,99,104). Since nuclear debris was observed in the lymphocyte-depleted areas, these cells were probably destroyed by tilorone (99). The depleted areas of spleen and lymph node became repopulated with lymphocytes and reverted to normal by 72 hr. Although no obvious bone marrow changes were observed histologically, it was reported that a single intraperitoneal dose of tilorone (80 mg/kg) depressed pluripotential-, granuloid-, and erythroid-committed cells in bone marrow of mice (92).

With repeated dosing of tilorone in rats and mice, a similar hematological and histological response was observed as with a single dose. The marked lymphopenia that occurred during the first 24 hr returned to control levels by 72-96 hr. Spleen- and lymph-node-depleted areas soon became repopulated with lymphocytes even on continued drug administration. After dosing for 2-3 weeks, a mild but definite lymphopenia was present; the histological appearance of the spleen and lymph nodes was normal, and at no time was the thymus or bone marrow noticeably affected (unpublished results).

Neither thymectomy, splenectomy, nor adrenalectomy prevented the hematological or histological changes induced by tilorone (13). A most interesting finding was that the adrenal corticosteroid, dexamethasone phosphate, given several hours before or concomitant with, but not after tilorone, completely prevented depletion of lymphocytes in T-cell areas of rats (99). Similar effects could be induced by nonspecific stress such as burns or fractures (99). The reason for this phenomenon is still unclear.

B. Effects on T and B Lymphocytes

The inhibition of cell-mediated immune responses in the face of enhancement of antibody production following tilorone administration suggested that the compound selectively suppressed T lymphocytes and enhanced B-lymphocyte activity. In nude athymic (nu/nu) mice which lack functional thymus tissue and are considered to be devoid of T lymphocytes, tilorone had no effect on the white blood cell count, whereas in the phenotypically normal mice (nu/+) a striking lymphopenia occurred (Fig. 3) (24).

The effect of tilorone on the B-lymphocyte population in the peripheral blood and spleen of mice was more directly shown using fluorescein-conjugated antimouse IgG prepared in rabbits (93). Consecutive administration of tilorone orally for 1, 3, and 9 days depressed the total white cell count 24 hr after the first dose with a return to control levels at 9 days even with continued dosing. Leukopenia was primarily a result of lymphopenia. Changes in the absolute number of B and T lymphocytes as shown with immunofluorescent tagging of IgG-bearing cells indicated that after the initial depletion of lymphocytes, which were predominantly T cells, the T cells in the peripheral blood were subsequently replaced by B cells in the return of the lymphocytes to control levels (Table 7) (93,98). Collins obtained similar results using antimouse IgG to tag B lymphocytes and anti-Thy 1.2 to tag T lymphocytes (60).

The increased B-cell population in peripheral blood was also reflected in the lymphocyte population of the spleen. When single cell suspensions of splenic lymphocytes were

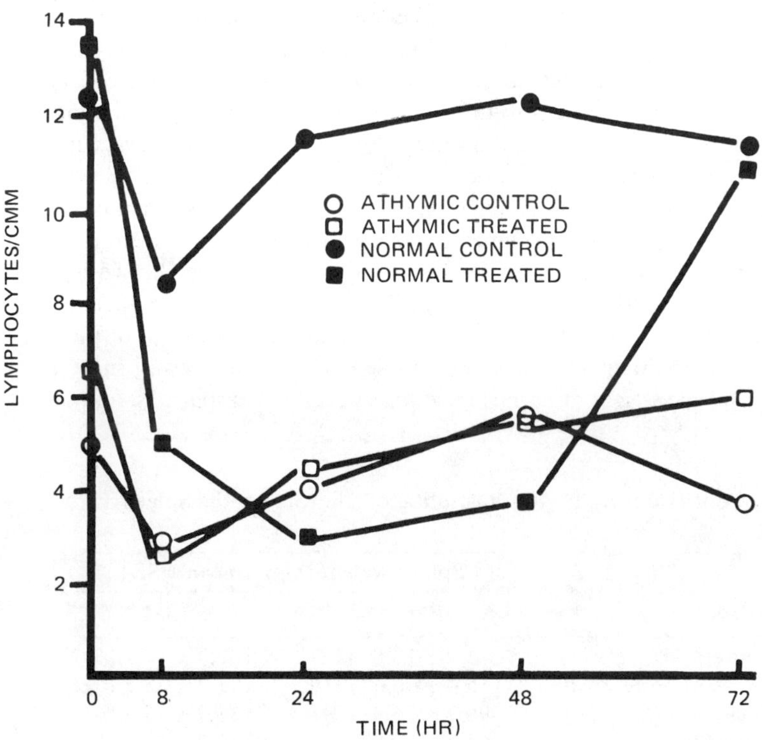

Figure 3 Effect of tilorone hydrochloride on peripheral lymphocyte count of athymic and phenotypically normal nude mice. (From Ref. 24.)

Table 7 Effect of Tilorone on Ig-Bearing Lymphocytes (B Cells) in the Peripheral Blood of Mice: Summary

Treatment	No. of days of tilorone administration	Lymphocytes × $10^3/mm^3$ (mean ± SD) Total lymphocytes	B cells	T cells and others
Control	—	7.08 ± 2.02	2.31 ± 0.7	4.73 ± 1.34
Tilorone	1	1.97 ± 0.45[c]	1.43 ± 0.33[b]	0.54 ± 0.12[c]
(100 mg/kg PO)	3	3.60 ± 0.75[c]	2.99 ± 0.62[a]	0.61 ± 0.12[c]
	9	7.08 ± 1.48	6.01 ± 1.26[c]	1.07 ± 0.22[c]

[a] $p < 0.05$.
[b] $p < 0.01$
[c] $p < 0.001$.
Source: Ref. 93.

reacted with fluoresceinated antimouse IgG, not only was the B-lymphocyte population increased by 15% following 9 days of treatment compared with the controls, but in addition the weight of the spleen increased by 30-40% (93).

C. Effect on Organ Weights

Another consistent finding in mice treated with tilorone was an increase in the weight of the spleen (71, 91,92) without any appreciable effect on thymus weights. This increase in splenic weight appeared to be a direct result of an increase in the numbers of lymphocytes in that organ (Megel and Raychaudhuri, unpublished results). Seidel and colleagues attributed this increase in spleen weight to that organ taking over hematopoietic function after tilorone administration (92). In studies where tilorone served as an adjuvant for antibody production, tilorone alone and antigen sensitization alone increased spleen weights, but had an additive effect in combination (71). To determine whether or not T lymphocytes played a role in this phenomenon, spleen weights were obtained from athymic and phenotypically normal mice after 11 daily doses of tilorone. In two separate experiments, the splenic weights of the phenotypically normal mice were significantly increased compared with the nontreated controls, whereas tilorone treatment of the athymic mice decreased the weight of the spleen (Table 8) (71). These results suggest that the increase in splenic weight of normal mice was dependent, in some fashion, on T lymphocytes.

Table 8 Effect of Continuous Daily Administration of Tilorone on the Spleen Weight of Nude Mice

Type of mouse	Spleen weight (mg) (mean ± SD) Exp. 1	Exp. 2
Phenotypically normal	76.2 ± 17.8 (12)[b]	109.7 ± 17.1 (6)
Phenotypically normal tilorone treated	115.4 ± 46.4[a] (10)	143.4 ± 38.5 (5)
Nude athymic vehicle control	90.1 ± 36.4 (9)	136.7 ± 35.8 (6)
Nude athymic tilorone treated	64.1 ± 16.8[a] (7)	110.3 ± 26.0 (5)

[a] $p < 0.05$
[b] ( ) = number of mice per group.
Source: Ref. 93.

D. Other Changes

After tilorone administration, intracellular cytoplasmic inclusions and occasional vacuoles were observed in circulating lymphocytes and granulocytes of mice, rats, dogs, and monkeys (83,120,121), in Kuppfer cells and hepatocytes of liver (83,120), in choroid cells of brain, and in distal convoluted tubules of kidney (103). These inclusions disappeared after a period off the drug (unpublished results). Electron microscopy revealed these inclusions to be aggregates of phospholipid membranes, often in myelinlike arrays or as fragments within lysosomes (122). Similar inclusions have been induced with many other drugs (123).

Nuclear inclusions in rat brain astrocytes have also been reported after tilorone administrations (124,125). These nuclear bodies were most obvious following brain trauma (burns) when inflammatory cells were present (124). The exact significance of these findings are not known.

VIII. CLINICAL EXPERIENCES

The safety and efficacy of tilorone and several analogs as antiviral and anticancer agents have been assessed in a limited number of clinical trials. The results of these studies have been reported in detail (9,12,126) but briefly will be summarized below.

A. Antiviral Activity

Tilorone given as a single oral dose to human male volunteers before inoculation with live rubella virus did not prevent the disease but shortened the length of illness (127). In a woman presenting with papovavirus-associated multifocal leukoencephalopathy 28 months after a renal transplant, neurological status and renal function were stabilized for 18 months after diagnosis by continued administration of prednisone and the replacement of azathioprine with tilorone (128). In diseases assumed to be induced by slow-growing viruses, tilorone effected a partial response in 2 of 4 children with subacute sclerosing panencephalitis (SSPE) (129), but did not alter the course of amyotrophic lateral sclerosis (ALS) in 16 patients (130).

No interferon has been detected in serum or tears of humans given tilorone orally or topically (131-133), and there was no effect on the number and function (PHA stimulation) of T lymphocytes in peripheral blood (134).

B. Anticancer Activity

Equivocal results were obtained in clinical trials in cancer patients, many of whom were in the terminal stages of the disease. Partial responses were noted in breast cancer (135), metastatic melanoma (136), renal cancer (137), and metastases to lung (138). Several investigators reported tilorone ineffective in metastatic melanoma (135), and in breast cancer when used alone (139) or in combination with other anticancer agents (140). Of interest is a recent report from China in patients with esophageal dysplasia that historically develop esophageal carcinoma (7-9%). Tilorone given in small doses (50 mg/day for 5 days every other week for 8 months) effected a significantly greater rate of remission (21 of 48 patients, 48.8%) than one would expect from a similar nontreated population (24%), and only 1 of 43 patients (2%) developed esophageal carcinoma (141).

C. Anti-Inflammatory Effects

Tilorone administered intraarticularly and RMI 11,002 given orally induced partial responses in subjects with severe rheumatoid arthritis (12). One of three subjects given tilorone showed a marked improvement lasting for 6 months in the injected knee but not in the knee that was not treated. In seven subjects given RMI 11,002 orally, four subjects completed a 3-week course of treatment of which two showed marked, and a third, slight, improvement.

D. Side Effects

The most common side effects reported were gastrointestinal and those of the central nervous system (nausea, vomiting, dizziness, diplopia) (129,136,139). These symptoms disappeared when the drug was stopped. Ocular changes as cloudy corneal epithelia, retinopathy, and keratopathy were reported in several patients whose cumulative intake of tilorone exceed 25 g; these changes were reversible and disappeared after the drug was discontinued (142,143). Tilorone was detected in corneal and conjunctival biopsy material (144,145). Abnormal inclusions similar to those described in Sec. VII. C were also observed in leukocytes after several doses of tilorone (136,138). These inclusions disappeared when the drug was stopped.

IX. SUMMARY AND CONCLUSIONS

The uniqueness of tilorone (and several of its analogs) is that it is a synthetic, orally active, small molecule demonstrating antiviral, antitumor, anti-inflammatory, and immunomodulatory activities primarily in mice and rats. Its role as an antiviral agent can be traced, in part, to interferon induction. Its antitumor activity may be a natural extension of its antiviral effects in preventing viral-induced malignant transformations, as well as result from the enhanced activities of NK cells and phagocytes that are cytotoxic to tumor cell growth.

As an anti-inflammatory agent, tilorone is effective in an immunologically induced complement-mediated model of inflammation (Arthus reaction). Tilorone does not appear to interfere with the formation of chemotactic factors by complement activation, but rather it may interfer with the chemotactic attraction of inflammatory cells. Tilorone, as are the nonsteroidal anti-inflammatory drugs (NSAID), is also effective in other more conventional models of inflammation that are not induced immunologically (carrageenan paw edema, carrageenan abscess). It differs from NSAID, however, in that it is most effective when given 24 hr prior to the phlogistic challenge; the NSAIDs are generally more effective when administered 1 hr before challenge. Many of the reported results, such as the effectiveness of tilorone as an anti-inflammatory agent, or in the suppression of GVH responses, could easily be misinterpreted if the temporal relationship between dosage of drug, route of drug administration, time of challenge, and the events being studied was not taken into account.

One of the more important aspects of tilorone activity in rats and mice was its paradoxical effect on the immune system. It enhanced antibody production, whereas it suppressed a variety of cell-mediated immune responses. A rather simplistic explanation for its immunomodulatory actions is that it preferentially depletes or destroys T lymphocytes from peripheral blood and lymphoid organs, and these cells are not available at the appropriate time to respond to antigen-presenting cells (APS) or to serve as effector cells.

B lymphocytes, on the other hand, are not appreciably altered and still can respond to APS. The B-cell population, in fact, appeared to increase as a concomitant of T-cell depletion. A more subtle role of tilorone on T-lymphocyte regulatory mechanisms must await further research in defining its effect on T-cell subsets (suppressor, helper, cytotoxic, DTH) and cellular interactions.

The effects of tilorone were not definitive in the limited number of studies carried out in man. Interferon induction could not be demonstrated. Antiviral and anticancer activity were equivocal; many cancer patients were in the terminal stages of the disease. Partial responses were observed with tilorone and RMI 11,002 in the treatment of rheumatoid arthritis in subjects that failed to respond to other therapeutic agents. The lack of definitive responses in man as opposed to mice may reside, in part, in the difference between the two species. For example, the lymphocyte/neutrophil ratio in peripheral blood of man is the reverse of that found in mice; mice have a greater percentage of lymphocytes. Man is relatively resistant, whereas the mouse is sensitive, to the lympholytic actions of corticosteroids (146). It is possible that the side effects encountered in man prevented sufficiently high concentrations of drug necessary to achieve desired responses. It is also possible that the dosage regimens were not optimal or of sufficient duration to achieve the desired results. More recently, lower doses for longer periods of time have been reported to effectively reduce esophageal dysplasia in a susceptible population (141). We feel that, in man, orally active molecules with tiloronelike biological profiles as observed in animals, would be useful contributions to the drug armamentarium in prolonging allograft survival, in the treatment of viral infections and cancer, and in inflammation as a consequence of certain cell-mediated autoimmune diseases.

REFERENCES

1. R. F. Krueger and G. D. Mayer, *Science*, *169*:1213 (1970).
2. G. D. Mayer and R. F. Krueger, *Science*, *169*:1214 (1970).
3. H. Megel, A. Raychaudhuri, S. Goldstein, C. R. Kinsolving, I. Shemano, and J. G. Michael, *Fed. Proc.*, *32*:1021 (1973).
4. H. Megel, A. Raychaudhuri, S. Goldstein, C. R. Kinsolving, I. Shemano, and J. G. Michael, *Proc. Soc. Exp. Biol. Med.*, *145*:513 (1974).
5. H. Megel, A. Raychaudhuri, I. Shemano, L. L. Thomas, and T. H. Beaver, *Proc. Soc. Exp. Biol. Med.*, *149*:89 (1975).
6. D. A. Stringfellow and L. A. Glasgow, *Antimicrob. Agents. Chemother.*, *2*:73 (1972).
7. P. Chandra and G. J. Wright, *Top. Curr. Chem.*, *72*:125 (1977).
8. G. D. Mayer, *Pharmacol. Ther.*, *8*:173 (1980).
9. G. D. Mayer and R. F. Krueger, in *Interferon and Interferon Inducers. Clinical Applications* (D. A. Stringfellow, ed.), Marcel Dekker, New York/Basel, 1980, pp. 187-221.
10. W. Regelson, *Pharmacol. Ther.*, *15*:1 (1981).
11. R. H. Levine, *Aldrichimica Acta*, *12*:77 (1979).
12. R. H. Levine and W. L. Albrecht, *Progress in Medical Chemistry*, *Vol. 18*, Elsevier/North Holland, Amsterdam, 1981, pp. 135-190.
13. S. Levin, J. P. Gibson, and H. Megel, *Proc. Soc. Exp. Biol. Med.*, *146*:245 (1974).
14. S. Levin, R. Sowinski, and W. L. Albrecht, *Toxic. Appl. Pharmacol.*, *40*:137 (1977).
15. E. De Clercq and T. C. Merigan, *Virology*, *42*:799 (1970).
16. C. E. Buckler, H. G. Du Buy, R. R. Rafajko, and S. Baron, *Int. Collog. on Interferon and Interferon Inducers, Leuven, Belgium*, 1971.

17. B. C. Cole, J. C. Overall, Jr., P. S. Lombardi, and L. A. Glasgow, *Infect. Immunol., 12*: 1349 (1975).
18. D. A. Stringfellow, E. R. Kern, D. K. Kelsey, and L. A. Glasgow, *J. Infect. Dis., 135*:540 (1977).
19. J. Wietzerbin, R. Falcoff, L. Catinot, and E. Falcoff, *Ann. Immunol., 128*:699 (1977).
20. J. Wietzerbin, S. Stephanos, R. Falcoff, and E. Falcoff, *Tex. Rep. Biol. Med., 35*:205 (1977).
21. J. S. Youngner and S. B. Salvin, *J. Immunol., 111*:1914 (1973).
22. R. Falcoff, *J. Gen. Virol., 16*:251 (1972).
23. M. Valle, G. W. Jordon, S. Haahr, and T. C. Merigan, *J. Immunol., 115*:230 (1975).
24. J. P. Gibson, H. Megel, K. P. Camyre, and J. G. Michael, *Proc. Soc. Exp. Biol. Med., 151*:264 (1976).
25. P. Chandra and M. Wolterdorf, *Febs. Lett., 41*:169 (1974).
26. P. Chandra and M. Wolterdorf, *Biochem. Pharmacol., 25*:877 (1976).
27. F. D. Miller, C. Lin, and J. H. VanDeSande, *J. Histochem. Cytochem., 29*:969 (1981).
28. M. Green, A. Rankin, G. F. Gerard, D. P. Grandgenett, and M. R. Green, *J. Natl. Cancer Inst., 55*:433 (1975).
29. M. Green and G. F. Gerard, *Progress in Nucleic Acid Research and Molecular Biology, Vol. 14* (W. E. Cohn, ed.), Academic Press, New York, 1974, pp. 225-334.
30. K. P. Camyre, J. W. Groelke, and W. L. Albrecht, Presentation at Am. Soc. Microbiol. Meeting, Miami Beach, Fla., 1973.
31. D. J. Giron, J. P. Schmidt, and F. F. Pindak, *Antimicrob. Agents Chemother., 1*:78 (1972).
32. G. L. Wampler and W. Regelson, in *Modulation of Host Immune Resistance in the Prevention or Treatment of Induced Neoplasias* (M. A. Chirigos, ed.), U.S. Government Printing Office, Washington, D.C., 1977, pp. 123-29.
33. E. V. Turner and J. H. Wallace, *Proc. Soc. Exp. Biol. Med., 167*:536 (1981).
34. A. E. Munson, J. A. Munson, W. Regelson, and G. L. Wampler, *Cancer Res., 32*:1397 (1972).
35. A. D. Barker, M. S. Rheins, and H. E. Wilson, *Proc. Soc. Exp. Biol. Med., 137*:981 (1971).
36. M. W. Rana and H. Pinkerton, *Anat. Rec., 178*:444 (1974).
37. D. G. Johns, S. M. Sieber, and R. H. Adamson, in *Modulation of Host Immune Resistance in the Prevention or Treatment of Induced Neoplasias* (M. A. Chirigos, ed.), U.S. Government Printing Office, Washington, D.C., 1977, pp. 117-21.
38. S. T. Yancey and W. A. Bleyer, *Cancer Res., 34*:1866 (1974).
39. S. E. Walker and M. R. Anver, *Clin. Res., 22*:612A (1974).
40. P. S. Morahan, J. A. Munson, L. G. Baird, A. M. Kaplan, and W. Regelson, *Cancer Res., 34*:506 (1974).
41. A. F. Gazdar, A. D. Steinberg, and S. Baron, Presentation at Int. Collog. on Interferon and Interferon Inducers, Leuven, Belgium, 1971.
42. G. R. Burleson and M. Pollard, *Fed. Proc., 35*:624 (1976).
43. A. F. Gazdar, A. D. Steinberg, G. F. Spahn, and S. Baron, *Proc. Soc. Exp. Biol. Med., 139*:1132 (1972).
44. A. F. Gazdar, *J. Natl. Cancer Inst., 49*:1435 (1972).
45. B. Fisher and M. Gebhardt, *Cancer Treat. Rep., 62*:1919 (1978).
46. W. A. Basley, R. C. Rees, J. A. Greager, and R. W. Baldwin, *Chemotherapy, 27*:44 (1981).
47. T. P. Waalkes, K. Sanders, R. G. Smith, and R. H. Adamson, *Cancer Res., 34*:385 (1974).
48. R. A. Dicloccui and B. I. S. Srivastava, *J. Natl. Cancer Inst., 60*:533 (1978).
49. G. E. Friedlaender, M. B. Mosher, and M. S. Mitchell, *Cancer Res., 34*:304 (1974).

50. M. Gidlund, A. Orn, H. Wigzell, A. Senik, and I. Gresser, *Scand. J. Immunol.*, *8*:156 (1978).
51. M. Gidlund, E. A. Ojo, A. Orn, H. Wigzell, and R. A. Murgita, *Scand. J. Immunol.*. *9*:167 (1979).
52. A. Senik, I. Gresser, C. Maury, M. Gidlund, A. Orn, and H. Wigzell, *Transplant. Proc.*, *11*:993 (1979).
53. A. Senik, I. Gresser, C. Maury, M. Gidlund, A. Orn, and H. Wigzell, *Cell. Immunol.*, 44:186 (1979).
54. P. Huguenin, A. Brownbill, P. Dukor, and A. R. Schuerch, *Experientia*, *36*:747 (1980).
55. L. Levy, F. Aizer, H. Ng, and T. M. Welch, *Lepr. Rev.*, *49*:215 (1978).
56. D. J. Giron, J. P. Schmidt, R. J. Ball, and F. F. Pindak, *Antimicrob. Agents Chemother.*, *1*:80 (1972).
57. R. Gruenewald and S. Levine, *Infect. Immun.*, *13*:1613 (1976).
58. E. T. Glaz, *Ann. Trop. Med. Parastiol.*, *73*:83 (1978).
59. F. M. Collins, *Antimicrob. Agents Chemother.*, *7*:447 (1975).
60. F. M. Collins, *Infect. Immunol.*, *30*:289 (1980).
61. P. F. Hoffman and H. W. Ritter, *J. Reticulo. Soc.*, *9*:638 (1971).
62. P. F. Hoffman, H. W. Ritter, and R. F. Krueger, in *Advances in Antimicrobial and Antineoplastic Chemotherapy* (M. Hejzlar, M. Semonaky, and S. Masak, eds.) Urban & Schwarzenberg, Munich, 1971, pp. 217-220.
63. T. Diamantstein, *Immunology*, *24*:771 (1973).
64. W. Regelson, *Ann. NY Acad. Sci.*, *277*:269 (1976).
65. J. R. Kettman, *Immunopharmacology*, *1*:29 (1978).
66. X. Y. Xu, Y. Li, and J. Xu, *Yao Hsueh Hsueh Pao*, *14*:443 (1979).
67. J. Cottney, J. Bruin, and A. J. Lewis, *Agents and Actions*, *10*:48 (1980).
68. Y-H. Chang and W. W. Hoffman, *Pharmacologist*, *17*:226 (1975).
69. Y-H. Chang and C. M. Pearson, *Arthritis Rheum.*, *21*:169 (1978).
70. G. D. Mayer, R. F. Krueger, and S. Yoshimura, Presented at Am. Soc. Microbiol. Meeting, Philadelphia, Pa., 1972.
71. H. Megel, A. Raychaudhuri, I. Shemano, and J. P. Gibson, in *Modulation of Host Immune Resistance in the Prevention or Treatment of Induced Neoplasias* (M. A. Chirigos, ed.), U.S. Government Printing Office, Washington, D.C., 1977, pp. 103-11.
72. D. G. Harrington, H. W. Lupton, C. L. Crabbs, L. E. Bolt, F. E. Cole, Jr., and D. E. Hilmas, *Proc. Soc. Exp. Biol. Med.*, *166*:257 (1981).
73. K. W. Eberly and J. Gavin, *Fed. Proc.*, *37*:838 (1978).
74. D. H. Katz, *Clin. Allergy*, *9*:609 (1979).
75. M. H. Flax and B. H. Waksman, *J. Immunol.*, *89*:496 (1962).
76. H. Megel, Presented at International Symposium on New Antiinflammatory Drugs, Pisa, Italy, 1976.
77. H. Megel, A. Raychaudhuri, M. Bayer, and T. H. Beaver, *Agents and Actions*, *8*:218 (1978).
78. R. J. Wojnar, R. J. Brittain, and E. Dzelzkalns, *J. Pharm. Sci.*, *68*:12 (1979).
79. J. R. Kettman, *Immunopharmacology*, *1*:21 (1978).
80. R. M. Massanari, *Clin. Res.*, *25*:380A (1977).
81. D. C. Argentieri, J. R. Mezzatesta, Jr., and R. P. Carlson, *Fed. Proc.*, *37*:604 (1978).
82. J. P. Donahoe, J. Giambrone, O. J. Fletcher, and S. H. Kleven, *Am. J. Vet. Res.*, *38*:2013 (1977).
83. G. Zbinden and E. Emch, *Acta Haematol.*, *47*:49 (1972).
84. L. E. Mobraaten, E. DeMaeyer, and J. DeMaeyer-Guignard, *Transplantation*, *16*:415 (1973).
85. A. Wildstein, L. E. Stevens, and G. Hashim, *Transplantation*, *21*:129 (1976).
86. A. Wildstein, L. Stevens, H. Applebaum, R. E. McCabe, G. Hashim, and H. Fitzpatrick, *Proc. Clin. Dial. Trans. Forum*, *5*:47 (1975).

87. A. Wildstein, L. E. Stevens, H. Applebaum, R. E. McCabe, G. A. Hashim, and H. Fitzpatrick, *Transplantation*, *22*:205 (1976).
88. W. Zschiesche, E. Slavina, and I. Leipunskaya, *Arch. Immunol. Ther. Exp.*, *25*:725 (1977).
89. W. Zschiesche, E. Slavina, and I. Leipunskaya, *Acta. Biol. Med. Ger.*, *36*:107 (1977).
90. H. Megel, A. Raychaudhuri, and L. L. Thomas, *Transplantation*, *21*:81 (1976).
91. H. Megel, A. Raychaudhuri, and J. P. Gibson, in *Control of Neoplasia by Modulation of the Immune System* (M.A. Chirigos, ed.), Reven Press, New York, 1977, pp. 409-420.
92. H. J. Seidel, U. Opitz, and L. Kreja, *Cancer Chemother. Pharmacol.*, *5*:49 (1980).
93. A. Raychaudhuri and H. Megel, *J. Reticulo. Soc.*, *20*:127 (1976).
94. P. Y. Paterson, E. D. Day, and C. C. Whitacre, *Immunol. Rev.*, *55*:89 (1981).
95. P. Y. Paterson, W. P. Richardson, and D. G. Drobish, *Cell. Immunol.*, *16*:48 (1975).
96. L. Ortiz-Ortiz and W. O. Weigle, *J. Exp. Med.*, *144*:604 (1976).
97. L. Ortiz-Ortiz, R. W. Nakamura, and W. O. Weigle, *J. Immunol.*, *117*:576 (1976).
98. S. Levine and E. J. Wenk, *Am. J. Pathol.*, *47*:61 (1965).
99. S. Levine, in *Modulation of Host Immune Resistance in the Prevention or Treatment of Induced Neoplasias* (M. A. Chirigos, ed.), U.S. Government Printing Office, Washington, D.C., 1988, pp. 89-96.
100. S. Levine and R. Sowinski, *Proc. Soc. Exp. Biol. Med.*, *156*:457 (1977).
101. S. Levine and R. Sowinski, *Arch. Int. Pharmacodyn. Ther.*, *230*:309 (1977).
102. S. Levine and R. Sowinski, *Am. J. Pathol.*, *82*:381 (1976).
103. S. Levine and R. Sowinski, *Toxic. Appl. Pharmacol.*, *40*:147 (1977).
104. D. Englert and K. Hempel, *Int. Arch. Allergy Appl. Immunol.*, *66*:326 (1981).
105. M. S. Mitchell, M. B. Mosher, and G. E. Friedlaender, in *Modulation of Host Immune Resistance in the Prevention or Treatment of Induced Neoplasias* (M. A. Chirigos, ed.), U.S. Government Printing Office, Washington, D.C., 1977, pp. 97-101.
106. M. Gidlund, A. Orn, H. Wigzell, A. Senik, and I. Gresser, *Nature*, *273*:759 (1978).
107. W. Regelson, A. E. Munson, J. A. Munson, G. D. Mayer, and R. F. Krueger, Presentation at International Meeting of the Reticuloendothelial Society, Freiburg, Germany, 1970.
108. N. Ackerman, A. Tomolonis, L. Miram, J. Kheifets, S. Martinez, and A. Carter, *J. Pharmacol. Exp. Ther.*, *215*:588 (1980).
109. C. A. Winter, E. A. Risley, and G. W. Nuss, *Proc. Soc. Exp. Biol. Med.*, *111*:544 (1962).
110. S. A. Metz, *Med. Clin. North. Am.*, *65*:713 (1981).
111. Y-H. Chang, *J. Pharmacol. Exp. Ther.*, *203*:156 (1977).
112. R. D. Sofia, L. Danielsen, and H. B. Vasser, *Pharmacol. Res. Comm.*, *11*:179 (1979).
113. A. W. Ford-Hutchinson, J. P. Bolam, and J. R. Walker, *J. Pharm. Pharmacol.*, *28*:790 (1976).
114. Y-H. Chang and W. Hoffman, *Arthritis Rheum.*, *20*:1507 (1977).
115. G. E. Davies, *Immunology*, *6*:561 (1963).
116. C. M. Pearson and F. D. Wood, *Arthritis Rheum.*, *2*:440 (1959).
117. B. H. Waksman, C. M. Pearson, and J. T. Sharp, *J. Immunol.*, *85*:403 (1960).
118. C. M. Pearson and Y. H. Chang, *Ann. Rheum. Dis.*, *38*:102 (1979).
119. L. R. Pflum and M. L. Graeme, *Agents and Actions*, *9*:184 (1979).
120. M. W. Rohovsky, J. W. Newberne, and J. P. Gibson, *Toxic. Appl. Pharmacol.*, *17*:556 (1970).
121. J. P. Gibson, *Vet. Pathol.*, *12*:71 (1975).
122. G. A. Leeson, S. A. Biedenbach, K. Y. Chan, J. P. Gibson, and. G. J. Wright, *Drug Metab. Dispos.*, *4*:232 (1976).
123. H. Lullman, K. Lullman-Rauch, and O. Wassermann, *Biochem. Pharmacol.*, *27*:1103 (1978).

124. S. Levine, R. Sowinski, and E. M. Hoenig, *Am. J. Pathol.*, *78*:319 (1975).
125. W. L. Thelmo and S. Levine, *Am. J. Pathol.*, *91*:355 (1978).
126. M. Cawein, B. C. Lampkin, I. Tsukimoto, G. Mayer, W. Regelson, and G. Schiff, Presentation at Symposium on Antivirals with Clinical Potential, Stanford, Calif., 1975.
127. G. M. Schiff, C. C. Linnemann, T. Rotte, G. Mayer, and S. Trimble, *Clin. Res.*, *21*:882 (1973).
128. J. B. Selhorst, K. F. Ducy, J. M. Thomas, and W. Regelson, *Neurology*, *28*:337 (1978).
129. G. M. Fenichel, G. Saavedra, and H. N. Cooper, Presented at Child Neurology Society Conference, Monterey, Calif., 1976.
130. W. H. Olson, J. A. Simons, and. G. W. Halaas, *Neurology*, *28*:1293 (1978).
131. H. E. Kaufman, Y. M. Centifanto, E. D. Ellison, and D. C. Brown, *Proc. Soc. Exp. Biol. Med.*, *137*:357 (1971).
132. H. Kaufman and Y. Centifanto, Presentation at International Congress of Chemotherapy, Prague, 1971.
133. H. E. Kaufman, E. D. Ellison, and Y. M. Centifanto, *Am. J. Ophthalmol.*, *74*:89 (1972).
134. C. A. Kauffmann, J. P. Phair, C. C. Linneman, Jr., and G. M. Schiff, *Infect. Immun.*, *10*:212 (1974).
135. P. Richter, G. L. Wampler, M. Kuperminc, and W. Regelson, in *Modulation of Host Immune Resistance in the Prevention or Treatment of Induced Neoplasias* (M. A. Chirigos, ed.), U.S. Government Printing Office, Washington, D.C., 1977, pp. 141-43.
136. G. L. Wampler, M. Kuperminc, and W. Regelson, *Cancer Chemother. Rep.*, *57*:209 (1973).
137. P. Richter, G. L. Wampler, M. Kuperminc, and W. Regelson, in *Modulation of Host Immune Resistance in the Prevention or Treatment of Induced Neoplasias* (M. A. Chirigos, ed.), U.S. Government Printing Office, Washington, D.C., 1977, pp. 139-40.
138. L. Israel, P. Miller, and R. Edelstein, in *Modulation of Host Immune Resistance in the Prevention or Treatment of Induced Neoplasias* (M. A. Chirigos, ed.), U.S. Government Printing Office, Washington, D.C., 1977, pp. 145-62.
139. M. Kuperminc and R. Gelber, *Proc. Am. Assoc. Cancer Res.*, *17*:260 (1976).
140. F. J. Cummings, R. Gelman, R. T. Skeel, M. Kuperminc, L. Israel, J. Colsky, and D. Tormey, *Cancer, 48*:681 (1981).
141. H. Cai, Y. Shu, G. Wang, A. Wu, P. Lin, S. Liu, and M. Li, *Chung Hua Chung Liu Tsa Chin*, *2*:92 (1980).
142. J. N. Weiss, R. S. Weinberg, and W. Regelson, *Am. J. Ophthalmol.*, *89*:46 (1980).
143. J. N. Weiss, A. L. Ochs, S. Abedi, and J. B. Selhorst, *Am. J. Ophthalmol.*, *90*:846 (1980).
144. R. V. Blake, J. J. Saady, D. C. Drummond, and J. N. Weiss, *J. Anal. Toxicol.*, *3*:206 (1979).
145. J. N. Weiss, R. S. Weinberg, and W. Regelson, *Invest. Ophthalmol. Vis. Sci.* (*Suppl.*), *29*: April (1980).
146. H. A. Claman, *N. Engl. J. Med.*, *287*:388 (1972).
147. R. H. Adamson, *J. Natl. Cancer Inst.*, *46*:431 (1971).
148. A. R. Rhoads, W. L. West, and H. P. Morris, *Res. Commun. Chem. Path. Pharmacol.*, *6*:741 (1973).
149. N. S. Doherty, *Fed. Proc.*, *40*:696 (1981).
150. N. S. Doherty, *Int. J. Immunopharm.*, *4*:67 (1982).
151. W. Zschiesche, B. Fahlbusch, I. Schumann, and E. Tonew, *Agents Actions, 8*:515 (1978).

152. W. Zschiesche, B. Fahlbusch, I. Schumann, and E. Tonew, *Curr. Chemother. Proc. Int. Congr. Chemother.*, *1*:315 (1978).
153. W. Zschiesche, *J. Reticulo. Soc.*, *25*:293 (1979).
154. B. Fahlbusch, W. Zschiesche, and W. Romer, *Acta. Biol. Med. Ger.*, *40*:147 (1981).
155. E. Katz, E. Margalith, and B. Winer, *Antimicrob. Agents Chemother.*, *9*:189 (1976).

7

Lipoidal Amines

William W. Hoffman Pfizer Inc., Groton, Connecticut

I. BACKGROUND

Initial host reactions to infection often involve nonspecific responses by cells of the immune system. As described in this volume, some relatively simple molecules appear to embody the necessary chemical features to evoke similar nonspecific responses and to facilitate the generation of immunological reactions to microorganisms and transformed or infected cells. One class of such substances, lipoidal amines, was discovered in the early 1970s and was shown to induce nonspecific viral resistance mediated by interferon (IFN) (1). A variety of these amphipathic basic lipids have been synthesized in the past decade, and some have been found to possess additional biological properties, notably antitumor (2,3) and adjuvant activity (4,5). Studies with many of these compounds indicate that all activities are not necessarily present in a given molecule and that, when present, the various activities are often not related mechanistically or temporally. This review will discuss the biological properties of lipoidal amines and the structural requirements that are associated with their expression of nonspecific and specific immunological activity.

II. PHYSICOCHEMICAL PROPERTIES

A. Structures

Lipoidal amines comprise a group of amines that are linked in various ways to a pair of hydrocarbon chains containing 8 to 20 carbons. The compounds include mainly, but not exclusively, diamines connected by relatively simple aliphatic or aromatic groups. Figure 1 shows members of four representative classes. The spectrum of their effects on host defenses can best be appreciated by first reviewing the properties of two prototypes that are

CP-20,961

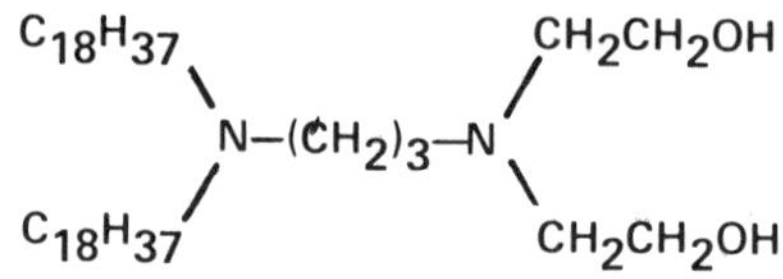

N,N-dioctadecyl-N′,N′-bis(2-hydroxyethyl)propanediamine

CP-28,888

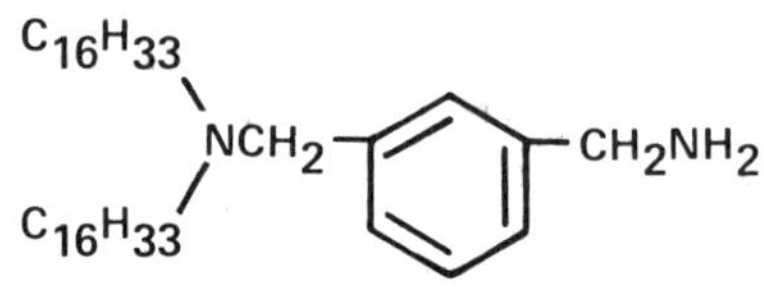

N,N-dihexadecyl-m-xylylenediamine

CP-34,315

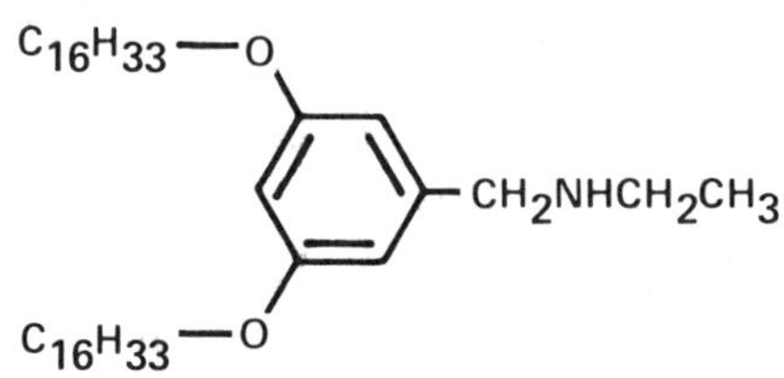

3,5-dihexadecyloxy-n-ethylbenzylamine

CP-46,665

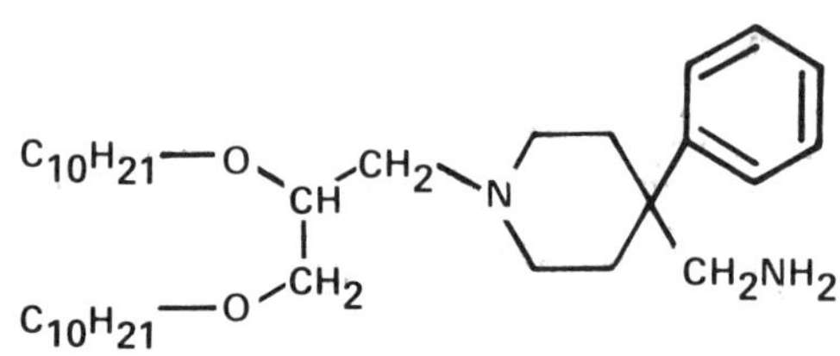

4-aminomethyl-1-(2,3-(di-n-decyloxy)-n-propyl)-4-phenylpiperidine

Figure 1 Structures of lipoidal amines.

on nearly the opposite ends of the physicochemical spectrum and which differ in the profile of their biological effects. These compounds are CP-20,961 [N,N-dioctadecyl-N′,N′-bis(2-hydroxyethyl)-propanediamine] and CP-46,665 [4-aminomethyl-1-(2,3-(di-n-decyloxy)-n-propyl)-4-phenylpiperidine]. CP-20,961 is a water-insoluble compound that was initially found to be an IFN inducer and was subsequently shown to be an immunological adjuvant, as potent as complete Freund adjuvant (CFA) with certain antigens. CP-46,665 is a water-soluble compound with a shorter didecyloxy, lipophilic moiety and is most active as an antitumor agent and macrophage activator. However, although CP-46,665 does not induce IFN, it has adjuvanting capacity; CP-20,961 shares the antitumor and macrophage-activating features of CP-46,665, albeit at higher doses. In many other lipoidal amines, possessing intermediate physicochemical characteristics, these properties are present to varying extents.

B. Preparation for Biological Testing

Because of their insolubility in water, certain of the lipoidal amines require preparation in suspension forms for evaluation in biological systems. The initial preparations of CP-20,961 were made with equal amounts of the surfactant, polysorbate 80, and glycerin in buffered saline (TG) (1). Physically, these formulations were fine milky suspensions, containing the lipoidal amine in particles of 1-2 μm in diameter. These preparations were studied in both animals and man for antiviral effects. CP-20,961 has also been incorporated into a soybean oil lipid emulsion, Intralipid (IL, Cutter Laboratories, Fairfield, New Jersey) (4), and has been dissolved or suspended in oils (6). In combination with 0.5 mol of synthetic lecithin, dimyristoylphosphatidyl choline, CP-20,961 can form small unilamellar liposomes (L) (unpublished observations). This preparation has been studied for antiviral (7) and adjuvant activity (8-10). Other lipoidal amines have been formulated by the same procedures. CP-46,665, because it is water-soluble, does not require special formulation. However, it has generally been administered intravenously in Intralipid to improve toleration (2). In those cases in which the biological activity of the lipoidal amines has been profoundly influenced by the method of formulation, this effect will be emphasized.

III. BIOLOGICAL ACTIVITIES

A. CP-20,961

1. Antiviral Activity and Interferon Induction in Animals

CP-20,961 was initially recognized to have antiviral activity in mice infected with RNA and DNA viruses (1,11). The compound was most effective when given by intraperitoneal (IP), subcutaneous (SC), and intramuscular (IM) routes, and less effective by the intravenous (IV) route; oral (PO) antiviral activity was not detected. Although IP or intranasal (IN) administration of the compound did not protect mice against lethal IN challenge (10 LD_{50}) with influenza virus or pnemonia virus of mice (1), six SC doses (first dose at -3 hr) over a 3-day period partially prevented changes in the lung weight of mice exposed to sublethal challenge (1/100 LD_{50}) with influenza virus (12). Local intravaginal application of CP-20,961 (L) to guinea pigs, 48 and 24 hr before local virus challenge, prevented lesion development caused by human herpes simplex virus, type 2 (7). In other studies, guinea pigs were completely protected from a footpad challenge with foot and mouth disease virus by 10 mg of CP-20,961 (L), given intracardially 1 hr before virus, and these animals were resistant to a second lethal challenge 2-4 weeks later (R. Knudsen, personal communication).

The mechanism of action of CP-20,961 was associated with induction of a partially acid-labile IFN which has been characterized in monkey sera to cross react with antibody against human IFNα (M. Langford and D. Slate, personal communications). No direct virucidal activity was found in cell culture systems, and efforts to achieve IFN induction in murine macrophages or peripheral blood leukocytes in vitro have been unsuccessful (1,11). However, peritoneal exudate cells (PECs), harvested from mice that were treated IP with CP-20,961 5 hr earlier, released more IFN into the medium after 24 hr in culture than PECs from untreated mice (4). The difficulty in finding in vitro cell systems that produce IFN in response to CP-20,961 may indicate a subtle collaborative interaction between macrophage and lymphoid cells in vivo (11). However, in vitro incubation of CP-20,961 with human nasal epithelial cells (13) or human fibroblast cells (R. Mason, personal communication) caused an antiviral state in the cells that could be partially reversed by anti-IFNα antibody. Also, the low IFN background detected in human lymphoblastoid (Namalva) cell cultures after 24 hr of incubation (2-4 U/ml) could be increased (32 U/ml) by a 4-hr preincubation with 30-50 μg/ml of CP-20,961 (L) (D. Slate, personal communication).

2. Clinical Antiviral Studies

In rhinovirus challenge studies with CP-20,961, its antiviral effect was extended to man and induced IFN was detected in 50% of nasal secretions (up to 60 U/ml in saline nasal washes) after drug treatment (14-19). When nasal sprays containing 50 mg of CP-20,961 (TG) were administered to volunteers both before (day −1, t.i.d.) and shortly after (day 0, b.i.d.) rhinovirus challenge, the predominant effect was a decrease in symptom intensity and duration, compared with placebo-treated controls (15-17,19). Illness rate was diminished in two studies (16,19) and virus shedding in one (16). Although symptoms were decreased, this did not alter the normal rate of seroconversion (60-79%) in volunteers (19). Treatments (q.i.d.) begun 2 days before challenge and continued for 5 days after challenge (14), were as effective as the 2-day regimen. However, no protective effects were seen when treatment was begun after challenge (17,19). Pretreatments with CP-20,961 at doses that stimulated nasal IFN production did not protect volunteers against experimental infection with influenza A2/England/42/72 (H_3N_2) (20). The authors suggest that the maximal levels of IFN calculated to occur at the nasal mucosa (3200 U/ml, when corrected for nasal wash dilution) may have been insufficient, since 10^6 U of exogenous IFN had failed to fully protect volunteers against influenza infections (21). Finally, the decrease in symptom severity that was objectively measured in challenge studies with defined serotypes of rhinovirus did not extend to field studies against a natural cross section of agents, including mild influenza, that cause common cold symptoms (18). This absence of effects in the latter studies may have resulted from reliance on subjective assessments of symptom severity and emphasis upon scoring disease incidence.

Studies of different lipid amine structures in mice led to the development of CP-28,888 (Fig. 1) as a more potent IFN inducer. In contrast to CP-20,961, CP-28,288 induced IFN in the rat and reduced symptoms of influenza A virus infection in hamsters (unpublished observations). In spite of these effects in animal systems, CP-28,888 proved to be less effective than CP-20,961 in inducing nasal IFN or lessening rhinovirus symptoms in volunteers (22). These results emphasized the species variation in responses to IFN inducers, even among structurally related compounds.

The sporadic recovery of IFN in nasal washes in clinical experiments and the poor correlations of IFN levels with clinical effectiveness led some investigators to suggest that IFN induction was not the only mechanism of action for these compounds (14,15,18).

3. Adjuvant Activity

CP-20,961 has been found to be an adjuvant for a number of antigens, including sheep red blood cells (4), viruses (4,5,10), tumor cells (2,4,23,24), and proteins (4,9). In addition, CP-20,961 can replace *Mycobacterium* in complete Freund adjuvant (CFA) and induce a disease that is indistinguishable from adjuvant arthritis in the Lewis strain of rats (6,24).

The drug dissolved in mineral oil (10 mg/0.2 ml) produced the disease, whereas oil alone or other interferon inducers, poly I, poly C, or tilorone, in oil were ineffective. The animals showed no skin hypersensitivity reaction to CP-20,961 in oil, suggesting that induction of the disease did not involve an immune response to the compound itself, but was, perhaps, an enhanced response to an endogenous immunogen (6). In support of this concept, the drug-induced arthritis could be suppressed specifically by type II collagen coupled to spleen cells (25). Since this procedure also suppressed disease caused by immunization of rats to type II collagen, this finding suggests that native type II collagen may be the endogenous immunogen responsible for drug-induced disease. The ability to induce arthritis is not common to all the lipoidal amines. Compounds CP-46,665, CP-28,888, and CP-34,315 (Fig. 1) in oil were all inactive in this regard (26). Even with CP-20,961 the formulation was important. This lipid amine (10 mg) was as arthritogenic as CFA when dissolved in mineral oil, but was less so when dissolved in olive oil or when suspended in mineral oil (6). At the same dose (10 mg), in a suspension formulation (TG), it was nonarthritogenic (D. Larson, personal communications).

In several studies, CP-20,961 showed adjuvant activity comparable with or superior to CFA for humoral responses and did not produce any CFA-like reactions at the injection site. In guinea pigs, the humoral response to sheep red blood cells (SRBCs) was greater with 3 mg of CP-20,961 in Intalipid (IL) as the adjuvant than with CFA (4). Similar intensities of delayed skin reactivity were observed for both adjuvants, but the site of IM immunization in the thigh showed only minor swelling when CP-20,961 was used, compared with swelling and granuloma formation of the limb after immunization using CFA. In mice immunized with formalin-inactivated Venezuelan equine encephalitis virus (VEE), 0.01-1.0 mg of CP-20,961 (IL), as an adjuvant, resulted in higher antibody titers than with CFA and produced equivalent or better protection from challenge (5). CP-20,961 (IL) greatly enhanced antibody titers to IM Rift Valley fever (RVF) virus vaccine in cynomolgus monkeys (10). Both oral and enteric vaccination in rats and mice led to an enhanced secretory immune response with reovirus, cholera, and *Streptococcus mutans*. In the latter case, increased salivary IgA antibody levels to *S. mutans* in rats were associated with decreased dental plaque (9). In pregnant pigs, immunized 6 and 2 weeks before farrowing, a subunit vaccine of transmissible gastroenteritis (TGE) virus and CP-20,961 (IL) produced higher antibody titers in serum and milk than the subunit combined with $Al(OH)_3$ or the subunit alone. Nursing piglets of the dams immunized with CP-20,961 as the adjuvant were completely protected against a challenge with virulent TGE, whereas the challenge was lethal to 38 and 62% of the piglets suckled on dams immunized with TGE and $Al(OH)_3$ or TGE subunit, respectively (P. Gough, personal communication). The adjuvant action of CP-20,961 is not always superior to CFA and may depend substantially upon the antigen. Thus, compared with CFA, CP-20,961 (IL) was a weak adjuvant for primary immunization with influenza B vaccine (4). Also, 3 mg of CP-20,961 (IL) mixed with 1.25 mg of myelin protein was not an effective immunogen in rabbits for inducing experimental allergic neuritis. In contrast, immunization with myelin mixed with CFA led to disease symptoms (D. Ziegler, personal communication).

In *Aotus* monkeys, 3 mg of CP-20,961 (IL) was an effective adjuvant for *Plasmodium falciparum*, merozoite vaccine derived from blood of infected monkeys (27). Animals were protected against challenge and showed minimal parasitemia. Results were comparable with those with CFA and 6-0-stearoyl-muramyldipeptide. The IM injection site showed transient swelling in the monkeys receiving the lipid amine, compared with the granulomatous abscesses formed after immunization with CFA. In contrast, when the parasite antigen was prepared from long-term in vitro cultures, vaccination using CFA, but not CP-20,961, protected monkeys from subsequent challenge (28).

Rats have been immunized IP against Ehrlich-Lette ascites carcinoma (EL4) cells using 20 mg of CP-20,961 dissolved in oil as an adjuvant (6). Both humoral antibody response and spleen cell killing of tumor cells were augmented to levels comparable with those found with CFA. Mice challenged with L1210 tumor cells survived longer if they had been vaccinated with CP-20,961 (IL) mixed with x-irradiated tumor cells (4).

The mechanism of adjuvant action of CP-20,961 is multifaceted. The lipoidal nature of the compound may provide a depot for antigen at the injection site, and its particulate nature may enhance processing by mononuclear phagocytes. In studies with VEE vaccine and CP-20,961 (IL), the complex of lipid emulsion, CP-20,961, and antigen was recognized in macrophages at the injection site and, 14 days after immunization, brown-pigmented macrophages were found both in local sites and in the epithelioid crescents near germinal follicles of the draining lymph nodes (5). The macrophages were observed to contain iron under light microscopy, and under electron microscopy, contained liposomelike membrane whorls (29). Typical of adjuvants and demonstrated by the use of labeled cells, CP-20,961 increased lymphocyte traffic both through the antigen depot and through the lymph nodes. Administration of antigen in vehicle alone led to only modest changes in this cellular traffic (5). CP-20,961 increases [^{125}IUdR] incorporation into spleen cell DNA to about the same extent as CFA (4). However, CP-20,961 is not a general mitogen like concanavalin A (ConA) since its mitogenic effects, like those of CFA, are confined to the spleen, whereas ConA increases [^{125} IUdR] incorporation into both spleen and liver (4). With enteric immunization, the adjuvant effects of CP-20,961 on the immune response were accompanied by both enlargement and increased number of Peyer's patches (9).

The adjuvant activity of CP-20,961 has recently been associated with an augmentation of dendritic cells (30). Injection of antigen with CP-20,961 into the footpad or thigh of rats stimulated the output of lymphocytes into the thoracic duct lymph. The proportion of lymphoblasts, monocytes, and dendritic cell precursers in the lymph was also increased. This effect reached a maximum 14 days after injection and was similar to that of CFA, but was less prominent. With both adjuvants, increased numbers of dendritic cells were observed to be associated with macrophages and dividing cells in the deep cortex of draining lymph nodes. Since dendritic cells appear to be more efficient than macrophages as antigen presenters, modulation of these cells could contribute significantly to the adjuvant activity of CP-20,961.

B. CP-46,665

1. Antitumor Activity

In addition to their adjuvant effects as components of vaccines, lipoidal amines exhibit nonspecific antitumor activity when given without antigen. This activity of the water-soluble compound, CP-46,665, in several murine tumor models recently has been reviewed (31).

2. Mechanism of Action

Indirect Evidence. The mechanism(s) responsible for the antitumor effect of CP-46,665 has been investigated. Interferon was apparently not involved, since none could be detected in the sera of mice given an IP dose of 50 mg/kg of the compound, and there was no evidence of antiviral protection in drug-treated mice subsequently challenged with encephalomyocarditis (EMC) virus (23). Distribution studies in rats with [^{3}H/CP] 46,665 showed that radioactivity preferentially accumulated in organs of the reticuloendothelial system such as lymph nodes, lung, spleen, and liver. The livers of chronically dosed animals contained histiocytic cells or Kupffer cells with foamy vacuoles that took up lipid stains (2). Autoradiographic studies in mice given IV drug showed moderate accumulations in alveolar macrophages at 2 hr and heavy accumulation by 24 hr (32).

CP-46,665 (1.25 mg/kg, IP) could maintain hypersensitivity to the contact-sensitizing agent, oxazolone, in mice bearing L1210 leukemia when given 3 days after tumor (31). Although the course of the disease was not altered, the drug effect suggested that this lipoidal amine could alter an anergic state in a tumor-bearing host.

Macrophage Activation. PECs removed from mice 3 days after IP injection of as little as 0.62 mg/kg of CP-46,665 (IL) became highly cytotoxic to B16 tumor cells (2). At an effector-to-target ratio of 12.5:1, PECs from mice treated with this drug level caused net lysis of 46% of B16 tumor cells (net lysis = percent [^{125}IUdR] release, treated − percent release, controls). Although CP-46,665 (IL) was directly cytotoxic to tumor cells at 5×10^{-5} M (IC_{50}), the observation of maximum cytotoxicity at 3 days after drug treatment suggested that a direct cytotoxic effect of the drug was not the only mechanism involved (2).

In normal mice, as little as 0.3 mg/kg of CP-46,665 (IL) given IV led to the appearance of tumoristatic macrophages in the lungs of treated mice (32). The effect was similar to that observed at a dose of 6 mg of *Corynebacterium parvum*, but occurred maximally at 2 days after drug treatment rather than after 5-9 days for *C. parvum*. The macrophage tumoristatic activity was associated with the ability of the macrophages to secrete prostaglandin (PGE_2). Although the relationship of the two effects was not determined, the augmented alveolar macrophage tumor stasis and increased peritoneal macrophage killing suggested a macrophage-mediated effector mechanism for the observed antitumor activity. Neither CP-46,665 nor *C. parvum* enhanced natural killer (NK) cell activity in the lungs or spleens of mice after IP treatment. However, IP inoculation of *C. parvum* enhanced spleen NK activity 2 days after treatment, whereas IP inoculation of CP-46,665 had no effect (33).

C. Structure Activity Relationships

1. Comparisons within Lipoidal Amine Classes

Closely related compounds from classes represented by CP-20,961, CP-28,888, and CP-46,665 (Tables 1-3) have been compared for their ability to produce IFN-mediated antiviral protection in mice and to prolong survival after IP implantation of sarcoma 180J (S180J) tumor (3,23). To test for antiviral activity, the drug was given IP 24 hr before SC EMC virus challenge. This regimen was used in order to maximize the protective effect of induced IFN. To determine activity against S180J, the tumor cells were inoculated IP 24 hr before IP drug treatment. Since S180J is an allogeneic tumor, the antitumor activity was not specific and may represent direct toxic effects, allograft rejection, PEC activation, or a combination of these effects. Tables 1-3 show similar patterns of activity for each class. In general, antiviral and anti-S180J activities were parallel for unsubstituted compounds with side chains of 14 and 16 carbons. However, compounds with shorter side chains (C8-C12) retained the anti-S180J activity, but lost the antiviral activity. On the other hand, the compounds with the longest chains (C18-C20) appeared to have more antiviral and less anti-S180J activity. Among the CP-20,961-like compounds (Table 1),

Table 1 Anti-EMC and Anti-S180J Activity of Alkyldiamines

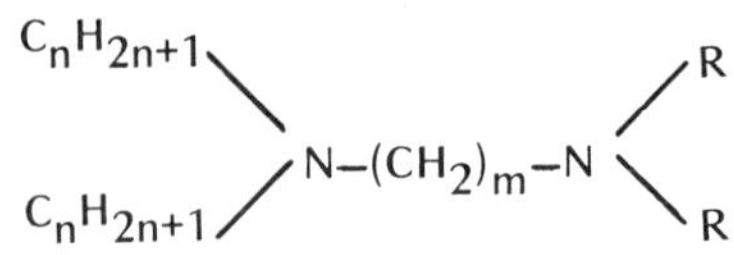

R	n	m	Anti-EMC[a] (% ES) 5 mg/kg	Anti-EMC[a] (% ES) 50 mg/kg	Anti-S180J[b] (% ILS) 5 mg/kg	Anti-S180J[b] (% S) 50 mg/kg
CH_2CH_2OH	18	2	–	40	–	–
CH_2CH_2OH	18	3	39	57	3	73 (16)
CH_2CH_2OH	18	4	8	51	35	61
CH_2CH_2OH	18	5	0	32	–	–
CH_2CH_2OH	18	6	5	20	16	14
H	18	3	13	37	33 (16)	73
CH_2CH_2OH	12	3	–	0	–	–
CH_2CH_2OH	14	3	–	60	63 (33)	120 (67)
CH_2CH_2OH	16	3	–	60	50	63 (16)
CH_2CH_2OH	20	3	–	0	27	13
CH_2CH_2OAc	18	3	0	0	16	39 (16)

[a]Compound was given IP 24 hr before SC challenge with 20 LD_{50} of encephalomyocarditis virus (EMC); % ES = excess survival (% survival in experimental group – % survival in virus control group).
[b]Compound was given IP 24 hr after IP injection of 1 million sarcoma 180J tumor cells (S180J); % ILS = % increased life span [(survival time in experimental group/survival time in control group × 100) – 100] % S = % survival after 40 days in groups of six mice.

the spacing between the nitrogens was optimum at 3-4 carbons for both activities. Acetylation of the hydroxyl groups was especially detrimental to the antiviral activity. In the aromatic series (Table 2), the p-isomer of CP-28,888 was equally potent, while the o-isomer was slightly less effective. Alkylation or acetylation of the primary amine decreased both activities. Although the above substitutions increased basicity, this did not appear to be a determining factor for activity, since the more basic amidine compound was highly effective in both tests.

These results showed that although certain structural changes alter both activities, changes in chain length caused the most obvious separation of antiviral effects from anti-S180J activity. Since the lower chain length compounds were more soluble and more cytotoxic, a direct effect on tumor cells may be involved. A similar relationship seemed to exist in the CP-46,665 series between cytotoxicity toward B16 cells in vitro and activation of PECs to kill B16 tumor cells (23).

2. Comparisons Among Lipoidal Amines Types

The relationship of various activities of lipoidal amines to one another can be appreciated by comparison of the profiles of the compounds that are representative of four structural classes shown in Fig. 1 (Table 4). As previously demonstrated, IFN induction was a property restricted to compounds with long lipophilic chains (C12-C20) and was, therefore not a property of CP-46,665. The values for CP-20,961, CP-28,888, and CP-34,315 are

Table 2 Anti-EMC Activity and Anti-S180J Activity of Xylylenediamines

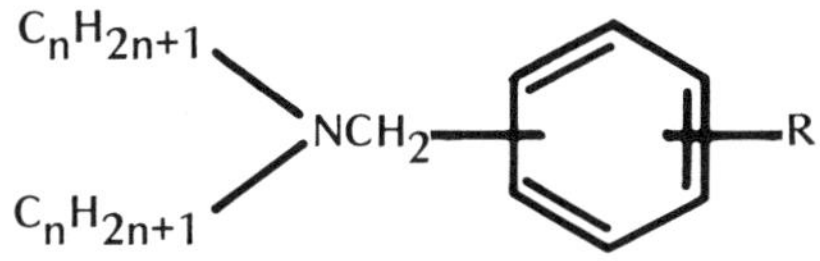

R	n	Isomer	Anti-EMC[a] (% ES) 5 mg/kg	Anti-EMC[a] (% ES) 15 mg/kg	Anti-S180J[b] (% ILS) 5 mg/kg	Anti-S180J[b] (% S) 15 mg/kg
CH_2NH_2	10	m	0	0	12	119 (50)
CN_2NH_2	12	m	0	–	46	90 (50)
CN_2NH_2	14	m	39	44	34	80 (33)
CN_2NH_2	16	m	45	56	83	111 (50)[c]
CH_2NH_2	18	m	35	45	16	100 (67)
CH_2NH_2	20	m	55	50	14	10
CH_2NH_2	16	o	30	50	14	34 (16)
CH_2NH_2	16	p	65	75	16	85 (33)
CH_2NHEt	16	m	55	55	11	24
CH_2NEt_2	16	m	12	17	8	2
$CII_2NMe_3^+$	6	m	33	38	15	0
CH_2NHAc	16	m	0	0	–	–
$C(NH_2)=NH$	16	m	55	60	44	137 (100)

[a]See footnote a, Table 1.
[b]See footnote b, Table 1.
[c]Dose was 25 mg/kg, IP.

Table 3 Anti-EMC and Anti-S180J Activity of Aminomethylphenyl Piperidines

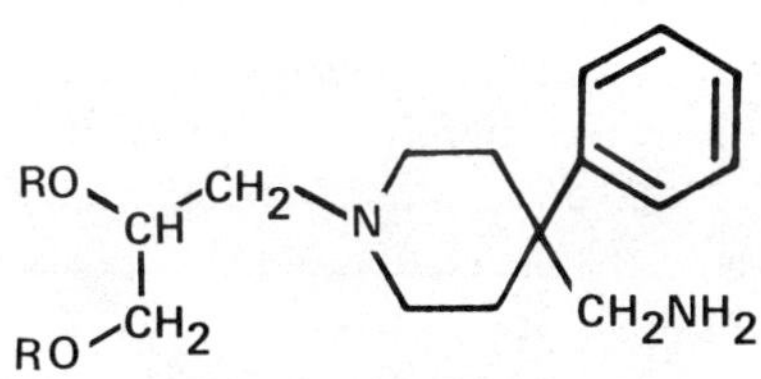

CP No.	R	Anti-EMC[a] (% ES) 5 mg/kg	Anti-EMC[a] (% ES) 15 mg/kg	Anti-S180K[b] (% ILS) 5 mg/kg	Anti-S180K[b] (% S) 15 mg/kg
46,487	C_8H_{17}	–	–	74 (67)	T
46,665	$C_{10}H_{21}$	0	10	89 (83)	110 (100)
41,919	$C_{14}H_{29}$	85	65	40 (33)	110 (100)
40,335	$C_{16}H_{33}$	65	78	52 (16)	76 (33)
41,175	$C_{18}H_{37}$	35	45	16 (0)	68 (33)

[a]See footnote a, Table 1.
[b]See footnote b, Table 1.

Table 4 Summary of Activities of Lipoidal Amines of Four Structural Types

	Anti-EMC[a] IP MED (mg/kg)	Macrophage activation[b] IP MED (mg/kg)	Anti-S180J[c] IP MED (mg/kg) (% ILS)	(% S)	L1210 Vaccine[d] IP MED (mg/kg)	Arthritogenicity[e] subplantar effect of 10 mg in oil
CP-20,961	3	1	25	75	30	+
CP-28,888	1	10	25	225	25	−
CP-34,315	5	15	Inactive		ND[f]	−
CP-46,665	Inactive	0.6	5	5	3	−

[a]See footnote a, Table 1; MED = minimum effective dose (1 and W. Hoffman, unpublished observations).
[b]Drugs were administered 3 days before harvesting of peritoneal macrophages; cytotoxicity against B16 melanoma target cells (4 and 26).
[c]See footnote b, Table 1, (26).
[d]Mice were vaccinated with drug plus 1.6 × 10^6 x-irradiated L1210 leukemia cells on day −7; challenged with 10^5 live L1210 cells (2,3).
[e]Drugs were injected into the footpad of Lewis rats on day 0; adjuvant arthritis was measured on day 16 (6).
[f]ND = not determined.

minimum effective doses (MEDs) for antiviral protection, when given 24 hr before an EMC virus challenge. The lower MEDs are generally associated with higher maximum IFN levels. For example, CP-20,961 given IP to mice at 25 mg/kg induced 50-200 U IFN/ml of serum, whereas CP-28,888 induced up to 300 U/ml (3). When up to 50 mg/kg of CP-46,665 was given to mice, no antiviral effect or IFN levels were found. All four compounds activate PECs in vivo, but CP-20,961 and CP-46,665 were more potent than the other two. In tumor models, CP-46,665 was more potent than any of the other compounds by a factor of at least 15. For example, when given IP with a vaccine of x-irradiated L1210 cells 7 days before challenge, CP-46,665 was 10 times more potent than CP-20,961 or CP-28,888. When given IP 1 day after IP challenge with S180J tumor, CP-46,665 was also more potent in producing tumor-free survivors than CP-20,961 or CP-28,888. CP-34,315, although an IFN inducer and PEC activator, was inactive (26). These IP systems examined treatment at the site of challenge and might be expected to measure a combination of direct effects of drug as well as activation of resident or elicited cells. Although CP-46,665 stimulates the tumoristatic activity of alveolar cells (31), activity in this system relative to CP-20,961 has not been determined. In any event, the comparisons described above suggest that activation of macrophages may be only part of the mechanism for the antitumor effects of CP-46,665.

The capacity of the compounds to cause adjuvant arthritis in rats was restricted to certain formulations of CP-20,961. The other three compounds administered in formulation that were most efficacious with CP-20,961 were all ineffective.

IV. TOLERATION

Lipoidal amines have been generally well tolerated at doses substantially above those that are optimal for activity. For example, CP-20,961 (TG), an effective IP IFN inducer at 5-10 mg/kg IP, has an IP LD_{50} of greater than 2000 mg/kg (1). The IV LD_{50} for this material was 70 mg/kg; a similar preparation at a daily IV dose of 5 mg/kg, was tolerated in dogs for 28 days (34). CP-20,961 (L) has an IV LD_{50} in mice of 145 mg/kg (unpublished observation). In humans, topical nasal application of 50 mg CP-20,961 (TG) t.i.d. for 4 days was accompanied by slight irritation, but that was also seen with vehicle and waned with continued dosing (17). The other most studied compound, CP-46,665 (IL), displays antitumor activity at an optimum dose in mice of about 2.5 mg/kg or less. The acute IV LD_{50} is 60-70 mg/kg in mice and rats. Treatment at 12.5 mg/kg for 14 days in rats showed no evidence of toxicity (2). Dogs received 25 mg/kg in Intralipid IV every 4 days for 3 months and showed only slight changes in hematological parameters and blood chemistries. Toleration studies in clinical populations of dogs and cats with various spontaneous tumors indicated that weekly doses of 5 mg/kg IV were without side effects even after 30 weeks (2).

V. SUMMARY AND PERSPECTIVES

Lipoidal amines are synthetic, relatively simple compounds that resemble natural membrane lipids in their amphipathic nature and solubility properties. The maximum effects of the compounds require, or are facilitated by, incorporation into lipid vehicles or inclusion into the lipid phase of oil-in-water suspensions. This method of delivery favors distribution to organs of the RES, and the particulate nature of these vehicles would suggest an initial interaction with cell surfaces prior to cellular uptake. In animal systems, the compounds stimulate host defenses that lead to anti-infective, antitumor, and adjuvant effects. These effects are associated with increased humoral and cell-mediated immunity, as well as stimulation of nonspecific host mechanisms such as IFN induction and macrophage-mediated killing of target cells. In animal models, a particular effect often depends upon the physical association and timing of drug presentation as well as the nature of the antigen, pathogen, or tumor cell. Thus, several mechanisms may be envisioned to operate at different times, often complicating interpretation in lengthy experiments.

Lipoidal amines have only been applied clinically as topical, nasally administered IFN inducers against respiratory infections. However, this experience and recent animal data suggest that other topical antiviral applications, such as antiherpetic use, could be practical. The use of IFN in the treatment of neoplasia is being intensively investigated. The combination of IFN induction and other antitumor properties in lipoidal amines might provide a useful alternative or adjunct to exogenous IFN. Lipoidal amines, like CP-20,961, could find application as adjuvants for vaccines that require the effectiveness of CFA, but for which CFA cannot be used because of its local and systemic toxic sequelae. Also, the oral adjuvant use of this lipoidal amine suggests additional potential for applications with a variety of microbial antigens and tumor cell components.

Further studies are required to more clearly define the mechanism(s) of action of lipoidal amines and the protocols most appropriate for their use. Multiple variables in formulation and dosage regimens will need to be investigated with each clinical indication. As with other immune modulating agents, frequent administration of high doses does not appear to be the most efficient or effective path to therapeutic success.

REFERENCES

1. W. W. Hoffman, J. J. Korst, J. F. Niblack, and T. H. Cronin, *Antimicrob. Agents Chemother.*, *3*:498-502 (1973).
2. J. S. Wolff, III, G. R. Hemsworth, A. R. Kraska, W. W. Hoffman, S. K. Figdor, D. O. Fisher, R. M. Jakowski, J. F. Niblack, and K. E. Jensen, *Cancer Immunol. Immunother.*, *12*:97-103 (1982).

3. A. R. Kraska, G. R. Hemsworth, W. W. Hoffman, and J. S. Wolff, III, in *Current Chemotherapy and Infectious Disease*, Vol. 2 (J. D. Nelson and C. Grassi, eds.), Am. Soc. Microbiol., Washington, D.C., 1980, pp. 1605-1607.
4. J. F. Niblack, I. G. Otterness, G. R. Hemsworth, J. S. Wolff, III, W. W. Hoffman and A. R. Kraska, *J. Reticuloendothel. Soc.*, *26*:655-666 (1979).
5. A. O. Anderson and J. A. Reynolds, *J. Reticuloendothel. Soc.*, *26*:667-680 (1979).
6. Y.-H. Chang, C. M. Pearson, and C. Abe, *Arth. Rheum.*, *23*:62-71 (1980).
7. Z. M. Zheng, D. R. Mayo, and G. D. Hsiung, *Antiviral Res.*, *3*:275-283 (1983).
8. A. O. Anderson, A. Plotner, and D. H. Rubin, *N. Y. Acad. Sci. Conf. Secretory Immune Systems*, Abst. P-1-2 (1982).
9. S. M. Michalek, A. O. Anderson, and D. H. Rubin, *N. Y. Acad. Sci. Conf. Secretory Immune Systems*, Abst. P-2-16 (1982).
10. D. D. LaBarre, C. L. Crabbs, and R. A. Reynolds, *82nd Ann. Meet. Am. Soc. Microbiol.*, Abst. E61 (1982).
11. E. T. Glaz and M. Talas, *Acta Microbiol. Acad. Sci. Hung.*, *25*:87-96 (1978).
12. M. R. Boyd and M. F. Beeson, *J. Antimicrob. Chemother.*, *1*(*Suppl.*):43-47 (1975).
13. M. W. Harmon, S. B. Greenberg, and P. E. Johnson, *82nd Ann. Meet. Am. Soc. Microbiol.*, Abst. T25 (1982).
14. R. G. Douglas, and R. F. Betts, *Infect. Immun.*, *9*:506-510 (1974).
15. B. G. Gatmaitan, E. D. Stanley, and G. G. Jackson, *J. Infect. Dis.*, *127*:401-407 (1973).
16. C. Panusarn, E. D. Stanley, V. Dirda, M. Rubenis, and G. G. Jackson, *N. Engl. J. Med.*, *291*:57-61 (1974).
17. E. D. Stanley, G. G. Jackson, V. A. Dirda, and M. Rubenis, *J. Infect. Dis. 133* (*Suppl*): A121-A127 (1976).
18. J. F. Niblack, *Tex. Rep. Biol. Med.*, *35*:528-534 (1977).
19. R. H. Waldman and R. Ganguly, *J. Infect. Dis.*, *138*:531-535 (1978).
20. R. G. Douglas, Jr., R. F. Betts, R. L. Simons, P. W. Hogan, and F. K. Roth, *Antimicrob. Agents Chemother.*, *8*:684-687 (1975).
21. T. C. Merigan, S. E. Reed, T. S. Hall, and D. A. J. Tyrrell, *Lancet*, *i*:563-567 (1973).
22. R. G. Douglas, R. H. Waldman, R. F. Betts, and R. Ganguly, *Antimicrob. Agents Chemother.*, *15*:269-272 (1979).
23. A. R. Kraska, V. A. Pollack, W. W. Hoffman, J. S. Wolff, and G. R. Hemsworth, *21st Interscience Conf. Antimicrob. Ag. Chemother.*, Abst. 329 (1981).
24. Y. -H. Chang, and C. M. Pearson, *Arth. Rheum.*, *21*:169-170 (1978).
25. D. E. Trentham and R. A. Dynesius-Trentham, *Arth. Found., Fellows Conf.*, Tarpon Springs, Abst. (1981).
26. I. G. Otterness, J. F. Niblack, J. S. Wolff, III, W. W. Hoffman, and A. R. Kraska, *4th Int. Cong. Immunol.*, Abst. 17.3.40 (1980).
27. W. A. Siddiqui, S. -C. Kan, K. Kramer, S. Case, K. Palmer, and J. F. Niblack, *Nature*, *289*:64-66 (1981).
28. W. A. Siddiqui, *Int. J. Immunopharm.*, *4*:309 (1982).
29. A. O. Anderson, *4th Int. Cong. Immunol.*, Abst. 17.3.02 (1980).
30. A. O. Anderson and J. T. Warren, *Adv. Exp. Biol. Med.*, *149*:671-680 (1982).
31. K. E. Jensen, J. F. Niblack, J. S. Wolff, III, A. R. Kraska, I. G. Otterness, W. W. Hoffman and G. R. Hemsworth, in *Human Cancer Immunology*, Vol. 3, Elsevier, Amsterdam, Chap. 4, 1982, pp. 55-63.
32. J. D. Gangemi and J. Hightower, *18th Natl. Reticuloendothel. Soc. Meet.*, Abst. 27 (1981).
33. J. D. Gangemi, R. A. Jackson, R. Blanding, and K. Jensen, *81st Ann. Meet. Am. Soc. Microbiol.*, Abst. E10 (1981).
34. J. F. Niblack, J. S. Wolff, III, G. R. Hensworth, A. R. Kraska, R. M. Jakowski, S. K. Figdor, and K. E. Jensen, in *Progress in Cancer Research and Therapy*, Vol. 16, *Augmenting Agents in Cancer Therapy* (E. M. Hersh, M. A. Chirigos, and M. J. Mastrangelo eds.), Raven Press, New York, 1981, p. 391.

Section B

Natural Products, Extracts, and Lower Molecular Weight Components

8

Thymosin, Peptidic Moieties, and Related Agents

Teresa L. K. Low and Allan L. Goldstein The George Washington University School of Medicine and Health Sciences, Washington, D.C.

I. INTRODUCTION

The effect of thymic extracts on various biological systems was extensively investigated long before the physiological role and biological function of thymus gland became fully understood. Crude thymic extracts from thymus of various species have been reported to stimulate such diverse processes as calcium and phosphorus metabolism (1,2), gonadal growth (3), and glucose metabolism (4). Thymic extracts were also found to modify animal growth and development (3,5-7), produce lymphocytosis (4), and influence lymphoid tissues (8-10). However, it was not until 1961 that the contribution of the thymus to the ontogenesis and maintenance of the lymphoid system was fully recognized. Miller (11), Good et al. (12), and others (compare 13) found that neonatal thymectomy was associated with severe depletion in the lymphocyte populations resulting in major immunological defects. These early studies established that the thymus was necessary for the normal development of the immune response. Subsequent studies by other investigators on the effects of thymus grafts in cell-impermeable Millipore diffusion chamber (14-18) and the effects of cell-free thymic extracts (10,19-23) helped to establish the endocrine function of the thymus.

The thymus gland is a bilobed lymphoid organ located immediately beneath the breast bone in the chest. The involution of the thymus is among the first noticed indications of aging (24). As shown in Fig. 1, numerous immunological studies have demonstrated that there is a concurrent decrease in cellular immunity with increasing age and a corresponding general increase in the incidence of the diseases of aging. Moreover, decrease in thymic function with advancing age causes senescence in T-cell immunity directly correlated with an increase in the incidence of cancer.

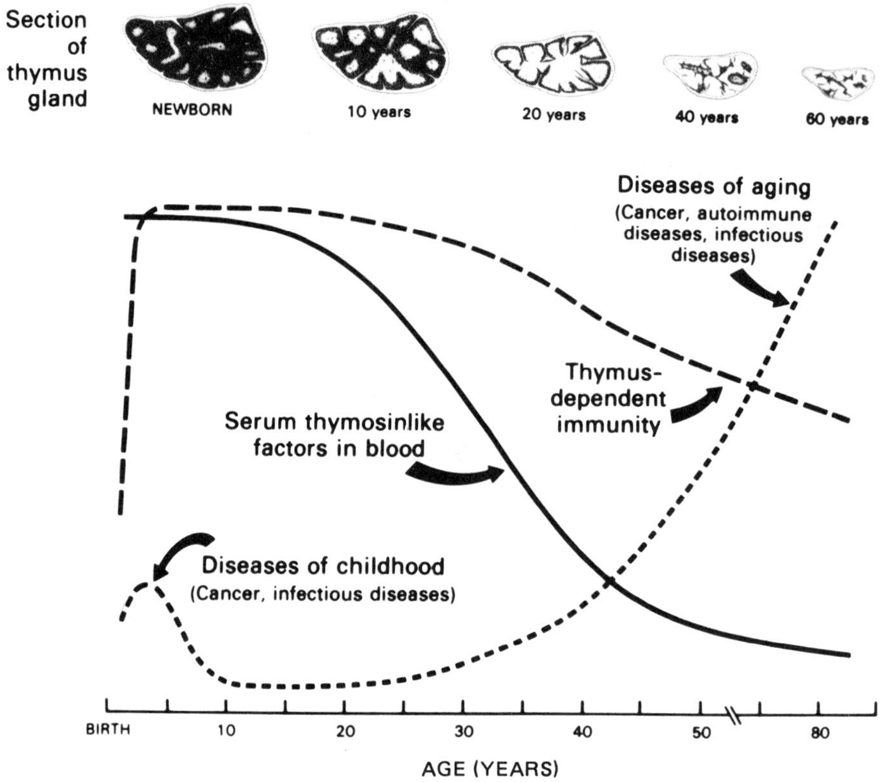

Figure 1 Involution of the thymus with the increasing age of the individual. Thymic factors in the blood and cellular immune mechanisms are shown to decline in similar fashion. The incidence of age-related diseases increases in inverse proportion to the shrinkage of the thymus and to the decrease of thymic-dependent immunity.

For the past several years a large research effort has been directed toward the isolation and identification of the thymic factors or hormones responsible for the physiological functions of the thymus gland. The most widely studied partially purified thymic preparation termed thymosin fraction 5 (F5) has been shown to be a potent immunopotentiating agent (25). Thymosin F5 corrects a number of the deficiencies resulting from lack of thymic function in animal models (26-28) as well as in humans with primary immunodeficiency diseases (29-32) and in immunosuppressed cancer patients (33-38). It has been shown that thymosin α_1 (one of the purified peptides isolated from F5) decreases with age in mouse and in man (39). These observations and documented defects in T-cell immunity with aging (40) suggest that a number of the diseases of the aged may be directly associated with the inability of the thymus gland to produce normal amounts of thymic hormones.

As illustrated in Fig. 2, endocrine thymus produces thymosin (41,42) and other thymic factors (43-46) which control the development of the thymic-dependent lymphoid system and the process of immune regulation. Impairment of lymphoid elements by

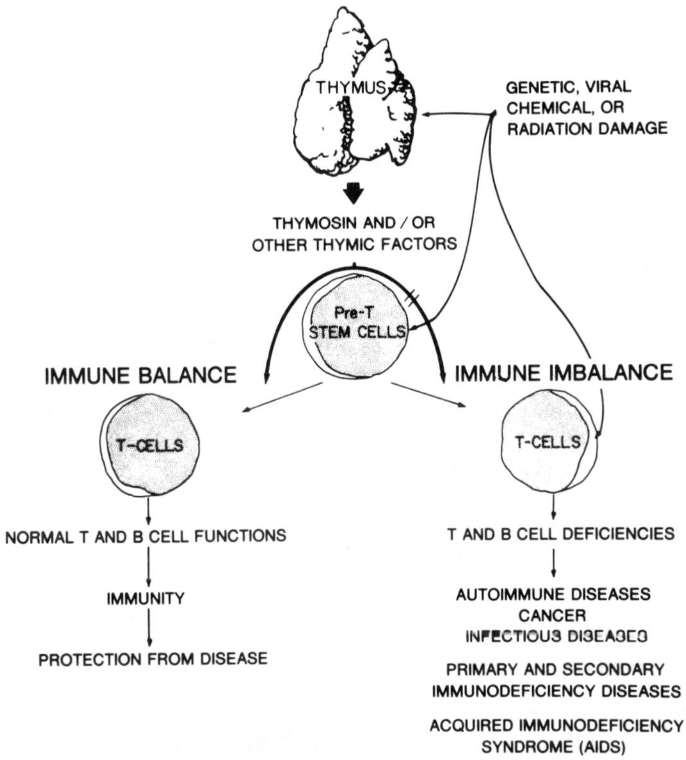

Figure 2 Thymus contribution to immunity. Impairment of lymphoid elements, including the thymus and immunocompetent cells, by various deleterious agents causes deficiencies in immunity which may lead to a variety of disease manifestations. These conditions may in part be the result of a malfunctioning thymus and inadequate levels of thymic secretions.

various deleterious agents causes deficiencies in immunity which may lead to a variety of disease manifestations.

Our ongoing studies have provided evidence that the partially purified thymosin F5 consists of a family of biologically active polypeptide components with hormonal-like activities (47). These peptides may act at different sites and on different subsets of T cells and contribute to the normal maintenance of immune function and balance. In addition to the thymosins, a number of factors with thymic hormone-like activity have been isolated from thymus tissue (compare 48), blood (46), and thymic epithelial supernatants (49,50). These preparations are in various stages of characterization.

In this chapter, we will summarize the progress being made in the chemical and biological characterizations of the thymosins. We will also briefly review our studies on the development of a radioimmunoassay for thymosin α_1, the identification of the epithelial cells in the thymus that produce thymosin polypeptides, and the therapeutic applications of thymosin. In addition, we will describe the chemical and biological properties of other well-defined thymic preparations and related agents. We will not attempt to review the extensive historical literature on thymic hormones and factors which are covered adequately in a number of comprehensive review articles (41,48,51-53).

II. ISOLATION AND BIOLOGICAL PROPERTIES OF THYMOSIN

Our studies on thymosin were initiated in 1964 in the laboratory of Dr. Abraham White at the Albert Einstein College of Medicine. These studies led to the isolation and identification of a lymphocytopoietic factor in rat and mouse thymus extracts (22,23). Later, a stable form of the biologically active fraction was prepared from calf thymus which was termed thymosin (54).

A. Preparation of Thymosin Fractions 5 and 5A

Thymosin F5 is prepared from calf thymus as described previously (25). As shown in Fig. 3, the preparation is obtained by homogenization of thymus tissue, followed by an 80°C heat denaturation step, an acetone precipitation step, and fractionation with ammonium sulfate. The 25-50% ammonium sulfate precipitate is further subjected to ultrafiltration in Amicon DC-2 hollow fiber system to yield F5. The 50-95% ammonium sulfate cut is also collected and processed through DC-2 and Sephadex G-25 to yield fraction 5A (F5A). Fraction 5 contains polypeptides with molecular weight ranging from 1000 to 15,000. There are detectable and identifiable amounts of carbohydrate, but they are essentially free of nucleotide. Fraction 5A similarly contains multiple polypeptide components with molecular weight under 15,000.

B. Nomenclature of Thymosin Polypeptides

On an isoelectric focusing gel, F5 is shown to consist of 30 or more individual polypeptide components. We have proposed a nomenclature system for thymosin peptides based on this isoelectric focusing pattern. As shown in Fig. 4, the separated protein bands are divided into three regions. The α region consists of polypeptides with isoelectric points below 5.0; the β region, 5.0-7.0; and the γ region, above 7.0. The subscript number $\alpha_1, \alpha_2, \beta_1, \beta_2$, and so forth, are used to identify the polypeptides from each region in the order that they are isolated. For comparative purposes, some other well-defined thymic factors such as FTS (facteur thymique serique), thymopoietin, and THF (thymic humoral factor) are also shown on the gel at appropriate positions according to their reported isoelectric points. The chemistry and biology of these thymic factors will be discussed in more detail in Sec. VII.

On the same isoelectric focusing gel system, thymosin F5A appears to contain mostly the β-region peptides and very few peptides from the α region (data not shown). It appears that F5A is a better source for isolation of β-region peptides, such as β_1 (55) and β_4 (56).

C. Biological Properties of Thymosin

Thymosin F5 exhibits activities in many biological systems. However, based on our limited biological data for thymosin F5A, it appears that this fraction is not active in some bioassays, indicating that it is devoid of some of the biologically active components of F5. Table 1 summarizes the major biological properties of thymosin F5. Thymosin has been found to induce T-cell differentiation and enhance immunological functions in genetically athymic mice (26), in adult thymectomized mice (26), in NZB mice with autoimmune reactions (16,27), in tumor-bearing mice (28,57,58), and in mice with casein-induced amyloidosis (59). It is also effective in inducing the differentiation of specific subclasses of T lymphocytes (60,61) and certain cell markers (terminal deoxynucleotidyl transferase, Thy 1, and Lyt) and functional expressions of lymphocytes maturation (60,62-66). In

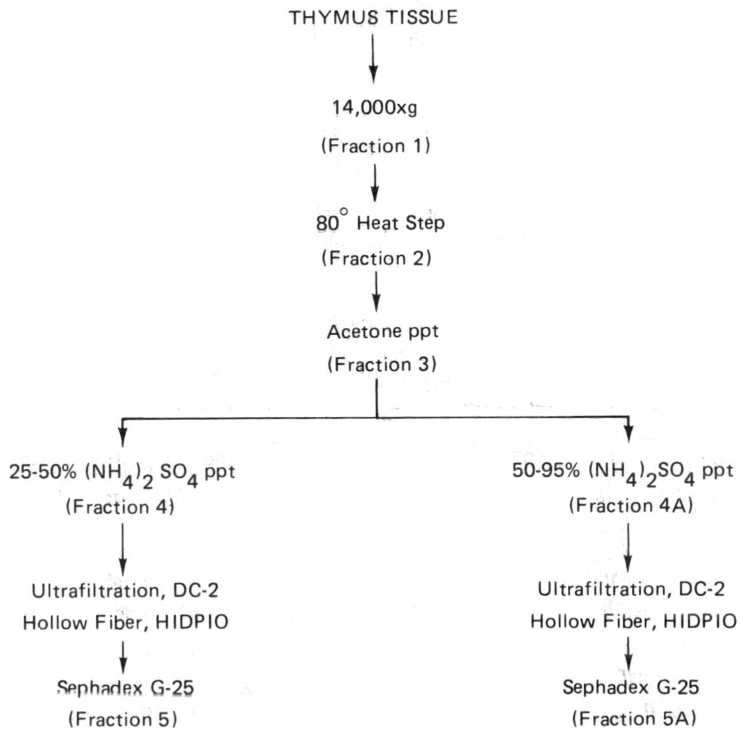

Figure 3 Purification of bovine thymosin fraction 5 and fraction 5A. One kilogram of thymus tissue homogenized in 3 L NaCl provides the sample to initiate the procedure.

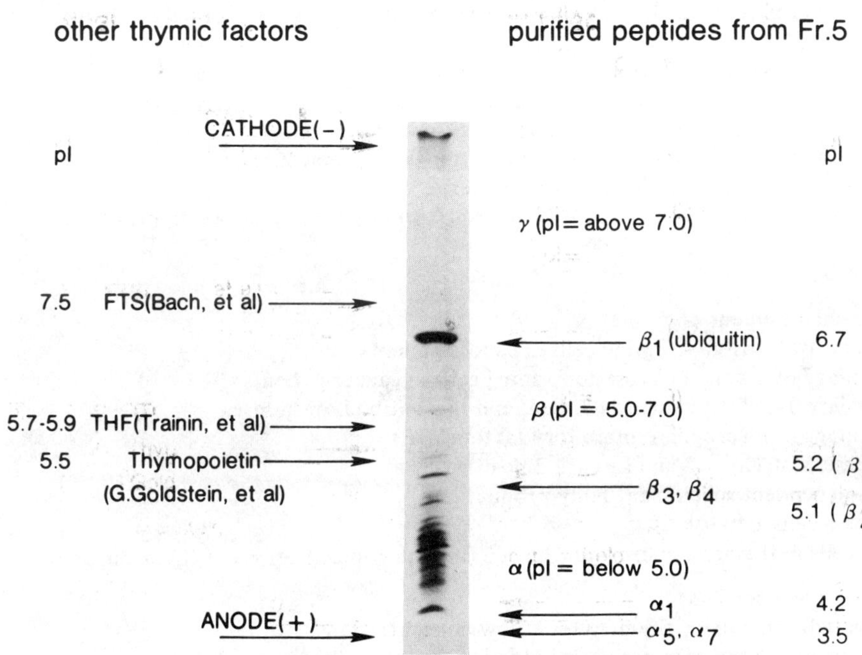

Figure 4 Isoelectric focusing of thymosin fraction 5 in LKB PAG plate (pH 3.5-9.5). Purified thymosin peptides from the α, β, and γ regions are identified. The isoelectric points of several other well-characterized thymic factors are illustrated for comparison.

Table 1 Major Biological Properties of Thymosin Fraction 5 and Its Component Polypeptides

Thymosin fraction 5

In vitro enhancement of:

- Number of azathioprine-sensitive E-rosette-forming spleen cells from adult, thymectomized mice
- Appearance of phenotype T-cell markers on mouse spleen and bone marrow cells
- Responsivity to mitogens
- Mixed lymphocyte reaction
- Conversion of bone marrow cells into cells reactive in the graft vs. host reaction in vivo
- Production of suppressor T cells
- Production of macrophage inhibitory factor
- Production of antibody to sheep erythrocytes by spleen cells of normal and thymectomized mice
- Intracellular cyclic GMP levels of mouse spleen cells
- Terminal deoxynucleotidyl transferase (TdT) activity
- Specific antibody production of tetanous, meningococcal, and gonococcal antigens
- LRF and LH production by medial basal hypothalamus and pituitary

In vivo enhancement of:

- Lymphocytopoiesis in normal, germ-free, adrenalectomized, neonatally thymectomized, and athymic mice
- Rate of allograft rejection in normal and neonatally thymectomized mice
- Resistance to progressive growth of Moloney virus-induced sarcoma in normal mice
- Mixed lymphocyte reaction (in vivo-in vitro) by lymphoid cells from normal or neonatally thymectomized mice
- Lymphoid cell response to mitogens (in vivo-in vitro) by cells of normal and athymic mice
- Resistance to growth of allogeneic and xenogeneic tumors in athymic mice
- Delay of abnormal thymocyte differentiation (loss of suppressor function) in NZB mice
- Antibody production in sheep erythrocytes (in vivo + in vitro)
- Survival in tumor-bearing mice (in conjunction with chemotherapy)
- Interferon production following viral challenge
- Adrenocorticotropin (ACTH), cortisone, and β-endorphin production in primates

Thymosin α_1

In vitro enhancement of:

- Numbers of E-rossete-forming cells in cancer patients
- Percentage of autologous rosette-forming cells in cancer patients
- Secondary T-cell-dependent IgG, IgM, and IgA antibody responses
- Percentage of macrophage inhibitory factor (MIF)
- Expression of Thy 1.2 and Lyt 1,2,3 positive cells
- T-cell-dependent specific antibody production
- Helper T-cells activity
- TdT^+ cells in the bone marrow and spleen (at high concentrations of thymosin α_1)

In vitro suppression of:

- TdT activity in murine thymocytes at low concentrations
- Elevated $T\gamma/T\mu$ ratios in peripheral blood of cancer patients

In vivo enhancement of:

- Lymphoid cell responses to mitogens (in vivo + in vitro)

Table 1 (continued)

Lymphotoxin production (in vivo + in vitro)
Survival in tumor-bearing mice
Interferon production
Corticosterone production in mice
MLR (mixed lymphocyte reaction) response and diseasefree interval in patients with lung cancer

Thymosin α_7

In vitro enhancement of:
Suppressor T cells
Expression of Lyt 1,2,3 positive cells

In vivo suppression of interferon production

Thymosin β_3 and β_4

In vitro and in vivo induction of TdT in separated bone marrow cells from normal or athymic mice
In vivo induction of TdT levels in thymocytes of immunosuppressed mice
In vitro stimulation of LRF and LH secretion
In vivo induction of LH production

aged mice, thymosin administration in vivo has been found to significantly increase hemagglutinin responses against sheep red blood cells (SRBCs), antihapten responses to TNP trinithophenyl (67), and delayed hypersensitivity responses to oxazolone (68). In vitro, thymosin has been found to correct the cell cycle of lymphocytes from again thymectomized rats (69).

D. Purification and Chemical and Biological Characterization of the Component Polypeptides in Thymosin Fraction 5

1. Thymosin α_1

Isolation and Chemical Characterization. The first thymosin polypeptide isolated from F5 has been termed thymosin α_1 (55). The isolation procedure for thymosin α_1 from F5 includes column chromatography on ion-exchangers CM-cellulose and DEAE-cellulose and gel filtration on Sephadex G-75. Thymosin α_1 migrates as a single band on analytical polyacrylamide gels at pH 8.3 and 2.9 and as a major band with an isoelectric point of 4.2 on an isoelectric focusing slab gel of pH range 3-5. The yield of thymosin α_1 from F5 is about 0.6%. The amino acid sequence of thymosin α_1 has been elucidated (70) and is shown in Fig. 5. It is composed of 28 amino acid residues with a molecular weight of 3108. The amino terminus of thymosin α_1 is acetylated. Using parameters for the prediction of protein conformation described by Chou and Fasman (71), it would appear that the C-terminal half of the molecule has a high helical potential.

Biological Properties. The biological activities of thymosin α_1 have been studied in many assay models. Thymosin α_1 has been demonstrated to be a potent immunologically

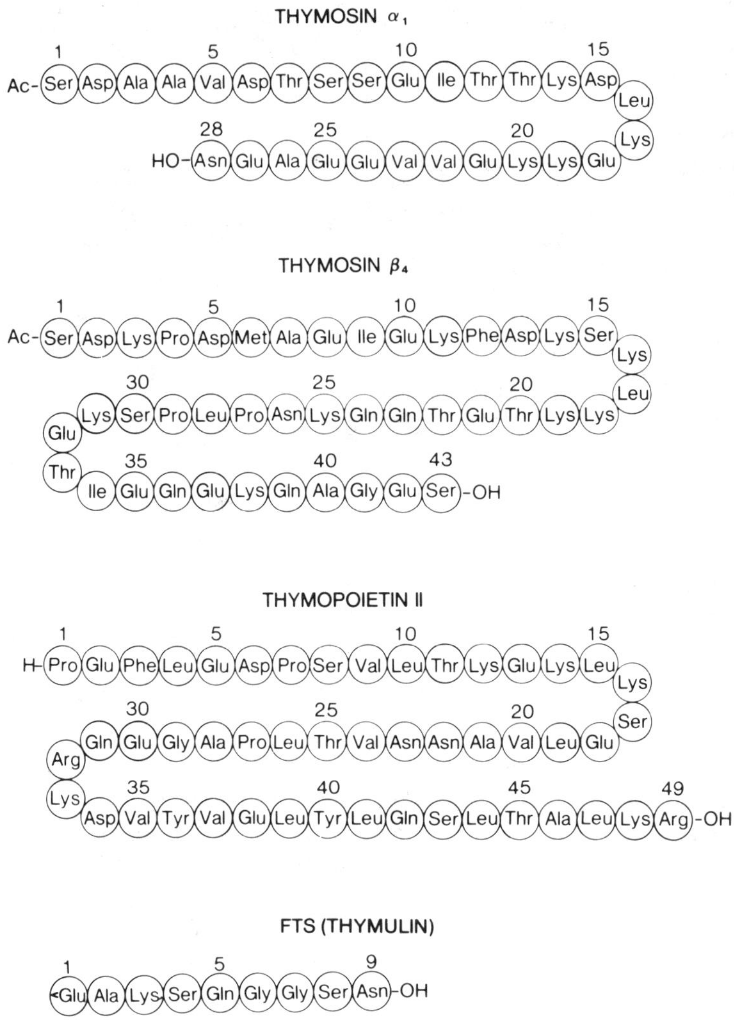

Figure 5 Amino acid sequence of purified thymic factors: thymosin α_1; thymosin β_4; thymopoietin II and FTS (thymulin).

active thymic polypeptide. It is 10-1000 times as active as the parent thymosin F5 in several biological models. As shown in Table 1, it induces the expression of certain T-cell markers Thy 1.2, Lyt 1,2,3 (42), and functional activity associated with lymphocyte maturation (helper T-cell activity, specific antibody production, production of macrophage inhibitory factor, etc.) (55,60,72). At high concentrations of α_1, it increases TdT-positive cells in the bone marrow and spleen (73). It also suppresses TdT activity in murine thymocytes in vitro at low concentration (66). Furthermore, incubation of thymocytes in vitro with thymosin F5 or α_1 results in an increase in the percentage of glucocorticoid-resistant cells (74) and in vivo enhances survival in tumor-bearing mice (75) and immunosuppressed mice with lethal candidal infection (76). Most recently, we have found that intercerebral injection of α_1 in mice stimulates corticosterone production (77).

2. Thymosin β_4

Isolation and Chemical Characterization. Thymosin β_4 is the first of the biologically active polypeptides from the β region of thymosin F5 to be completely characterized (56). Thymosin β_4 is composed of 43 amino acid residues with an acetyl group at the N-terminal end. It has a molecular weight of 4963 and an isoelectric point of 5.1. The complete amino acid sequence of thymosin β_4 is shown in Fig. 5.

A computer search for possible sequence homology between the sequence of thymosin β_4 and other published protein sequences has been conducted at the National Biomedical Research Foundation, Washington, D.C. The results do not indicate a statistically significant relationship of thymosin β_4 to any other sequenced protein currently stored in the data bank. However, there is an interesting internal duplication between residues 18-30 and 31-43, as illustrated in Fig. 6. Using data for prediction of protein conformation, described by Chou and Fasman (71), two regions were identified to contain high helical potential. As shown in Fig. 7, residues 4-12 and 32-40 were identifiable to be helical regions. No region suggestive of β-sheet structure was found.

Biological Properties. Thymosin β_4 has been found to induce TdT expression in TdT-negative murine bone marrow cells in vivo and in vitro (78). It also increases TdT activity in thymocytes from hydrocortisone-immunosuppressed mice in vivo (66). Thus, it appears that thymosin β_4 is acting on lymphoid stem cells and may influence the early stages of the maturation process of thymus-dependent lymphocytes.

Furthermore, thymosin β_4 was found to inhibit macrophage migrations (72). Preliminary studies indicate that this molecule acts directly on the macrophages to inhibit their migration. However, the possibility that they act on lymphocytes and induce them to release a macrophage migration inhibitory factor (MIF) has not been completely ruled out.

Most recently, thymosin β_4 was shown to stimulate secretion of luteinizing hormone-releasing factor (LRF) from superfused medial basal hypothalami of female rats (79). In addition, luteinizing hormone (LH) was released from pituitary glands superfused in sequence with hypothalami (79) and when injected directly into the ventricles of male mice (80). These data provide the first evidence of a direct effect of the endocrine thymus on the hypothalamus and suggest a potentially important role for thymic peptides in reproductive function.

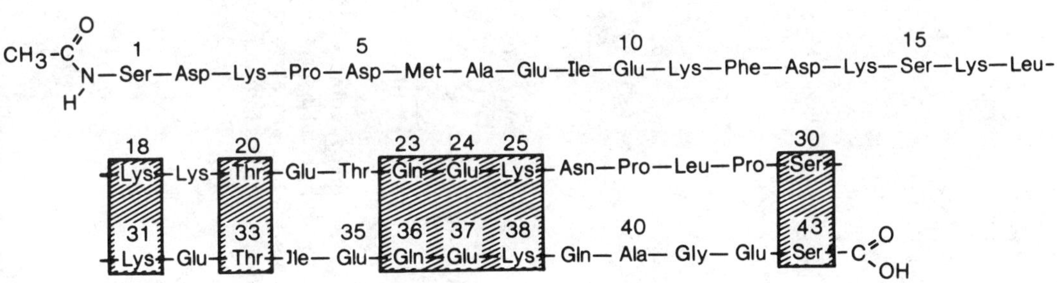

Figure 6 Regions of internal duplication in thymosin β_4. Residues 31-43 are aligned with 18-30, and six identities are identified by shaded areas.

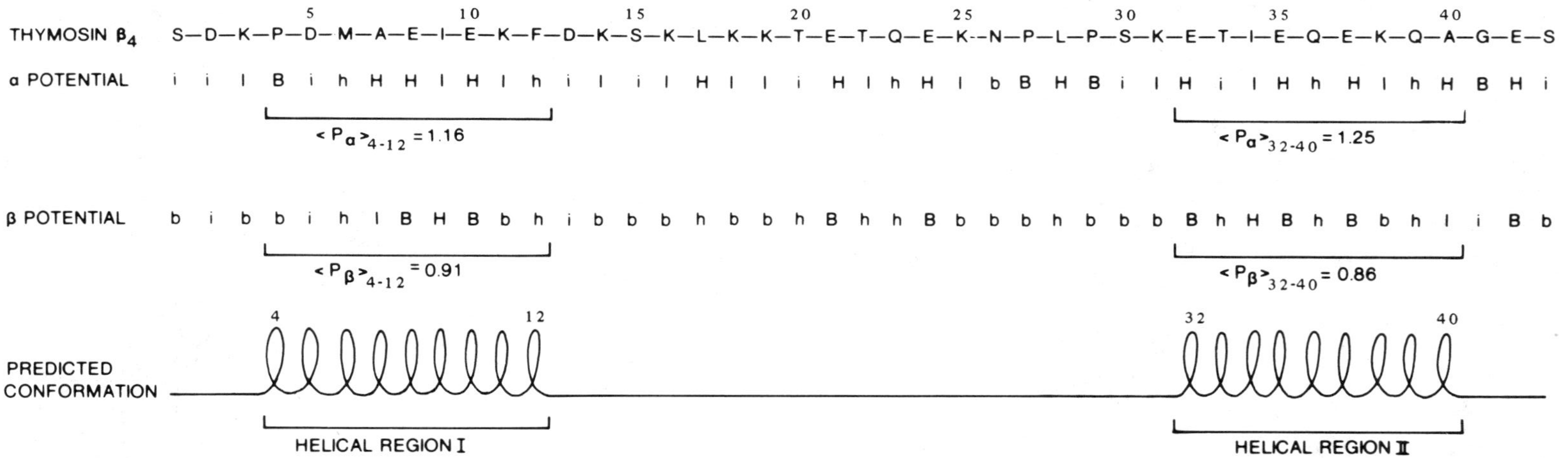

Figure 7 Prediction of protein conformation using the method of Chou and Fasman (71). Assignments of amino acids as formers, breakers, and indifferent for helical and β-sheet regions based on conformational parameters, $P\alpha$ and $P\beta$, are indicated as *H*, strong former; *h*, former; *I*, weak former; *i*, indifferent; *b*, breaker, and *B*, strong breaker. Two regions (residues 4-12 and 32-40) were identified to contain high helical potential. No potential β-sheet was found in the molecule. [The one-letter notation of amino acids used for thymosin β_4 is from Dayhoff, M. O., (ed.) (1972) *Atlas of Protein Sequence and Structure*, National Biomedical Research Foundation, Washington, D.C.]

3. Thymosin α_7

Thymosin α_7 was isolated from thymosin F5 by ion-exchange chromatography on CM-cellulose and DEAE-cellulose and gel filtration on Sephadex G-75 (Low and Goldstein, unpublished). It is highly acidic with an isoelectric point around 3.5. Thymosin α_7 is a partially purified preparation and can be resolved into several components by high-performance liquid chromatography on a reversed phase column (Low and Goldstein, unpublished). Purification of these components is now in progress.

Biologically, thymosin α_7 has been shown to be a potent inducer of suppressor cells in humans (S. Horowitz, personal communication) and in mice (60) and is also active in inducing T-cell markers (60).

4. Polypeptide β_1

Polypeptide β_1 is the predominant band on the isoelectric focusing gel of F5 (see Fig. 3). It was isolated from thymosin F5A as described (55). It has a molecular weight of 8451 and an isoelectric point of 6.7. The amino acide sequence of β_1 has been determined (70) and has revealed that this molecule is identical to ubiquitin and a portion of protein A24, a nuclear chromosomal protein. Polypeptide β_1 does not show biological activity in our bioassay systems, indicating that it is not an important molecule for T-cell maturation. Ubiquitin was found to be identical with APF-1, the polypeptide cofactor of ATP-dependent protein degradation (81). This defines the important biological role of the molecule which is unrelated to the specific function of the thymus. Furthermore, its role in protein degradation explains the ubiquitous nature of this molecule (82).

5. Other Peptides

Several peptides isolated from thymosin F5 have structures closely related to thymosin β_4. Thymosin β_3 has an isoelectric point of 5.2 and a molecular weight of approximately 5500. Preliminary studies (Low and Goldstein, unpublished) indicate that thymosin β_3 shares an identical sequence to β_4 through most of its amino terminal portion and differs only at the carboxyl terminal ends. However, the complete sequence of this molecule has not been determined. Like thymosin β_4, thymosin β_3 induced the expression of TdT in TdT-negative murine bone marrow cells in vivo and in vitro (78). It also increases TdT activity in thymocytes from hydrocortisone-immunosuppressed mice in vivo (66). In addition, thymosin β_3 inhibits macrophage migration independent of antigen (72).

Recently, Hannappel et al. (83) reported the isolation of two new peptides, thymosin β_8 and β_9, from calf thymus. As shown in Fig. 8, the amino acid sequences of thymosin β_8 and β_9 were found to be homologous to thymosin β_4.

Of the 38 amino acid residues present in thymosin β_8, 31 are identical to the corresponding residues in thymosin β_4. Thymosin β_9 is identical to thymosin β_8 except for the presence of an additional dipeptide, -Ala-Lys-OH, at the carboxyl terminus. However, no biological function was defined for either molecule.

E. Thymosin α_1 from Other Species

To evaluate the species variation of thymosin polypeptides, we have prepared F5 from thymus tissues of human, pig, sheep, chinchilla, and mouse. The human thymus tissue was excised during open heart surgery and from selected autopsies. Biological studies (48) on human, porcine, ovine, and murine F5 indicated that they possess similar activities as

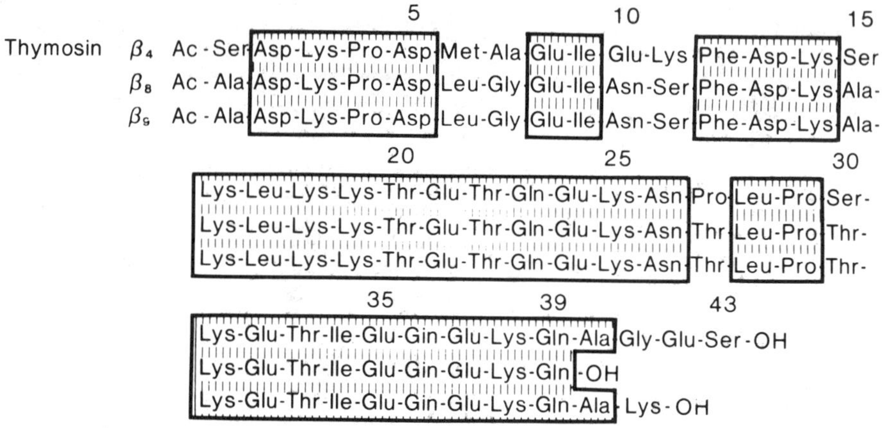

Figure 8 Sequence homology of thymosin β_4-β_8 and β_9. The residues that are identical with those in thymosin β_4 are shaded.

bovine F5 in a mixed lymphocyte reaction (MLR) assay (85), a mouse mitogen assay (86), a macrophage migration inhibitory factor (MIF) assay (72), and a human E-rosette assay (30). Thymosin α_1 from several species was prepared from F5, using a modification of the extraction and fractionation procedures developed for the isolation of bovine α_1. Human (48), porcine, and ovine (84) thymosin α_1 have also been partially sequenced. From the results obtained, they appear to have an identical sequence to bovine α_1. Most recently, thymosin F5 preparations were analyzed by high-performance liquid chromatography (HPLC) on a μBondapak C_{18} (Waters) reverse phase column (87). Fractions were collected around the region where bovine α_1 was eluted. These fractions were analyzed by radioimmunoassay for thymosin α_1 (39). In each case, the immunoreactive peak coelutes with the protein peak at the rention time of bovine α_1. The results indicated that each of the F5 preparations examined consists of a peptide with similar or identical structure to bovine α_1. On the other hand, chromatographic analysis of fresh rat and calf thymus extracts using similar HPLC system did not reveal a detectable protein peak at the α_1 position. These observations suggest that α_1 may be synthesized in a precursor form in animal tissues which supports the report of Hannappel et al. (88). Freire et al. (89) have translated messenger RNA from fresh calf thymus and carried out synthesis in a cell-free wheat germ system. A peptide of 16,000 daltons that was immunoprecipitable with antisera against thymosin fractions was analyzed and found to contain tryptic peptides corresponding to fragments of thymosin α_1. Thus, the 16,000-dalton peptide appears to be a precursor of thymosin α_1.

III. SYNTHETIC ANALOGS OF THYMOSIN α_1 AND β_4

A. Thymosin α_1

Thymosin α_1 has been synthesized by several laboratories, including Wang et al. (90), Birr and Stollenwerk (91), and Abiko et al. (92), using solution synthesis procedures, and Folkers et al. (93), Wang et al. (94), Wong and Merrifield (95), and Colombo (96), using solid phase procedures.

The synthetic material prepared by Wang et al. (90) migrated as a single spot on acrylamide gel isoelectric focusing (pH 3.5-9.5) and on high-voltage silica gel thin-layer electrophoresis (pH 1.9 and 5.6), and was indistinguishable from the natural thymosin α_1. As shown in Fig. 9, the synthetic polypeptide migrates to the same position as the natural thymosin α_1 preparation on LKB PAG plate with pH range 3.5-9.5. The synthetic material has been tested in our laboratories for biological activities, and has been found to be similar to the natural α_1 in TdT assay (66) and MIF assay (72).

Thymosin α_1 has also been synthesized utilizing recombinant DNA procedures (97). In this important new development, the gene for thymosin α_1 was synthesized. The gene was inserted under lac operon control into the plasmid and expressed as part of a β-galactosidase chimeric protein. The plasmid is then cloned in a strain of *Escherichia coli.* The structure of the N^{α}-desacetyl thymosin α_1 was confirmed by sequence analysis. The molecule was found to be as active as the chemically synthesized α_1 (90) in an MIF assay (72) and a TdT assay (66). A method for amino-acetylation of the N^{α}-desacetyl thymosin α_1 has been reported by Kido et al. (98), using a transacetylase associated with a wheat germ ribosomal preparation.

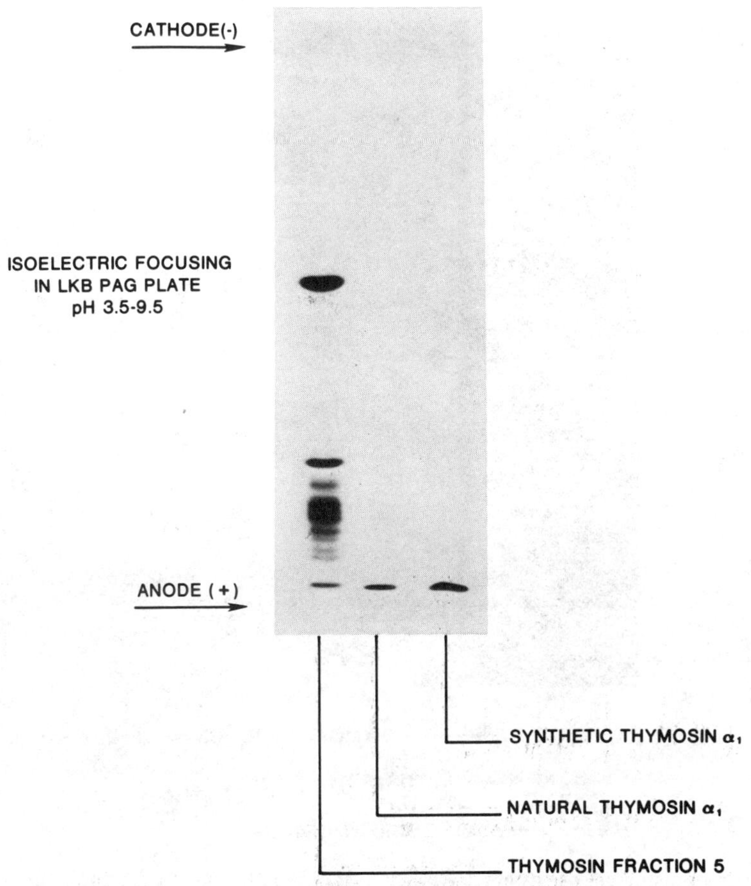

Figure 9 Isoelectric focusing in polyacrylamide gel (LKB PAG plate, pH 3.5-9.5). The gel was fixed in 20% trichloroacetic acid and then stained with 0.1% coomassie blue to reveal the protein bands. The amounts loaded on the gel were 200 μg of thymosin fraction 5 and 100 μg each of natural and synthetic thymosin α_1.

Most recently, Ciardelli et al. (99) have found that several synthetic C-terminal fragments (spanning positions 17-28) of α_1 possess activity in azathioprine E-rosette inhibition assay (100). They suggest that a basic-acidic-lipophilic sequence character is a possible essential feature of a molelcular signal for T-cell differentiation.

B. Thymosin β_4

The chemical synthesis of thymosin β_4 using a solid phase procedure has been accomplished (101). The synthetic material was shown to be identical to the natural thymosin β_4 by tryptic peptide mapping and amino acid compositional analyses. As shown in Fig. 10, on an LKB PAG plate at pH 3.5-9.5, the synthetic thymosin β_4 moves to the similar position as the natural material with pI of 5.1. Biologically, synthetic thymosin β_4 was found to be as active as the natural compound in a TdT assay (see Table 2) and an MIF assay (see Table 3). Thus the proposed structure (56) of this peptide hormone was confirmed by chemical synthesis.

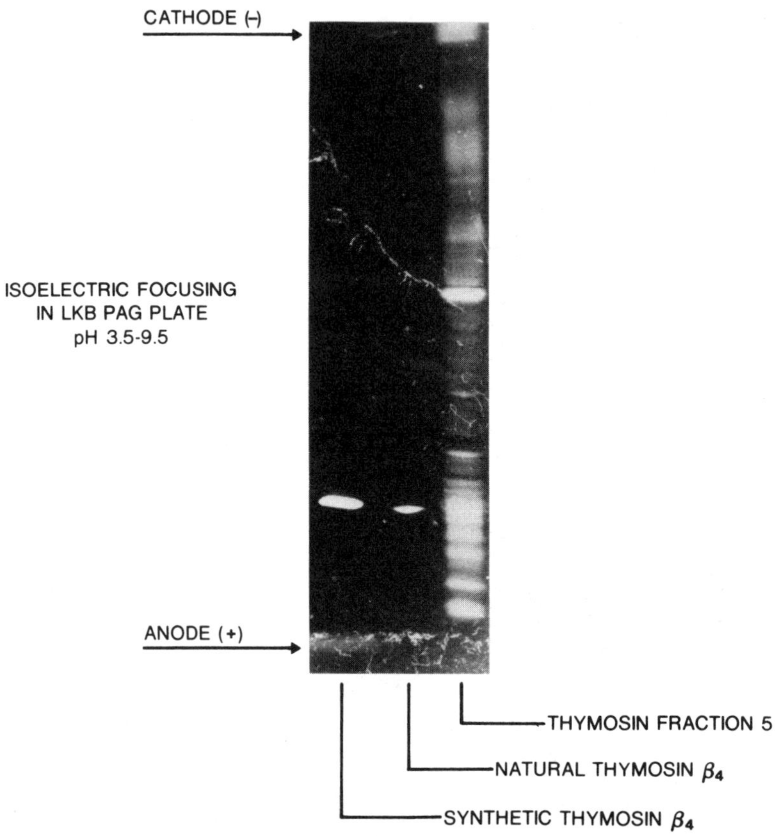

Figure 10 Isoelectric focusing gel of thymosin fraction 5, bovine thymosin β_4, and synthetic thymosin β_4 on LKB PAG plate at pH 3.5-9.5. The amount loaded on the gel were 200 μg each of thymosin fraction 5 and synthetic thymosin β_4 and 50 μg of natural thymosin β_4. The gel was fixed in 20% trichloroacetic acid for 1 hr to reveal the protein bands as shown in this picture.

Table 2 In Vivo Induction of TdT by Thymosin in Thymocytes from Hydrocortisone Acetate-Treated C57B1/6J Mice

Treatment[a]	Dose (μg)	TdT specific activity[b]	Increase (%)
Saline	–	38.3	–
Thymosin F5	100	51.0	33.2
Spleen F5	100	42.2	10.1
Natural thymosin β_4	1	52.5	37.1
Natural thymosin β_4	0.1	46.7	21.9
Synthetic thymosin β_4	1	54.2	41.5
Synthetic thymosin β_4	0.1	47.5	24.0

[a]Mice were treated with 1.25 mg of hydrocortisone acetate, followed by daily injection of the indicated agents for 11 days. Amount used per injection is given in the dose column.
[b]Specific activity is expression as nmol of dGTP incorporation per 10^8 cells per hour.

IV. RADIOIMMUNOASSAY FOR THYMOSIN

A sensitive and specific radioimmunoassay (RIA) has been developed in our laboratory to measure thymosin α_1 in human blood and tissue extracts (39). Antiserum to thymosin α_1 was produced in rabbits by immunization with synthetic thymosin α_1 (90) coupled to hemocyanin. A synthetic analog, N-Ac-(Tyr)-thymosin α_1 was radioiodinated by using Na ^{125}I and soluble lactoperoxidase. A calibration curve was generated for highly purified synthetic α_1 standard which had a minimal detectable dose of 30-50 pg and an ED_{50} (50% response) of 150-400 pg. Using the RIA, we have found a high immunological cross reactivity of thymosin α_1 in the thymus extracts of all species examined, including humans, cattle, sheep, pig, rat, mouse, and guinea pig. In humans, thymosin α_1 concentrations are

Table 3 Effect of Thymosin Polypeptides in the Macrophage Migration Inhibition (MMI) Assay[a]

Preparation tested	Concentration (nmol/ml)	Specific MMI response to PPD (% inhibition)	Nonspecific migration inhibition (%)
Synthetic thymosin α_1	5×10^{-1}	36	None[b]
Natural thymosin β_4	5×10^{-1}	None	35
	5×10^{-2}	None	32
	5×10^{-3}	None	23
	5×10^{-4}	None	23
	5×10^{-5}	None	20
	5×10^{-6}	None	18
Synthetic thymosin β_4	5×10^{-1}	None	45
	5×10^{-2}	None	34
	5×10^{-3}	None	32
	5×10^{-4}	None	25
	5×10^{-5}	None	33
	5×10^{-6}	None	26

[a]See Thurman et al., 1981 (72) for details of the assay.
[b]Less than 15% inhibition.

highest in the fetal circulation (2-4 ng/ml) and decline significantly with age (39). In mice, thymosin α_1 levels appear to be maximal between 10 and 18 days of age and also decrease significantly with age. These studies reflect the capacity of the thymus to regulate immune balance.

Development of radioimmunoassay for thymosin β_4 and thymosin α_7 is now in progress in our laboratory, using the antisera prepared against synthetic thymosin β_4 and partially purified thymosin α_7.

V. LOCALIZATION OF THYMOSIN IN THYMIC EPITHELIAL CELLS

Immunohistochemical studies by Kater et al. (102) and van den Tweel et al. (103), using antithymosin fraction 6 (a partially purified thymosin fraction containing mostly acidic peptides in F5) antiserum on tissue cultures, have shown localization of thymosin in thymic epithelial cells. Furthermore, using the antisera to synthetic thymosin α_1 and natural thymosin β_4, the site of synthesis of thymosin has been studied by Hirokawa et al. (104) in the thymus glands of human individuals ranging in age from newborn to 62 years old. An indirect fluorescent antibody technique was employed in these studies. The sections were first incubated with antithymosin antiserum followed by incubation with fluorescein-isothiocyanate-labeled goat antirabbit gamma globulin. Thymosin α_1 was detected specifically in thymic epithelial cells of the medulla and in cells covering the cortical surface. Hirokawa et al. (104) have found that the number of thymosin-α_1-positive medullary epithelial cells decreased progressively with age beginning at around 13 years. On the other hand, thymosins β_3 and β_4 were detected almost exclusively in cells covering the subcapsular cortex. These findings are compatible with the known biological activity of thymosins α_1 and β_3, β_4 in the induction and suppression of TdT (66,78), and further demonstrates the role of thymosin in T-cell differentiation. It appears that the TdT-negative prothymocytes may migrate to the thymic cortex and become high TdT-containing cortical thymocytes under the influence of thymosins β_3 and β_4. It is possible that some of these thymocytes then move to the thymic medulla and become TdT-negative, more mature thymocytes under the influence of thymosin α_1.

Most recently, Haynes et al. (personal communication) have found that thymosin-α_7 antiserum localizes specifically on the epithelial cells of the medulla that comprise the Hassall's corpuscles.

VI. THERAPEUTIC APPLICATIONS OF THYMOSIN

Most clinical studies on thymosin have been performed with bovine thymosin F5. More recently, some trials have been initiated with synthetic thymosin α_1. The patients who have been treated with thymosin include immunodeficiency and autoimmune diseases, as well as cancer. The clinical trials of thymosin have been summarized by Low and Goldstein (105). Some of these trials are briefly described below.

A. Immunodeficiency Patients

Over 100 children have received thymosin F5 for a variety of primary immunodeficiency diseases (29-32,106). These patients have been treated with injections of thymosin up to 400 mg/m^2 for periods over 6 years (usually daily for 2-4 weeks, then once per week maintained injections). Most of the patients have received 60 mg/m^2 thymosin by subcutaneous injection. There has been no evidence of serious toxicity due to thymosin administration. A close correlation was found between the number of patients whose cells responded in vitro in the E-rosette assay and those patients who have also responded in vivo with increased absolute T-cell numbers and clinical improvement. In recent studies, Barrett et al. (106) and Wara et al. (31) have found that a good correlation between changes in mixed lymphocyte culture (MLC) reactivity with thymosin can be used as an indicator of the in vivo efficacy of thymosin to enhance T-cell function.

B. Autoimmune Disorders

To date, six patients with autoimmune diseases have been treated with thymosin F5 for periods ranging from 4 to 16 months using phase I protocols (107). Five of the patients had systemic lupus erythematosus (SLE) and the sixth rheumatoid arthritis (RA). While receiving thymosin, significant elevation in T-cell percentage and decrease in null cell percentage were noted. There was also a major decrease in a cytotoxic serum factor that causes the lysis of murine thymocytes in the presence of complement and is present in many patients with autoimmune diseases.

Although the possible mechanism of immune reconstitution with thymosin fraction 5 in patients with SLE is not as yet defined, it may be related to induction of a subpopulation of thymosin-activated suppressor or regulator T cells. Such a population of cells can be induced in vitro by incubation of periphenol blood lymphocytes (PBL) from SLE patients with thymosin or cultured thymic epithelium (108). Based upon a lack of toxicity and positive immunological responses, phase II randomized trials in SLE and RA have been initiated to establish efficacies.

C. Phase I and Phase II Cancer Trials

More than 200 cancer patients have been treated according to phase I or phase II protocols. No major side effects have been seen in the majority of patients treated with thymosin F5.

Phase I cancer trails of thymosin were first initiated in 1974 at the University of Texas Medical Branch in Galveston. Greater than 75% of the phase I cancer patients who responded to thymosin in vitro have shown increased numbers of T cells following thymosin treatment (33-35,109). Furthermore, the first efficacy trial of thymosin has now been completed in patients with nonresectable small cell carcinoma of the lungs by Chretien and M. Cohen and their associates (36-38). In this trial, thymosin F5 was found to significantly prolong the survival of cancer patients when given in conjunction with intensive chemotherapy. Thymosin effects in cancer patients might be due to an increase in mature T cells, which would enhance endogenous antitumor activity. In addition, thymosin may function in immunosuppressed cancer patients to increase T-cell reactivity and thus help in reducing the high incidence of infection that often accompanies treatment with radiotherapy and chemotherapy.

Most recently, the National Cancer Institute (NCI) has initiated a number of phase I and phase II clinical trials with thymosin F5 and α_1 as part of their new Biological Response Modifier Program (BRMP). A list of these trials and the regimens being studied are shown in Table 4.

VII. OTHER THYMIC FACTORS

In addition to the thymosins, a number of factors with thymic hormonelike activity have been isolated from thymus tissue, blood, and thymic epithelial cell cultures. These

Table 4 NCI Biological Response Modifier Program (BRMP) Thymosin Trials

Individual/institution	Treatment	Study design	Dosage (s)	Duration of treatment
R. Schulof/George Washington University Medical Center	Thymosin α_1	1. 2 X week dosing	900 $\mu g/m^2$	2 doses/week for 52 weeks
		2. Intensive load dose	900 $\mu g/m^2$	14 daily doses + 2 doses/week for 50 weeks
		3. Control	Placebo	14 daily doses + 2 doses/week for 50 weeks
C. Pinsky/Memorial Sloan–Kettering Cancer Center	Thymosin F5	Escalating doses X 10	0.6 mg/m^2, 6 mg/m^2 60 mg/m^2, 600 mg/m^2	Single dose, 1-week rest, 3 doses/week for 2 weeks
W. Wara/ U.C. San Francisco	Thymosin F5	Escalating 30-mg/m^2 doses	60 mg/m^2, 90 mg/m^2 120 mg/m^2, 150 mg/m^2 180 mg/m^2, 210 mg/m^2	Daily X 15 days
R. O. Dillman/ U.C. San Diego	Thymosin F5	Escalating doses (100%)	60 mg/m^2, 120 mg/m^2 240 mg/m^2, 480 mg/m^2 960 mg/m^2, 1920 mg/m^2	Single dose
	Thymosin α_1	Escalating doses (100%)	600 $\mu g/m^2$, 1.2 mg/m^2 2.4 mg/m^2, 4.8 mg/m^2	Single dose
	Thymosin α_1		9.6 mg/m^2, 1.2 mg/m^2	3 X week/2 weeks
A. Fefer and R. Goldberg/ Fred Hutchinson Cancer Research Center	Thymosin F5	Escalating doses (100%)	60 mg/m^2, 120 mg/m^2 240 mg/m^2, 480 mg/m^2 960 mg/m^2	Daily X 7, 3-weeks rest [patients exhibiting no progression or toxicity will receive the next dose daily (7 days, etc.)]
	Thymosin α_1	Escalating doses (100%)	600 $\mu g/m^2$, 1.2 mg/m^2 2.4 mg/m^2, 4.8 mg/m 9.6 mg/m^2, 19.2 mg/m^2 38.4 mg/m^2	Same as above

preparations are in various stages of characterization. Table 5 summarizes their reported chemical and biological properties. Some of the better characterized preparations will be described in some detail below.

A. From Thymus Tissue

1. Thymopoietin

Thymopoietin was first isolated from bovine thymus by Goldstein (43,110) and was initially named thymin. The bioassay used to isolate thymopoietin was the detection of delayed neuromuscular impairment in mice following the injecton of thymic extracts or purified polypeptides. This assay was derived from basic experimental studies related to myasthenia gravis. This disease is characterized by a deficit in neuromuscular transmission and thymic malfunction.

The purification procedures include homogenization, ultrafiltration on Amicon H10 X 100 and Diaflo UM2, a heat step (70°C), gel-filtration on Sephadex G-75 and G-50, and ion-exchange chromatography on QAE-Sephadex. Two related peptides, thymopoietins I (TP-I) and II (TP-II), were isolated by this procedure. They were immunologically cross-reactive and had indistinguishable biological activities. The complete amino acid sequence of TP-II was determined (44). Most recently, a revised sequence of TP-II along with the sequences of TP-I and TP-III were reported (111). TP-III was isolated from bovine spleen with similar procedures. The sequence of TP-II is shown in Fig. 5. TP-I and TP-II differed by only three amino acid residues at positions 1 (Gly), 2 (Gln), and 43 (His). Likewise, TP-III and II are mostly identical except for amino acid substitutions at position 34, Asp (TP-II) versus Glu (TP-III), and position 43, Ser (TP-II) versus His (TP-III). Although TP-I and TP-II have indistinguishable biological activities in induction of early T-cell differentiation and modulation of mature lymphcoytes (112-114), no biological study has been reported for TP-III. There is precedent for the isolation of identical or closely related polypeptides at different anatomical sites, such as cholecystokinin (115) and enkephalin and endorphins (116). However, the functional significance of these variations is not clear.

Chemical synthesis of a tridecapeptides of thymopoietin (see Fig. 5, residues 29-41) has been reported (117). This molecule was found to have 3% activity in comparison with thymopoietin in inducing T-cell differentiation. The synthesis of the entire molecule of TP-II was reported (118) by Fujino and co-workers using a conventional liquid phase coupling method. The synthetic material was found to induce Thy 1 on prothymocytes. Bliznakov et al. (119) also reported the total synthesis of thymopoietin by solid phase methodology on a Beckman 990 peptide synthesizer.

2. Thymic Humoral Factor (THF)

Trainin and his colleagues at the Weizmann Institute of Science in Israel have prepared cell-free thymic extracts that conferred immune competence to spleen cells from neonatally thymectomized mice (120,121). The preparation was named thymic humoral factor (THF). The initial bioassay was an in vitro model of the graft versus host reaction. The method used for the isolation of THF involved prolonged dialysis of crude bovine thymic homogenates against cold distilled water. More recently, THF has been purified to homogeneity judging by isoelectric focusing on polyacrylamide gels. The procedure involves successive chromatographic steps on Sephadex G-10 and G-25 and DEAE-Sephadex A-25.

Table 5 Thymic Preparations and Their Biological Effects

Thymic preparations	Principal investigators	Chemical properties	Biological effects
From thymus tissue			
Thymosin fraction 5	Hooper, A. Goldstein, et al.	Family of heat-stable, acidic polypeptides, mol wt 1000-15,000	Induces T-cell differentiation and enhances immunological function in animal models and in humans
Thymosin α_1	Low, A. Goldstein et al.	Polypeptide of 28 residues, mol wt 3108, pI 4.2, sequence determined	Increases mitogenic responsiveness of murine lymphocytes; induces enhancement of MIF and interferon production, increases Thy 1.2 and Lyt 1,2,3 positive cells and helper T cells; modulates TdT activity
Thymosin β_4	Low, A. Goldstein et al.	Polypeptide of 43 residues, mol wt 4963, pI 5.1, sequence determined	Induces TdT in vivo and in vitro in bone marrow cells from normal and athymic mice; in vivo induction of TdT in thymocytes of immunosuppressed mice; increase in LRF and LH secretion
Thomosin α_7	Low, A. Goldstein et al.	Acidic polypeptide, mol wt 2500 pI $\sim$3.5	In vitro enhancement of suppressor T-cell expression of Lyt 1,2,3 positive cells; in vivo suppression of interferon production
Thymic humoral factor (THF)	Trainin et al.	Polypeptide of mol wt 3200, pI 5.7, amino acid composition determined	Restoration of ability of spleen cells from neonatally thymectomized donors to induce an in vivo graft vs. host reaction; enhancement of ability of normal spleen cells to respond to PHA and ConA
Thymopoietin	G. Goldstein et al.	Polypeptide of 49 residues, mol wt. 5562, pI 5.5, sequence determined	Causes delayed impairment of neuromuscular transmission in vivo; induces bone marrow cells to develop intrathymic lymphocytes
Thymic polypeptide preparation (TP)	Milcu, Potop et al.	Mixture of polypeptides and amino acids	Elevation of serum calcium concentration and decrease in serum inorganic phosphate; stimulation of antibody synthesis in immunized, x-ray-irradiated rabbits
Thymosterin	Potop et al.	Lipids or lipoproteins, one purified component termed IIB_3 is C_{28} steroid with methyl groups at C-21 and C-28	Antiproliferative action on KB tumor cells in culture; repairs the specifically altered metabolism of normal or thymectomized tumor-bearing animals
Thymic factor X (TFX)	Aleksandrowicz, Skotnicki, et al.	Polypeptide, mol wt 4200, amino acid composition reported	In vitro restoration of the azathioprine sensitivity of spleen rosette-forming cells from adult thymectomized mice; in vivo increase in blood T-cell number and return of delayed hypersensitivity
Thymostimulin (TS)	Falchetti et al.	Mixture of polypeptides	Induced markers and specific functions of lymphocytes both in immunosuppressed animals and in immunodeficient patients; stimulated interferon production in mice following challenge with Poly I:Poly C

Procine thymic hormone (PTH)	Jin et al.	Mixture of polypeptides, mol wt 9000-68,000, pI 5.0-7.5	Increased rosette formation in fetal thymocytes
Bovine thymic preparation	Liu et al.	Mixture of polypeptides	Increased rosette formation in umbilical cord blood lymphocytes
Homeostatic thymic hormone (HTH)	Comsa et al.	Glycopeptide, mol wt 1800-2500	Suppression of deleterious consequences of thymectomy in young guinea pigs; restoration of delayed hypersensitivity of thymectomized rats
Lymphocytopoietic factors (LSH_h and LSH_r)	Luckey et al.	Polypeptides, mol wt 80,000 (LSH_r) and 15,000 (LSH_h); amino acid composition of LSH_r is available	Enhances antibody production to sheep erythrocytes and induces a lymphocytosis
Hypocalcemic and lymphocytopoietic substances (TP_1 and TP_2	Mizutani et al.	Polypeptides	Enhances production of antibody to sheep erythrocytes in neonatal mice; hypocalcemic activity in normal rabbits
From blood			
Thymulin (FTS-Zn)	Bach, Dardenne et al.	Nonapeptide, mol wt 857, pI 7.5, sequence determined	Enhancement of the generation of effector cytotoxic T cells both in vitro and in vivo; inhibition of contact sensitivity in normal mice
Protein fraction from human plasma	White et al.	Protein, mol wt $\bar{5}7,700$, properties analogous to prealbumin	Enhances ability of neonatally thymectomized mice to reject an allogeneic skin graft, enhances MLR of mouse spleen cells incubated with the blood fraction
Human serum factor (SF)	Astaldi et al.	Adenosine (possibly other small molecular weight components)	Increases the intracellular cyclic AMP level of human and mouse thymocytes; increases the population of hydrocortisone-resistant cells
From thymic epithelial supernatants			
Thymic epithelial supernatant (TES)	Kruisbeek et al.	Crude extract, chemical nature not characterized	Augments the proliferative responses of rat thymocytes to PHA or ConA; stimulates mixed lymphocytes reactivity and antibody production to sheep erythrocytes by spleen cells from nude mice
Human thymic epithelial medium (HTEM)	Kater et al.	Crude extract, chemical nature not clear	Augments the mitogen responsiveness of thymocytes

The molecule was determined to be a heat-stable polypeptide with a pI of 5.7-5.9 and a molecular weight of around 3000 (45). It has been reported (122) that this molecule is composed of 31 amino acid residues. However, its primary structure has not been delineated.

THF was shown to increase the cytotoxic reactivity of lymphoid cells against syngeneic tumors in vitro and in vivo (123,124). It was also shown to restore cellular graft versus host (GvH) reactivity and the ability of spleen cells from neonatal thymectomized mice to produce a primary immune response to sheep red blood cells (122,125,126).

3. Porcine Thymic Hormone (PTH)

The isolation of porcine thymic hormone was first reported by Jin et al. (127) using a similar purification procedure as thymosin F5 with some modifications. The preparation was shown to increase rosette formation in fetal thymocytes. Recently, two polypeptides, T_1 and E_1, were further purified from porcine thymic hormone preparation by ion-exchange chromatography on CM-cellulose and preparative isoelectric focusing (128). T_1 has a molecular weight of 13,000 with an isoelectric point of 4.6. The molecular weight of E_1 is around 68,000 with pI of 5.2. Both peptides are highly active in the rosette assay. From the amino acid composition, it appears that these two peptides differ from all the thymic hormones reported. PTH has been widely used in clinical trials in China (127) on patients with autoimmune disorders, virus hepatitis, leprosy, and other diseases. Preliminary results indicate that PTH is effective in treating various autoimmune disorders, including Sjögren syndrome, SLE, and rheumatoid arthritis. Encouraging results were also obtained for the treatment of severe-type virus hepatitis, chronic hepatitis, and lepromatous leprosy.

B. From Blood

1. Thymulin (FTS-ZN)

Using the azathioprine-rosette assay, Bach and his colleagues (46) isolated an active factor from pig serum which they termed FTS. The purification included ultrafiltration, gel filtration on Sephadex G-25, and ion-exchange chromatography on CM-cellulose. The active factor, FTS, has a molecular weight of 847 and an isoelectric point of 7.5 (129,130). FTS has been characterized as a nonapeptide (129). The amino acid sequence of this molecule is shown in Fig. 5.

Recently, it has been reported (131) that FTS requires zinc for its biological activity. They have renamed the active form of FTS thymulin (FTS-Zn). It was shown (131) that FTS lost its biological activity in a rosette assay (100) after treatment with a metal ion-chelating agent. The activity was restored by the addition of zinc salts.

FTS has been shown to enhance mitogen response in cells of nude mice in vitro (132), to induce suppressor T cells in NZB mice (133), and to normalize the abnormally high level of autologous erythrocyte-binding cells in adult thymectomized mice (134).

FTS was chemically synthesized using solid phase techniques (135). Bliznakov et al. (136) also reported the synthesis of FTS and a dodecapeptide analog of FTS (Val-Lys-Arg-Gln-Ala-Lys-Ser-Gln-Gly-Gly-Ser-Asn-Asn) on a Beckman 990 peptide synthesizer. Both synthetic peptides were found to reverse the marked suppression of the primary humoral hemolysin immune response in old mice.

2. Porcine Fraction from Human Plasma

Burton and his colleagues (137) isolated an active component from human plasma that stimulated azathioprine-sensitive rosettes. Purification included ammonium sulfate fractionation, gel filtration on Sephadex G-150, and preparative gel electrophoresis. The amino acid composition, amino terminal end group analysis, and subunit structure of the final purified product were identical with authentic prealbumin (137). No chemical relationship of prealbumin to FTS is apparent.

VIII. PERSPECTIVES

Our basic research on the chemical characterization of thymosin has demonstrated that thymosin F5 is a mixture of many components. Furthermore, our biological studies have indicated that individual active polypeptides in F5 are acting on different subpopulations of T cells in the maturation sequence. As shown in Fig. 11, thymosin α_1 appears to act at both early and late stages of thymocyte maturation. Thymosin α_7 converts immature T cells to cells with suppressor function. Thymosins β_3 and β_4 appear to act at very early stages of the maturation sequence on TdT-negative bone marrow stem cells to form TdT-positive prothymocytes. From the various thymic preparations discussed in this chapter, it is evident that a great multiplicity of apparently unique thymic factors exist which are capable of promoting thymic-dependent immune responses. Although the precise relationships among the various hormonal-like factors are still not defined, a number of generalizations can be made regarding their biological properties:

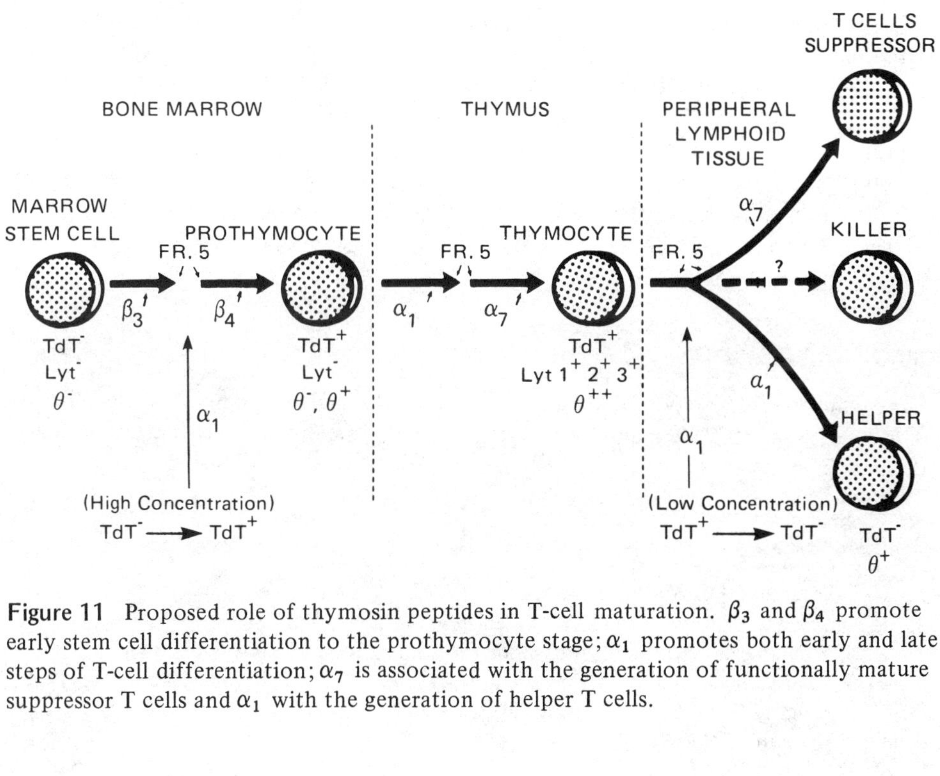

Figure 11 Proposed role of thymosin peptides in T-cell maturation. β_3 and β_4 promote early stem cell differentiation to the prothymocyte stage; α_1 promotes both early and late steps of T-cell differentiation; α_7 is associated with the generation of functionally mature suppressor T cells and α_1 with the generation of helper T cells.

1. In a murine system, thymic factors can induce the appearance of T-cell surface antigens (e.g., Thy, Ly 1,2,3) from precursor cells in vitro.
2. Thymic factors tend to induce the proportions and absolute numbers of human E-rosette-forming cells in vitro. The magnitude of the effect correlates inversely with initial T-cell levels.
3. Thymic factors can affect the expression of TdT on precursor T cells.
4. Thymic preparations exhibit a wide range of immune restorative properties in vivo.

The most important contribution of thymic hormone research resides in its application to the clinical management of thymus-dependent diseases. Our ongoing clinical trials of thymosin have suggested that thymosin has a major role in restoring immune responsiveness and augmenting specific lymphocyte activities in children with hypothymic function and in patients with secondary T-cell deficiencies resulting from a variety of disorders, including cancer and autoimmune disease.

Most of the clinical trials with thymosin have been carried out using thymosin F5. The complete elucidation of the structure of thymosin α_1, thymosin β_4, and other thymic factors and successful chemical synthesis of these molecules renders the clinical trials of purified thymic polypeptide hormones feasible.

In anergic cancer patients, thymosin or other thymic hormones may be of importance as an adjunct to conventional treatments by increasing T-cell function in response not only to tumor cells, but also to pathogens, thus reducing the high incidence of infection that often accompanies cancer treatment.

With an increasing number of clinical trials using thymosin or other thymic preparations, it will help to establish the optimal conditions for employing thymic hormones as a therapeutic modality in the treatment of cancer and other diseases associated with immune deficiency.

Furthermore, our studies on the interrelationships of thymus and the central nervous system (138,139), as well as the reproductive system (79,80), will provide possible new approaches for treatment of many endocrine disorders with thymic peptides. The acquisition of a full understanding of the biological function of thymosin peptides will make possible the treatment of different diseases with different components or a combination of them. This approach should prove to be extremely useful in the area of immunotherapy and immunopharmacology.

ACKNOWLEDGMENTS

The thymosin studies reported herein were supported in part by grants from the NIH (CA24974 and AI17710) grants and/or gifts from Hoffmann-LaRoche, Inc. and Alpha 1 Biomedics, Inc.

REFERENCES

1. V. Eskelund and C. M. Plum, *Acta Endocrinol.*, *12*:171 (1953).
2. H. Schwartz, M. Price, and C. A. O'Dell, *Metabolism, 2*:261 (1953).
3. L. G. Rowntree, J. H. Clark, and A. M. Hanson, *JAMA*, *103*:1425 (1934).
4. C. Bomskov and L. Sladovic, *Dtsch. Med. Wochenschr.*, *66*:589 (1940).
5. H. G. Goslar, *Exp. Pathol. Pharmakol.*, *233*:201 (1958).
6. W. W. Nowinski, *Biochem. Z.*, *226*:415 (1930).
7. W. W. Nowinski, *Biochem. Z.*, *259*:182 (1933).
8. J. Comsa, *C. R. Soc. Biol.*, *133*:24 (1940).

9. J. Comsa, *Am. J. Med. Sci.*, *250*:79 (1955).
10. J. Comsa, *Ann. Endocrinol.*, *17*:777 (1956).
11. J. F. A. P. Miller, *Lancet*, *2*:748 (1961).
12. R. A. Good, A. P. Dalmasso, C. Martinez, O. K. Archer, J. C. Pierce, and B. W. Papermaster, *J. Exp. Med.*, *116*:773 (1962).
13. J. D. Sherman, M. M. Adner, and W. Dameshek, *Blood*, *23*:375 (1964).
14. D. Osoba and J. F. A. P. Miller, *J. Exp. Med.*, *119*:177 (1964).
15. A. C. Aisenberg and B. Wilkes, *Nature*, *205*:716 (1965).
16. R. T. Schaller and J. K. Stevenson, *Proc. Soc. Exp. Biol. Med.*, *124*:199 (1967).
17. R. H. Levey, N. Trainin, and L. W. Law, *J. Natl. Cancer Inst.*, *31*:199 (1963).
18. R. H. Levey, N. Trainin, L. W. Law, P. H. Black, and W. P. Rowe, *Science*, *142*:483 (1963).
19. S. Roberts and A. White, *J. Biol. Chem.*, *178*:151 (1949).
20. D. Metcalf, *Br. J. Cancer*, *10*:442 (1956).
21. P. DeSomer, P. Denys, and R. Leyten, *Life Sci.*, *2*:810 (1963).
22. J. J. Klein, A. L. Goldstein, and A. White, *Proc. Natl. Acad. Sci. USA*, *53*:812 (1965).
23. J. J. Klein, A. L. Goldstein, and A. White, *Ann. N.Y. Acad. Sci.*, *135*:485 (1966).
24. W. L. Duckworth, in *Galen on Anatomical Procedures, The Later Books* (M. C. Lyons and B. Towers, eds.), Cambridge Univ. Press, London and New York, 1962.
25. J. A. Hooper, M. C. McDaniel, G. B. Thurman, G. H. Cohen, R. S. Schulof, and A. L. Goldstein, *Ann. N.Y. Acad. Sci.*, *249*:125 (1975).
26. G. B. Thurman, A. Ahmed, D. M. Strong, M. E. Gershwin, A. D. Steinberg, and A. L. Goldstein, *Transplant. Proc.*, *7*:299 (1978).
27. M. J. Dauphinee, N. Talal, A. L. Goldstein, and A. White, *Proc. Natl. Acad. Sci. USA*, *71*:2637 (1974).
28. M. A. Hardy, M. Zisblatt, N. Levine, A. L. Goldstein, F. Lilly, and A. White, *Transplant. Proc.*, *3*:926 (1971).
29. D. Wara and A. J. Ammann, *Transplant. Proc.*, *10*:203 (1978).
30. D. W. Wara, A. L. Goldstein, A. L. Doyle, and A. J. Ammann, *N. Engl. J. Med.*, *292*:70 (1975).
31. D. W. Wara, D. J. Barret, A. J. Ammann, and M. J. Cowan, *Ann. N. Y. Acad. Sci.*, *332*:128 (1980).
32. A. L. Goldstein, D. W. Wara, A. J. Ammann, H. Sakai. N. S. Harris, G. B. Thurman, J. A. Hooper, G. H. Cohen, A. S. Goldman, A. S. Costanzi, and M. C. McDaniel, *Transplant. Proc.*, *7*:681 (1975).
33. L. A. Schafer, A. L. Goldstein, J. U. Gutterman, and E. M. Hersh, *Ann. N.Y.Acad. Sci.*, *277*:609 (1976).
34. L. A. Schafer, J. U. Gutterman, E. M. Hersh, G. M. Mavligit, K. Dandridge, G. H. Cohen, and A. L. Goldstein, *Cancer Immunol. Immunother.*, *1*:259 (1976).
35. L. A. Schafer, J. U. Gutterman, E. M. Hersh, G. M. Mavligit, and A. L. Goldstein, in *Progress in Cancer Research and Therapy* (M. A. Chirigos, ed.), Raven Press, New York, 1977.
36. D. S. Lipson, P. B. Chretien, R. Makuch, D. E. Kenady, and M. H. Cohen, *Cancer*, *43*:863 (1979).
37. P. B. Chretien, S. D. Lipson, R. Makuch, D. E. Kenady, M. H. Cohen, and J. D. Minna, *Cancer Treat. Rep.*, *62*:1787 (1978).
38. M. H. Cohen, P. B. Chretien, D. C. Ihle, B. E. Fossicek, R. Makuch, P. A. Bunn, A. V. Shackney, M. J. Matthews, S. O. Lipson, D. E. Kenady, and J. D. Minna, *JAMA*, *241*:1813 (1979).
39. J. E. McClure, N. Lameris, D. W. Wara, and A. L. Goldstein, *J. Immunol.*, *128*:368 (1982).
40. A. L. Goldstein, J. A. Hooper, R. S. Schulof, G. H. Cohen, G. B. Thurman, M. C. McDaniel, A. White, and M. Dardenne, *Fred. Proc.*, *33*:2053 (1974).

41. A. L. Goldstein, A. Asanuma, and A. White, *Recent Prog. Horm. Res.*, *26*:505 (1970).
42. A. L. Goldstein, T. L. K. Low, G. B. Thurman, M. M. Zate, N. Hall, J. Chen, S. Hu, P. Naylor, J. E. McClure, *Recent Prog. Horm. Res.*, *37*:369 (1981).
43. G. Goldstein, *Nature*, *247*:11 (1974).
44. D. H. Schlesinger and G. Goldstein, *Cell*, *5*:361 (1975).
45. A. I. Kook, Y. Yakir, and N. Trainin, *Cell Immunol.*, *19*:151
46. J. F. Bach, *Ann. Rev. Pharmacol. Toxicol.*, *17*:281 (1977).
47. T. L. K. Low, G. B. Thurman, C. Chincarini, J. E. McClure, G. D. Marshall, S. K. Hu, and A. L. Goldstein, *Ann. N.Y. Acad. Sci.*, *332*:33 (1979).
48. T. L. K. Low and A. L. Goldstein, in *The Year in Hematology*, (R. Silber, J. Lobuc, and A. S. Gordon, eds.), Plenum, New York, 1978.
49. A. M. Kruisbeck, G. C. B. Astaldi, M. J. Blankwater, L. A. Ziglstra, L. A. Leverb, and A. Astaldi, *Cell. Immunol.*, *35*:134 (1978).
50. L. Kater, R. Oosterom, J. E. McClure, and A. L. Goldstein, *Int. J. Immunopharmacol.*, *1*:273 (1979).
51. N. Trainin, *Physiol. Rev.*, *54*:272 (1974).
52. J. F. Bach and C. Carnaud, *Prog. Allergy*, *21*:418 (1976).
53. A. L. Goldstein, G. B. Thurman, T. L. K. Low, J. L. Rossio, and G. E. Trivers, *J. Reticuloendothel. Soc.*, *23*:253 (1978).
54. A. L. Goldstein, F. D. Slater, and A. White, *Proc. Natl. Acad. Sci. USA*, *56*:1010 (1966).
55. T. L. K. Low, G. B. Thurman, M. McAdoo, J. E. McClure, J. L. Rossio, P. H. Naylor, and A. L. Goldstein, *J. Biol. Chem.*, *254*:981 (1979).
56. T. L. K. Low and A. L. Goldstein, *J. Biol. Chem.*, *257*:1000 (1982).
57. M. Zisblatt, A. L. Goldstein, F. Lilly, and A. White, *Proc. Natl. Acad. Sci. USA*, *66*: 1170 (1970).
58. B. A. Khaw and A. H. Rule, *Br. J. Cancer*, *28*:288 (1973).
59. M. A. Scheinberg, A. L. Goldstein, and E. S. Cathcart, *J. Immunol.*, *116*:156 (1976).
60. A. Ahmed, D. M. Wong, G. B. Thurman, T. L. K. Low, A. L. Goldstein, S. J. Sharkis, and I. Goldschneider, *Ann. N.Y. Acad. Sci.*, *332*:81 (1979).
61. G. D. Marshall, G. B. Thurman, J. L. Rossio, and A. L. Goldstein, *J. Immunol.*, *1*:26 (1981).
62. M. P. Scheid, M. K. Hoffman, K. Komuro, H. Hammerling, E. A. Boyse, G. H. Cohen, J. A. Hooper, R. S. Schulof, and A. L. Goldstein, *J. Exp. Med.*, *138*:1027 (1973).
63. A. Ahmed, A. H. Smith, and K. W. Sell, in *Immune Modulation and Control of Neoplasia by Adjuvant Therapy* (M. A. Chirigos, ed.), Raven Press, New York, 1978.
64. A. Ahmed, A. H. Smith, D. M. Wong, G. B. Thurman, A. L. Goldstein, and K. W. Sell, *Cancer Treat. Rep.*, *62*:1739 (1978).
65. N. H. Pazmino, J. N. Ihle, and A. L. Goldstein, *J. Exp. Med.*, *147*:708 (1978).
66. S. K. Hu, T. L. K. Low, and A. L. Goldstein, *Mol. Cell. Biochem.*, *41*:49 (1981).
67. G. D'Agostaro, D. Frasca, M. Garavini, and G. Doria, *Cell. Immunol.*, *53*:207 (1980).
68. M. Bruley-Rosset, I. Florentin, N. Kiger, J. Schulz, M. Davigny, and G. Mathe, in *The Immune System, Functions and Therapy of Dysfunction* (H. Faraitre, ed.), Academic Press, New York, 1979.
69. M. P. Dabrowski and A. L. Goldstein, *Immunol. Commun.*, *5*:695 (1976).
70. T. L. K. Low and A. L. Goldstein, *J. Biol. Chem.*, *254*:987 (1979).
71. P. Y. Chou and G. D. Fasman, *Biochemistry*, *13*:211 (1974).
72. G. B. Thurman, T. L. K. Low, J. L. Rossio, and A. L. Goldstein, in *Lymphokines and Thymic Hormones: Their Potential Utilization in Cancer Therapeutics* (A. L. Goldstein and M. A. Chirigos, eds.), Raven Press, New York, 1981.
73. I. Goldschneider, A. Ahmed, F. J. Bollum, and A. L. Goldstein, *Proc. Natl. Acad. Sci. USA*, *78*:2469 (1981).

74. P. L. Osheroff, *Cell. Immunol.*, *60*:376 (1981).
75. M. M. Zatz, M. Glaser, C. M. Seals, and A. L. Goldstein, in *Lymphokines and Thymic Hormones: Their Potential Utllization in Cancer Therapeutics* (A. L. Goldstein and M. A. Chirigos, eds.), Raven Press, New York, 1981.
76. F. Bistoni, P. Marconi, L. Frati, E. Bonmassar, and E. Garaci, *Infect. Immun.*, *36*:609 (1982).
77. G. V. Vahouny, E. Kyeyne-Nyombi, J. McGillis, N. S. Tare, K. Y. Huang, R. Tombes, A. L. Goldstein, and N. R. Hall, *J. Immunol.*, *13*:791 (1983).
78. N. H. Pazmino, J. H. Ihle, R. N. McEwan, and A. L. Goldstein, *Cancer Treat. Rep.*, *62*:1749 (1978).
79. R. W. Rebar, A. Miyake, T. L. K. Low, and A. L. Goldstein, *Science*, *214*:669 (1981).
80. N. R. Hall, J. P. McGillis, B. Spangelo, E. Palazynski, T. Moody, and A. L. Goldstein, in *Current Concepts in Human Immunology and Cancer Immunomodulation* (B. Serrou, ed.), Elsevier Press, New York, 1982.
81. K. D. Wilkinson, M. K. Urban, and A. L. Haas, *J. Biol. Chem.*, *255*:7529 (1980).
82. D. H. Schlesinger, G. Goldstein, and H. D. Niall, *Biochem.*, *14*:2214 (1975).
83. E. Hannappel, S. Davoust, and B. L. Horecker, *Proc. Natl. Acad. Sci. USA*, *79*:1708 (1982).
84. S. K. Hu, *Ph.D. dissertation*, The Univ. of Texas Med. Branch, Galveston, 1980.
85. G. H. Cohen, J. A. Hooper, and A. L. Goldstein, *Ann. N.Y. Acad. Sci.*, *249*:145 (1975).
86. G. B. Thurman and A. L. Goldstein, in *The Biological Activity of Thymic Hormones* (D. W. van Bekkum, ed.), Kooyker Scientific Publ., Rotterdam, 1975.
87. T. L. K. Low, J. E. McClure, P. H. Naylor, B. L. Spangelo, and A. L. Goldstein, *J. Chromatogr.*, *266*:533 (1983).
88. E. Hannappel, S. Davoust, and B. L. Horecker, *Biochem. Biophys. Res. Commun.*, *104*:266 (1982).
89. M. Freire, E. Hannappel, M. Rey, J. M. Freire, H. Kido, and B. L. Horecker, *Proc. Natl. Acad. Sci. USA*, *78*:192 (1981).
90. S. S. Wang, I. D. Kulesha, and D. P. Winter, *J. Am. Chem. Soc.*, *101*:253 (1978).
91. C. Birr and U. Stollenwerk, *Angew. Chem.*, *91*:422 (1979).
92. T. Abiko, I. Onodera, and H. Sekino, *Chem. Pharm. Bull.*, *28*:3542 (1980).
93. K. Folkers, J. Leban, N. Sakura, G. Rampold, E. Lundanes, J. Dahmen, M. Lebek, J. Ohta, and C. Y. Bowers, in *Polypeptide Hormones* (R. F. Beers and E. G. Bassett, eds.), Raven Press, New York, 1980.
94. S. S. Wang, R. Makofske, A. Bach, and R. B. Merrifield, *Int. J. Pept. Protein Res.*, *15*:1 (1981).
95. T. W. Wong and R. B. Merrifield, *Biochem.*, *19*:3233 (1980).
96. R. Colombo, *J. Chem. Soc. Chem. Comm.*, *19*:1012 (1981).
97. R. Wetzel, H. L. Heyneker, D. V. Goeddel, P. Jhurani, J. Shapiro, R. Crea, T. L. K. Low, J. E. McClure, and A. L. Goldstein, *Biochemistry*, *19*:6096 (1980).
98. H. Kido, A. Vita, E. Hannappel, and B. L. Horecker, *Arch. Biochem. Biophys.*, *208*:95 (1981).
99. T. L. Ciardelli, G. S. Incefy, and C. Birr, *Biochemistry*, *21*:4233 (1982).
100. M. Dardenne and J. F. Bach, in *Biological Activity of Thymic Hormones* (D. W. van Bekkum, ed.), Kooyker Scientific Publ., Rotterdam, 1975.
101. S. S. Wang, T. L. K. Low, and A. L. Goldstein, *Biochemistry*, *22*:733 (1983).
102. L. Kater, R. Oosterom, J. E. McClure, and A. L. Goldstein, *Int. J. Immunopharmacol.*, *1*:273 (1979).
103. J. G. van den Tweel, C. R. Taylor, J. McClure, and A. L. Goldstein, *Adv. Exp. Med.* *114*:512 (1979).

104. K. Hirokawa, J. E. McClure, and A. L. Goldstein, *Thymus, 4*:19 (1982).
105. T. L. K. Low and A. L. Goldstein, in *Maturation Factors and Cancer* (M. A. S. Moore, ed.), Raven Press, New York, 1982.
106. D. J. Barrett, D. W. Wara, A. J. Ammann, and M. J. Cowan, *J. Pediatr., 97*:66 (1980).
107. M. T. Lavastida and J. C. Daniels, *Fed. Proc. Am. Soc. Exp. Biol., 37*:1669 (1978).
108. S. Horowitz, C. O. Borcherding, A. V. Moorthy, R. Chesney, H. Schulte-Wisserman, and R. Hong, *Science, 197*:4307 (1977).
109. A. L. Goldstein, G. B. Thurman, J. L. Rossio, and J. J. Costanzi, *Transplant. Proc., 9*:1141 (1977).
110. G. Goldstein, *Ann. N.Y. Acad. Sci., 249*:177 (1978).
111. T. Audhya, D. H. Schlesinger, and G. Goldstein, *Biochemistry, 20*:6195 (1981).
112. R. S. Basch and G. Goldstein, *Ann. N.Y. Acad. Sci., 249*:290 (1975).
113. M. P. Scheid, G. Goldstein, and E. A. Boyse, *J. Exp. Med., 147*:1727 (1978).
114. G. H. Sunshine, R. S. Basch, R. G. Coffey, K. W. Cohen, G. Goldstein, and J. W. Hadden, *J. Immunol., 120*:1594 (1978).
115. A. M. Buchan, J. M. Polak, E. Solcia, C. Capella, D. Hudson, and A. G. E. Pearse, *Gut, 19*:403 (1978).
116. J. M. Polak and S. R. Bloom, *Miles Int. Symp. Ser., 12*:371 (1980).
117. D. H. Schlesinger, G. Goldstein, M. P. Scheid, and E. A. Boyse, *Cell, 5*:367 (1975).
118. M. Fujino, W. Shinagawa, T. Fukuda, M. Takaoki, H. Kawaji, and Y. Sugino, *Chem. Pharm. Bull., 25*:1486 (1977).
119. E. G. Bliznakov, Y. Wan, D. Chang, and K. Folkers, *Biochem. Biophys. Res. Commun., 80*:631 (1978).
120. N. Trainin, A. Bergerano, M. Strahilevitch, D. Goldring, and M. Small, *Israel J. Med. Sci., 2*:549 (1966).
121. N. Trainin, M. Burger, and A. Kaye, *Biochem. Pharmacol., 16*:711 (1967).
122. N. Trainin, M. Small, D. Zipori, T. Umiel, A. I. Kook, and V. Rotter, in *Biological Activity of Thymic Hormones* (D. K. van Bekkum, ed.), Kooyker Scientific Publ., Rotterdam, 1975.
123. C. Carnaud, D. Ilfeld, I. Brook, and N. Trainin, *J. Exp. Med., 138*:1521 (1973).
124. N. Trainin, V. Rotter, Y. Yakir, R. Leve, Z. Handzel, B. Shohat, and R. Zaizov, *Ann. N.Y. Acad. Sci., 332*:9 (1979).
125. P. Lonai, B. Mogilner, V. Rotter, and N. Trainin, *Eur. J. Immunol., 3*:21 (1973).
126. N. Trainin, M. Small, and A. Globerson, *J. Exp. Med., 130*:765 (1969).
127. Y. Jin, X. Xu, J. Zhu, Y. Wang, A. Zhu, and H. Zhang, *J. Nanking Univ., 1*:115 (1979).
128. Y. Jin, X. Xu, and G. Tang, *Acta Biochim. Biophys. Sinica, 12*:133 (1980).
129. J. F. Bach, M. Dardenne, and J. M. Pleau, *Nature, 266*:55 (1977).
130. J. F. Bach, M. Dardenne, J. M. Pleau, and M. A. Bach, *Ann. N.Y. Acad. Sci., 246*:186 (1975).
131. M. Dardenne, J. *M*. Pleau, B. Nabarra, P. Lefrancier, M. Derrien, J. Choay, and J. F. Bach, *Proc. Natl. Acad. Sci. USA, 79*:5370 (1982).
132. M. A. Bach, C. Fournier, and J. F. Bach, *Ann. N.Y. Acad. Sci., 249*:316 (1975).
133. M. A. Bach, and P. Niaudet, *Immunology, 117*:760 (1976).
134. J. Charrier and J. F. Bach, *Proc. Natl. Acad. Sci. USA, 72*:3201 (1975).
135. R. B. Merrifield, *J. Am. Chem. Soc., 85*:2149 (1963).
136. E. G. Bliznakov, Y. Wan, D. Cahng, and K. Folkers, *Biochem. Biophys. Res. Commun., 80*:631 (1978).
137. P. Burton, S. Iden, K. Mitchell, and A. White, *Proc. Natl. Acad. Sci. USA, 75*:823 (1978).
138. N. R. Hall, in *Molecular and Behavioral Neuroendocrinology* (C. B. Nemeroff and A. J. Dunn, eds.), Spectrum, New York, 1981.
139. N. R. Hall and A. L. Goldstein, in *Psychoneuroimmunology* (R. Ader, ed.), Academic Press, New York, 1981.

9

Corynebacterium parvum and Its Fractions

Cecil S. Cummins Virginia Polytechnic Institute and State University, Blacksburg, Virginia

I. THE RETICULOSTIMULATORY ACTIVITY OF *CORYNEBACTERIUM PARVUM*

The organism commonly called *Corynebacterium parvum* is one of a fairly large number of biological agents which have been used in cancer therapy in the hope of enhancing the immunological reactivity of the host against his tumor. It is also one of the few mycobacterium bovis [Bacillis Calmette-Guérin (BCG) is another] where the idea of reticulostimulatory activity has become firmly associated with the name of a particular microorganism, and this may have given it an aura of mystery and specificity which it does not entirely deserve.

Investigations in this laboratory have been more concerned with the chemical nature of the reticulostimulatory material and its location in the bacterial cell than with details of the cellular and humoral responses in the experimental animal. The present article will reflect this bias, and it is not proposed to review in any detail the evidence for or against the involvement of any particular cell line in the process of reticulostimulation or tumor rejection.

The activities of *C. parvum* have been reviewed several times in recent years (100, 152) and have been the subject of at least one complete book (68). The basic facts about the antitumor and other activities of these vaccines are therefore not in doubt. In addition, many general aspects of immunomodulation by bacteria and bacterial products have been covered in recent reviews and reports of conferences (36,57,72), so it seems unnecessarily repetitious to cover the ground again. For the same reason, the clinical use of *C. parvum* vaccines has not been discussed, nor has (except incidentally) their relationship with BCG. Both of these subjects, if covered adequately, would require more space than is available. I have therefore concentrated on some aspects of the use of *C. parvum* vaccines (including the name) which seem to be less frequently discussed. For earlier work on the subject of *C. parvum* and other anaerobic coryneforms see the 1960 review by Prévot (115).

II. HISTORICAL BACKGROUND

The organism was first described by Mayer in 1926 as *Corynebacterium parvum infectiosum,* a small gram-positive anaerobic rod-shaped organism isolated from a chronic and ultimately fatal infection in a woman whose illness started after childbirth (98). Mayer also reported in the same paper the isolation of the same or a very similar organism from another 23 cases, mostly puerperal infections. No details of the range of properties of individual strains were given, and the original description of the organism was meager.

It appears that Prévot was the first to use the more correct binomial *Corynebacterium parvum.* He and his colleagues in a number of publications from 1948 onwards (115) described a group of strains of anaerobic *Corynebacteria* isolated from the blood or tissues of patients with diseases of the reticuloendothelial system. Heat-killed suspensions of some of these strains produced a striking degree of reticulostimulation in the rabbit, especially of the liver and spleen, and repeated injections led to the death of the animals. One of these strains, designated *C. parvum* 936 B, was found by Halpern et al. to be particularly active in inducing increased clearance of carbon particles from the blood of the mouse (69). The same strain was later used by Halpern et al. (70) to produce inhibition of tumor growth in mice.

Prévot and his colleagues at that time recognized 10 species of anaerobic coryneforms (115), and it was known that strains with a number of different specific names might show reticulostimulatory activity and that not all strains in a particular species were active. Thus, in the earlier literature strains labeled *C. granulosum, C. anaerobium,* or *C. acnes,* for example, have been described as active in addition to *C. parvum.* However, the firm association of the name *C. parvum* with the phenomenon of reticulostimulation is probably due to the use of such a strain by Halpern, whose early investigations quickened interest in the material as a possible antitumor agent. Another factor is undoubtedly the generosity of the Burroughs-Wellcome Company which over a considerable period has provided many investigators with suspensions of *C. parvum* CN 6134. It should be mentioned for the record, without I hope adding to the confusion, that this strain (CN 6134) was originally *C. anaerobium* 4685 from the Pasteur Institute (10).

III. TAXONOMY

All of these organisms were originally classified in the genus *Corynebacterium* because of their morphology, and they were collectively described as "anaerobic corynebacteria," "anaerobic diphtheroids," or "anaerobic coryneforms." In all, 12 named species were recognized by Prévot and Fredette, including *C. acnes* (116). However, these strains all differ in a number of important attributes from the classical *Corynebacteria* as exemplified by *Corynebacterium diphtheriae* (see Table 1). On the other hand, they have a number of characters in common with the *Propionibacteria*, especially the production of propionic acid as a major end product of metabolism (47,103). An examination of a large number of strains (79) showed that three broad groups could be recognized, now described as the three species *P. acnes, P. granulosum,* and *P. avidum* (26). These three species were originally defined on the basis of cell wall composition and DNA homology groupings, but can be distinguished by physiological tests (Table 2). In the course of

Table 1 Comparison of Anaerobic Coryneforms with Classic *Corynebacteria*

Characteristic	Anaerobic coryneforms	Classical *Corynebacteria*
Relation to oxygen	Microaerophilic to anaerobic	aerobic
Presence of mycolic acids	–	+++
DAP isomer in cell walls	LL– (occ. DL–)	DL–
Presence of arabinogalactan	–	+++
Characteristic fatty acids in cell lipids	C15 branched	C14, C16, C18

Source: Ref. 40.

these investigations 59 strains labeled *C. parvum* were examined, and 52 of them were found to be *P. acnes,* 3 were *P. granulosum,* and 3 *P. avidum.* The remaining strain was probably *Actinomyces naeslundii* (41). On the basis of these results, it was suggested that *C. parvum* be regarded as a synonym for *P. acnes.*

These points have been labored at some length for several reasons. First, it should be appreciated that *C. parvum* is not some strange organism with mystical properties, but, as *P. acnes,* is a predominant organism in the human skin flora. This may have important immunological implications for its use as a reticulostimulant in man, since most adolescents and adults have detectable antibody to it (160). Second, the organisms of the acne group do not have the arabinogalactan, peptidogylcolipids (Wax D), or the trehalose-dimycolate complexes which play an important part in the adjuvant properties of the classic *Corynebacteria* and especially the *Mycobacteria* such as *Mycobacterium bovis* (BCG).

As will be evident from the above introductory paragraphs, the taxonomy of these organisms has been the subject of some controversy. It is also evident that the name *C. parvum,* although representing an organism that is identical with *P. acnes,* is firmly entrenched in the immunological literature. In the present article the organisms will be referred to generally as *P. acnes, P. avidum,* and *P. granulosum,* or the acne group, but other names (including C. *parvum*) may be used if necessary in quoting published work.

It should be pointed out also that a number of strains originally described as *C. granulosum* appear to be *P. acnes,* so that *C. granulosum* is not necessarily equivalent to *P. granulosum* as defined here. A further complication is that at least one commercial *C. parvum* vaccine (that from the Institut Merieux, Lyon, France) is actually *P. avidum* (26,42).

Table 2 Physiological Tests to Separate *P. acnes, P. avidum,* and *P. granulosum*

Organism	Glucose	Sorbitol	Maltose	Sucrose	Esculin Hydrolysis	Indole Production	Gelatin Liquefaction	Nitrate Reduction
P. acnes I	+	+or–	–	–	–	+	+	+
P. acnes II	+	–	–	–	–	+	+	+
P. avidum I	+	–	+	+	+	–	+	–
P. avidum II	+	–	+	+	+	–	+	–
P. granulosum	+	–	+	+	–	–	–	–

Source: Ref. 40

IV. DISTRIBUTION OF RETICULOSTIMULATORY ACTIVITY AMONG DIFFERENT GROUPS OF BACTERIA

A. Acnes Group Strains

The association of reticulostimulatory activity with a strain of anaerobic coryneform identified as *C. parvum* led to a search for activity among other similar organisms, and it was soon found that not all strains were equally active—and indeed that some were virtually inactive. Moreover, it was found that strains which were originally highly active may lose their activity (199,125). It must be noted that activity in this context has generally meant ability to cause an increase in carbon particle clearance, or to produce hepatosplenomegaly.

Because of the different system of nomenclature used for strains reported in earlier work (*C. parvum, C. anaerobium, C. granulosum,* etc.), many of which are probably *P. acnes* (79), it is not always easy to compare these with later results. However, in terms of the three species *P. acnes, P. granulosum,* and *P. avidum,* it is very generally agreed that strains of *P. granulosum* are without activity as far as splenomegaly production or carbon clearance tests are concerned (10,42,84,94,111). The antitumor activity of *P. granulosum* strains is also usually reported to be low or nonexistent (85,94). However, antitumor activity may depend on the method of administration. Both McBride et al. (94) and Ko et. al. (85) gave vaccine intraperitoneally, while the tumor inoculum was given either subcutaneously or intravenously. We (Cummins et al., unpublished) have found that when vaccine is given intramuscularly together with the tumor inoculum, strains of *P. granulosum* can give excellent protection against a methylcholanthrene-induced fibrosarcoma in BALB/C mice (see Sec. IX.B).

In comparing strains of the other two species, *P. acnes* and *P. avidum,* it is evident from the tests reported on two large series of strains by Cummins et al. (44) and Ko et al. (85) that *P. acnes* is superior to *P. avidum* both in the proportion of strains giving good or excellent reticulostimulation and in the level of stimulation produced by active strains. For example, in the series published by Ko and his colleagues (85), 19 of 135 strains (approximately 1 strain in 7) of *P. acnes* gave a spleen weight/20 g body weight of over 400 mg while the highest spleen weight produced by any of 33 *P. avidum* strains tested was 337 mg. Similar results were obtained by Cummins and Linn (42). The reason for the considerable differences in activity found between different strains of *P. acnes* has not received much attention. In terms of splenomegaly production it was reported (42) that some *P. acnes* type II strains were more effective than type I strains, but this was by no means always the case. Early investigations by Prévot and Thouvenot (119a) indicated that lysogenic strains of anaerobic coryneforms were inactive (by carbon clearance tests). Assuming that most of the strains used were *P. acnes,* the observation is an interesting one, as it seems possible that such strains could undergo some autolysis in the later stages of growth (i.e., in postlog phase cultures). This partial autolysis could make them more susceptible to intracellular destruction by phagocytes. Other than lysogenicity, no cultural characters have been reported that will distinguish active from inactive strains. However, no large series of strains have yet been compared for antitumor activity.

The recognition that the acnes group of organisms had many similarities with the classic *Propionibacteria* from cheese has led to the testing of some of the latter for reticulostimulatory ability. For example, O'Neill et al. (111) tested one strain of each of *P. freudenreichii, P. arabinosum, P. jensenii,* and *P. rubrum,* and found none were able to cause a significant rise in phagocytic index (carbon clearance test). Similar results were obtained by McBride et al. (94) with a single strain of *P. freudenreichii*; they also found that the antitumor activity of the strain was very low.

B. Organisms in Other Groups

The name and reputation of *C. parvum* as a reticulostimulatory agent may be partly responsible for the fact that there has been relatively little systematic testing of the reticulostimulatory or antitumor activity of other gram-positive bacteria. However, the idea of using bacteria or their products as antitumor agents goes back to the days before Lister and Koch, when it was noted that the severe streptococcal infections prevalent in those preantiseptic days occasionally led to the resolution and total disappearance of extensive tumors [e.g., Busch (1868), quoted in 136]. One of the best documented series of attempts to treat human tumors with bacterial products is that of Coley (see Nauts et al., 105). Coley's "mixed toxins" were mixtures of uncertain composition prepared in various ways, but, broadly speaking, appear to have been a mixture of *Streptococcus pyogenes* and *Serratia marcescens* killed by gentle heat (70°C). The method of preparation suggests that endotoxin from *Serratia marcescens* was a major active component, augmented perhaps by cell wall components (peptidoglycan ?) from the *Streptococcus*. Some spectacular cures were recorded over the years between 1893 and 1936 (105), but the material does not seem to have been investigated systematically in experimental animals using inbred lines and modern immunocytological techniques. It may be noted in passing that one of the features of the clinical use of this material was an insistence on the value of repeated injections. Treatment frequently extended over 6 months and sometimes over 1-2 years.

In more recent years there have been several reports of the antitumor action of bacteria other than those of the acnes group. For example, *Lactobacilli* (81), *Bifidobacteria* (87), and *Streptococci* (136) have all been reported to have an antitumor effect. In some cases (*Bifidobacteria*) the bacterial suspension was given mixed with the tumor cell inoculum; in others (*Lactobacillus*) the tumor cells were given subcutaneously and the bacterial vaccine given IV or IP. Growth of a hepatocarcinoma in guinea pigs was stopped and the tumors regressed in animals given repeated intratumoral injections of killed suspensions of *E. coli*, *Streptococcus mutans*, *Listeria monocytogenes*, and *P. acnes* (25,97).

The above examples refer specifically to the antitumor activity of various bacterial strains. However, the original clues to the potential antitumor activities of *P. acnes* vaccines arose out of the demonstration that these vaccines were powerful reticulostimulatory agents, inducing increased phagocytic activity and considerable hepatosplenomegaly. In this respect, it seems that ability to cause marked splenomegaly is rare among gram-positive organisms. Out of 15 strains designated *Bifidobacterium*, *Actinobacterium*, *Propionibacterium*, *Catenabacterium*, and *Ramibacterium* examined by Breuillard et al. (22), only 3 (2 *Bifidobacterium* and 1 *Actinobacterium*) showed an increase in the size of liver and spleen which was apparently significant. In this laboratory (Bishop and Cummins, unpublished) we have examined 65 strains of gram-positive bacteria (other than *P. acnes*) for ability to produce hepatosplenomegaly. The only strains in the groups which produced a rise in the splenic index to 3 or over were four strains of *Bifidobacterium*. (Splenic index = spleen weight in test group/spleen weight in control group.) Heat-killed vaccines were given intraperitoneally at 1.4 mg/mouse and the spleen weight determined 14 days after injection. These results, coupled with those of Kohwi et al. (87) on the antitumor effect of strains of *Bifidobacterium*, seem to indicate that this group of organisms would repay further investigation.

Reticulostimulatory and antitumor activities are of course not confined to gram-positive bacteria, and several gram-negative bacteria such as *Bordetella pertussis* have been used as adjuvants (19,20). However, it is not proposed to discuss these here, or to consider the activities of extracted lipopolysaccharide (LPS, endotoxin) which also has powerful antitumor activity under certain conditions.

V. EFFECTS PRODUCED BY ADMINISTRATION OF *P. ACNES* VACCINES TO NORMAL ANIMALS

The convenient word "activity" has of necessity been used fairly frequently throughout this article, as it has in other reviews. However, a rather large number of different activities has been attributed to the administration of *P. acnes* vaccines in experimental animals, and some brief discussion of these will be necessary. A list of the principle effects so far described is given in Table 3, but the major ones can be grouped under three general headings.

1. Macrophage activation, increased particle clearance, and development of hepatosplenomegaly.
2. Modulation of both humoral and cellular aspects of the immune response
3. Effects on liver enzymes

To some extent (perhaps to a large extent) the separation of the various phenomena produced is artificial, because of the two-way interactions between the various cells of the reticuloendothelial system. The grouping is also partly historical, since in earlier work with

Table 3 Effects Produced by Administration of *P. acnes*

Effect	References
Increased clearance of carbon particles: hepatosplenomegaly	7,69,93,111
Increased resistance to bacterial, protozoal, or viral infections	32,37-39,52,59, 83,83a,164
Production of lymphocyte trapping	58
Stimulation of B-cell function: adjuvant activity	76
Induction of suppressor macrophages and suppressor T cells	82,90
Activation and induction of cytotoxicity in macrophages	62
Inhibition of T-cell functions such as PHA reactivity, mixed lymphocyte reaction, and GVH activity	139
Induction of NK cell activity	139
Fall in body weight, decrease in size of thymus, anemia, thrombocytopenia, fall in plasma iron, diminution in hematocrit value	23,31,92
Recovery of hemopoiesis in lethally irradiated mice	132
Increased production of interferon(s)	50
Production of prostaglandins	67
Activation of complement	94,156
Increased histamine sensitivity	5
Increased sensitivity to endotoxin (LPS)	54,64
Production of tumor necrosis factor	29
Increased sensitivity to anesthetics	51,104
Increased glucose-6-phosphate dehydrogenase in liver	64
Protection against artifically induced tumors	Numerous Refs., see review, Ref. 100

these vaccines activity was largely measured by increase in particle clearance and the development of hepatosplenomegaly.

A. Particle Clearance, Macrophage Activation, and Production of Hepatosplenomegaly

Increased clearance of foreign particles from the blood was the criterion largely used as a determinant of activity in earlier investigations. This was generally done by the determination of the phagocytic index (K values) based on the disappearance of carbon particles from the bloodstream after IV injection (69,93,111).

The maximum increase in the rate of carbon clearance is not found until at least the fourth day after vaccine injection (10), and the maximum increase in size of the liver and spleen is found at 2-3 weeks (30,31). There is also considerable stimulation of macrophage production in the bone marrow (16,33). The hepatosplenomegaly may therefore be due in part to local multiplication of macrophages in these organs and in part to recruitment of fresh macrophages from the bone marrow. This is perhaps related to the phenomenon of lymphocyte trapping (the sequestration of lymphocytes in lymphoid organs which is actively stimulated by *P. acnes*) (58).

Examination of sections of liver soon after IV injection of fluorescein-labeled vaccines gives the impression that very large numbers of bacteria have been taken up by Kupffer cells (142; Cummins and Bishop, unpublished). The high concentration of vaccine in the liver after systemic injection is confirmed by studies using organisms labeled with ^{99m}Tc or ^{3}H (14,135). However, the mechanisms by which a suspension of one bacterium (e.g., *P. acnes*) induces a six-or sevenfold degree of splenomegaly, while that of another (e.g., *P. granulosum*) fails to do so, remain almost totally obscure. It is also uncertain how these effects are related to the numerous rather dramatic effects on liver enzymes which are described below.

Techniques for separating Kupffer cells from other cellular elements of the liver are available (150,158), and a detailed examination of the fate of active and inactive vaccines in the liver should prove interesting.

B. Modulation of the Immune Response

As an adjuvant in the classic sense (i.e., increasing the antibody response to a given antigen), *P. acnes* vaccines have been reported to stimulate a moderately increased response to a number of thymus-dependent antigens such as sheep red blood cells (SRBCs) (30,31). In some cases, as with bovine serum albumin in rabbits, a substantial increase in secondary response was reported (113). On the other hand, a *P. acnes* vaccine was found to depress rather than increase the antitoxic response to tetanus toxoid (84).

It appears that in general these vaccines are not as efficient in stimulating antibody production as mycobacterial products, and the type of response is different (111,158,159). This is illustrated in Table 4 (158). Bomford (19,20) concluded that "*C. parvum* is a promising candidate adjuvant for promoting cell mediated immunity without recourse to water-in-oil emulsions," but the vaccine used was not found to be particularly active in promoting antibody production.

In terms of the effects of *P. acnes* on the cellular aspects of the immune response, a bewildering number of reactions of one kind or another have been described, involving virtually all kinds of reticuloendothelial cells (see Table 3). Since the present discussion is principally concerned with the nature of the active substance or substances in the bacteria which may produce effects in the host, I do not propose to review the cellular aspects in

Table 4 Comparison of the Immunological Actions of *Mycobacteria* and Anaerobic Coryneforms

Adjuvant effect	*Mycobacteria*	Anaerobic coryneforms
Antibody		
Precipitin	+++ (up to fivefold)	+ (two- and threefold)
Ig	2	1
CFT	+++ (over fivefold)	–
Cytophilic 2 at 3 weeks	+	–
α-glob at 7 days	+	–
Cell-mediated hypersensitivity		
Skin, guinea pig	+++	--
Cornea, guinea pig	+++	–
Granuloma	Large, with necrosis mixed macrophages, epitheloid and giant cells, lymphoid foci with germinal centers	Inconspicuous, no necrosis, macrophages
Macrocytostimulant effects		
Chemotaxis	No direct effect, indirect on neutrophilis and macrophages	Direct effect, specific for macrophage
Phagocytic index	+	+
Increase of acid hydrolases	+++	++ to ±

Source: Ref. 9.

detail here, especially since it has been done elsewhere (11,100). Cytotoxic and cytolytic activities are obviously of more importance in antitumor studies, and therefore the activation of macrophages, cytolytic T cells, and natural killer cells (NK cells) are of most interest. No doubt the recent demonstration that NK cells are active producers of highly reactive oxidant groups such as the superoxide radicle (13,129) will increase interest in their activities.

C. Effects on Liver Enzymes

Another group of effects which follows the systemic administration of *P. acnes* vaccines is concerned with hepatic microsomal enzyme activity. Decreased tolerance for anesthetics and prolonged barbiturate sleep time were found in mice and rats (51,95,104). Depression of O-demethylation, N-demethylation, p-hydroxylation, and ring hydroxylation were reported (71,95). Green and Dobrjansky (64) found that microsomes from livers of *C. parvum*-treated mice had significantly decreased cytochrome P450, aminopyrine demethylase, and lipid peroxidase. However, glucose-6-phosphate dehydrogenase activity in the livers of the treated mice was considerably increased (1500% of controls).

In addition, thrombocytopenia, decreased plasma fibrinogen, and anemia have been described in mice (102), and a marked fall in plasma iron coupled with anemia, reticulocytosis, and hepatosplenomegaly in rats (23). In the latter case the liver and spleen were shown to contain mononuclear cell infiltrates, granulomata, and giant cells. These effects on liver enzymes are associated with decreased drug-metabolizing activity in the liver, which may be responsible for the enhanced tumor inhibition found when vaccine is given together with cyclophosphamide (71).

The administration of *P. acnes* vaccines renders mice extremely sensitive to endotoxin [lipopolysaccharide (LPS)] (54,65; Cummins, unpublished). This is also mediated through effects of the vaccines on the liver and is associated with pronounced hypoglycemia and raised aspartate transaminase levels. According to Ferluga et al. (54) mononuclear cells recruited into the liver by the action of vaccine release soluble factors toxic for hepatocytes when exposed to LPS. These factors may be prostaglandins or free radicles liberated during prostaglandin synthesis, since inhibitors such as indomethacin considerably ameliorate the symptoms.

It is probable that the tumor necrosis factor (TNF), which is produced when LPS is given to animals already primed by *P. acnes* or other reticulostimulants, comes from activated macrophages in liver and spleen (29).

VI. NATURE OF THE RETICULOSTIMULATORY MATERIAL

A. Location in the Cell

The reticulostimulatory activity of *P. acnes* vaccines is obviously associated with some firmly bound component of the cell, since it is not removed by thorough washing of suspensions. It was suggested by Prévot et al. (118) that the cell wall was the location of the active material, and subsequent work by a number of investigators points clearly to the wall as the source of activity. For example, Riveros-Moreno and Niblock (126) stated that "the relevant stimulatory principle in *C. parvum* is of carbohydrate nature, and most probably present on the surface of the bacterium," and Adlam and his colleagues (7,9) concluded that either peptidogylcan or a peptidoglycan-polysaccharide complex was essential for activity, thus firmly locating material in the wall.

Further evidence that the bacterial wall is the site of active material comes from a consideration of the effect of antibiotics on the development of reticulostimulatory activity. Ability to cause splenomegaly does not normally develop until late in the logarithmic phase of bacterial growth and is shown best in the postlogarithmic phase (44). Cultures harvested at 12 and 24 hr (early and middle log phase with *P. acnes*) have little or no activity, whereas 48-hr (postlog phase) cultures are fully active. However, activity develops quickly if chloramphenicol is added to early log phase cultures (e.g., 16 hr) (121). Moreover, this early development of activity can be prevented if penicillin is added soon after chloramphenicol. Since cell wall synthesis is the only major activity of the cell not inhibited by chloramphenicol, but specifically inhibited by penicillin (130), these results point clearly to the wall as the site of active material.

B. Nature of the Active Material

If splenomegaly production is used as a measure of activity, the active material has the general properties shown in Table 5. This combination of properties suggests very strongly that the active material is polysaccharide in nature. Moreover, these properties might be regarded as further evidence that the site of the material is the bacterial wall, since it is difficult to imagine any location in the cell other than the wall for material which can resist extraction with phenol at 65°C or 10% sodium lauryl sulfate at 100°C.

The two major polysaccharide elements of the bacterial wall in gram-positive bacteria are *peptidoglycan* and *extractable polysaccharide*, and the main features of each are considered below.

Table 5 General Properties of Material in *P. acnes* Vaccines Which Produce Splenomegaly

Property	References
Resistant to:	
Heating at neutral pH	9,44
Heating in dilute alkali	44
Phenol extraction (45% phenol at 68°C)	9,28,44,126
Extraction with lipid solvents	9,28,44,126
Extraction with hot SLS (100°C)	44
Treatment with proteolytic enzymes	9,42,44
Treatment with nucleases	9
Sensitive to[a]:	
Periodate oxidation	28,44,126,127
Extraction with TCA at 56°C	44
Heating in dilute acid	44,126
Extraction with hot formamide (165-170°C)	Cummins, unpublished
Acetylation	44
Dilute HNO_2 at 0°C	44

[a]After these treatments the ability to induce splenomegaly is lost.

1. Peptidoglycan

The peptidoglycan is the principal structural element of the wall, consisting of a hexosamine backbone, cross-linked by peptide side chains which are attached to the lactic acid group of muramic acid.

The structure of peptidoglycan has been reviewed in numerous publications because of its interest as a substrate for bacteriolytic enzymes and as being the site of action of important antibiotics such as penicillin. A classic description of the variations to be found in peptidoglycan structure in different bacteria is given in a review by Schleifer and Kandler (138). Modern descriptions of peptidoglycan structure in all its aspects can be found in Rogers et al. (130), and in Tipper and Wright (150). The general structure of the peptidoglycans found in *P. acnes* and *Mycobacterium bovis* BCG is shown in Fig. 1. It should be appreciated that this is an idealized structure, and in practice not every peptide chain is cross-linked. The number of free amino groups in the chain is a measure of cross-linkage; in *propionibacteria*, for example, about 25% of peptide chains are not linked (137).

The peptidoglycan composition of *P. acnes* and other members of the acnes group (*P. granulosum* and *P. avidum*) consists of the usual hexosamine backbone of N-acetyl glucosamine and N-acetyl muramic acid, with a peptide side-chain of L-alanine, D-glutamic acid, LL-diaminopimelic acid, and D-alanine. Two possible structures have been suggested for this (Fig. 1, A and B), depending on whether or not glycine is regarded as taking part in the interpeptide linkage (8,137,80a;Kandler, personal communication). In a few strains of *P. acnes* and *P. avidum* the meso-isomer of DAP is found in place of the LL-isomer, and these strains lack glycine (8,79; Cummins, unpublished; Kandler, personal communication).

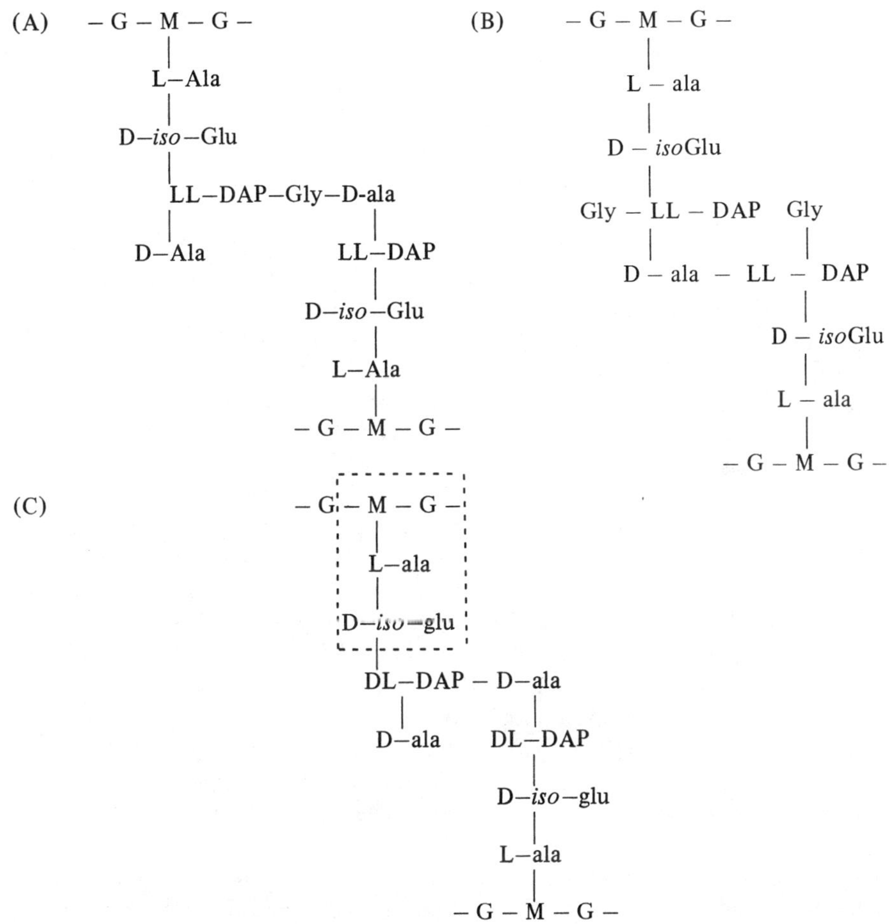

Figure 1 (A), (B) Alternative peptidogylcan structures in *P. acnes.* G = N-acetylglucosamine, M = N-acetylmuramic acid, LL-DAP = LL-diaminopimelic acid. (C) Peptidoglycan structure in *Mycobacterium bovis* BCG. Portion within the dotted line = Muramyldipeptide (MDP). DL-DAP = DL-diaminopimelic acid.

2. Extractable Polysaccharide

The kinds of polysaccharides found in the walls of gram positives are many and varied, and the variations cannot be detailed here. Almost all are extractable (without too much degradation) by such procedures as hot dilute acid (e.g., N/20 HCl or 1% acetic acid at 100°C), trichloroacetic acid at temperatures varying from 4 to 55°C, or hot neutral formamide at 165-170°C. Enzymic cleavage of the peptidoglycan can also be used to liberate the polysaccharides, if suitable enzymes can be found. The classic muralytic enzyme lysozyme, which attacks the hexosamine backbone of peptidoglycan, often cannot be used because it will lyse the walls of relatively few gram-positive bacteria. *P. acnes* and other members of the acnes group, for example, are resistant to lysozyme. However, a number of other enzymes are available which will attack peptidoglycan at various points in a number of organisms (62a).

In the case of *P. acnes* the extractable polysaccharide of the wall is composed of hexosamine and some combination of glucose, galactose, and mannose (7,40,79). The components vary depending upon the serological type; in *P. acnes* type I, the neutral sugars found are glucose, galactose, and mannose while in *P. acnes* type II the polysaccharides contain only glucose and mannose. In both types the hexosamines are glucosamine and galactosamine. The qualitative compositions of polysaccharides extracted from strains of *P. acnes*, *P. granulosum*, and *P. avidum* are given in Table 6. The detailed composition of these polysaccharides has yet to be established, and since they are acidic (Cummins, unpublished) other components, perhaps uronic acids, are almost certainly present; however, they contain little or no phosphate and are not teichoic acids. A rather different type of polysaccharide, containing galactose, glucose, fucose, hexosamines, sialic, and uronic acids, was described in *P. acnes* by Dawes et al. (45). This was found as a soluble antigen in 7-day cultures. Its relationship to the cell wall polysaccharides extracted by trichloroacetic acid is not clear. Acidic polysaccharides in culture supernates of *P. acnes* have also been described by Belsheim et al. (17).

The results of the tests outlined in Table 5 do not enable us to decide clearly whether the polysaccharide or the peptidoglycan part of the wall is primarily concerned with activity. In general terms, peptidoglycan is responsible for the integrity of the wall, and there is evidence that some quality of peptidoglycan is closely connected with the stimulatory ability of the vaccines. For example, activity of whatever kind (splenomegaly induction or antitumor activity, see Table 7) appears to require postlog phase bacteria (48-hr cells): log phase cells (12-18 hr in the case of *P. acnes*) have little or no activity in either case. Electron microscopy shows that while postlog phase bacteria persist apparently unchanged within macrophages for quite long periods, log phase cells quite soon show gross distortion and disorganization (Pringle and Cummins, 122). This suggests that the walls of log phase cells, unlike those of mature bacteria, are quite rapidly destroyed by lysosomal enzymes, perhaps because the peptidoglycan in log phase walls is not as fully cross-linked. The importance of the degree of cross-linkage (and hence, perhaps the ability to persist intracellularly) is underlined by the effects of chloramphenicol and penicillin on the development of activity in log phase cells noted above (Pringle and Cummins, 121). However, it must be remembered that an inefficiently assembled wall could be deficient in other respects (e.g., polysaccharide might not be tightly bound to the peptidoglycan backbone, and activities dependent on polysaccharide would therefore not be elicited). Since the cell wall is so obviously implicated in the reticulostimulatory activity,

Table 6 Sugars and Amino Sugars Present in Cell-Wall Polysaccharides of Acnes Group Organisms

	Components	
Organisms	Sugars	Amino sugars[a]
P. acnes type I	Glucose, galactose, mannose	Glucosamine, galactosamine
type II	Glucose, mannose	Galactosamine
P. avidum type I	Glucose, galactose, mannose	Galactosamine
Type II	Glucose, mannose	Galactosamine
P. granulosum	Galactose, mannose (trace glucose)	Galactosamine, trace glucosamine

[a]All strains also contain 2,3-diamino-2,3-dideoxygluconic acid (44a).
Source: Cummins, 1975 and unpublished.

Table 7 Comparison of Antitumor Activity with Ability to Cause Splenomegaly[b]

Vaccine material	Antitumor activity (BALB/C mice)	Splenomegaly production (CBA mice)
48 hr 0009, heat killed	++++[a]	++++
Log phase 0009	– to +	–
48 hr 0009, periodate treated	++++	–
48 hr 0009, TCA extracted	++++	–
48 hr 0009, formamide extracted	++++	–
48 hr 0009, acetylated	++++	–
48 hr 0009 CW suspension	– to +	–
48 hr CN 5888 vaccine	+++	–
48 hr 6500 vaccine	++++	–

[a]++++ = all animals in group of five protected; +++ = four of five animals survived; – to + = 0-1 animals survived; – = no survivors.
[b]Technical details: Splenomegaly production: see Ref. 44. Antitumor tests: 500 μg vaccine material + 10^4 tumor cells in a total of 0.1 ml in left hind leg intramuscularly on day 0. Survival followed for a minimum of 58 days. Tumor was a methylcholanthrene-induced fibrosarcoma synergenic in BALB/C mice. Periodate treatment and acetylation: see Ref. 44; (periodate treatment was for 1 hr). Details of strains: 0009 = *P. acnes* serological type I; CN 5888 = *P. granulosum*; 6500 = *P. granulosum*; (Cummins et al., unpublished).

the effect of lysozyme on vaccine activity was investigated, even though *P. acnes* is not lysed by that enzyme (44). It was found that treatment of vaccines by high concentration of lysozyme (1 mg/ml) significantly reduced their ability to cause splenomegaly when the vaccines were given intraperitoneally. If given intravenously, no reduction in activity was noted. Similar results were obtained with other basic proteins such as histones or poly-L-lysine, and it was assumed that the results were due, not to enzymic action, but to lysozyme acting as a basic protein and influencing the surface charge of bacteria. This seemed clear also from the fact that the action of lysozyme could be reversed by subsequent treatment with trypsin. Lysozyme, although producing a marked effect on activity, did so for what appear to be nonenzymic reasons. A large number of other glycosidases were without effect (44), but recently a lytic enzyme preparation from molluscs has been found to have an inactivating effect on *P. acnes* [Stimpson (1982), Ph.D. thesis, Virginia Polytechnic University and State University]. The fact that loss of activity accompanies lysis is once again evidence that a primary requirement for activity of any kind is an intact bacterial cell envelope.

C. Lipid Extracts

Lipid extracts of *P. acnes* have been described with reticulostimulatory and chemotactic properties (52,53,134). However, the general finding has been that bacterial cells after extraction with neutral solvents (e.g., chloroform/methanol) have lost litte if any of their reticulostimulatory activity (9,28,42). A somewhat different type of extract has been reported (89,152) in which an active vaccine (Burroughs Wellcome CN 6134) was extracted several times with pyridine at 37°C. The extract had antitumor effects, produced macrophage and NK cell activation, and induced the production of interferon. It did not induce splenomegaly. The bacterial residue after extraction, however, still had all the biological activities of the original vaccine, including the ability to produce splenomegaly. The question of the activity and mode of action of lipid extracts of *P. acnes* is further complicated by the demonstration of prostaglandinlike materials in ethyl acetate extracts (1-3,73). The exact nature of this prostaglandinlike material is not yet known, nor is it known whether it occurs in all strains. Of all materials extracted by lipid solvents, the pyridine extracts seem to be the most promising, but the composition of the material has not yet been reported. It seems possible that it may contain peptidoglycan intermediates and thus be related to muramyl dipeptide.

VII. INTACT CELLS VERSUS CELL WALLS

It has been emphasized earlier in this article that all the evidence points to the cell wall as being the site of reticulostimulatory activity. The logical course of action therefore in an investigation of the nature of the reticulostimulatory material would be to prepare and test cell wall fractions, in the expectation that these would contain the active principle in concentrated form. Unfortunately, in the hands of most investigators this has proved not to be the case, and cell wall fractions have been found to have little or no ability to induce hepatosplenomegaly or to prevent development of tumors. In gram-positive bacteria from stationary-phase cultures it may be assumed that the cell walls make up 15-20% of the dry weight of the cell. Assuming a figure of 20%, one might expect a fivefold increase in activity per unit weight if cell walls are used in place of whole bacteria, yet nothing of the kind has been reported. For example, Riveros-Moreno et al. (128) tested cell wall preparations from the Burroughs-Wellcome strain CN 6134 for lymphoreticular stimulation and antitumor effects in CBA-T6T6 mice. They found that cell wall preparations could not induce splenomegaly, and on a dry weight basis the ability of the walls to induce cytotoxicity in peritoneal macrophages, or to suppress tumor outgrowth (M4 fibrosarcoma), was less than 10% of that of the original vaccine. This was despite the fact that the distribution and persistence of radiolabeled cell walls (^{125}I) after IP injection were similar to that of labeled whole cells. Cantrell and Wheat (28) using material from the same strain report similar findings: cell walls could not induce splenomegaly and "the percentage of mice protected from tumor growth by cell walls was markedly less than that by whole cells. . . ." Experience in this laboratory bears this out: cell wall preparations washed free of whole cells by differential centrifugation were totally unable to induce splenomegaly (44), despite the fact that the whole cells recovered from the same disintegrate were fully active. This latter observation seems to indicate clearly that the lack of activity of cell wall fragments is not due to inactivation by autolytic or other enzymes liberated during disintegration of the cells. Moreover, we have found that if a highly active vaccine is mechanically disintegrated so that no intact cells remain, the resulting disintegrate is now almost inactive, although nothing has been removed from it (Cummins, unpublished). Similar results have been reported by Buck and Kelly (27) and by Cantrell and Wheat (28) who found that a recombination of cell walls and protoplasm did not restore either the reticulostimulatory or the antitumor activities. We have also found that cell wall suspensions will not protect BALB/C mice against an inoculum of fibrosarcoma cells, although the original vaccine was highly active (see Table 7).

It has been reported by Riveros-Moreno and Niblock (127) that if bacteria are disrupted under reducing conditions (in the presence of dithiothreitol) the cell walls are able to induce splenomegaly and cause regression of tumors. However, we have been unable to produce splenomegaly in CBA mice with cell wall preparations which were produced under stringent anaerobic conditions during disruption and washing (Pringle and Cummins, unpublished).

Assuming that the cell wall is the location of the active material in bacterial vaccines, it seems as if this must be presented to the body cells in the form of intact bacteria. The fact that cell wall fragments will not trigger the reaction may be due to size or to the fact that new surfaces which become exposed on fracture are in some way inhibitory. Examination of the charged groups at the surface of both intact cells and cell wall fragments from an active strain of *P. acnes* revealed that -COOH and $-NH_2$ groups were solely responsible for the surface charge in both cases, but the charge density on cell wall fragments was considerably lower at all pH values (121). However, it might be assumed that the detailed configuration of the groups is different on the edges and inner surfaces of the wall. It appears that in the case of *Staphylococcus aureus* wall fragments are as readily phagocytosed as are whole cells (104). We have found that the same is true of cell wall fragments of *P. acnes*, which are avidly phagocytosed by mouse peritoneal macrophages in vivo. Assuming that phagocytosis of vaccine material is the initial stage in any response, it does not seem that lack of activity of cell wall fragments is due to failure to be ingested. However, as pointed out in Sec. XIII it may be cell contact, rather than phagocytosis that is important.

In short, the almost total loss of activity following mechanical disruption of active vaccines is a considerable paradox, and from the practical point of view has made the investigation of the active material much more difficult. One cannot help feeling that the difference between the response to intact bacteria and that to cell wall fragments holds an important clue to the primary mechanism of action of these vaccines.

VIII. ANTITUMOR ACTIVITY OF *P. ACNES*

One of the main reasons for the sustained and still-continued interest in *C. parvum* vaccines is their antitumor activity, but the mechanism for this still elude explanation.

The phenomenon was first described almost simultaneously by Woodruff and Boak (162) and by Halpern et al. (70) in 1966, following earlier work in which Halpern et al. (69) had demonstrated the intense stimulation of the reticuloendothelial system caused by the agent. In both investigations a sarcoma and a carcinoma in mice were used, and the best protection (90% survival) was noted by Halpern in the case where an Ehrlich ascites tumor in Swiss male mice was treated with repeated intraperitoneal injections of the vaccine. Intravenous injections were much less effective against the Ehrlich tumor. It is of interest also to note that in these early investigations Halpern found that killed suspensions of *Salmonella typhi* given by repeated intraperitoneal injection were as effective as *P. acnes*. Live BCG suspensions, on the other hand, were almost totally without effect.

Since these two early papers, a large amount of work has confirmed that under certain conditions these vaccines do indeed have a powerful antitumor activity. Depending on the method and time of administration of the vaccine, and the kind of tumor, this may be shown by the ability to prevent an inoculum of tumor cells from causing the formation of a tumor, by ability to cause existing tumors to regress, or by ability to prevent or diminish the development of metastases.

The background to the antitumor activity of *C. parvum* vaccines has been thoroughly reviewed by Milas and Scott (100). Similarly the question of the effect by bacterial vaccines on immunoregulation and their role in the immunotherapy of cancer have been considered more recently by Baldwin and Byers (11). Therefore, it is not proposed here to give more than a general outline of the major mechanisms which may operate in particular situations.

In operational terms, two basic experimental designs have been most often employed.

1. The vaccine is given systemically (intravenously or intraperitoneally) at a site distant from the tumor site.
2. The vaccine is given at the tumor site, either at the same time as a live tumor inoculum or into the tumor after the latter has started to develop.

In another variation, killed (irradiated) tumor cells are used mixed with vaccine, and the animals subsequently challenged with a live tumor inoculum.

It is probable that systemic administration produces a generalized nonspecific immunostimulation, while local administration is likely to give a more specific cell-mediated immune response, either against the bacterial antigen or the tumor cells. Intraperitoneal injection is usually considered as systemic administration, but may be more equivalent to local administration if the tumor is also given intraperitoneally (e.g., Ehrlich ascites tumor and intraperitoneal administration of vaccine).

A. General Systemic Immunostimulation

One of the first two papers demonstrating the antitumor activity of *P. acnes* vaccines (162) showed that vaccine given IV caused significant dealy in the development of a subcutaneously injected tumor inoculum (a mammary carcinoma).

Since then, many examples have been recorded of systemically administered vaccines inhibiting the growth of various kinds of tumors (100,141). For these systemic injections of vaccine to be successful the material must be given intravenously or intraperitoneally; subcutaneous or oral administration is ineffective.

It seems almost certain that antitumor activity following systemic administration is largely due to a generalized and nonspecific activation of macrophages in the reticuloendothelial system (16). This activation is probably also associated with the increased activity of clearance mechanisms (increased carbon clearance) and with the development of hepatosplenomegaly, which are also found after systemic administration of vaccines.

B. Cell-Mediated Immune Responses

1. Specific Antitumor Immunity

One important mechanism by which rejection can occur following the injection of *P. acnes* vaccines is by the induction of tumor-specific immunity. Two examples from the literature will suffice to illustrate this.

Likhite (91) showed that tumor-specific protection in mice induced by *C. parvum* could follow (a) inoculation of tumor cells mixed with vaccine or (b) injection of vaccine into an already growing tumor. He used two similar but antigenically distinct adenocarcinomata in DBA/2 mice. The immunity induced in each case was tumor specific, and no protection was afforded against inoculation with cells of the other tumor. It may be noted that Likhite used vaccine provided by the Institut Merieux, Lyon, France, in which the organism is *P. avidum* and not *P. acnes* (42,133).

Dye et al. (48) and Mills et al. (101) showed that injection of tumor cells mixed with vaccine into the hind footpad of the mouse caused development of a tumor which grew for a time and then regressed. The regression was associated with the development of a tumor-specific T-cell-mediated immunity that would cause regression of an untreated tumor of the same type growing at a distant site. However, the effect against the distant tumor was limited to cases where the tumors were immunogenic; tests with two nonimmunogenic tumors did not induce inhibition at the distant site.

2. Antitumor Effect of Response to Bacterial Antigens

There is very good evidence that cell-mediated immunity specific for bacterial antigens in the vaccine may under certain circumstances be lethal to tumor cells present at the reaction site. For example, Tuttle (15) and Tuttle and North (153) showed that the induction of delayed-typed hypersensitivity against vaccine material in the footpad of the mouse would prevent the outgrowth of a normally lethal dose of tumor cells given into the footpad together with the eliciting dose of vaccine. Similarly, in sensitized mice, injection into the tumor of a dose of vaccine produced marked regression of tumor growth if given during the sensitive period (maximum about 9 days after the sensitizing dose).

Tuttle and North (153) suggested that the cellular mechanism for tumor rejection produced by this method was the induction of activated macrophages, and noted that it seemed to be associated with the persistence of intact bacteria within phagocytes at the site of the injection.

IX. RELATIONSHIP OF ANTITUMOR ACTIVITY TO ABILITY TO CAUSE SPLENOMEGALY: EFFECTS OF CHEMICAL TREATMENT OF VACCINES

The early measurements of activity of *C. parvum* vaccines used increased particle clearance and the development of splenomegaly as indicators. When interest in the antitumor activity of these vaccines developed, it was generally assumed that the ability of the vaccines from various strains to cause hepatosplenomegaly ran parallel with their ability to cause tumor regression. There is good evidence in the literature that this is usually so (9,85,94), although only a relatively small number of strains have been tested for antitumor activity compared with the large numbers surveyed for ability to cause splenomegaly (42,85).

The assumed relationship between antitumor activity and general ability to stimulate the reticuloendothelial system was based on the use of vaccines which had been killed by formalin or heat, but not otherwise treated except for washing. If vaccines treated chemically in various ways are used, the picture is somewhat different, as can be seem from Table 7. These results would appear to indicate that induction of antitumor activity and induction of splenomegaly may be due to two separate mechanisms, since it appears clear that several treatments which abolish the ability to cause splenomegaly leave the antitumor activity unimpaired. Riveros-Moreno and Niblock (127) have also suggested that splenomegaly production and antitumor activity are due to different substances, since they found that treatment with low concentrations of periodate (2 mM) would abolish splenomegaly but leave antitumor activity unimpaired. However, higher periodate concentrations (20 mM) abolished both activities.

The results in Table 7 have a number of interesting features.

1. Log phase cells and cell wall suspensions are quite ineffective in both types of test. However, this was known from previous work (see section on cell walls versus whole cells).
2. Treatments which might be expected particularly to modify the polysaccharide part of the wall [i.e., acetylation, trichloroacetic acid (TCA) or formamide extraction, or treatment with periodate] remove the ability to cause splenomegaly but do not affect antitumor activity.

3. The two strains of *P. granulosum* are almost as effective in antitumor tests as is *P. acnes* 0009.

There seems to be a clear indication here that the extractable polysaccharide of the wall is in some way responsible for the induction of splenomegaly, while the peptidoglycan skeleton alone may be sufficient to induce antitumor activity. However, for the polysaccharide to exert its effect, it seems that it must be part of an intact, or at least an unbroken, bacterium. Extracted polysaccharide in solution has no reticulostimulatory effect (27; Cummins, unpublished), and cell wall fragments, although containing polysaccharide, are without activity. Another point is that the action of polysaccharide in inducing hepatosplenomegaly can apparently be affected in two ways: chemical alteration in situ (e.g., periodate oxidation, or acetylation) or physical removal (TCA or formamide extraction).

The effect of periodate in low concentrations for short periods of time is primarily to attack unsubstituted 1,2-glycol groupings or amino groups (80). Cantrell and Wheat (28) reported that there was a large decrease in galactose content of polysaccharides from strain CN 6134 on treatment with periodate. This is perhaps to be expected, since other evidence from limited hydrolysis in dilute acid (79) suggests that galactose is an end-sugar in the structure. However, good splenomegaly has been produced by strains of *P. acnes* type II, whose polysaccharides do not contain galactose (7,42), so that galactose does not appear to be a key component for this type of activity. The activity of periodate-treated vaccines can be restored to some extent by borohydride reduction, suggesting that perhaps the aldehyde groups resulting from periodate treatment are inhibitory (44) for splenomegaly production.

The effect of acetylation in abolishing the ability to cause splenomegaly is also unexplained. Acetyl groups may be expected to attach to unsubstituted -NH_2 groups on both polysaccharide and peptidoglycan, but it is not clear whether the presence of acetyl groups is inhibitory or whether they act by making -NH_2 groups unavailable. The suggestion that some specific groupings in the cell wall polysaccharide are responsible for splenomegaly induction, while peptidoglycan is concerned with antitumor activity, is in keeping with the results obtained for *P. granulosum* strains. The polysaccharide in these strains is immunologically quite distinct from *P. acnes* polysaccharides, and also differs in qualitative composition in having galactose and mannose but virtually no glucose (40). However, the peptidoglycan composition is generally similar to that from *P. acnes*, although the alanine content may be somewhat higher (7).

Finally, in comparing antitumor activity with ability to cause splenomegaly, the route and timing of administration of both vaccine and tumor inoculum may play a role. For example, it appears from our recent work (Table 7) that vaccines of *P. granulosum* are as effective as *P. acnes* if given together with the tumor inoculum at the same site, yet Riveros-Moreno and Niblock (127) gave *P. granulosum* CN 5888 vaccine 2 days after the tumor inoculum in the footpad, and found it to be without effect. In tests utilizing inhibition ofmetastases, where vaccine is administered systemically (IV) and lung metastases are counted, the evidence has generally been that *P. granulosum* vaccines are ineffective compared with *P. acnes* (7,21,85). It appears (21) that the elimination of lung metastases is due to radiation-resistant cells (i.e., macrophages), and does not require an immune response to either vaccine or tumor antigens. If this is so, then the fact that *P. granulosum* vaccines are inactive in this respect would suggest that *P. acnes* polysaccharide, rather than peptidoglycan, is important for macrophage activation, since the polysaccharides of the two organisms are so different.

X. PEPTIDOGLYCAN OR MURAMYL DIPEPTIDE?

The results surveyed in the preceding paragraphs have suggested that while the extractable polysaccharides of the wall are important for splenomegaly production, the peptidoglycan is responsible for antitumor activity, at least when vaccine is given mixed with tumor inoculum. This immediately raises the question. Is the activity of the peptidoglycan due simply to the muramyl dipeptide moiety?

Muramyl dipeptide (MDP: N-acetyl-muramyl-L-alanyl-D-isoglutamine) is now recognized as the minimal structure of bacterial peptidoglycan that can replace *Mycobacteria* in Freund complete adjuvant. Historically, the material dervies from a detailed structural analysis of mycobacterial cell walls, primarily by Lederer and his colleagues (4,34,49) in France and Kotani et al. (83) in Japan. However, the fragment which is active (MDP) occurs in almost all bacteria which have peptidoglycan as a backbone for their wall structure. A few organisms (e.g., *Corynebacterium poinsettiae*) have glycine instead of L-alanine as the residue attached to muramic acid and hence do not exhibit the MDP structure (138,150).

Since *P. acnes* peptidoglycan contains as part of its structure the MDP moiety (Fig. 1), it is legitimate to ask what part this may play in the adjuvant and other properties of *P. acnes* vaccines. As noted above (see section on cell walls versus whole cells) the immediate answer might be "not very much," since cell wall fragments have little or no activity either for production of splenomegaly or in antitumor tests. The structure shown in Fig. 1A is somewhat conventionalized and shows glycine occurring as a linking amino acid between DAP on one peptide chain and D-ala on the other. Recent information (80a) suggests that this may not be the case, and that glycine, although attached to DAP, does not take part in the linkage (see Fig. 1B). There are numerous possible substituents or variations which have not been explored, such as the degree of acylation; the nature of the acyl groups present; the presence or absence of amidation on the α-carboxyl of glutamic acid; the degree of cross-linkage between tetrapeptides, and hence the number of free DAP or glycine groups; and so on.

MDP in vitro will stimulate macrophages to show various signs of activation such as increase in collagenase production, prostaglandin synthesis, glass adherence, fibroblast stimulation factor, and so on (154). MDP in vivo appears to induce somewhat paradoxical effects in the reticuloendothelial system, since it causes lymph node hyperplasia but depression of the reaction of spleen cells (24). Although it influences a number of macrophage functions, it does not appear to have antitumor effects in vivo probably because it is a small molecule, rapidly eliminated from the body after injection (about 90% eliminated in 1 hr) (34). However, if given encased in liposomes it induced tumoricidal activity in murine alveolar macrophages and could cause the regression of spontaneous pulmonary metastases (55). This would seem to indicate that packaging of potentially stimulatory material is very important in determining activity, possibly by ensuring that it reaches the correct cell in a state suitable for endocytosis or cell contact by whatever means. The occurrence of the MDP structure in the peptidoglycan of *P. acnes* is of course no direct indication that any of the activities of the original vaccine are due to it. The intact peptidoglycans of different bacteria often differ greatly in reticulostimulatory and adjuvant activity [see review by Stewart-Tull (147)], and Goguel et al. (63a) have shown that the peptide structure in peptidoglycan and its route of administration can influence its antitumor activity. Nevertheless, repeated extraction with, for example, hot formamide will leave only peptidoglycan as the major insolube residue of the cell, and since the antitumor activity of the residue seems unimpaired (Table 7), the role of muramyl dipeptide in its activity obviously needs to be determined.

XI. ANTIBODIES TO *P. ACNES* IN MAN AND ANIMALS: ACTIVATION OF COMPLEMENT

P. acnes is usually present in large numbers on the human skin, and antibodies to it are found in humans even in the absence of acne vulgaris, especially after puberty. Levels estimated by agglutination of bacterial suspensions usually vary from 1:20 to 1:320. In patients with acne they are higher, 1:40 to 1:1280 (124,160). Studies do not seem to have been made to determine whether antibodies to *P. acnes*, *P. granulosum*, and *P. avidum* are all present, and if so, whether they are directed against all serological types.

For other animals information is scanty and somewhat contradictory. Webster et al. (156) failed to find *P. acnes* on the skin of a number of animal species (mice, guinea pigs, rabbits, dogs, cats), although the organisms were found in the anal gland of the guinea pig. This accords with our own experience (McDonald and Cummins, unpublished). However, anaerobic coryneforms (unspecified as to group) have been reported from the skin of rabbits (144). No systematic search has been made for organisms of the acnes group in other anatomical situations in these animals, such as the mouth or the intestine.

Although *P. acnes* was reported from the anal gland of the guinea pig (156), McBride et al. (94) did not detect antibody to *C. parvum* in a sample of pooled guinea pig sera (25 animals). However, Wolberg et al. (160) reported titers of 1:32-1:64 in guinea pigs (five animals). In mice, moderate background titers (1:4-1:32) have been reported by both Woodruff et al. (163) and Wolberg (160), which presumably reflect some previous exposure to the antigens.

The presence of moderate to substantial levels of antibody to *P. acnes* in man is of more than theoretical importance if these vaccines are to be used therapeutically. It has been shown that *P. acnes* suspensions can activate complement by both the classic and alternate pathways (156,94), and it seems likely that in the case of the classic pathway this is due to the presence of anti-acnes antibodies.

McBride et al. (93) showed that washed suspensions of *C. parvum* would cause consumption of complement in human or guinea pig sera. In human sera which contain antibody to *C. parvum* (= *P. acnes*), it was assumed that the classic pathway was activated. In guinea pig sera, in which no antibody was found, the alternate pathway was found to operate. Webster et al. (155) have recently shown that the complement-activating material in *P. acnes* is carbohydrate and probably not peptidoglycan. In mice, circulating immune complexes were detected after *P. acnes* injection, and after repeated injections a diffuse proliferative glomerulonephitis developed (Mitcheson et al., 102). Hematuria and proteinuria were detected in 24 of 28 patients treated with *P. acnes* vaccines intravenously and evidence of circulating immune complexes was found in 16 of them, although it was possible that some of this effect was due to antitumor antibodies.

Cleavage of C_3 may be one method of macrophage activation by vaccines. Since activated macrophages will in turn cleave more C_3, a small amount of initial cleavage by vaccine will produce a rapid chain reaction (21). Ghaffer (61) has shown that if C_3 levels in mice were reduced by either sodium cyanate or cobra venom, *P. acnes* vaccines failed to generate cytotoxic macrophages, thus making it very likely that C_3 is important in this process.

It seems somewhat ironic that almost exactly similar studies of complement consumption have been done in relation to the reticulostimulatory activity to *C. parvum* and in the field of acne pathogenesis, except that in the latter case the organism is referred to as *C. acnes* or *P. acnes* (Webster et al., 155).

XII. DISCUSSION

There are still many anomalies and contradictions which obstruct attempts to explain the action of *C. parvum* vaccines, both in considering the nature of the vaccine material and in the sequence of events by which effects are produced in the animal body. In considering the nature of the active material, one of the major anomalies is the fact that suspensions of cell wall fragments show little activity of any kind, despite the solid weight of evidence pointing to the wall as the site of the reticulostimulating substance. A further curiosity which badly needs investigation is the lack of activity of log phase cells, although the evidence seems persuasive that this is connected with the degree of cross-linkage in peptidoglycan. There is also the rather dramatic loss of ability to induce splenomegaly, sensitivity to LPS, and (presumably) other similar activities when the vaccine is acetylated. Studies to compare the distribution of untreated and acetylated vaccine would be of interest here, but the difference may of course lie in the inability of acetylated vaccines to trigger some essential cellular mechanism. Neither of these points has been investigated as yet.

In reading the literature of the last 15 years it seems that a great deal of effort (often successful) has been expended in determining which cell type is activated by the administration of *C. parvum* vaccine. However, only peripheral attention has been paid to the actual fate of the bacteria comprising the vaccine material, especially during the first few hours after injection. It is presumably just at this period that they are coming into intimate contact with, or being phagocytosed by, cells that play some vital part in subsequent events. For example, it would be interesting to know whether any of the material is phagocytosed by polymorphonuclear leukocytes and, if so, what its subsequent fate is. Is it destroyed and lost to subsequent reactions, processed to form an essential intermediate, or merely liberated again to be rephagocytosed by macrophages?

It seems most reasonable to assume that the primary cell in any chain of events is a phagocytic, actively mobile cell (i.e., a macrophage or polymorph which will have the best chance of coming into contact with injected material). There is presumably a sequence in which the primary event, contact, and/or phagocytosis of bacterial particles by some cell is followed by secondary events in which other cells become involved due to the production of lymphokines, prostaglandins, or other messenger substances. Such messenger substances will introduce a considerable local multiplication of effect by being able to move through tissue fluids fairly rapidly. In the case of the macrophage, some very interesting evidence has been provided by Ögmundsdóttir and Weir and their colleagues (63, 107-109) concerning the conditions governing activation of host cells by contact with the bacteria in the vaccine. They showed that cells of *P. acnes* bound strongly to normal mouse peritoneal macrophages, while cells of *P. freudenreichii* (inactive) bound only very weakly. They also demonstrated that bacteria did not bind to T cells, and the presence of T cells was not necessary for phagocytosis by macrophages. However, in the absence of T cells, the macrophages would not become activated by the bacteria (uptake of myo-^{3}H-inositol). Similarly, in the absence of at least a small number of macrophages (about 5%)

the bacteria could not activate T cells (uptake of [^{3}H]-thymidine). This indicated clearly a back-and-forth interreaction between macrophage and T cell, with surface attachment of bacteria to macrophage, presentation to T cells and their activation, followed by activation of macrophages. In the experiments the macrophages phagocytosed the bacteria, but phagocytosis of particles alone was not sufficient for activation, since phagocytosis of latex beads, carbon particles, or *Staphyloccocus albus* cells was not sufficient to cause macrophage activation even in the presence of T cells. In any case, attachment of bacteria occurred at 4°C, although phagocytosis did not take place until the mixture was warmed up to 37°C. Ögmundsdóttir and Weir have also shown that the receptors on macrophage membranes to which *P. acnes* cells bound were probably carbohydrate, and demonstrated that some individual sugars which were components of the bacterial cell wall polysaccharide (glucose, galactose) would inhibit binding at a concentration of 10 mM. However, they also noted inhibition with other sugars (rhamnose, arabinose) which are not normally found in the wall.

These results emphasize that specificity of binding to host cells may be extremely important as a first step in producing the many effects attributable to *P. acnes* vaccines. If this is so, the nature of the bacterial surface is obviously as important as that of the host cell. As noted previously, an investigation of the surface charge on *P. acnes* and the groups responsible has been made (121), but it did not reveal any striking differences between active and inactive strains. However, such an examination can only measure overall charge, and cannot give details of specific charge patterns. Our investigations of the surface charge arose out of the observation that lysozyme and other basic proteins appeared to diminish the activity of *P. acnes* vaccines by coating the bacterial surface, thus suggesting that the value of the surface charge was important for activity. It would obbiously be of considerable interest to determine the degree of binding of bacteria to macrophages after the bacteria had been subjected to various chemical treatments.

Finally, at the risk of committing *lèse-majesté*, the question must be asked, Is *P. acnes* (in the guise of *C. parvum*) so unusual as a reticulostimulant? It can undoubtedly produce some dramatic effects both in vitro and in vivo. T cells, B cells, macrophages, NK cells, and suppressor cells of different kinds can be activated and animals protected against inocula of tumor cells which would otherwise always kill them. It can induce tremendous splenomegaly in suitable experimental animals, and make them very susceptible to drugs which the liver normally detoxifies. Yet (leaving aside *Mycobacteria* and related organisms), there is evidence that similar activity may reside in other groups of bacteria, *Bifidobacterium* for example (see p. 167). If organisms in other groups unrelated to *Propionibacterium* can be found which show the same degree of reticulostimulatory activity, a comparison in detail of their cell wall structures with those of *P. acnes* will make it easier to determine the active groupings. The same argument holds for antitumor tests. It would probably be helpful to test a wide range of bacteria for antitumor activities, since a determination of the common structure that is shared by those strains that are active may give important clues to the basis for the activity. *C. parvum* has served immunologists well as a reticulostimulant, but perhaps it would be better if it were taken off its pedestal and thoroughly examined chemically. It is, after all, not a rare and mystical organism, but the bacillus of acne, and probably the most common bacterium in the skin flora of man.

XIII. SUMMARY

Although a great deal has been learned about the cellular reactions which *P. acnes* (*C.*

parvum) vaccines will cause in the animal body, the nature of the initial stimulus caused by the vaccine is still obscure. All the evidence points to the cell wall as being the site of the active material, although it seems that the wall polysaccharide is important in causing hepatosplenomegaly and increased particle clearance, while the peptidoglycan portion is important in antitumor activity, especially when vaccine is given locally rather than systemically.

Although all evidence points to the cell wall as the site of activity, a major paradox still to be explained is the almost total lack of activity of suspension of cell wall fragments.

The crucial primary event determining activity of vaccines is probably the nature of the initial cell contact between bacteria in the vaccine suspension and some host cell. At this point the nature of the bacterial surface may determine the subsequent course of events.

REFERENCES

1. S. Abrahamsson, K. Green, L. Hellgren, and J. Vincent, *Experientia, 36*:58 (1980).
2. S. Abrahamsson, R. J. Gryglewski, L. Hellgren, J. Splawinski, J. Vincent, and B. Wojtaszek, *Experientia, 37*:164 (1981).
3. S. Abrahamsson, L. Hellgren, and J. Vincent, *Experientia, 34*:1446 (1978).
4. A. Adam, R. Ciorbaru, F. Ellouz, J. F. Petit, and E. Lederer, *Biochim. Biophys. Res. Comm., 56*:561 (1974).
5. C. Adlam, *J. Med. Microbiol., 6*:527 (1973).
6. C. Adlam, E. S. Broughton, and M. T. Scott, *Nature* (*New Biol.*), *235*:219 (1972).
7. C. Adlam and D. E. Reid, in *Developments in Biological Standardization*, Vol. 38 (A. H. Griffiths and R. H. Regamey, eds.), S. Karger, Basel, 1978, p. 115.
8. C. Adlam, D. E. Reid, A. J. Marshall, and P. Torkington, *J. Med. Microbiol., 12*:429 (1979).
9. C. Adlam, D. E. Reid, and P. Torkington, in *Corynebacterium Parvum: Applications in Experimental and Clinical Oncology* (B. Halpern, ed.), Plenum Press, New York, 1975, p. 35.
10. C. Adlam and M. T. Scott, *J. Med. Microbiol., 6*:261 (1973).
11. R. W. Baldwin and V. S. Byers, in *Immunostimulation* (L. Chedid, P. A. Miescher, and H. J. Müller-Eberhard, eds.), Springer-Verlag, New York, 1980, p. 73.
12. R. W. Baldwin and M. V. Pimm, *Adv. Cancer Res., 28*:91 (1978).
13. B. M. Barbior and D. W. Parkinson, *Nature, 298*:511 (1982).
14. R. F. Barth and O. Singla, in *Developments in Biological Standardization*, Vol. 38 (A. H. Griffiths and R. H. Regamey, eds.), S. Karger, Basel, 1978, p. 129.
15. R. C. Bast, B. S. Bast, and H. J. Rapp, *Ann. N.Y. Acad. Sci., 277*:60 (1976).
16. M. Baum and M. Breese, *Br. J. Cancer, 33*:468 (1976).
17. J. Belsheim, A. Dalen, H. Gnarpe, L. Hellgren, O. -J. Iversen, and J. Vincent, *Experientia, 35*:1587 (1979).
18. N. Bloksma, E. de Heer, H. van Dijk, and J. M. Willers, *Clin. Exp. Immunol., 37*:367 (1979).
19. R. Bomford, *Clin. Exp. Immunol., 39*:426 (1980).
20. R. Bomford, *Clin. Exp. Immunol., 39*:435 (1980).
21. R. Bomford and M. Olivotto, in *Corynebacterium Parvum: Applications in Clinical and Experimental Oncology* (B. Halpern, ed.), Plenum Press, New York, 1975, p. 268.
22. J. Breuillard, A. Lemoine, and M. A. Bertrand, *Rev. Inst. Pasteur* (*Lyons*), *9*:213 (1976).
23. B. Brozovic, V. S. Sljivic, and G. W. Warr, *Br. J. Exp. Path., 56*:183 (1975).
24. F. Brummer and D. A. Stevens, *Cell. Immunol., 59*:195 (1981).

25. M. J. Brunda, H. L. Mathews, H. R. Ferguson, J. K. McClatchy, and P. Minden, *Cancer Res.*, *40*:3211 (1980).
26. R. E. Buchanan and N. E. Gibbons, *Bergey's Manual of Determinative Bacteriology*, *8th ed.*, Williams and Wilkins, Baltimore, 1974, p. 633.
27. G. E. Buck and M. T. Kelly, *Infect. Immunol.*, *27*:620 (1980).
28. J. L. Cantrell and R. W. Wheat, *Cancer Res.*, *39*:3554 (1979).
29. E. A. Carswell, L. J. Old, R. L. Kassel, S. Green, N. Fiore, and B. Williamson, *Proc. Natl. Acad. Sci. USA*. *72*:366 (1975).
30. J. E. Castro, *Eur. J. Cancer*, *10*:121 (1974).
31. J. E. Castro, *Eur. J. Cancer*, *10*:115 (1974).
32. I. Cerutti, *C. R. Acad. Sci.*, (Paris), *279*:963 (1974).
33. M. J. B. Chase and M. Baum, in *Developments in Biological Standardization*, Vol. 38 (A. H. Griffith and R. H. Regamey, eds.), S. Karger, Basel, 1978, p. 195.
34. L. Chedid and E. Lederer, *Biochem. Pharmacol.*, *27*:2183 (1978).
35. L. Chedid, P. A. Miescher, and H. J. Müller-Eberhard, *Immunostimulation*, Springer-Verlag, New York, 1980.
36. M. A. Chirigos, M. Mitchell, M. J. Mastrangelo, and M. Krim (eds.), *Progress in Cancer Research and Therapy*, *Vol. 19*, Raven Press, New York, 1981.
37. R. H. Civil and A. A. F. Mahmoud, *J. Immunol.*, *120*:1070 (1978).
38. I. A. Clark, F. E. G. Cox, and A. C. Allison, *Parasitology*, *74*:9 (1977).
39. F. M. Collins and M. T. Scott, *Infect. Immun.*, *9*:863 (1974).
40. C. S. Cummins, in *Anaerobic Bacteria, Selected Topics* (D. W. Lambe, Jr., R. J. Genco, and K. J. Mayberry-Carson, eds.), Plenum Press, New York, 1980, p. 205.
41. C. S. Cummins and J. L. Johnson, *J. Gen. Microbiol.*, *80*:433 (1974).
42. C. S. Cummins and D. M. Linn, *J. Natl. Cancer Inst.*, *59*:1697 (1977).
43. C. S. Cummins and S. A. Stimpson, *Abstr. Ann. Meet. Am. Soc. Microbiol.*, *E33*:48 (1978).
44. C. S. Cummins, S. A. Stimpson, R. L. Tuttle, and C. J. Week, *J. Reticuloendothelial Soc.*, *29*:1 (1981).
44a. C. S. Cummins and R. H. White, *J. Bacteriol.*, *153*:1388 (1983).
45. J. Dawes, S. J. Tuach, and W. H. McBride, *J. Bacteriol.*, *120*:24 (1974).
46. M. M. C. Diesseldorf den Dulk, R. W. Crofton, and R. van Furth, *Immunology*, *37*:7 (1979).
47. H. C. Douglas and S. E. Gunter, *J. Bacteriol.*, *52*:15 (1946).
48. E. S. Dye, R. J. North, and C. D. Mills, *J. Exp. Med.*, *154*:609 (1981).
49. F. Ellouz, A. Adam, R. Ciorbaru, and E. Lederer, *Biochim. Biophys. Res. Commun.*, *59*:1317 (1974).
50. S. R. Evans and H. M. Johnson, *Cell. Immunol.*, *64*:64 (1981).
51. D. Farquhar, T. L. Loo, R. Reed, and M. Lana, *Lancet*, *1*:914 (1975).
52. R. M. Fauve, in *Corynebacterium Parvum*: *Application in Experimental and Clinical Oncology* (B. Halpern, ed.), Plenum Press, New York, 1974, p. 77.
53. R. M. Fauve and M. B. Hevin, *Proc. Natl. Acad. Sci. USA*, *71*:573 (1974).
54. J. Ferluga, A. Kaplun, and A. C. Allison, *Agents and Actions*, Barkhäuser Verlag, Vol. 9, Basel, 1979, p. 566.
55. I. J. Fidler, S. Sone, W. E. Fogler, and Z. L. Barnes, *Proc. Natl. Acad. Sci. USA*, *78*:1680 (1981).
56. J. Fishbach and L. A. Glasgow, *Infect. Immun.*, *11*:80 (1975).
57. H. Friedman, T. W. Klein, and A. Szentivanyi (eds.), *Immunomodulation by Bacteria and Their Products*, Plenum Press, New York, 1981.
58. P. Frost and E. M. Lance, in *Immunopotentiation* (G. E. W. Wolstenholme and J. Knight, eds.), Ciba Foundation Symposium, No. 18, Associated Scientific Publishers, Amsterdam, 1973, p. 29.

59. D. A. Gabrielson, J. A. Kelleher, and J. Varani, *Infect. Immun.*, *30*:791 (1980).
60. S. Gauthier-Raman, B. Halpern, and D. Besluau, in *Developments in Biological Standardization*, Vol. 38 (A. H. Griffiths and R. H. Regamey, eds.), S. Karger, Basel, 1977, p. 205.
61. A. Ghaffar, *J. Reticuloendothelial Soc.*, *27*:327 (1980).
62. A. Ghaffar, R. T. Cullen, N. Dunbar, and M. F. A. Woodruff, *Br. J. Cancer*, *29*:199 (1974).
62a. J-M. Ghuysen, D. J. Tipper, and J. L. Strominger, in *Methods in Enzymology*, Vol. VIII (S. P. Colowick and N. O. Kaplan, eds.), Academic Press, New York, p. 685.
63. E. Glass, J. Stewart, and D. M. Weir, *Immunology*, *44*:529 (1981).
63a. F. Goguel, G. Lespinats, and C. Nauciel, *J. Natl. Cancer Inst.*, *68*:657 (1982).
64. S. Green and A. Dobrjansky, *J. Natl. Cancer Inst.*, *63*:497 (1979).
65. S. Green, A. Dobrjansky, and M. A. Chiasson, *J. Natl. Cancer Inst.*, *59*:1519 (1977).
66. A. H. Griffiths and R. H. Regamey, *Developments in Biological Standardization*, Vol. 38, S. Karger, Basel, 1977.
67. W. Grimm, N. Seitz, H. Kirschner, and D. Gemsa, *Cell. Immunol.*, *40*:419 (1978).
68. B. Halpern (ed.), *Corynebacterium Parvum: Applications in Experimental and Clinical Oncology*, Plenum Press, New York, 1975.
69. B. N. Halpern, A. R. Prévot, G. Biozzi, C. Stiffel, D. Mouton, J. C. Morard, Y. Bouthillier, and C. Decreusefond, *J. Reticuloendothelial Soc.*, *1*:77 (1964).
70. B. N. Halpern, G. Biozzi, C. Stiffel, and D. Mouton, *Nature*, *212*:853 (1966).
71. C. W. Hamilton, R. L. DeAngelis, S. A. Gall, B. Fisher, and J. K. Whisnant, *Cancer Immunol. Immunothor.*, *8*:157 (1980).
72. E. M. Hersh, M. A. Chirigos, and M. A. Mastrangelo (eds.), *Augmenting Agents in Cancer Therapy*, *Progress in Cancer Research and Therapy*, *Vol. 16*, Raven Press, New York, 1981.
73. L. Hellgren, G. Selstam, and J. Vincent, *Experientia*, *35*:196 (1979).
74. R. G. Hirst and R. Campbell, *Infect. Immun.*, *17*:319 (1977).
75. R. G. Hirst and M. E. Wallace, *Infect. Immun.*, *14*:475 (1976).
76. J. G. Howard, G. H. Christie, and M. T. Scott, *Cell. Immunol.*, *7*:290 (1973).
77. J. G. Howard, M. T. Scott, and G. H. Christie, in *Immunopotentiation, Ciba Foundation Symposium No. 18* (G. E. W. Wolstenholme and J. Knight, eds.), Associated Scientific Publishers, Amsterdam, 1973, p. 101.
78. K. James, W. McBride, and A. Stuart (eds.), *The Macrophage and Cancer*, Univ. of Edinburgh, Scotland, 1977.
79. J. L. Johnson and C. S. Cummins, *J. Bacteriol.*, *109*:1047 (1972).
80. E. A. Kabat and M. M. Mayer, *Experimental Immunochemistry*, 2nd ed., Charles C. Thomas, Springfield, Ill., 1961, p. 542.
80a. K. Kamisango, H. Fuji, Y. Yanagihara, I. Mifuchi, and I. Azuman, *Microbiol. Immunol.*, *27*:635 (1983).
81. I. Kato, S. Kobayashi, T. Yakokura, and M. Mutai, *Gann*, *72*:517 (1981).
82. H. Kirschner, H. T. Holden, and R. B. Heberman, *J. Immunol.*, *115*:1212 (1975).
83. H. Kirchner, M. T. Scott, H. M. Hirst, and K. Munk, *J. Gen. Virol.*, *41*:97 (1978).
83a. F. Kierszenbaum, *Infect. Immunol.*, *12*:1227 (1975).
84. P. A. Knight and R. N. Lucken, in *Corynebacterium Parvum: Applications in Experimental and Clinical Oncology* (B. Halpern, ed.), Plenum Press, New York, 1975, p. 91.
85. H. L. Ko, W. Roszkowski, J. Jeljaszewica, and G. Pulverer, *Med. Microbiol. Immunol.*, *170*:1 (1981).
86. F. Kobayashi, T. Nagoya, T. Koshi, and Y. Saino, *Infect. Immun.*, *27*:391 (1980).
87. Y. Kohwi, K. Imai, Z. Tamura, and Y. Hashimoto, *Gann*, *69*:613 (1978).
88. S. Kotani et al., in *Immunomodulation by Bacteria and Their Products*

(H. Freidman, T. W. Klein, and A. Szentiranyi, eds.), Plenum Press, New York, 1981, p. 231.

89. A. Lichtenstein, R. Tuttle, J. Cantrell, and J. Zighelboim, *J. Nat. Cancer Inst.*, *69*:495 (1982).
90. A. Lichtenstein, R. Murahata, R. Sugasawara, and J. Zighelboim, *Cell. Immunol.*, *58*:257 (1981).
91. V. K. Likhite, in *Corynebacterium Parvum: Applications in Experimental and Clinical Oncology* (B. Halpern, ed.), Plenum Press, New York, 1975, p. 244.
92. W. H. McBride, J. Dawes, N. Dunbar, A. Ghaffar, and M. F. A. Woodruff, *Immunology*, *28*:49 (1975).
93. W. H. McBride, J. T. Jones, and D. M. Weir, *Br. J. Exp. Path.*, *55*:38 (1974).
94. W. H. McBride, D. M. Weir, A. B. Kay, D. Peace, and J. R. Caldwell, *Clin. Exp. Immunol.*, *19*:143 (1975).
95. C. M. McNee and R. H. Nimmo-Smith, in *Developments in Biological Standardization, Vol. 38* (A. H. Griffiths and R. H. Regamey, eds.), S. Karger, Basel, 1978, p. 427.
96. T. J. MacVittie, *J. Reticuloendothelial Soc.*, *26*:479 (1979).
97. H. L. Mathews, *Cancer Immunol. Immunother.*, *12*:81 (1981).
98. G. Mayer, *Zbl. Bakt. I. Abt. Orig.*, *98*:370 (1926).
99. L. Milas, *Lancet*, *i*:695 (1974).
100. L. Milas and M. T. Scott, *Adv. Cancer Res.*, *26*:257 (1978).
101. C. D. Mills, R. J. North, and E. S. Dye, *J. Exp. Med.*, *154*:621 (1981).
102. H. D. Mitcheson, P. Hilgard, A. McGraw, and J. E. Castro, *Br. J. Cancer*, *41*:117 (1980).
103. W. E. C. Moore and E. P. Cato, *J. Bacteriol.*, *85*:870 (1963).
104. B. Mosedale and M. A. Smith, *Lancet*, *i*:168 (1975).
105. H. C. Nauts, G. A. Fowler, and F. H. Bogatko, *Acta. Med. Scand.*, *45* (*suppl 256*):1 (1953).
106. R. S. Nussenzweig, *Exp. Parasitol.*, *21*:224 (1967).
107. H. M. Ögmundsdóttir and D. M. Weir, *Clin. Exp. Immunol.*, *26*:334 (1976).
108. H. M. Ögmundsdóttir, D. M. Weir, and B. P. Marmion, *Br. J. Exp. Path.*, *59*:1 (1978).
109. H. M. Ögmundsdóttir and D. M. Weir, *Immunology*, *37*:689 (1979).
110. E. Ojo, O. Haller and H. Wigzell, *Scand. J. Immunol.*, *8*:215 (1978).
111. G. J. O'Neill, D. C. Henderson, and R. G. White, *Immunology*, *24*:977 (1973).
112. A. A. Otu, R. J. Russell, and R. G. White, *Immunology*, *32*:255 (1977).
113. J. Parlebas and B. Halpern, in *Developments in Biological Standardization* (A. H. Griffiths and R. H. Regamey, eds.), S. Karger, Basel, 1978, p. 201.
114. P. K. Peterson, B. J. Wilkinson, Y. Kim, D. Schmeling, S. D. Douglas, P. G. Quie, and J. Verhof, *J. Clin. Invest.*, *61*:397 (1978).
115. A. R. Prévot, *Ergeb. Microbiol.*, *33*:1 (1960).
116. A. R. Prévot, J. Levatidi, P. Tordieux and O. Nazimoff, *Ann. Inst. Past.*, *Paris*, *88*:537 (1955).
117. A. R. Prévot, J. Levatidi, P. Tordieux and O. Nazimoff, *Ann. Inst. Past.*, *Paris*, *88*:537 (1955).
118. A. R. Prévot, T. Nguyen-Dang, and H. Thouvenot, *C. R. Acad. Sci.*, *267*:1061 (1968).
119. A. R. Prévot and J. Tran van Phi, *C. R. Acad. Sci.* (*Paris*), *258*:4619 (1964).
119a. A. R. Prévot and H. Thouvenot, *C. R. Acad. Sci.*, *259*:1447 (1964).
120. A. T. Pringle and C. S. Cummins, *Canad. J. Microbiol.*, *28*:375 (1982).
121. A. T. Pringle and C. S. Cummins, *Infect. Immun.*, *34*:734 (1982).
122. A. T. Pringle, C. S. Cummins, B. F. Bishop, and V. S. Viers, *Infect. Immun.*, *38*:371 (1982).
123. R. G. Pugh-Humphreys and A. W. Thompson, *Br. J. Exp. Path.*, *60*:259 (1979).

124. S. M. Puhvel, M. Barfatani, M. Warnick, and T. H. Sternberg, *Arch. Dermatol.*, *90*:421 (1964).
125. M. Raynaud, B. Kouznetzova, B. Bizzini, and J-C. Cherman, *Ann. Inst. Past.*, *122*: 695 (1972).
126. V. Riveros-Moreno and A. Niblock, *Immunology*, *36*:495 (1979).
127. V. Riveros-Moreno and A. Niblock, *Cancer Immunol. Immunother.*, *8*:265 (1980).
128. V. Riveros-Moreno, R. Bomford, and M. T. Scott, *J. Natl. Cancer Inst.*, *60*:653 (1978).
129. J. C. Roder, S. L. Helfand, J. Werkmeister, R. McGarry, T. J. Beaumont, and A. Duwe, *Nature*, *298*:569 (1982).
130. H. J. Rogers, H. R. Perkins, and J. B. Ward, *Microbial Cell Walls and Membranes*, 2nd ed., Chapman and Hall, New York, 1980.
131. W. Roszkowski, H. L. Ko, K. Roszkowski, S. Szmigielski, J. Jeljaszewica, and G. Pulverer, *Med. Microbiol. Immunol.*, *169*:1 (1980).
132. W. Roszkowski, S. Lipski, H. L. Ko, S. Szmigrelski, J. Jeljaszewica, and G. Pulverer, *Strahlentherapie*, *156*:729 (1980).
133. M. Roumiantzeff, M. C. Mynard, B. Cognet, C. Goldman, and G. Ayme, in *Corynebacterium Parvum: Application in Experimental and Clinical Oncology*, Plenum Press, New York, 1975, p. 11.
134. R. J. Russel, R. J. McInroy, P. C. Wilkinson, and R. G. White, *Immunology*, *30*:935 (1976).
135. T. E. Sadler, W. A. Cramp, and J. E. Castro, in *Developments in Biological Standardization*, Vol. 38 (A. H. Griffith and R. H. Regamey, eds.), S. Karger, Basel, 1978, p. 137.
136. Y. Sakurai, S. Tsukahoshi, H. Satoh, T. Akiba, S. Suzuki, and Y. Takagaki, *Cancer Chemother. Rep.*, *56*:9 (1972).
137. K-H. Schleifer, R. Plapp, and O. Kandler, *FEBS Lett.*, *1*:287 (1968).
138. K-H. Schleifer and O. Kandler, *Bact. Rev.*, *36*:407 (1972).
139. M. T. Scott, *Cell. Immunol.*, *5*:459 (1972).
140. M. T. Scott, *Cell. Immunol.*, *5*:469 (1972).
141. M. T. Scott, *Sem. Oncol.*, *1*:367 (1974).
142. M. T. Scott, in *Developments in Biological Standardization*, Vol. 38 (A. H. Griffiths and R. H. Regamey, eds.), S. Karger, Basel, 1978, p. 123.
143. M. T. Scott and L. Milas, *Cancer Res.*, *37*:1673 (1977).
144. A. Seto, S. A. Salehi, K. Miyanomae, T. Ushijima, and Y. Ho, *Oncology*, *37*:12 (1980).
145. N. A. Sher, S. D. Charapas, L. E. Greenberg, and S. Bernard, *Infect. Immun.*, *12*:1325 (1975).
146. L. F. Soyka, W. G. Hunt, S. E. Knight, and R. S. Foster, *Cancer Res.*, *36*:4425 (1976).
147. D. E. S. Stewart-Tull, *Ann. Rev. Microbiol.*, *34*:311 (1980).
148. C. Stiffel, D. Mouton, Y. Bouthillier, C. Decreusefond, and B. G. Biozzi, *J. Reticuloendothelial Soc.*, *7*:280 (1970).
149. S. A. Stimpson and C. S. Cummins, *Abstr. Ann. Meet. Am. Soc. Microbiol.*, p. 145 (1982).
150. D. J. Tipper and A. Wright, in *The Bacteria, Vol. VIII* (I. C. Gunsalus, ed.), Academic Press, New York, 1979, p. 291.
151. R. L. Tuttle, in *Developments in Biological Standardization*, Vol. 38 (A. H. Griffiths and R. H. Regamey, eds.), S. Karger, Basel, 1978, p. 189.
152. R. L. Tuttle and J. Cantrell, in *Augmenting Agents in Cancer Therapy* (E. M. Hersh, M. A. Chirigos, and M. J. Mastrangelo, eds.), Raven Press, New York, 1981, p. 53.
153. R. L. Tuttle and R. J. North, *J. Natl. Cancer Inst.*, *55*:1403 (1975).
154. S. M. Wahl, L. M. Wahl, J. B. McCarthy, L. Chedid, and S. E. Mergenhagen, *J. Immunol.*, *122*:2226 (1979).
155. G. F. Webster, U. R. Nilsson, and W. P. McArthur, *Inflammation*, *5*:165 (1981).

156. G. F. Webster, M. R. Ruggieri, and K. J. M. McGinley, *Appl. Environ. Micro.*, *41*:1269 (1981).
157. E. Wisse and D. L. Knook, *Kupffer Cells and Other Liver Sinusoidal Cells*, Elsevier/North-Holland, New York, 1977.
158. R. G. White, in *Corynebacterium Parvum*: *Applications in Experimental and Clinical Oncology* (B. Halpern, ed.), Plenum Press, New York, 1975, p. 148.
159. R. G. White, G. J. O'Neill, D. C. Henderson, J. Cater, and P. C. Wilkinson (eds.), in *Non-Specific Factors Influencing Host Resistance*, S. Karger, Basel, 1973, p. 285.
160. G. Wolberg, G. S. Duncan, C. Adlam, and J. K. Whisnant, *Infect. Immun.*, *15*:1004 (1977).
161. G. E. W. Wolstenholme and J. Knight (eds.), *Immunopotentiation, Ciba Foundation Symposium, No. 18*, Associated Scientific Publishers, Amsterdam, 1973.
162. M. F. A. Woodruff and J. L. Boak, *Br. J. Cancer*, *20*:345 (1966).
163. M. F. A. Woodruff, W. H. McBride, and N. Dunbar, *Clin. Exp. Immunol.*, *17*:509 (1974).
164. P. R. Wood and I. A. Clark, *Infect. Immun.*, *35*:52 (1982).

10

Cyclosporin A

Current Status, Including the Cape Town Experience

Peter Jacobs The University of Cape Town Medical School, and Groote Schuur Hospital, Observatory, Cape Town, South Africa

Linda Eglin The University of Cape Town Medical School, Cape Town, South Africa

I. INTRODUCTION

The well-being of the human race is constantly challenged by the presence of antigens in the environment; some may be foreign or extrinsic, such as bacteria or viruses, while others are intrinsic, being known as autoantigens. Although superficially different, the physiological response in each situation is linked by the functional integrity of the immune system. Historically, credit is due to the stimulating work of early immunobiologists, including Burnet (1), Billingham et al. (2), and Medawar (3), but it is the vast amount of work carried out in the last decade that forms the basis for understanding the physiology and pathology of the immune system (4,5). Under normal circumstances, the immunological response differs between antigen that is foreign, or non-self, and that which belongs, or self. The former elicits the activation of highly specific humoral and cell-mediated mechanisms which interact to remove the antigen, often involving a nonspecific immune process such as production of opsonins and phagocytosis. In contrast, the development of immune tolerance prevents the initiation of a similar process directed against host antigen.

The complex nature of the immune system is gradually being unraveled and disturbances, congenital or acquired, in the humoral or cellular components are being increasingly correlated with distinct clinical syndromes. Thus, failure of immune surveillance to distinguish self from non-self may lead to an autoimmune reaction exemplified by systemic lupus erythematosus. In addition, there is a whole new discipline developing in medicine in which foreign tissue is transferred from one individual to another, and in this process of transplantation, graft acceptance and subsequent function often depend upon the deliberate suppression of the immune response.

In parallel with the better understanding of the structure and function of the immune system and the disturbances that give rise to clinically important disease entities (5), manipulation of immune responsiveness has become the goal of therapy in many patients. Not surprisingly, there has followed the development of a large number of drugs and other agents whose effects vary from stimulation through modulation to immunosuppression. It is the latter that are of particular interest since they are most widely used in the treatment of autoimmune disease and are indispensable in tissue transplantation.

A. Immunosuppressive Drugs: Current Shortcomings

Agents for the suppression of immunologically mediated inflammatory processes are, as a group, nonselective. As a result, undesirable side effects are evident on practically every organ and tissue in the body, notably, the gastrointestinal tract and the hematopoietic system. For this reason, the ever present challenge is for the development of substances with clearly defined sites of action. In theory, these could be directed against the nonspecific immune process, interfering with phagocytosis of particulate antigen. Alternatively, the action could be restricted to specific or adaptive immunity influencing macrophages or different lymphocyte subpopulations.

Initially, drugs interfering with immune phenomena included the antihistaminics (6), the anti-inflammatory drugs (7), and the immunosuppressive agents themselves (8). Not only are the actions of these drugs still awaiting accurate characterization, but many have wide-ranging complications, including myelotoxicity (9), and their lack of specificity also predisposes the patient to the serious hazards of opportunistic infection (10) and the risk of malignant disease (11).

In view of these shortcomings, attention has increasingly been directed at improving specificity. The first step in this direction was the development and then the use in clinical practice of antilymphocyte globulin (12). The latter approach suffers from limitation in that there is relative lack of specificity since large numbers of lymphocyte subpopulations may be removed or their function destroyed. Subsequently, antithymocyte globulin (13) was developed in the hope that the target population could be narrowed to T lymphocytes. Further refinement has been the veritable explosion of monoclonal antibodies that followed the introduction of the hybridoma technique (14). While these biological reagents are becoming more abundant, and already whole libraries exist, their availability for therapy is still limited.

It is in this context that the unique and interesting antilymphocyte agent, cyclosporin A, needs to be judged.

B. Cyclosporin A: Historical Perspective

In the general quest to develop greater selectivity for immunosuppressive agents, one option is to identify those with an action predominantly against a specific lymphocyte subpopulation. Cyclosporin A meets this criterion, since the fungal metabolite appears to modify T-helper activity. Of special note is a surprising lack of bone marrow toxicity so that it already has an important role in clinical programs while, at the same time, attracting attention in the study of basic immunological phenomena.

Historically, the synthesis of the cyclosporins began with the isolation of a metabolite from a new strain of *Trichoderma*, one of the fungi imperfecti. In practice, the large-scale production is achieved by growing the fungi in submerged culture and then extracting the cyclosporin polypeptides from the mycelia since they are not released into the culture medium.

Based on this fermentation procedure, a series of developments took place in the laboratories of Sandoz in Switzerland and, while credit has been given to all those involved (15), Jean Borel stands out as the driving force in getting the product now known as cyclosporin A to clinical trial. It is interesting that the fungal extract has little fungistatic activity in vivo, but it was known that such metabolites of microbial origin may possess cytostatic or other pharmacological activities. Efforts were than made to define its properties, and particular attention was given to elucidating any immune suppressive effects (16,17).

In a long series of systematic studies, this latter property was compared with a variety of immunosuppressive, cytostatic, and other reference drugs, using several different models. These initial observations revealed two important properties of cyclosporin A, in that the immunosuppression was separable from more general cytotoxic side effects and that both humoral and cell-mediated pathways were affected (16,17).

Following purification, characterization by x-ray analysis (18,19), and synthesis, the pure product was further tested. Comparing murine splenic and mastocytoma cells, an interesting phenomenon was demonstrated (20): cyclosporin A, like hydrocortisone and antilymphocyte serum, had a selectivity for lymphoid cells, and this was in sharp contrast to conventional cytostatic drugs which, in this assay system, inhibited both cell types to a similar degree. Furthermore, the effect with the fungal metabolite was achieved without the usually associated myelotoxicity that characterized administration of equipotent doses of immunosuppressive drugs such as azathioprine. Further studies by Borel and his associates (21,22) showed that cyclosporin A was not lymphocytotoxic and had selectivity for the T-helper cells; an effect was also demonstrable on T-effector cells, but this was less evident and depended on the model used. Last, these actions were primarily evident during the induction phase of lymphoid cell proliferation and not during mitosis.

Although initially bedeviled by problems with absorption, the group at Cambridge (23-26) confirmed the claims for an immunosuppressive effect, using an animal heterotopic cardiac allograft model. Subsequently, similar series were reported in patients with mismatched cadaver kidney transplants (27) and following allogeneic bone marrow transplantation (28).

Clearly, then, cyclosporin A is a unique and potentially important new immunosuppressive agent. However, while it enjoys current widespread interest, there remain a number of important questions to be answered. What, for example, is its exact mechanism of action? In which body compartment, serum or red cells, should concentrations be measured? What minimal level in the plasma reflects optimal immunosuppression? Can peak and trough measurements in the serum, whether determined by radioimmunoassay or high-performance liquid chromatography, be used to monitor the development of short- or long-term toxicity? Is there a particular place for a natural killer cell assay in guiding therapy? What is the ultimate role of cyclosporin A in chronic inflammatory disease and organ transplantation? Should it be used as a single agent or in combination? If the latter, what combination and on what schedule?

Undoubtedly, we are on the threshold of a change in direction for the use of immunosuppressive agents. In this context, cyclosporin A represents an advance in specificity on antilymphocyte globulin comparable with the way in which that material, whatever its inherent limitations are, was a step forward from the use of the cytotoxic drugs where myelotoxicity often limited adequate therapy.

To place in perspective what is currently known about cyclosporin A, we have reviewed the available information and, where relevant, integrated new data from our own experience.

II. CHEMISTRY

A. Origin

Cyclosporin A is a fungal cyclic undecapeptide $C_{62}H_{111}O_{12}$, isolated from *Tolypochladium inflatum Gams.*

B. Structure (Fig. 1)

The compound has several N-methylated amino acids and one novel C_9-amino acid. It has a molecular weight of 1202.6 daltons, and its structure is shown in Fig. 1 (18,19,29).

C. Properties

The peptide is neutral, rich in hydrophobic amino acids, insoluble in water and n-hexane, but very soluble in all other organic solvents and lipids. Cyclosporin A may be crystallized to a white hydrophobic powder, and this property has given rise to some of the difficulties in its preparation for clinical use.

Originally, animal experiments were carried out, suspending the active principal in 0.5% tragacanth, but more recently a solution in ethanol and Tween has been developed.

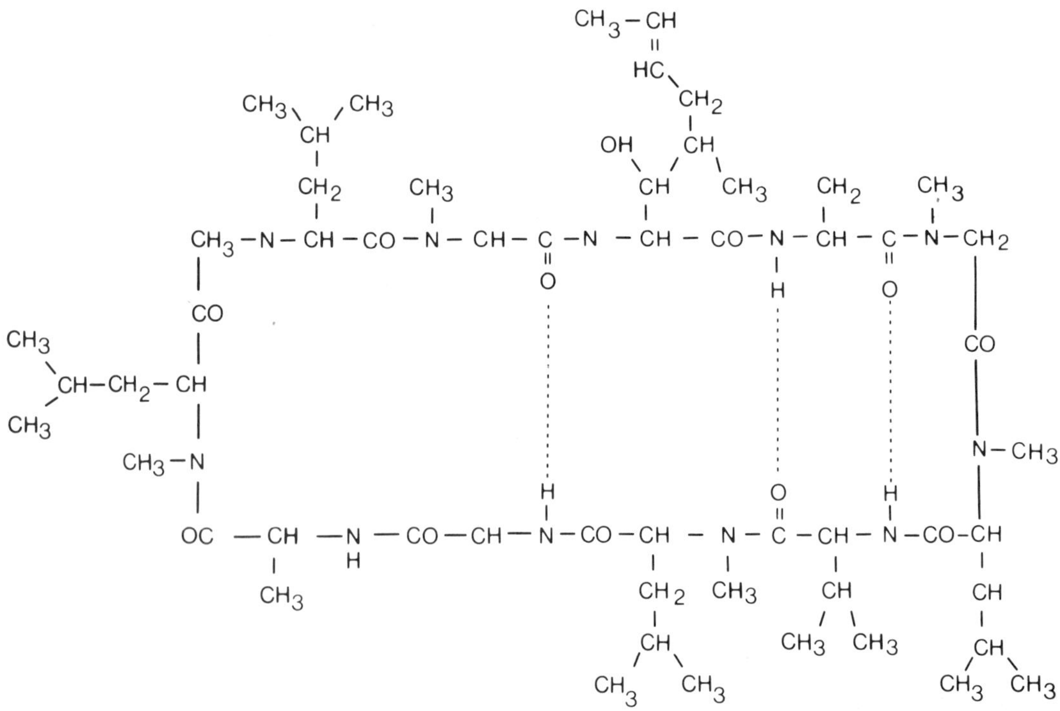

Figure 1 The chemical structure of cyclosporin A. The molecule is thought to exist partly as an open loop and partly as a β-pleated sheet. The β-hydroxy group in the C_9-ENE side chain forms a hydrogen bond with the carbonyl oxygen atom of the same amino acid and may account for the immunosuppressive activity of this fungal metabolite. (From Ref. 19.)

Both preparations are well tolerated by experimental animals and when given, using an olive-tipped gastric cannula, dependable administration schedules are easily possible. In clinical trials, a recently formulated drinking solution is well tolerated, particularly in a taste-disguising milk solution to which chocolate, cocoa, or Caotina has been added.

Injectable forms are available, prepared by dissolving cyclosporin A in a mixture containing ethanol and Miglyol, and subcutaneous, intramuscular, and intravenous routes in both experimental animals and patients, in our experience, have been used without any local side effects.

D. Assay Methods

1. High-Performance Liquid Chromatography (HPLC)

The determination of cyclosporin A (OL 27-400) is possible in human plasma and urine, using high-performance chromatographic separation in a reversed phase mode and ultraviolet absorption detection at 210 nm. At this wavelength, the compound has an extinction epsilon of 45,000 with an e_{max} of 66,000 at 195 nm in methanol. The internal standard used is cyclosporin D (33-804), differing only slightly from cyclosporin A in structure and chromatographic properties. The detection limit is 20 ng/ml, and the method has a linear calibration curve in the concentration range of 25-2000 ng/ml. Precision is good, and metabolites do not interfere with determination of the parent compound so that this is a reliable technique with high specificity (30,31).

This method has been further examined and its sensitivity confirmed (32). These workers have emphasized the higher levels obtained with radioimmunoassay when compared with HPLC, which may be attributed to cross reactivity of the antibody with metabolites of the cyclosporin. The generally poor correlation between the level of cyclosporin A in the plasma when determined by the radioimmunoassay and development of toxicity emphasizes a role for HPLC as a means to monitor the parent compound. Similarly, this technique provides the only method for measuring metabolites in the various compartments that include blood cells, biopsy material, and from detailed postmortem studies.

2. Radioimmunoassay (RIA)

Cyclosporin A (OL 27-400) can be determined by radioimmunoassay, using an antiserum raised in rabbits to cyclosporin C (Threonyl) hemisuccinate coupled to free amino acid groups of guinea pig immunoglobulin (IgG). The antiserum reacts primarily with cyclosporin A and cross reacts with the metabolites, dihydrocyclosporin A, and dihydrocyclosporin C (33,34).

Based on the continuous use and development of this assay in our laboratory, we have found the standard curve to be reproducible between 0.125 and 4 ng/tube, with linearity from 0.50 to 4 ng/tube, the assay to be sensitive to a lower limit of 62.5 ng/ml, with an interassay variation of less than 5%.

We have not personally evaluated the assay for cross reactivity with metabolites, although this has been reported (33,35). Abisch (33) has confirmed the specificity of the assay and tested metabolites designated 1, 8, 17, and 21 for cross reactivity with the antiserum 031180. The highest concentration for these compounds was 40.5, 122, 8, and 64 ng/0.1 ml, respectively. Cross reaction with cyclosporin C and dihydrocyclosporin C is 100%, because cyclosporin C was the hapten used to raise the antibodies.

The detection range with 2-μl samples is 40-2000 ng/ml plasma: but 10 μl of unknown plasma is needed to detect between 10 and 400 ng with any precision.

We consider the radioimmunoassay a dependable method for determining the parent substance and its metabolites in the serum and urine of experimental animals and in patients on clinical trial. It is, however, necessary to appreciate its limitations which are largely the result of cross reaction with metabolites. The question of distribution between the different cellular components in blood and the plasma phase is another theoretical consideration in using RIA.

3. Correlation and Perspective between HPLC and RIA

The correlation between high-performance liquid chromatography and radioimmunoassay in serum (36) has been examined in patients following allogeneic bone marrow transplantation (37), and the results compared by a linear regression analysis. In 50 observations over a 35-day period with the patients on oral administration, the coefficient of correlation was high ($r = .933$), with the value determined by RIA being 30-70% higher due to cross reacting metabolites.

These data confirm not only the reliability of both methods but establish their linear relationship. Nevertheless, the role of the two methods in monitoring clinical trials requires further attention, particularly since difficulties exist with inability to discriminate between therapeutic administration with optimal immunosuppression and inadequate or excessive treatment (35).

4. Cyclosporin A in Serum and Other Tissues

The distribution and binding to blood components have been reviewed (38), and in vitro studies have shown uptake predominantly by lipoproteins and erythrocytes. The lipoproteins, obtained by ultracentrifugation and fractionation, showed that over 60% of the drug was associated with this compartment independently of drug concentration. Uptake by erythrocytes was rapid and linear, accounting for 50% of the uptake by blood cells. In contrast, leukocytes bound only between 10 and 20%, but the kinetics of this phenomenon were nonlinear and the process was saturable.

Very little data are available at the present time on the distribution of cyclosporin A or its metabolites in different cellular compartments in the body, and a major deficit in our current knowledge is whether there is preferential binding, perhaps to lymphocytes, monocytes, or early hematopoietic precursors in the marrow, that may have profound immunological effects and where pharmacological monitoring by means of plasma levels may be inappropriate.

It may therefore be concluded, with regard to the assay methods currently available, that while radioimmunoassay is suitable for determining plasma levels in experimental animals and clinical studies, a great deal more essential information is required. Of particular importance will be the correlation of immunological effects with levels in the different tissue compartments and clarification on whether these effects and such toxicity as occurs correlate most closely with determination of parent substance or the total spectrum of metabolites determined immunologically by radioimmunoassay.

III. IN VITRO STUDIES

Current interest in the clinical use of cyclosporin A centers on its activity as a potent immunosuppressive agent. The available evidence suggests that these effects are mediated with little or no bone marrow toxicity. For these reasons it is logical to review first what has been established about the effects that this novel antifungal metabolite exerts on lymphoid cells in vitro. In reviewing what is rapidly becoming a voluminous literature, it is clear that results may, in some studies, have been affected by technical variations. The most notable of these is that since cyclosporin A is an extremely hydrophobic substance, its solubility is critical in standardizing preparation of material for in vitro studies. At the present time, it would seem prudent to follow in minute detail recommendations for its preparation (22). Furthermore, in all studies appropriate solvent control must be included.

A. Nucleic Acid Synthesis

The biological effects of cyclosporin A are its specificity for lymphocytes, a critical dependency on time of administration, and suppression of both humoral and cellular immunity in the laboratory animals (39). The further exploration of these effects (22) was undertaken in vitro in both mouse spleen cells and human peripheral blood lymphocytes. Both the incorporation of tritiated thymidine into DNA and the uptake of radiolabeled uridine into RNA were inhibited by cyclosporin A in doses between 30 and 1000 ng/ml, which are in the range currently achieved in many therapeutic trials. This phenomenon was critically time dependent, requiring addition of cyclosporin A at the same time as the mitogens, concanavalin A or phytohemagglutinin; the later addition of the cyclosporin A to the culture failed to have any inhibitory effect. Furthermore, and of note, was that this phenomenon was reversible, not easily by washing, but by elution over a 24-hr period. This reversibility, occurring without loss of cells in the culture, established a lack of lymphotoxicity (26,40).

These results show a primary effect of this agent directed toward early cellular events in which lymphocytes, in response to mitogenic stimulation, are prevented from undergoing blastogenesis. The cells do not lose their proliferative ability since, following elution of cyclosporin A, this function is again evident. It appears likely that the lymphoid cells are arrested in the G_0-phase of the cell cycle and that this is a physiological phenomenon explaining the reversibility of this effect.

B. Effect on Lymphocyte Subpopulations

The mixed lymphocyte reaction (MLR) and cell-mediated lymphocytotoxicity (CML) have been used in the study of porcine, canine, and human lymphocytes.

In the pig studies (26), in vitro assay of T-cell proliferation and mixed lymphocyte reaction demonstrates a dose-dependent inhibition in the presence of cyclosporin A.

In dogs (41), the results from the MLR indicate that cells reactive to histocompatibility antigens persist but are suppressed in the presence of cyclosporin A, whereas recognition of foreign antigen occurred predictably in the absence of cyclosporin A in the culture system under controlled circumstances. Similarly, a suppressive effect could be demonstrated when cultures were carried out in the serum from dogs treated with cyclosporin A, with the effect evident as early as 1 hr after oral administration to the animal. Of note was the persistence of the suppressor effect, in two dogs, for as long as 10-12 days after cyclosporin A administration. CML demonstrated the ability of lymphocytes from cyclosporin-treated dogs to generate cytotoxic effector cells against suitable target cells when the assay was carried out in normal pooled serum, but when the cultures were performed in the serum from cyclosporin-A-treated dogs, this cytoxicity was suppressed completely. These results suggest that the effects do not occur through either clonal deletion or a suppressor cell mechanism, but that the action is abrogated or suppressed in the presence of cyclosporin A.

The results of MLR and CML assays carried out on lymphocytes derived from human subjects provide support for the animal data (42,43). Thus, cyclosporin A does not favor generation or induction of suppressor cell lymphocytes; it spares them while inhibiting other subpopulations, resulting in an imbalance in the immune system with consequential profound immunosuppression. This phenomenon may results from the inhibition or killing of T-helper subpopulations. Cyclosporin A interferes with memory cell recognition on a short-term basis, reflected in disturbances in the recognition phase of the mixed lymphocyte reaction. In vitro human lymphocyte responses studied in the MLR showed that the induction of cytotoxic or cytolytic lymphocytes was markedly suppressed by minimal amounts of cyclosporin A, whereas that of alloantigen-activated suppressor cells was much less inhibited, results favoring the induction of suppressor cell mechanisms as opposed to cytolytic effector cells in the primary MLR (44). The latter investigators suggest that a state of specific operational tolerance may be induced in vitro which accords with their earlier in vivo data (45). This is thought to occur without clonal elimination, and this altered immunological state was considered to be induced or maintained by an active suppressor cell which could be identified by its adherence to nylon wool.

C. Molecular Basis of Cyclosporin A Activity

A review of the data reported for the in vitro effects of cyclosporin A in animals and in humans does not support clonal deletion, and while opinion is not uniform on the generation or induction of suppressor cell lymphocytes, the profound immunosuppression that this novel agent has appeared to center on T-helper subpopulations (22,42) and is reflected ultimately in diminished activity of cytolytic or effector lymphocytes.

Studies in mice (22) showed that cyclosporin A effectively inhibited plaque-forming cells when assayed using the Mishell and Dutton technique (46). These results provide evidence of an anti T-helper cell action for this agent. The selective effect on functional B-cell subsets (47) showed that T-dependent and certain T-independent antigens, the TI-1 mitogens, the TI-2 agents, are exquisitely sensitive. These studies emphasize the value of cyclosporin A in analyzing lymphocyte subpopulations, but it is uncertain whether these observations have clinical relevance. If any extrapolation is possible and B and T cells from humans respond in a similar way to mouse cells, then cyclosporin A should have little impact on established antibody responses and therefore be of limited use for suppression of autoantibody production. Furthermore, cyclosporin A should inhibit some primary antibody responses but leave others unaffected, as might occur with bacterial infection.

The central role played by T lymphocytes raised the theoretical consideration that the various observations could be united through an effect on the interleukins or factors that modulate the activation of lymphocytes. In this regard, it has been shown (48) that concanavalin A-activated suppressor T cells respond to T-cell growth-factor stimulation and exert their suppressor function by absorbing this material, with a consequent decrease in its concentration.

The molecular basis for this action of cyclosporin A on T-cell proliferation is explicable by the interleukins which provide communication between different populations of leukocytes. There are two molecules designated Interleukin 1 and Interleukin 2. The first is a monokine, generated at the time antigen is processed by the Ia^+ macrophage and has an effect on the T-helper cell. The latter, simultaneously in all probability, senses the first signal for antigen presentation from the macrophage. The net result of the presentation of processed antigen to the T-helper cell as well as with the second signal from Interleukin 1, is to permit differentiation of the immature helper T-cell with the subsequent release of Interleukin 2 (Fig. 2) (49). Interleukin 2 facilitates further interaction between the antigen bearing cell and lymphocytes with the proliferation of suppressor and cytotoxic T lymphocytes.

Based on this model, researchers (50,51) have presented evidence that cyclosporin A may interfere with the release of Interleukin 1 from macrophages and the release of Interleukin 2 from activated T-helper cells. A word of caution is necessary since the in vivo or physiological significance of these molecules has not yet been clearly defined, but the hypothesis remains an attractive one and compatible with data previously reported by Borel and his co-workers (20,22). It is also not clear what importance must be attached to reports that cyclosporin A inhibits migration-inhibition factor (52), macrophage-activating factor, and other lymphokines (53).

Cyclosporin A has also been studied in vitro on a number of isolated lymphoid cell populations. In general terms, a direct effect is less clearly demonstrable on the B lymphocytes (20). In vitro, cyclosporin A inhibits immunoglobulin secretion in response to pokeweed mitogen-induced B-cell activation. However, this phenomenon is T-cell dependent (54), and its inhibition may be the result of T-cell inactivation. Similarly, it appears that cyclosporin A specifically deletes or at least inactivates the cytotoxic T-cells normally responsible for the in vitro regression of Epstein-Barr virus lines, so that it may be reasonably speculated that the emergence of lymphoma in patients receiving renal allografts may occur on this basis. There is, however, no evidence that this immunosuppressive agent, in its own right, causes lymphoma.

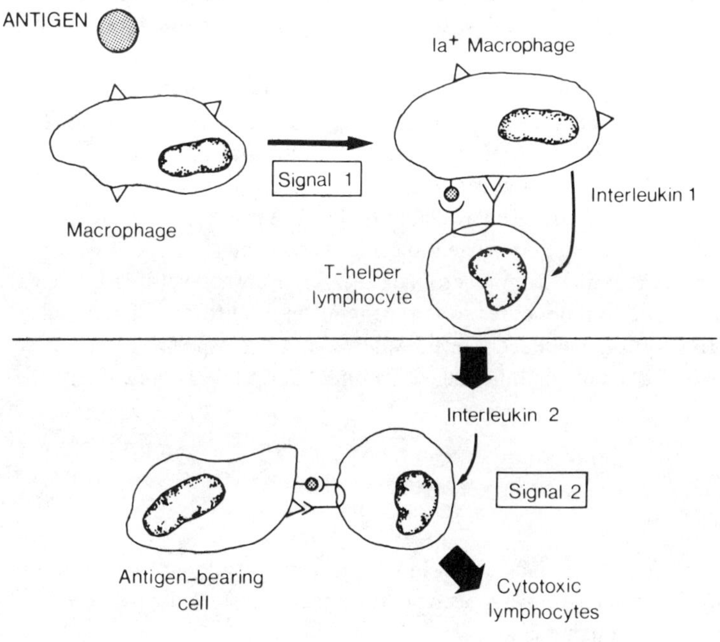

Figure 2 Putative scheme for the release of Interleukin 1 and Interleukin 2, based on the two-signal concept. (From Ref. 49.)

It has also been shown (55) that cyclosporin A will suppress both T- and B-lymphocyte blastogenesis, and the data have been interpreted by these workers as reflecting immunosuppression due to a direct effect on the blast cell rather than being mediated via a third-party accessory cell. This is an interesting study and provides some support for the controversial "decloning" hypothesis suggested as a possible mode of action for cyclosporin A in vivo (56,57). This evidence would suggest that, at least in humans, cyclosporin A is capable of directly inhibiting certain B-cell activation mechanisms, irrespective of whether these are normally dependent or independent of T-cell activation.

Of interest are the effects that cyclosporin A may have on killer cells, and here the evidence remains debatable. In assays using human lymphocytes in mixed lymphocyte culture, cyclosporin A was shown to efficiently prevent the development of cytotoxic T cells directed against target cells expressing the phenotype of the stimulator cells. This occurred without preventing an increase in the natural killing (NK) activity measured against tumor targets (58). In contrast, cyclosporin A has been shown to inhibit human natural killer activity (59), while another study (60) has shown inhibition of natural killing by cyclosporin A to be rapid, dose dependent, and not requiring the presence of T cells, B cells, or macrophages. These workers interpret the data as direct depression of NK activity with cyclosporin A and could find no evidence that this was mediated through suppressor cells.

These effects occur without marked reduction in lymphoid tissue, notably the spleen, and are in contrast to the effects of other immunosuppressive agents such as cyclophosphamide and azathioprine. The findings are consistent with cyclosporin A producing its effect by interference with stimulation or proliferation of lymphoid cells in the spleen. Similarly, for the thymus (61), data show that the immunosuppressive effects produced by cyclosporin A in vivo are not mediated by the pituitary-adrenal gland system and the results are, therefore, in line with those found in mesenteric lymph nodes and spleen.

What conclusions may be drawn from all this data? The in vitro effects of cyclosporin A are the basis for understanding the observations both in experimental models and in clinical trials. Although results from many studies are not uniform, a number of conclusions are possible. Cyclosporin A acts at a very early stage in the immunologically mediated response to foreign antigens. The available evidence suggests that the major action is on T-lymphocyte-mediated help. The molecular basis is most likely to be by blocking the release of Interleukin 1 from macrophages and thereby preventing the release of Interleukin 2 from T-helper lymphocytes so that generation of cytotoxic T-lymphocytes does not take place. In addition, evidence is accumulating that cyclosporin A has a direct effect both on cytotoxic T and natural killer cells. Its direct action on B cells, if any, awaits clarification.

D. Effects on Nonlymphoid Cells

1. In Vitro Marrow Culture

The most striking observation to be made about in vitro assessment of cyclosporin A on both hematopoiesis and lymphocytopoiesis, using culture techniques, is the paucity of data on which to base any reasonable assessment.

Myelopoiesis in humans has been assessed, using an in vitro culture technique (62,63). These studies have limited relevance for the clinical situation since doses between 5 and

10 μg/ml were studied, whereas in therapeutic terms, doses around 1 μg would be much more realistic. Nevertheless, a clearcut reduction in granulocyte-macrophage: colony-forming units in culture (GM:CFU_c) was observed, being most obvious at the higher level. In the data reported by Gordon and Singer (63), the T lymphocytes were affected much more than B lymphocytes or hematopoietic precursor cells in the range of 1-5 μg/ml.

Our experience differs from this since the in vivo situation was more closely approximated by using serum from patients containing between 500 and 1000 ng/ml. Control studies were run in parallel using stored serum from the same patients before starting cyclosporin A administration. There was a clearcut uniform suppression of erythroid colony formation, but granulocyte and macrophage growth was normal. These findings, furthermore, correlated with reduced erythropoiesis in the marrow, reflected in low reticulocyte counts and persisting mild anemia while granulopoiesis and megakaryopoiesis were apparently normal. Confirmatory experiments are in progress.

In studies carried out on T-lymphocyte colony formation from peripheral blood and bone marrow (64), it was shown that the effect was most marked on peripheral blood lymphocytes with bone marrow cells being less sensitive, suggesting that this may contribute to the role of this agent in treating graft-versus-host disease in humans.

2. Peripheral Blood Hematology

In mice (39), comparison of cyclosporin A with other immunosuppressive agents showed much less leukopenia, although lymphocytes were approximately 20% below control values. Platelets were not affected. Evaluation of changes in the peripheral blood are difficult to interpret since, for the most part, this immunosuppressive agent is used in patients undergoing allogeneic bone marrow transplantation, of which most are already pancytopenic. However, in a group of patients receiving cyclosporin A as the primary form of treatment for severe acute aplastic anemia, where there was no transplantation option, we have been unable to document any significant changes in peripheral blood hematology.

3. The Phagocytic System

In vitro studies on phagocytic cells (55) failed to show any effect, suggesting that immunocompetent lymphocytes are affected rather than the adherent, radiation-resistant, Ia-bearing accessory population.

Similarly, in serial studies on patients following transplantation or those with marrow aplasia receiving cyclosporin A as a primary form of therapy, we have demonstrated no effect on random migration, chemotaxis, phagocytosis, and intracellular killing.

4. Malignant Cells

Tumor cells studied in vitro are of interest. Available results show that the major activity in all the assay systems tested appears directed at T-cell tumors with very little effect on nonlymphoid lines. The common factor appears to be the presence of recognizable T-cell-associated surface antigens, and on this basis cyclosporin A would appear to selectively recognize a series of differentiation antigens on lymphoid cells and their malignant counterparts. It is of further interest that inhibition of permanently growing cell lines requires much higher concentrations than are necessary to produce similar quantitative effects in mitogen-induced T-cell proliferation.

IV. PHARMACOLOGY

A. Human

A single 600-mg oral dose of drinking solution of cyclosporin A, equivalent to approximately 10 mg/kg lean body mass, has a maximal plasma concentration between 242 and 1246 ng/ml when determined by high-performance liquid chromatography. This peak is reached in 3-4 hr after administration and is characterized by a lag time of 0.65 hr, after which, oral absorption is fairly rapid with a half-life of about 1 hr. There are two recognizable disposition phases with an α component having a half-life of 1.2 hr and the β clearance curve having a half-life of 27 hr. The maximum concentration is reached in the peripheral compartment after 8 hr; within 12 hr there is roughly eight times more cyclosporin A in this pool than was present in the blood (65).

In a further series of studies reported by the same authors, nine patients undergoing allogeneic bone marrow transplantation had serum levels of cyclosporin A determined after initial intramuscular or continuous intravenous infusion at total doses of 20 mg/kg/day, followed by maintenance at a dose of 12.5 mg/kg/day. These patients showed similar kinetics to the six patients who received a single 600-mg oral dose (65).

In a series of eight studies (66), the clearance of cyclosporin A from plasma was measured, using radioimmunoassay (Fig. 3) and a maximum concentration was found between 2 and 4 hr, with the peak at 2 hr. All patients received oral cyclosporin A as a drinking solution. These studies provide information only for absorption and clearance from the plasma.

The pharmacology is best explained by a two-compartment open model (65) which proposes that cyclosporin A, which is lipophilic, will leave the plasma and distribute itself widely in the tissues of the body, collectively designated as the peripheral compartment. While the validity of this hypothesis awaits confirmation, it has the attraction of emphasizing the need to measure cyclosporin A in tissues other than just the plasma. Our own studies (66) confirm reports that red cell or whole blood levels may be higher than those found in plasma (67). The exact relationship between cyclosporin A levels determined by radioimmunoassay for serum and whole blood hemolysate remains to be established. In this regard, it is theoretically possible that the immunosuppressive level needed may be reflected best by whole blood concentration of cyclosporin A; in contrast, monitoring of plasma concentration may provide a basis for avoiding dose-dependent and reversible renal dysfunction.

The detailed metabolism of cyclosporin A is unknown. However, in pooled plasma collected between 2 and 8 hr after patients had received cyclosporin A in olive oil, 27% of the radioactivity remained present as the parent drug at concentrations of 210 ng/ml. Of importance was the demonstration that 12 separate radioactive components could also be detected, but none was considered to be of major importance. Furthermore, the mean cumulative urinary excretion of radioactivity in a 96-hr period corresponded to 6% of the original dose together with 15 radioactive analogs. These data demonstrate that ^{3}H-OL 27-400 is rapidly and extensively metabolized in man to provide a qualitatively similar pattern of metabolites in both plasma and urine.

Further studies on the distribution and binding of ^{3}H-OL 27-400 show that over 60% of the drug is associated with lipoproteins and that this distribution occurs independently of drug concentration. The second major blood component that takes up the cyclosporin A are the erythrocytes. At plasma concentrations between 25 and 500 ng/ml, this population will account for approximately 50% of cellular binding and shows a linear

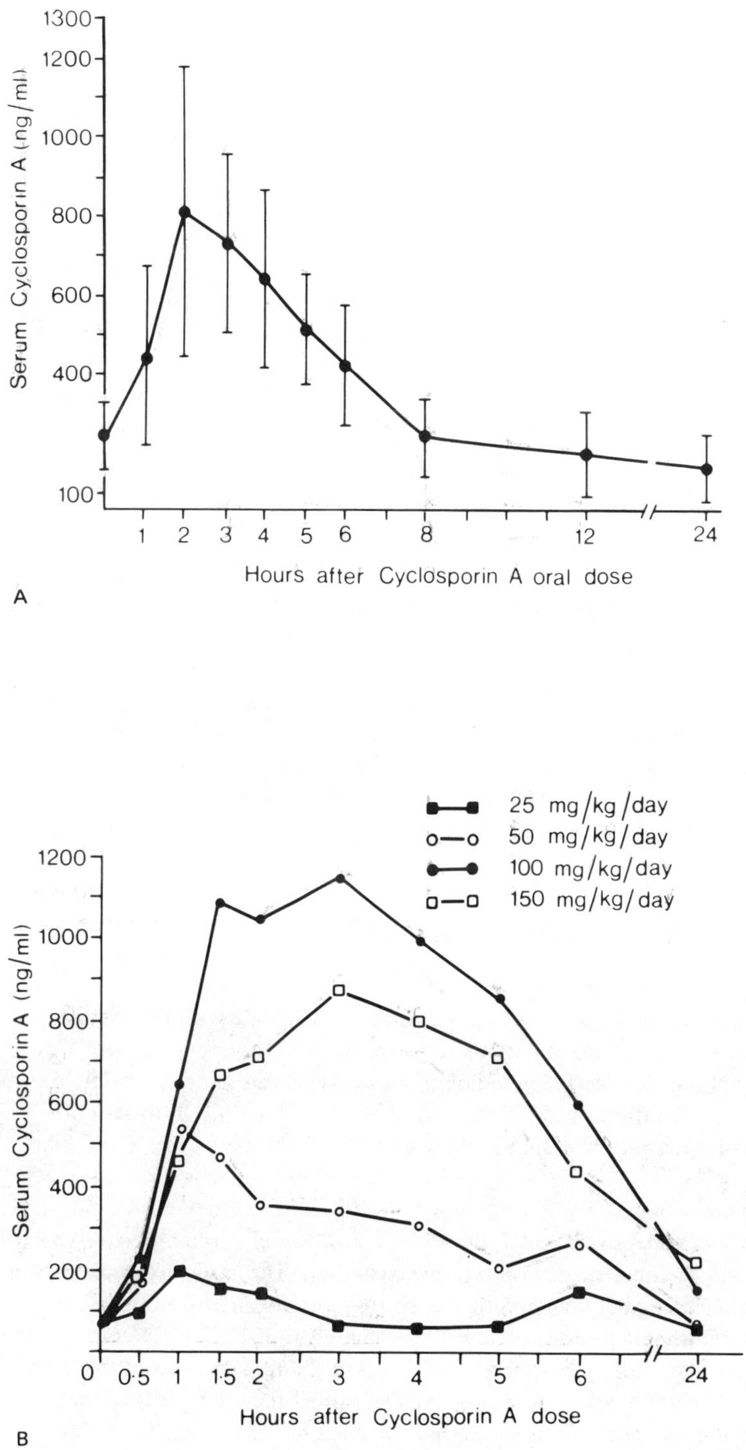

Figure 3 Mean plasma level from eight studies, showing peak at 2 hr. (From Ref. 66.)

distribution with dosage. The leukocyte accumulation varies between 10 and 20% and appears to be a saturable process. The importance of this compartment may be underestimated if only binding capacity is considered, but it may play an important role if there is differential distribution between the various leukocytes. Thus, should the major concentration occur in monocytes and lymphocytes, a greater effect on the immune process becomes a theoretical consideration.

It is this distribution pattern between the lipoproteins in the plasma compartment and the cells, notably the erythrocytes, that raises the important question of the best material for assay to monitor cyclosporin A doses. One approach would be to use radioimmunoassay to detect all immunologically related analogs and to avoid underestimating total body content by measuring levels in whole blood hemolysate.

B. Experimental Animals

Pharmacokinetic studies, including biotransformation, have been carried out in rat, dog, and monkey. In these experiments, tritium-labeled drug was used to examine absorption, distribution, and excretion characteristics, and the data are based on partitioning of total radioactivity.

In rats, absorption was low (12%) when given orally in a solution of Myglyol, with the drug eliminated mainly by the biliary route. Both oral and intravenous administration levels of radioactivity were higher in the tissue of peripheral compartment than in the blood, suggesting tissue affinity for the unchanged drug or its metabolites.

In dogs, oral absorption from a Myglyol solution was again poor, but reached 50% when administered in olive oil, with peak levels between 2 and 3 hr. Biotransformation was extensive, with only trace amounts of parent drug being detectable in the urine.

In rhesus monkeys, absorption characteristics were essentially the same as in dogs, with about 20% of the drug excreted by the kidneys and the biliary route accounting for the majority.

In rabbits, absorption was poor from polyethylene glycol. The presence of a major metabolite and absence of parent drug in the urine were evidence in favor of extensive biotransformation.

In our rabbit studies, we were able to confirm the poor absorption of cyclosporin A when given as the drinking solution. Even on a twice-daily schedule with doses studied systematically between 50 and 300 mg/kg, there was a relatively poor correlation between intake and plasma levels. Using radioimmunoassay, it was seldom possible to achieve consistent concentrations in the plasma in excess of 500 ng/ml. Furthermore, both time- and dose-response curves showed a peak for the rabbit between 1½ and 2 hr (Fig. 4).

The isolation and characterization of the metabolites have been extensively studied (67). The isolation was undertaken on DEAE A25 Sephadex and chromatography on amberlite XAD-2 with the final extraction into diethyl ether. The crude components were purified by liquid chromatography and defined spectroscopically and by amino-acid analysis. The four major metabolites which were designated 1, 8, 17, and 21 contain the intact oligopeptide structure of cyclosporin A, with minor modifications resulting from hydroxylation and N-demethylation reactions. Analysis of all the available information on the metabolism of cyclosporin A indicates that the main biotransformation takes place along a pathway leading to the production of one polar, water-soluble, metabolite designated peak 1, which has not yet been definitively characterized, and a number of associated metabolites extractable with organic solvents such as diethyl ether.

DOSE mg/kg	PRE	0.5	1.0	1.5	2.0	3.0	4.0	5.0	6.0	24.0	
		HR AFTER CYCLOSPORIN-A DOSE									
25	62	62	175	190	175	62	62	62			
	62	120	210	120	110	62	62	62	150	62	
Mean	62	91	192	155	142	62	62	62	150	62	
50	62	115	340	410	320	340	205	85			
	62	215	725	525	380	330	410	330	260	62	
Mean	62	165	532	467	350	335	307	207	260	62	
100	62	62	125	205	950	85					
	62	360	1200	1675	1000	1075	850	775	410	190	
	62	105	525	1075	1400	1650	1050	975	925	170	same rabbit at beg.
	62	385	850	1375	1650	1750	1075	825	440	62	& end of 1 week of
Mean	62	228	649	1082	1043	1140	991	858	592	140	CSA
150	62	135	700	925	950	700	490	155	62	62	
	62	225	245	380	470	925	1250	1475	825	315	same rabbit at beg.
	62	170	435	75	700	1000	650	525	500	270	& end of 1 week of
Mean	62	176	460	663	706	875	796	718	441	215	CSA

Figure 4 Rabbit studies showing relationship between peak levels and time at different oral doses of cyclosporin A. The dose approximation in serum levels between the 100 and 150 kg/mg/day curves suggests that an absorption maximum may operate for oral cyclosporin A.administration. (From Ref. 66.)

In the light of this information, it should be realized that the pharmacokinetic data which are based on radioactive measurements do not, therefore, differentiate between the parent drug and its major, closely related, derivatives.

In summary, it can be stated, first, that absorption is critically dependent upon the composition of the oral dosage form with Myglyol being a less satisfactory vehicle than when ^{3}H-OL-27-400 is dissolved in olive oil. In the former situation, absorption ranges between 2 and 12%, but this may approach 50% in olive oil. It appears that the absorption in humans, when cyclosporin A is given in olive oil, approximates that in dogs. It is of note that the time to achieve peak concentration is also shorter with olive oil, being in the range 2-4 hr, but as long as 24 hr with Myglyol.

Second, the blood levels, which may usefully be compared using the β phase, are seen to have a half-life between 27 hr for humans and approximately 50 hr for monkey, with dog being intermediate. This latter point is of particular interest, since it raises important considerations for scheduling a therapeutic dosage of cyclosporin A.

Third, excretion, when studied after a single dose of cyclosporin A, is influenced by route, formulation, and dose. A fairly consistent pattern is demonstrable between all the animal species studied and humans, with approximately 10% appearing in the urine (range 1.1=23.2%) within the first 96 hr and the remainder demonstrable in feces (range 43.1= 90.6%) in the same time period. It therefore appears that renal excretion is only a minor pathway of elimination in all the species tested and is lowest when it is administered in the form of either Myglyol or polyethylene glycol (PEG 200). The major route is via the bile, as indicated by the recovery of radioactivity in the feces. In dog and monkey, excretion is incomplete following an intravenous administration, whereas 80-90% of the radiolabel can be recovered in all species after oral administration. This inconsistency again focuses attention on the differential distribution that cyclosporin A may achieve between compartments and emphasizes the need for further studies on biotransformation.

Fourth, such biotransformation data as are available are most complete for rabbit, dog, and humans, where similar metabolite patterns have been demonstrated in plasma and in urine.

Finally, protein binding, particularly in the therapeutic concentration range, shows partition between lipoprotein and red cells, but it is clear that data for the different metabolites are as yet incomplete. This latter consideration may have important bearing on not only assay methods but choice of compartment and cyclosporin level selected to monitor therapy.

C. Dosage and Drug Monitoring

Based on the pharmacokinetic data, no uniform recommendation can be made about cyclosporin A administration in humans. Three generalizations are possible. First, sufficient drug must be given for an adequate period of time to allow equilibration between plasma lipoprotein and other compartments before patients are transferred to maintenance programs. Second, the monitoring of plasma levels by high-pressure liquid chromatography provides different information from that derived by radioimmunoassay. The former measures parent substance only, whereas the latter would include immunologically identifiable analogs, some of which share immunosuppressive properties, albeit less than the parent substance. In this regard, it is not yet known which assay method is preferable, particularly since the relative toxicity of the parent substance and metabolites has not been defined. Thus, the relationship between the administered material and its metabolites with immunological reactivity and toxicity require clarification. Third, the relative value of plasma as opposed to red cell or leukocyte concentration has not been fully explored. Initial data using radioimmunoassay show a discrepancy between plasma and red cell levels.

In our studies (66), the red cell levels are consistently higher, so that tissue binding may be underestimated by measurements of plasma level alone. Thus far, we have not been able to clearly define a constant relationship, at any one moment, between levels obtained by radioimmunoassay of serum or red cell hemolysate in patients receiving therapeutic doses of cyclosporin A.

In this state of uncertainty, a sound principle would appear to be the administration of sufficient cyclosporin A to achieve a predetermined plasma level by radioimmunoassay. This dose would then be decreased in the presence of toxic effects or increased with the development of escape phenomena such as rejection or emergence of graft-versus-host disease. Our current practice is to correlate serum levels with those in the peripheral tissue compartment, as reflected in red cell cyclosporin A concentration determined by the same assay.

Four additional points require emphasis. First, in the field of organ transplantation, it has not been established what considerations other than dosage and plasma levels need to be incorporated into the design of immunosuppressive schedules. For example, bearing in mind the time taken to achieve plasma levels following oral administration and the absence of data defining the rate at which tissue compartments are saturated, the period before transplantation in which the recipient should be treated is unknown. Furthermore, at least in the case of allogeneic bone marrow transplantation, the question of pretreating the donor cannot be ignored.

Second, the question of cyclosporin A and drug interaction is still confused. When combined with glucocorticosteroids in vitro, there is experimental evidence to support combination therapy. However, despite studies in a variety of animal species and using differing experimental models to examine this problem in the allografting of kidney, heart, lung, and bone marrow, there is no uniformity of opinion. Thus, at the present time, the role of cyclosporin A as a single agent or in combination with other drugs or radiotherapy to achieve safe but optimal immunosuppression awaits clarification.

The situation in humans (27) has raised questions about adding prednisolone and a cyclosphosphamide derivative to cyclosporin A therapy in patients thought to be rejecting their kidneys. Here, too, the relative merits of this agent alone or in combination continue to be actively debated.

Third, consideration needs to be given to the immunosuppressive properties of cyclosporin A in predisposing patients to severe bacterial and viral infections and, undoubtedly, the risk would be increased when combined with other immunosuppressive agents. Similarly, the theoretical possibility exists that cyclosporin A, either singly or in combination with other effective agents, may predispose patients to the emergence of second tumors. Concern, for example, about emergence of lymphomas has already been expressed (68); but the specific situation in the patient with chronic renal disease may be different (69), and there is need for caution to avoid prematurely incriminating this drug in the pathogenesis of second malignancies.

Last, the nephrotoxicity associated with cyclosporin A emphasizes the risk of interaction with other drugs potentially likely to impair renal function. These include the aminoglycoside antibiotics which may be present in plasma concentrations not normally considered dangerous. A similar argument applies to some of the diuretics, and these assume importance in many of the clinical situations where cyclosporin A is given to severely ill patients whose renal function is compromised in consequence of their underlying disease.

Drug interaction with cyclosporin A is clearly important. It is incumbent upon physicians using this agent to be fully informed of the theoretical hazards. On the one hand, there is the need to constantly monitor the patients for the adequacy of cyclosporin levels present in plasma or tissue compartment. On the other hand, one should pay attention to additional complications that may arise in consequence of drug interaction, especially the early biochemical changes of deteriorating renal function.

V. TOXICOLOGY

In experimental models and clinical studies, a number of side effects have been reported. The majority are dose related, being reversible with reduction in cyclosporin A dosage.

A. Experimental Studies

Acute toxicity has been examined in mouse, rat, and rabbit, following oral and intravenous injections. Wide differences were found among species, with 14 day LD_{50} being, respectively, 107, 25.4, and greater than 10 mg/kg/day for intravenous route and approximately 2500, 1500, and greater than 1000 for oral administration. Dyspnea, tachypnea, cramplike movements, stupor, pilo-erection, and death occurred within 3 hr after intravenous injection and up to 9 days with oral administration, diarrhea was a prominent sign with enteral administration.

Chronic studies in rats at oral doses of 14 mg/kg/day showed reduced circulating lymphocytes and a generalized atrophy of lymphoid tissue. At higher doses of 45 and 90 mg/kg/day, death resulted from hepatic and renal toxicity, but in animals surviving after discontinuation of cyclosporin A administration, biochemical tests of hepatic and renal function returned to normal. There was associated cloudy swelling of renal tubular epithelium and single cell necrosis in the liver. It is noteworthy that the red cell series was reduced.

In dogs, low doses of 5 and 15 mg/kg/day were tolerated without toxicity, but diarrhea and conjunctival hyperemia were encountered at 45 mg/kg/day, food intake was irregularly reduced, and weight decreased. The hematology was altered by an increased erythrocyte sedimentation rate, anemia, and decrease in white cell and platelet counts.

In rabbits, three extensive toxicity studies (66) using New Zealand White males with a starting weight of 3 kg have been completed. The animals were individually housed in stainless steel cages in a temperature-controlled vivarium. Water and complete rabbit diet (Epol, Johannesburg) were allowed freely.

The animals in the first study received a single daily oral administration of cyclosporin A (OL 27-400, Sandoz) in a volume of 3 ml, with a loading dose of 25 mg/kg/day in the first week and 12.5 mg/kg/day in the ensuing 12 weeks. At the end of this period, dosage escalation was undertaken with half the animals being maintained at 25 mg/kg/day and the other half at 50 mg/kg/day for 8 weeks; in a further 8-week period, doses were doubled to 50 and 100 mg/kg/day in the two groups, respectively. In all the animals, blood count, chemistry, and radioimmunoassay for cyclosporin A were undertaken weekly. During this study, all the animals gained weight consistently to an average of 4 kg by day 62. Regular monitoring of plasma cyclosporin A levels showed a peak absorption at 1½ hr following oral dosage and maintenance of plasma levels between 100 and 400 ng/ml that had returned to baseline by 6 hr (Fig. 4). No toxic effects were demonstrable on hematopoiesis, but transient elevations in hepatic enzymes were documented at dosage levels above 50 mg/kg/day. The only consistent abnormality was an increase in plasma creatinine, which promptly reversed on discontinuing therapy.

In a second toxicity study, cyclosporin A was given at doses of 50 and 100 mg/kg/day for 17 weeks. There was a consistent fall in hemoglobin, down to a mean of 10 g/dl, and some minor reduction in platelet count that was not statistically significant. Detailed examination of autopsy material showed generalized bone marrow hyperplasia, focal areas of hepatic necrosis, and cloudy swelling with acute tubular necrosis in the kidneys of some animals.

In the third study, higher doses of 75 mg/kg were given twice a day in a deliberate attempt to define any acute toxic effects that may develop within 6 weeks. In a subsequent 6-week period, doses were doubled, in a stepwise manner, to 300 mg/kg/day on a split schedule. In these animals, the pattern of toxicity was essentially the same as that found at the lower doses. At these higher doses, the absorption peak is delayed and elimination is slower (Fig. 4).

The rabbit studies may be summarized by stating that oral administration of cyclosporin A results in demonstrable serum levels when measured by radioimmunoassay, and even at high dosage, minimal clinical toxicity is found over prolonged periods of study. The only two constant hematologic observations were mild to moderate reduction in hemoglobin level in the presence of a normocellular bone marrow with an intact maturation sequence and variable reduction in blood lymphocyte count. At all dosage levels, reversible biochemical changes of renal dysfunction occurred, reflected by elevations in serum creatinine level, although blood urea usually remained normal. Histological examination of the kidneys showed cloudy swelling and, in occasional animals, acute tubular necrosis. Lymph nodes and spleen had general reduction of lymphoid tissue following prolonged periods of administration, and this was associated with an increased rate of infection late in the course of those animals receiving high doses of cyclosporin A.

Studies on carcinogenesis in a variety of animals have failed to demonstrate embryotoxicity or teratogenicity in nontoxic doses. Similarly, mutagenicity using *Salmonella typhimurium* as an indicator organism was unsuccessful. Tumors did not develop in any of our rabbits.

B. Clinical Trials

1. Patient Tolerance

Both the presently available drinking solution (Sandoz, Basel) and the intravenous preparation are tolerated without any gastrointestinal tract discomfort. With experience now in excess of 3 years, we can endorse the recommendation that the cyclosporin A be given in milk containing a taste-disguising additive such as cocoa, chocolate, or Caotina.

2. Nephrotoxicity

The major side effect of cyclosporin A administration is nephrotoxicity, but many of the studies in humans are difficult to interpret because the drug has been used following kidney grafting or after major surgery for pancreatic or hepatic transplantation (70). A similar problem arises when it is administered either to facilitate engraftment or to control graft-versus-host disease in patients receiving allogeneic bone marrow grafts (28).

In patients undergoing renal grafting, data reporting the effect of long-term cyclosporin A on renal function (71) at a dosage level of 5.9 mg/kg body weight (range 4.0-8.6) were compared with a posttransplantation regimen containing corticosteroids and azathioprine. This study included three renal biopsies which showed nonspecific changes of interstitial nephritis which may reflect low-grade graft rejection or cyclosporin A toxicity. It is noteworthy that plasma cyclosporin A levels are not reported, although the authors indicate that this is desirable. Similarly, cyclosporin A is reported as a feasible immunosuppressive agent in patients with oliguric acute tubular necrosis (72), and this group has initiated a randomized prospective study comparing prednisone with cyclosporin A with prednisone, azathioprine, and antilymphocyte globulin for recipients of either cadaver or live related renal grafts.

Reports on the effects of cyclosporin A in the liver and kidney transplants from America (73) confirm nephrotoxicity between 13 and 22 days of therapy in patients receiving 16.3 ± 2.9 (SEM) mg/kg/day of cyclosporin A, but that kidney function returned to normal with dosage reduction to 9.2 ± 2.3 (SEM) mg/kg/day. Of note was the fact that 4 of 66 patients were switched from cyclosporin A to azathioprine after 4-8 months because of persisting unsatisfactory renal function; in 3 of them graft function improved. The experience of this group is that cyclosporin A is nephrotoxic but that this is easily reversed even after many months of treatment. This study is again limited by the fact that plasma cyclosporin A levels were not used in the decision-making process.

It would appear that the nephrotoxicity is due to a tubular effect (74), although other renal biopsy studies have shown no significant glomerular or tubular lesions (75), and this author has commented on possible protective effects of a mannitol-induced diuresis. Apart from mild and transient elevations of blood urea, nitrogen, and creatinine, glomerular thromboses and severe tubular damage have been reported (76) to correlate with both the clinical course and laboratory findings of severe renal failure in three recipients of allogeneic marrow grafts who were given prophylactic cyclosporin A. These workers emphasized that rising creatinine concentration, accompanied by thrombocytopenia, microangiopathic anemia, and hypertension, suggests cyclosporin A nephrotoxicity and that kidney biopsy at the onset of renal failure may help elucidate the early principal lesions, since autopsy data probably represent a combination of effects.

Our studies (66) would suggest that cyclosporin A is toxic to renal tubules in a dose-dependent and reversible manner. In a series of patients receiving cyclosporin A as primary immunosuppressive therapy for severe acute aplastic anemia, without prior allogeneic bone marrow transplantation, a predictable increase in biochemical parameters of renal function correlates with increasing administration of the drug. Creatinine is affected more than the urea level, although both bear a linear relationship to peak and trough cyclosporin A levels measured by radioimmunoassay in serum samples (66). Based on these studies, we endorse the observations of the Swiss group (77) that any increase in serum creatinine levels, particularly while still within the normal range, should be treated by oral administration of loop-acting diuretics. Our practice is to commence 40 mg of furosemide in the morning and, if the biochemical changes have not stabilized or started to reverse within 24 hr, to add a second dose in the evening. Further increase in creatinine level on this regimen is managed by 25% reduction in cyclosporin A dosage while monitoring plasma levels. Used in this way, we have found nephrotoxicity related to cyclosporin A an easily controllable problem. Red cell RIA is now recommended as preferable to plasma assay.

These observations have been extended to patients following allogeneic bone marrow transplantation and, to date, such meticulous control of dosage with regular biochemical monitoring has resulted in equal ease of control of cyclosporin A toxic effects.

Two points require additional comment. The administration of cyclosporin A with other potentially nephrotoxic drugs, notably, the aminoglycoside antibiotics, results in deteriorating renal function despite antibiotic levels being monitored and remaining in the supposedly nontoxic range (78). Our own practice has therefore been to avoid any agent with the potential for interfering with renal function. Currently, antibiotics of choice are third-generation cephalosporins, and their use has virtually abolished our previous experience of renal failure related to drug administration.

Second, with regard to histological changes, those evident on light microscopy (76) are supplemented by ultrastructural changes (79) which suggest that cyclosporin A, or its metabolites, may interfere with mitochondrial metabolism.

3. Hepatoxicity

Biochemical evidence of liver dysfunction, in which the hyperbilirubinemia may progress to jaundice, has been reported in association with cyclosporin A administration (80,81). It is, however, necessary to bear in mind that in many of these patients, notably those following allogeneic bone marrow transplantation, other factors such as graft-versus-host disease (GVHD), septicemia, and drugs known to be hepatotoxic may, independently of cyclosporin A administration, produce similar changes. The way in which cyclosporin A compounds the problem remains unresolved. It has been suggested (80) that hyperbilirubinemia is a toxic consequence of cyclosporin A therapy rather than the cause, and it has been postulated (78) that because cyclosporin A is excreted in the bile there may be competition with the pathway used for bilirubin clearance. If this is correct, then any factor inhibiting the excretory pathway of the latter may impair excretion of cyclosporin A, leading to increased plasma levels.

Our experiences with patients undergoing allogeneic bone marrow transplantation and with those receiving cyclosporin A as a primary form of treatment for severe acute aplastic anemia, where no bone marrow transplantation option exists, show a clear temporal relationship between rising cyclosporin A levels and the development of hyperbilirubinemia, as reported by others (81). It appears that cyclosporin A-induced hyperbilirubinemia occurs with trough levels that are consistently above 400 ng/ml; accordingly, there is a need to monitor plasma levels three times a week. We have found that reduction of cyclosporin A levels will lead to a decrease in bilirubin level, provided this is not raised for some other reason, of which we have found septicemia to be the most common.

To further define the possible mechanism, an isolated rat liver model has been used (82). In this in vitro study, a variety of biochemical techniques have consistently failed to demonstrate cyclosporin A in association with ligandin or the Y-transport protein in hepatic cytosol. This evidence would suggest that competition between bilirubin and cyclosporin A for hepatic proteins is not the mechanism by which their efflux is regulated. The finding of cyclosporin A in association with the 15,000-dalton fraction is compatible with hepatic excretion via the minor or Z-protein-mediated pathway. However, a number of other enzymes, peptides, and low molecular weight proteins found in the same area have made it impossible to definitively incriminate cyclosporin A competitive binding even in this quantitatively less important route for bilirubin excretion.

It therefore appears that hepatotoxicity, and particularly hyperbilirubinemia, is a consequence of a rising plasma cyclosporin A level which, in our experience, invariably follows biochemical evidence for impaired renal function. The mechanism by which cyclosporin A exerts its hepatotoxicity is presently unknown, but direct competition with the bilirubin transport system along the lingandin pathway in the liver seems unlikely.

4. Hypertension

In patients receiving cyclosporin A, systemic hypertension and convulsions have been reported (83) and, while the pathogenesis is not clear, the available data suggest that impaired renal function causes fluid retention which promotes these events. The complications seem directly related to cyclosporin A blood levels, with younger patients being more susceptible to the toxic effects of this drug.

5. Infection

In the immunosuppressed patient following cyclosporin A administration, herpes simplex, herpes zoster, and cytomegalovirus infections have been reported (70). In the Cape Town clinical experience, the incidence of viral or bacterial infections in patients receiving cyclosporin A for aplastic anemia, who have not undergone allogeneic bone marrow transplantation, is no different from the control population. Furthermore, this finding holds true for patients undergoing allogeneic bone marrow transplantation whether they received methotrexate immunosuppression or only cyclosporin A.

6. Immunosuppression and Neoplasms

Breast lumps have been reported in two patients (84). The question of malignant disease in patients receiving cyclosporin A is complicated by the immunosuppressive effects that may be associated with end-stage renal disease and cell-mediated immunity in these patients (85). Nevertheless, concern about lymphoma developing in patients on cyclosporin A started with the report of the Cambridge group (70). Subsequently, this risk has been reemphasized (54,68,86) and, since there is a sound immunological basis for considering this possibility, caution is necessary (69).

7. Other Toxicities

We have not encountered gastrointestinal tract intolerance, pancytopenia, lymphocytopenia, or gingival hypertrophy. Hirsutism has been seen in 1 of 50 patients, and extrapyramidal signs of neurotoxicity elicited by careful examination in 5 of 50 patients, but this was short-lived in 4 and required drug dosage reduction in only 1.

VI. EXPERIMENTAL MODELS

A. Kidney Allografts

A number of experimental animal systems have established, in broad terms, the effectiveness of cyclosporin A administration in maintaining graft function and survival despite histoincompatibility. Apart from species differences, other important variables are dosage, scheduling, and mechanisms by which tolerance is induced.

In rats (87-89), cyclosporin A conferred a clear dose-related advantage to survival of kidneys transplanted from DA to Lewis strains, despite the existence of a strong histocompatibility barrier. Histological studies showed the presence of mononuclear cell infiltration, although function remained excellent. This evidence would suggest that the lymphocytotoxin or humoral antibody-mediated response, leading to acute rejection, was suppressed, whereas the cell-mediated cytotoxicity, reflected in the mononuclear cell infiltration, was little altered.

A second consideration is the presently unexplained way in which this immunosuppressive advantage is lost at high dose. Thus, although plasma levels are not quoted, when cyclosporin A was administered intravenously at 5 mg/kg/day for 14 days (90) or orally (91), levels high enough to impair renal or hepatic function lead to a paradoxical loss of immunosuppression, but it is not clear whether this represents an effect on the donor kidney or an alteration in the host immune response. These observations were extended by studying renal allograft survival in which the recipients had been previously sensitized by skin grafting for up to 5 weeks prior to kidney transplantation (88). The studies showed the drug to be relatively ineffective in suppressing rejection of a renal allograft in a previously sensitized recipient. Of particular importance is the scheduling of the immunosuppressive agent in relation to the transplantation procedure. Thus, neither pretreatment alone nor commencement after a delay of 4 days following transplantation appears effective in suppression of rejection (89,92).

In rabbits, confirmatory data have been reported. At 25 mg/kg/day by mouth, 18- or 28-day courses prolong survival of renal allografts (56,93), while untreated animals died from renal failure associated with acute rejection. In an autografted group from the same study, the survival was not statistically different from those receiving cyclosporin A. Of note was the fact that 6-mercaptopurine was less effective than cyclosporin A in maintaining graft survival. In addition, the latter agent had the unusual property of its immunosuppressive effect persisting in the rabbits after therapy had been discontinued, and this was equivalent whether given by the intramuscular or oral route.

To define the specificity of this tolerance (94-96) experiments using both skin grafts and second kidney transplants from the original or third-party donors were carried out. The accumulated results of the studies were not uniform. One group (94) interpreted the data as reflecting donor but not tissue specificity while another (96) considered the tolerance to be nonspecific. It was pointed out (97) that the discrepancies may in part be explained by the delayed appearance of donor-specific tolerance which is known to occur in the rat (57,98) and in part by the different assay methods used.

In the rabbit, mononuclear cell infiltrates were found in kidney biopsies; but their interpretation remains controversial, and Green (99) raised the possibility that cyclosporin A may have attenuated mainly the humoral antibody response or alternatively could have inhibited migration of lymphocytes. Furthermore, the author questioned whether the cells were T helper in nature or whether the phenomenon was a concentration effect because there were insufficient lymphocytes to mount an aggressive attack and destroy the organs. The latter would be a manifestation of the quantum theory (100) so that the kidneys simply underwent slow attrition over a period of many months.

In dogs (101), early studies demonstrated the immunosuppressive properties of cyclosporin A and showed these were superior to azathioprine but were less spectacular than in rats and rabbits, despite which, some animals survived for long periods after cessation of all therapy (99). In subsequent systematic studies (102), the effects were confirmed, and rejection was completely suppressed with a clear dose-response relationship (103). Of note was the fact that rejection occurred approximately 2 weeks after withdrawal of the cyclosporin A, and this response differed from that observed in the rat. Another point of distinction between species was the observation that cyclosporin A combined with prednisolone did not result in the adverse effects in dogs that had been noted in rabbits (104) and, furthermore, conversion of the immunosuppressive regimen from cyclosporin A to conventional drugs such as azathioprine or prednisone was possible (105,106).

Perhaps surprisingly, reversal of acute rejection could also result from cyclosporin A administration 4 days after allografting (107) which differs from the analagous experiment in rats and rabbits (99).

B. Allogeneic Bone Marrow Transplantation and Graft-Versus-Host Disease

In mice, Borel et al. (17) demonstrated a capacity for cyclosporin A to allow reconstitution of hematopoietic and lymphoid tissues by incompatible spleen cells and to delay the emergence of lethal graft-versus-host-disease.

In rats (45), cyclosporin A provides adequate immunosuppression both for graft acceptance and prevention of subsequent graft-versus-host disease. The animals develop a chimerism with normal immune response and repopulation of T-cell areas in lymphoid organs. The establishment of a chimeric state with specific tolerance to donor and recipient but not to third-party grafts may reflect the generation of a suppressive cell population (108,109).

In the rabbit, conflicting results have been obtained. Histoincompatible skin grafts were possible in a model where red Burgundy donor and outbred New Zealand White recipient animals were used but, at doses of 15 mg/kg subcutaneously, while engraftment occurred, graft-versus-host disease could not be prevented. The experience in Cape Town (110) is different. Using incompatible NZW and R strain animals, there is a statistically significant difference in animals receiving 10 mg/kg/day of cyclosporin A by intramuscular injection for 28 days after transplantation. Thus, at 40 days only 10% of allograft control animals were alive, whereas 44% of those receiving cyclosporin A survived. This difference was even more obvious at 100 days when none of the control animals survived but a third of those that were treated were still alive and well, with normally functioning donor grafts. Furthermore, the histologically recognizable features of graft-versus-host disease were present in all the control animals and in only 25% of those receiving cyclosporin A. It appears that in this animal model, species differences may be critical in trying to understand the differences between results obtained by the Swiss and the South African groups since, in most other respects, the experimental animal models were remarkably similar.

In dogs (41, 111-113) cyclosporin A increased the incidence of graft failure, although with engraftment median survival is prolonged and the onset of graft-versus-host disease is delayed, despite the failure to induce stable tolerance.

C. Skin Allografting

In mice (29), cyclosporin A was comparable with antilymphocyte serum for graft retention although in subsequent studies (114,115) the immunosuppressive action was demonstrable only as long as cyclosporin A was biologically active and rejection took place between 10 and 14 days after discontinuing the treatment. A similar dose-dependent prolongation of skin graft survival has been reported by other workers (116).

In rats (117), essentially the same phenomenon occurs but may be modified in animals receiving a heart graft. From this, it was suggested that when a large mass of foreign tissue is tolerated, this may be sufficient to block rejection of skin graft, whereas the smaller volume involved in transfer of skin only is incapable of exerting this effect (99).

D. Cardiac Allografts

In rats, heterotopic cardiac transplantation (118) established the potency of cyclosporin A with even short courses, preventing rejection for prolonged periods of time. Subsequently (23), attention was focused on this phenomenon, but these studies are difficult to interpret because information about plasma cyclosporin A concentration, or that found in other cellular compartments, is not available.

In rats, xenografting (119) from outbread Syrian hamsters to the renal vessels of Lewis rats results in modest prolongation of the donor heart while on an oral course of cyclosporin A of 35 mg/kg/day.

In nonhuman primate heterotopic grafting (120), it was established that cyclosporin A is superior to azathioprine and corticosteroid immunosuppression, but that prolonged treatment with this antifungal agent singly or in combination with other drugs may be necessary to maintain function.

In pigs, orthotopic grafting (24) is of particular interest since survival of control animals mismatched at the major locus was 6 days, whereas those animals to which cyclosporin A was administered at a dose of 24 mg/kg/day by intramuscular injection followed by oral maintenance had mean survival times of 265 days. The animals were healthy, without biochemical evidence of hepatic, renal, or hematologic abnormality, and established not only the effectiveness of immune suppression for cyclosporin A in this model but the fact that survival was possible for prolonged periods of time without additional treatment.

Nonhuman primate orthotopic cardiac allografting, which has important parallels for clinical practice, has been extensively studied (120-123). These experiments show that function is prolonged even in association with mononuclear cell infiltration and myocyte injury. As in the heterotopic grafting, cyclosporin A exerts a powerful immunosuppressive effect which is superior to other currently available agents; however, prolonged administration is necessary, and it may well be required in combination with other agents for optimal preservation of function.

E. Pancreatic Allografting

In rats, with segmental and pancreatic islet transplants (124-126) it has been demonstrated that cyclosporin A has a relatively modest effect, although another study (127) has been more successful in inducing long-term survival in the diabetic animals. An attempt to define reasons for both the differences found in these studies and also between results obtained with pancreas and other tissues has been made by exploring a possible role for the macrophage. Indefinite graft survival followed injection of 50 mg/100 g body weight of silica (128), suggesting that this cell system may play a special role in transplantation of this organ.

In dogs, allografting of the pancreas has been undertaken using vascularized segmental grafts, and prolonged survival is possible at high doses of cyclosporin A (129). While neither prednisolone nor azathioprine prolonged survival of animals compared with untreated grafted controls, cyclosporin A at a dose of 25 mg/kg/day orally extended the period of normoglycemia from a mean of 9 to 85 days, and of individual survival from a mean of 13 to a maximum of 129 with a mean of 72 days.

F. Lung Allografting

In dogs (130), it has been shown that survival of this organ for over 5 months was possible with cyclosporin A administered in oral doses of 17 mg/kg/day for 35 days, after which the drug was gradually reduced and given concurrently with low-dose azathioprine (2 mg/kg/day for 14 days). It was remarkable that rejection occurring while on this regimen was later in onset and more easily reversed by high-dose corticosteroids than that developing on standard immunosuppression.

Nonhuman primates (123) have a long survival following lung transplantation with cyclosporin A therapy and, apart from mild lymphocytic infiltration, rejection injury is minimal. This is particularly attractive because bacterial infection is reduced and healing mechanisms appear better preserved. It is currently necessary to define dosage and schedule, to establish whether simultaneous administration of other drugs including corticosteroids may confer additional advantages and, since malignant lymphoma may occur in the primates under these circumstances, to investigate the mechanism of tumor induction.

G. Corneal Allografting

In the rabbit (131,132), skin grafts were placed from the same donor 14 days later to ensure rejection of the cornea. In control animals, the corneal grafts were rejected promptly in contrast to a 50% survival when animals received cyclosporin A at a dosage level of 25 mg/kg by intramuscular route for 28 days from the time of the operation. With a shorter period of administration (14 days), the survival period was intermediate between control and 28-day administrations. Skin graft survival was also prolonged but invariably shorter than the cornea.

Topical application of cyclosporin A was not effective in preventing graft rejection, and it is speculated that this may be due to the scheduling of cyclosporin A and the provocative antigen. It also remains uncertain whether the physical and biological stability of the immunosuppressive agent is altered in the aqueous medium on the surface of the eye.

H. Skeletal Muscle

Cyclosporin A has been demonstrated to permit persistence of an allograft in A and CVA mice, whereas in the nontolerant hosts the allografts were rejected between the tenth and the twelfth day (133).

I. Nerve and Schwann Cells

It has been demonstrated (134) that both minor and major antigens evoke an immune response that prevents functional regeneration in nerve allografts. Nerve fibers, however, regenerate in immunosuppressed hosts. In an extension of these studies (135), it was demonstrated that cyclosporin A can prevent the rejection of nerve allografts with host axon regeneration through long nerve segments.

J. In Vivo Cell-Mediated Immune Reactions

The delayed hypersensitivity skin reaction to oxazolone in mice (20) defined by the suppressive index induced in the skin reaction was examined for both primary and secondary response. It emerged that when cyclosporin A, cyclophosphamide, and azathioprine were compared, the most favorable ratio between toxic and pharmacological effects was found with cyclosporin A.

In guinea pigs, the delayed skin reaction to tuberculin (21) showed a clear advantage for cyclosporin A over large doses of phenylbutazone and azathioprine. The data also supported differences in action between cyclosporin A and the anti-inflammatory agent, phenylbutazone, with the former inhibiting effector cells at clinically well-tolerated doses, whereas phenylbutazone produced severe side effects; azathioprine, although impairing the hypersensitivity reaction, was associated with deaths in some of the animals.

Cell-mediated cytolysis in mice (16) was characterized by clear dose-dependent inhibition of allogeneic target cell lysis by specifically sensitized lymphoid cells. In this assay system, cyclosporin A was compared with procarbazine, cyclophosphamide, the epipodophyllotoxin VP 16-213, and antilymphocyte serum. The results showed a general cytostatic action of procarbazine, cyclophosphamide, and the epipodophyllotoxin whereas cyclosporin A, in common with antilymphocyte serum, appeared primarily to affect lymphocytes at the stage of sensitization.

K. Immune Experimental Models

1. Experimental Allergic Encephalomyelitis (EAE)

In rats, primary sensitization with an emulsion containing spinal cord and killed dried *Mycobacterium* smegma caused the development of paralysis in control animals (39), and some 8-10 days later in those treated with cyclosporin A at the time of sensitization (39,136). A greater effect was obtained with oral doses of cyclosporin A between 50 and 100 mg/kg than was seen when azathioprine was given as a reference drug. It appears that in this particular test model, cyclosporin A inhibits sensitization and suppresses the effector phase but is not curative, since withdrawal of treatment is followed by development of symptoms after a lag period of 1-2 weeks.

In guinea pigs (137), cyclosporin A was highly effective in suppressing EAE at doses of 35 mg/kg, given on either a prophylactic or a therapeutic schedule. Of note was an unexplained sex difference in the response to drug, with the greater effect being evident in females. Predictably, prophylaxis was the more effective and such therepeutic benefit as occurred may reflect prevention of T-lymphocyte recruitment to perpetuate the inflammatory reaction.

In the rhesus monkey (138), paralysis killed control animals between day 22 and day 42. In the test group which received 50 mg/kg of cyclosporin A every alternate day, the disease was suppressed, and one animal relapsed but responded to intramuscular injections of the same dose. A similar finding was present in a second animal, while two others developed no neurological signs. Secondary challenge 204 days after beginning the experiment did not alter progression of the established disease. Of note is the finding that two of these aninals never developed the disease while on cyclosporin A, despite sensitization. The ability to mount a secondary response is seen as evidence that priming must have taken place, leading to the formation of memory cells.

The information obtained in these studies on experimental allergic encephalomyelitis is of relevance for similar demyelinating diseases in man, such as multiple sclerosis and postinfectious encephalomyelitis.

2. Freund Adjuvant Arthritis

In rats (21), when comparing the effects of cyclosporin A, phenylbutazone, and azathioprine on the prevention and treatment of arthritis, the most striking benefits were found when 30 mg/kg/day of cyclosporin A was given orally on a prophylactic schedule with some limited inhibition also occurring once the arthritis had become clinically manifest. On the preventive schedules, cyclosporin A appeared better than both phenylbutazone and azathioprine, but the expression of the ED^{50} on a milligram per kilogram basis may not be the most valid basis for comparison. Once arthritis was established, the drugs were given from days 14 to 20 inclusive, and here, azathioprine was not effective, while there was little to chose from between phenylbutazone and cyclosporin A. It was pointed out (21) that the peptide is inactive in the acute inflammatory process, and is without effect in carragenan paw edema and other such models.

3. Experimental Autoimmune Uveitis

In rats (139), cyclosporin A was effective when given concomitantly with the retinal S-antigen at 10 mg/kg, and caused partial prevention of uveitis down to 5 mg/kg/day. Even when the daily injections were started 7 days after immunization, treatment was effective, but here a higher dose of 40 mg/kg/day was needed to suppress the inflammatory process in the eye.

4. Lupus Erythematosus

In New Zealand mice, the classic model for the study of this autoimmune entity, proteinuria and mortality were the end points of a study (136) comparing the use of cyclosporin A with cyclophosphamide, and showed that at 20 mg/kg/day, cyclosporin A had no effect on proteinuria. This physical sign was, however, markedly suppressed when doses were increased to 60 mg/kg/day, and the result was the same as could be achieved with cyclophosphamide at 60 mg/kg/day given in a 10-day course. Mortality increased gradually through the 18 months of the study, with the first deaths occurring at 8 months and reaching 50% at 12 months. Cyclosporin A was less effective than cyclophosphamide in protecting animals from the autoimmune disease in this model, and therefore the interpretation and extrapolation of relatively incomplete data in humans would be inappropriate. Further detailed characterization is necessary, including patterns of response in other experimental animals. While potentially of value, the preliminary data suggest the need for caution in using cyclosporin A in patients with systemic lupus erythematosus.

5. Experimental Infections

Neither bacterial infections in mice nor fungal infestations in mice or guinea pigs appear to be adversely affected by cyclosporin A administration. Viral infections in mice and guinea pigs are marginally altered by cyclosporin A, but currently the evidence is insufficient to incriminate this substance in aggravating this risk.

An antimalarial effect has been reported for cyclosporin A in the mouse (140) in which cyclosporin A started concurrently with the inoculation of the *Plasmodium berghi* or *chabaudi* were less effective than treatment started when parasitemia was already established. The available evidence suggests that the antimalarial action results from direct toxic effect to the parasites.

In the mouse (141), cyclosporin A has been reported to exert an effect on *Schistosoma mansoni* by significantly reducing the number of mature and immature male, and to a greater extent female, worms.

VII. CLINICAL TRIALS

A. Renal Transplantation

The initial study with cyclosporin A in man (27) was in seven patients on dialysis with renal failure who were given kidneys from mismatched cadaver donors and immunosuppressed with intramuscular cyclosporin A for 3 postoperative days and then maintained on oral administration. While establishing clearly the value of cyclosporin A in clinical renal transplantation and the fact that this occurred without marrow toxicity, two other important points emerged. First, while there was no histological evidence for severe rejection, a number of patients had poorer function immediately after transplantation than had been anticipated, necessitating the addition of the other immunosuppressive agents, prednisolone and cytimum, on the basis that low-grade rejection was occurring. In these patients, neophrotoxicity, reflected in raised serum creatinine and urea levels, improved when cyclosporin A dosage was reduced or the drug was withdrawn.

The Cambridge experience was then extended (70), confirming the value of cyclosporin A in the immunosuppression of cadaveric organ grafts and drawing attention to the higher incidence of infection, often lethal, when cyclosporin A was combined with prednisolone or alkylating agents. The occurrence of lymphoreticular malignancy was noted in these patients (142). In addition, when this drug was used in patients who were well hydrated (143), 1-year graft survival was 86%; 11 of 32 patients retained good function for between 3 months and 2 years, never having received steroids; and 13 others required these agents for the treatment of rejection only. The nephrotoxicity associated with cyclosporin A can be anticipated from regular monitoring of plasma or whole blood levels with appropriate dosage adjustment if necessary.

In a controlled trial (97), cyclosporin A was compared with the established azathioprine, low-dose prednisolone regimen in diuresing patients who have received HLA-DR incompatible kidneys. With 35 patients studied, graft survival was comparable and, furthermore, this improved on conversion to azathioprine and prednisolone. The presence of cellular infiltrate in biopsy specimens has led these workers to consider steroids necessary in conjunction with cyclosporin A with the intention of avoiding longstanding renal damage from rejection.

At least two other clinical experiences can now be analyzed, since sufficient numbers of patients are available for study. In the United States (144,145), cyclosporin A has been combined with prednisolone, and again there have been graft survivals of approximately 80% at 1 year. These investigators consider it important to use corticosteroids in conjunction with cyclosporin A rather than the latter agent on its own.

On balance, there is little double that the experience in experimental animals applies also to allografting in humans. There is a consensus that cyclosporin A is effective, but the major unresolved issue is whether this should be used as a single drug or whether long-term benefit will accrue from combination with other agents, such as prednisolone, and perhaps in combination with azathioprine. To a lesser extent, but nevertheless of major importance, are the side effects. These include gum hypertrophy, hirsutism, tremor, and hepatoxicity with the problems of infection and the possibility of lymphoma in the immunocompromised host still to be defined.

B. Bone Marrow Transplantation

In the initial study (28), cyclosporin A was given to five patients with acute leukemia for the treatment of graft-versus-host disease, with poor results. In an extended study (146), cyclosporin A was used in conjunction with allogeneic sibling bone marrow transplantation to treat 23 patients, and 15 are reported to be in good health; 1 has developed florid graft-versus-host disease.

In Cape Town, the initial experience in a small number of patients treated with cyclosporin A alone for immunosuppression following allogeneic bone marrow transplantation showed no difference in the incidence of acute or the later development of chronic graft-versus-host disease. The one remarkable observation, however, was that where patients on cyclosporin A did develop acute graft-versus-host disease, this could be rapidly controlled with high-dose prednisolone, whereas we have previously been unsuccessful in managing fulminating GVHD with any currently available immunosuppressive agent.

On the basis of our experience, two considerations have arisen. The first of these is that time- and dose-response curves show a lag period of some 7 days before adequate trough levels are found in the plasma after oral administration of 25 mg/kg/day, suggesting that some time is necessary to saturate peripheral compartments. Under these circumstances, the rationale for giving cyclosporin A together with the donor marrow graft is suspect, and recipients therefore receive cyclosporin A long enough before the antigen to stabilize serum trough levels between 200 and 350 ng/ml and peak levels between 500 and 750 ng/ml.

A second and equally important consideration is whether the donor should be pretreated with cyclosporin A. On the basis that graft-versus-host disease, particularly the acute variant, may reflect transfer of immunologically competent lymphocytes to the recipient, we have followed this policy in the last six patients. All donors take cyclosporin A only after having been fully appraised of the risks and after having given informed consent. To date, no donor toxicity has been encountered, and it is remarkable that the last six consecutive transplant patients have been devoid of graft-versus-host disease. These initial observations require confirmation.

Experience with one patient was initially perplexing in that she developed GVHD on the regimen of donor and patient pretreatment with cyclosporin A where we would not have anticipated this. Plasma levels showed immeasurable quantities of cyclosporin A, and the patient was insistent that she was taking the drug. However, on admission to hospital, measurement of the dose-response curve showed a prompt oral absorption. Unfortunately, grade 1 cutaneous GVHD had emerged in a butterfly distribution on her face, and while this has not extended, it has also not resolved with continued cyclosporin A and prednisolone treatment. This finding is in keeping with our experience that reversal of established GVHD is less satisfactory than prophylaxis with cyclosporin A.

Two points are of particular interest. The first of these is the question of nephrotoxicity which we find to occur universally in our patients. We completely endorse the Swiss experience (147) that meticulous regular monitoring of plasma urea, creatinine, and clearance levels is mandatory. Any rise in the creatinine level, even while in the normal range, is managed by low-dose loop-acting diurectic and, under these circumstances, control is rapidly achieved providing peak and trough plasma levels are in the arbitrarily defined therepeutic range. Rarely is it necessary to reduce the cyclosporin A dosage in patients because of deteriorating renal function when early management to promote diuresis has been started. In one patient, failure to appreciate the graviity of a rising creatinine level required drug withdrawal and, on continuing diuresis, renal function returned to normal within 14 days. Creatinine clearance, corrected for surface area and renal biopsy, was normal, and the patient subsequently tolerated further cyclosporin A therapy without undue sensitivity to the drug.

We consider the concomitant use of nephrotoxic agents, notably aminoglycoside antibiotics, particularly hazardous. It has therefore been our policy to replace these with third-generation cephalosporins which are considerably less damaging to the kidney, and we are convinced that the drug interaction, leading to impaired renal function on the basis of cyclosporin A administration, has sharply decreased.

The second point is the development of hepatotoxicity, and we have yet to see our first patient where this has occurred ahead of renal failure. When biochemical disturbances in liver function arise, the release of hepatic enzymes into the plasma usually occurs and, in our opinion, reflects GVHD. Hyperbilirubinemia occurs in occasional patients where cyclosporin A administration is improperly controlled or where adequate management of deteriorating renal function has not taken place. Two patients managed with less frequent clinic visits than we consider optimum, because of domestic circumstances, have had transient periods of jaundice. In both, renal function has sharply deteriorated, cyclosporin A levels were high, and in both, drug discontinuation, forced diuresis, and correction of plasma levels of cyclosporin A resulted in bilirubin returning to normal within 21 days. These patients remain on cyclosporin A without the development of GVHD and without further complications, but require close clinical supervision.

On the basis of our pilot study we believe that pretreatment of donor with cyclosporin A to a standardized plasma or preferably whole blood level can be achieved with minimal side effects and may beneficially influence incidence and severity of acute GVHD. To define this schedule further it is presently being randomly and prospectively compared to a control group in which donors are not pretreated; the recipients in both arms of the trial start CSA 14 days before autograft and continue for at least 180 days.

C. Liver Transplantation

Clinical experience (70,143,144) has been encouraging and doses of 10 mg/kg have not been associated with major hepatotoxicity. However, rejection remains a problem, and it has been concluded (144) that cyclosporin A must be combined with prednisone.

D. Pancreas Transplantation

To date, clinical experience has been limited (70), but the attraction of an immunosuppressive agent which would make it unnecessary to use corticosteroids with their profound effects on carbohydrate metabolism cannot be denied. The published data are insufficient to be able to see the procedure of vascularized segmental pancreatic allografting in any role other than developmental, but the preliminary experience with cyclosporin A (99) in immunosuppressive therapy is encouraging.

E. Nontransplantation Experience

1. Rheumatoid Arthritis

In this condition (148), data are insufficient for any critical evaluation. However, it is interesting that gastrointestinal tract intolerance with reversible nephrotoxicity occurs and that some degree of hepatoxicity is reported. It is difficult, however, to establish the time sequence between toxic effects on the kidney and on the liver in this study.

2. Severe Acute Aplastic Anemia

In Cape Town, a prospective randomized clinical evaluation has been carried out in patients who meet the internationally defined criteria for severe acute aplastic anemia, but who lack a donor option, to compare cyclosporin A with cyclosporin A in combination with antilymphocyte globulin. The patients were evaluated immunologically with cell membrane surface marker studies and for in vitro erythroid colony growth in the presence of the immunosuppressive agent. By such parameters, no response to cyclosporin A has been obtained. Of particular note has been the opportunity to study, over a mean period of 2 years (range 6 months to 3 years), cyclosporin A toxicity in these patients whose course is not complicated by the severe morbidity of allogeneic bone marrow transplantation.

Quite clearly, nephrotoxicity occurs on a reversible basis. Early recognition of a rising plasma creatinine, while peak and trough plasma cyclosporin A levels are still in an established therapeutic range, can often avert progression by the addition of small doses of loop-acting diuretics. In two patients who followed this course and then underwent renal biopsy, only nonspecific changes were found. Hyperbilirubinemia was encountered in three patients where very high cyclosporin A levels were present in the plasma and where renal function was severely compromised. In each of these, renal function returned to normal within 28 days following the start of diuretics and adjustment of cyclosporin A plasma levels, and bilirubin level returned to normal more slowly but did not remain elevated in any.

In the second phase of the same clinical trial, patients failing to improve on cyclosporin A, with or without antilymphocyte serum, are receiving a 6-month trial of additional anabolic androgen and corticosteroid therapy. None of these patients has improved, despite the longer period of treatment, and no additional toxicity has been noted. Perhaps surprisingly, hepatotoxicity associated with anabolic androgen administration has not been a problem.

In the second phase of the same clinical trial, patients failing to improve on cyclosporin A, with or without antilymphocyte serum, are receiving a 6-month trial of additional anabolic androgen and corticosteroid therapy. None of these patients has improved, despite the longer period of treatment, and no additional toxicity has been noted. Perhaps surprisingly, hepatotoxicity associated with anabolic androgen administration has not

3. Psoriasis

In psoriasis (149), there has been dramatic reduction reported in skin lesions, but these recur on discontinuing therapy.

4. Primary Biliary Cirrhosis

In primary biliary cirrhosis, a significant decrease in the ratio of helper to suppressor T cells has been reported (150); these changes are not seen in other forms of cholestatic liver disease but bear a close similarity to those described in chronic GVHD. In this study, the proportion of suppressor T lymphocytes and liver function improved in six patients, confirming the immunoregulatory action of cyclosporin A, but prolonged studies were precluded by nephrotoxicity.

VIII. COMMENTS

The scientific publications on the pharmacology, immunology, experimental studies in animals, and clinical trials of cyclosporin A increase daily. Despite all this work, a considerable time will need to elapse before the role that cyclosporin A comes to occupy among the immunosuppressive agents is defined. Nevertheless, the availability of this unique fungal metabolite represents an advance in current immunosuppressive therapy. In order to realize the potential that this agent has, both in basic immunology and in clinical practice, effort will be needed to resolve a number of important issues.

First, the specific action of cyclosporin A remains controversial. The bulk of evidence favors interference with a particular molecular event involving Interleukin 1 early in antigen recognition. This phenomenon finds its expression as impairment of those immunological responses that depend upon T-lymphocyte help for their optimum activity. Not surprisingly, both humoral and cell-mediated mechanisms have been reported as being defective in the presence of this agent. Of fundamental scientific interest is the need to disentangle the effect on lymphocyte subpopulations and their interactions with other cells of which the monocyte-macrophage system is of special interest.

Second, there is the question of pharmacology. While preliminary observations are available for experimental animals and for humans, it is still not known how best to monitor cyclosporin A therapy. Should plasma or whole blood measurements be used to anticipate the development of toxicity? What is the best method to recognize the maximal immunosuppressive effect that can be achieved? Superficially, these two considerations would appear to be related. However, there is currently no secure basis for the belief that a given plasma or whole blood level will directly correlate with optimum immune suppression of immune integrity. Thus, the current practice of determining plasma levels only provides evidence that the drug is being taken. Most investigators have established broad guidelines to integrate these observations with careful consideration of biochemical changes in renal and hepatic function to anticipate the development of toxic but reversible side effects. It remains to reach agreement on the relative merits of radioimmunoassay as opposed to high-performance liquid chromatography, the compartment to be sampled, and the therapeutic index for cyclosporin A.

Third, much of the toxicology requires confirmation. Although reversible nephrotoxicity is recognized, the correlation of functional with morphological changes, particularly at the ultrastructural level, is in its infancy. Serial studies in experimental animals and clinical studies are needed to define late sequelae and test proposals for drug scheduling where other nephrotoxic agents are unavoidable. A similar degree of uncertainty characterizes liver damage. It is not clear how changes in bilirubin level or enzymes are brought about. In marrow transplantation, there is the added problem of graft-versus-host disease disturbing hepatic biochemical function and how these two are to be separated with certainty. The temporal sequences relating disturbances in renal and hepatic function are not clear and, until the mechanisms are established, decisions made for patient management must remain largely anecdotal.

Fourth, the many experimental models used and the enormous variation in evaluating cyclosporin A have added to the confusion. Despite meticulous examination of the original experimental reports, painstaking reanalysis of data, graphs, and tables, and attempts to match results from different studies, many insoluble questions remain unanswered. For example, the formulation of the drug has changed during the course of these investigations so that route, schedule, and presentation are not uniform. Few, if any, of the studies have reported measurements of plasma levels, and no data are available on tissue concentrations. Despite these shortcomings, there is now a large block of information which supports an unequivocal immunosuppressive activity for cyclosporin A. Future studies will benefit from the availability of standardized assay techniques, and the experimental model remains a major source of information in urgently answering some of the questions. These would include, for example, the type of infection or the emergence of tumors that may occur in individuals immunosuppressed with cyclosporin A. Another question would be the schedule for allogeneic bone marrow transplantation and our suggestion that donor and recipient pretreatment may be the critical issue in abrogating graft-versus-host disease rather than restricting the agent to the recipient. The answer to these and other questions will in large part be derived from properly designed and meticulously executed studies, but attention must now be given to the inclusion of immunological and pharmacological monitoring in data reporting.

Fifth, the clinical trials are in many areas confirming encouraging results obtained from animal studies. Experience is limited, and many of the same reservations apply to humans as to experimental animals. Undoubtedly, clinical trials with cyclosporin A are now a reality, but results are not uniform. Again, interpretation is bedeviled by changes that have occurred with improvements in drug formulation, often the failure to correlate results with standardized plasma levels, and paucity of data on concurrent monitoring of changes in humoral and cell-mediated immunity. There would be little excuse for persistence with trials that failed to take into account such fundamental requirements. On this basis, a period of consolidation lies ahead. An issue that requires urgent attention is the value of cyclosporin A as a single agent or its role in combination with other immunosuppressive drugs, ranging from antithymocyte globulin through adrenocorticosteroids to cytotoxic agents. Sufficient time has now elapsed to pool experience to answer the question about emergence of infections or neoplasia. Of particular relevance at the clinical level is an urgent need to define a correlation between survival of the transplanted organ with some measurement that will reflect optimal immunosuppression and simultaneously predict for the risk of developing complications.

Clearly, much remains to be learned about cyclosporin A. It can, be concluded, however, that this simple substance is a most powerful immunosuppressive agent and is deserving of all the attention it has received to date. Futthermore, cyclosporin A is unique in exerting its effects without the profound suppression of the bone marrow that has, in the past, characterized drugs given to produce immunosuppression.

Finally, there exists the possibility that it may influence a very specific molecular event occurring early in the immunological response to foreign antigen. If this is confirmed, then cyclosporin A has considerable potential as a more selective immunosuppressive agent and may well be a real advance representing the first step in a new generation of agents for clinically effective immunosuppressive therapy.

ACKNOWLEDGMENTS

Supported by the University of Cape Town Leukaemia Centre and Staff Research Fund, the Medical Research Council, and the National Cancer Association. We thank Jackie Davies for typing, Jeanne Walker for illustrations, and Sheila Katcher for bibliographic assistance. The cyclosporin used in these studies was generously donated by Sandoz Limited, Basel, Switzerland. Jean Borel kindly reviewed the manuscript, and we are also indebted to Eric Wiskott, Tom Beveridge, and Carol Greenwood, all of Sandoz, for making available additional information. We record with appreciation the collaboration of our colleagues, Mr. Graham Manual and Mr. Keith Hart and staff of the university vivarium, in the animal studies reported. The human studies would not have been possible without the help of Senior Sister Lucille Wood and nursing staff in the transplant unit and intensive care unit at Groote Schuur Hospital. We thank the medical superintendent for permission to publish.

REFERENCES

1. M. Burnet, *The Clonal Selection Theory of Acquired Immunity*, Cambridge, Cambridge University Press, 1954.
2. R. E. Billingham, L. Brent, and P. B. Medawar, *Nature*, *172*:603-606 (1953).
3. P. B. Medawar, *The Uniqueness of the Individual*, London, Methuen, 1957.
4. E. J. Holborow and W. G. Reeves, *Immunology in Medicine. A Comprehensive Guide to Clinical Immunology*, London, Academic Press, 1977.
5. P. A. Meischer and H. J. Muller-Eberhard, *Textbook of Immunopathology*, 2nd ed., Vols. I and II, New York, Grune and Stratton, 1976.
6. B. Halpern, Antihistaminics in immunopathologic reactions, in *Testbook of Immuno-Pathology* (P. A. Meischer and H. J. Muller-Eberhard, eds.), 2nd ed., New York, Grune and Stratton, 1976, pp. 315-337.
7. T. G. Kantor, Anti-inflammatory drugs, in *Textbook of Immunopathology* (P. A. Meischer and H. J. Muller-Eberhard, eds.), 2nd ed., New York, Grune and Stratton, 1976, pp. 329-342.
8. P. A. Meischer, A. Gerebtzoff, and P. H. Lambert, Immunosuppressive therapy, in *Textbook of Immunopathology* (P. A. Meischer and H. J. Muller-Eberhard, eds.), 2nd ed., New York, Grune and Stratton, 1976, pp. 343-365.
9. J. L. Decker, *Arth. Rheum.*, *16*:89-91 (1973).
10. R. H. Rubin, Infection in the immunocompromised host, in *Scientific American Medicine* (E. Rubenstein and D. D. Federman, eds.), New York, Scientific American, 1982, Fas 7, pp. 1-28.
11. E. R. Hurd, Drugs affecting the immune response, in *Immunology in Medicine. A Comprehensive Guide to Clinical Immunology* (E. J. Holborrow and W. G. Reeves, eds.), London, Academic Press, 1977, pp. 1067-1099.
12. R. H. Rousell and B. I. Hoffbrand, *Prostgrad. Med. J.*, *52*:9-148 (Suppl. 5) (1976).
13. P. S. Russell and H. J. Winn, *N. Engl. J. Med.*, *282*: 786-793, 848-854 (1970).
14. G. Kohler and C. Milstein, *Nature*, *256*:495 (1975).
15. J. F. Borel, History of cyclosporin A and its significance in immunology, *Int. Symp. Cyclosporin A*, Cambridge, England, 1981.
16. J. F. Borel, *Immunology*, *31*:631-641 (1976).
17. J. F. Borel, C. Feurer, C. Magnee and H. Stahelin, *Immunology*, *32*:1017-1025 (1977).
18. A. Ruegger, M. Kuhn, H. Lichti, H-R. Loosli, R. Huguerin, C. Quiquerez, and A. von Wartburg, *Helv. Chim. Acta*, *59*:1075-1092 (1976).
19. H. J. Petcher, H. Weber, and A. Ruegger, *Helv. Chim. Acta*, *59*:1480-1489 (1976).

20. J. F. Borel and D. Wiesinger, Effect of cyclosporin A on murine lymphoid cells, in *Mechanisms in Lymphocyte Activation* (D. O. Lucas, ed.), New York, Academic Press, 1977, pp. 716-718.
21. J. F. Borel, D. Weisinger, and H. U. Gubler, *Eur. J. Rheum. Inflam.*, *1*:237-241 (1978).
22. D. Wiesinger and J. F. Borel, *Immunobiology*, *156*:454-463 (1979).
23. A. J. Kostakis, D. J. G. White, and R. Y. Calne, *IRCS Med. Sci.*, *5*:280-282 (1977).
24. R. Y. Calne, D. J. White, K. Rolles, D. P. Smith, and B. M. Herbertson, *Lancet*, *1*: 1183-1185 (1978).
25. D. C. Dunn, D. J. White, and J. Wade, *IRCS Med. Sci.*, *6*:464 (1978).
26. D. J. White, A. M. Plumb, G. Pawelec, and G. Brons, *Transplantation*, *27*:55-58 (1979).
27. R. Y. Calne, D. J. G. White, S. Thiru, D. B. Evans, P. McMaster, D. C. Dunn, G. N. Craddock, B. D. Pentlow, and K. Rolles, *Lancet*, *2*:1323-1327 (1978).
28. R. L. Powles, A. J. Barrett, H. K. Clink, H. E. M. Kay, J. Sloane, and T. J. McElwain, *Lancet*, *2*:1323-1327 (1978).
29. M. Dreyfuss, E. Harri, H. Hofman, H. Kobel, W. Pache, and H. Tscherter, *Eur. J. Appl. Microbiol.*, *3*:125-133 (1976).
30. W. Niederberger, Personal communication (1979).
31. W. Niederberger, P. Schaub, and T. Beveridge, *J. Chromatogr.*, *182*:454-458 (1980).
32. B. Leyland-Jones, P. Deesen, W. Kreis, R. O'Reilly, and C. W. Young, *ASCO Abstracts*, *1*:16 (April 1982).
33. E. Abisch, Personal communication (December 1980).
34. P. Donatsch, E. Abisch, M. Homberger, R. Traber, M. Trapp, and R. Voges, *J. Immunoassay*, *2*:19-32 (1981).
35. P. Keown, C. R. Stiller, R. A. Ulan, N. R. Sinclair, W. S. Wall, G. Carruthers, and W. Howson, *Lancet*, *1*:686-689 (1981).
36. E. Abisch and W. Niederberger, Personal communication (1981).
37. T. Beveridge, B. Speck, P. Cornu, and A. Gratwohl, Personal communication (April 1981).
38. N. Lemaire, Personal communication (December 1980).
39. J. F. Borel, C. Feurer, H. U. Gubler, and H. Stahelin, *Agents Actions*, *6*:468-475 (1976).
40. P. Leoni, R. C. Garcia, and A. C. Allison, *J. Clin. Lab. Immunol.*, *1*:67-72 (1978).
41. H. J. Deeg, R. Storb, L. Gerhard-Miller, H. M. Shulman, P. L. Weiden, and E. D. Thomas, *Transplantation*, *29*:320-325 (1980).
42. S. B. Leapman, R. S. Filo, E. J. Smith, and P. G. Smith, *Transplantation*, *30*:404-408 (1980).
43. S. B. Leapman, R. S. Filo, E. J. Smith, and P. G. Smith, *Transplantation Proc.*, *13*: 405-409 (1981).
44. A. D. Hess and P. J. Tutschka, *J. Immunol.*, *124*:2601-2608 (1980).
45. P. J. Tutschka, W. E. Beschorner, A. C. Allison, W. H. Berns, and G. W. Santos, *Nature*, *280*:148-151 (1979).
46. R. I. Mishell and R. W. Dutton, *Science*, *153*:1004-1005 (1966).
47. A. Kunkl and G. G. B. Klaus, *J. Immunol.*, *125*:2526-2531 (1980).
48. R. Palacios and G. Moller, *J. Exp. Med.*, *153*:1360-1365 (1981).
49. J. W. Mier and R. C. Gallo, *Proc. Natl. Acad. Sci. USA*, *77*:6134-6138 (1980).
50. D. Bunjes, C. Hardt, M. Rollinghoff, and H. Wagner, *Eur. J. Immunol.*, *11*:657-661 (1981).
51. L. Andrus and K. J. Lafferty, *Scand. J. Immunol.*, *5*:449-458 (1981).
52. L. H. Block. W. Siegenthaler, and J. Drews, *Klin. Wochenschr.*, *58*:739-742 (1980).
53. A. Grieder, D. Wiesinger, and A. Fontana, Inhibition of synthesis or secretion of lymphokines by cyclosporin A, *4th Int. Congr. Immunol.* (Abst.) Paris, 1980.
54. A. G. Bird and S. M. McLachlan, *Lancet*, *2*:418 (1980).
55. T. Paavonen, H. Jaervelaeinen, S. Kontiainen, and P. Hayry, *Clin. Exp. Immunol.*, *43*:342-350 (1981).
56. C. J. Green and A. C. Allison, *Lancet*, *1*:1182-1183 (1978).

57. W. P. Homan, J. W. Fabre, and P. H. Morris, *Transplantation*, *28*:439-441 (1979).
58. U. Landegren, U. Ramstedt, L. Axberg, A. Orn, and H. Wigzell, *Int. J. Cancer*, *28*: 725-730 (1981).
59. M. Introna, P. Allavena, F. Spreafico, and A. Mantovani, *Transplantation*, *31*:113-116 (1981).
60. R. H. Yanagihara and W. H. Adler, *Immunology*, *45*:325-332 (1982).
61. B. Ryffel, H. Deyssenroth, and J. F. Borel, *Agents Actions*, *11*:373-379 (1981).
62. A. Hellman and J. M. Goldman, *Transplantation*, *30*:386-387 (1980).
63. M. Y. Gordon and J. W. Singer, *Nature*, *279*:433-443 (1979).
64. R. Foa and D. Catovsky, *Clin. Exp. Immunol.*, *45*:371-375 (1981).
65. T. Beveridge, A. Gratwohl, F. Michot, W. Niederberger, E. Nuesch, K. Nussbaumer, P. Schaub, and B. Speck, *Curr. Ther. Res.*, *30*:5-18 (1981).
66. P. Jacobs and L. Eglin, Unpublished observations (1982).
67. G. Maurer and E. Schreirer, Personal communication.
68. D. H. Crawford, J. A. Thomas, G. Janossy, P. Sweny, O. N. Fernando, J. F. Moorhead, and J. H. Thompson, *Lancet*, *1*:1355-1356 (1980).
69. P. Jacobs and E. C. Gordon-Smith, *Lancet*, *2*:1296 (1980).
70. S. Thiru, D. B. Evans, P. McMaster, D. C. Dunn, G. N. Craddock, R. G. Henderson, S. Aziz, and P. Lewis, *Lancet*, *2*:1033-1036 (1979).
71. D. V. Hamilton, R. Y. Calne, D. B. Evans, R. G. Henderson, S. Thiru, and D. J. G. White, *Lancet*, *1*:1218-1219 (1981).
72. J. J. Rynasiewicz, D. E. Sutherland, R. L. Simmons, R. M. Ferguson, W. D. Payne, and J. S. Najarian, *Lancet*, *1*:276 (1981).
73. G. H. Klintmalm, S. Iwatsuki, and T. E. Starzl, *Lancet*, *1*:470-471 (1981).
74. P. Sweny, J. Hopper, M. Gross and Z. Varghese, *Lancet*, *1*:663 (1981).
75. R. Y. Calne, *Nephron*, *26*:57-63 (1980).
76. H. Shulman, G. Striker, H. J. Deeg, M. Kennedy, R. Storb, and E. D. Thomas, *N. Engl. J. Med.*, *305*:1392-1395 (1981).
77. B. Speck and A. Gratwohl, Personal communication (1982).
78. J. M. Hows, S. Palmer, S. Want, C. Dearden, and E. C. Gordon-Smith, *Lancet*, *2*: 145-146 (1981).
79. M. J. Mihatsch, W. Olivieri, U. Marbet, G. Thiel, F. Harder and H. U. Zollinger, *Lancet*, *2*:1162-1163 (1981).
80. R. Loertscher, M. Wenk, F. Harder, F. Brunner, F. Follath, and G. Thiel, *Lancet*, *2*:635-636 (1981).
81. A. Laupacis, P. A. Keown, A. Ulan, N. R. Sinclair, and C. R. Stiller, *Lancet*, *2*:1426-1427 (1981).
82. P. Jacobs and L. Eglin, In preparation (1982).
83. D. V. Joss, A. J. Barrett, J. R. Kendra, C. Lucas, and S. Desai, *Lancet*, *1*:906 (1982).
84. K. Rolles and R. Y. Calne, *Lancet*, *2*:795 (1980).
85. J. R. Curtis, *Br. Med. J.*, *1*:69-70 (1982).
86. J. Nagington, *Lancet*, *2*:196-197 (1981).
87. W. P. Homan, J. W. Fabre, P. R. Millard, and P. J. Morris, *Transplantation*, *29*:219-222 (1980).
88. W. P. Homan, J. W. Fabre, K. A. Williams, P. R. Millard, and P. J. Morris, *Transplantation*, *29*:361-366 (1980).
89. W. P. Homan, J. W. Fabre, P. R. Millard, and P. J. Morris, *Transplantation*, *30*:354-357 (1980).
90. W. P. Homan, J. W. Fabre, P. R. Millard, and P. J. Morris, *Transplantation* (in press).
91. M. H. Simms, J. K. Cruickshank, J. D. Blainey, A. H. Cameron, and A. D. Barnes, *Transplant Proc.*, *12*:256-260 (1980).
92. W. P. Homan, K. A. Williams, P. A. Millard, and P. J. Morris, *Transplantation*, *31*:423-442 (1981).

93. D. C. Dunn, D. J. White, B. M. Herbertson, and J. Wade, *Transplantation*, *27*:359-361 (1979).
94. C. J. Green, A. C. Allison, and S. Precious, *Lancet*, *2*:123-125 (1979).
95. D. C. Dunn, *Transplant. Proc.*, *13*:383 -385 (1981).
96. D. C. Dunn, D. J. G. White, and B. M. Herbertson, *Transplantation*, *29*:349-351 (1980).
97. P. J. Morris, *Transplantation*, *32*:349-354 (1980).
98. D. J. G. White, T. Nagao, and H. S. Davies, *13th Int. Congr. Transplant. Clin. Immunol.*, Amsterdam, Excerpta Medica (in press).
99. C. J. Green, Cyclosporin A, in *Immunosuppressive Therapy* (J. R. Salaman, ed.), Lancaster, MTP Press, 1981, pp. 75-109.
100. L. Brent and P. Medawar, *Proc. Roy. Soc.* (*Biol.*), *165*:281-307 (1966).
101. R. Y. Calne and D. J. G. White, *IRCS Med. Sci.*, *5*:595 (1977).
102. R. Y. Calne, D. S. G. White, B. D. Pentlow, K. Rolles, T. Syrakos, T. Ohtawa, D. P. Smith, P. McMaster, D. B. Evans, B. M. Herbertson, and S. Thiru, *Transplant. Proc.*, *11*:860-864 (1979).
103. W. P. Homan, M. E. French, P. R. Millard, T. G. Denton, J. W. Fabre, and P. J. Morris, *Surgery*, *88*:168-173 (1980).
104. D. C. Dunn, D. J. White, B. M. Herbertson, and K. Rolles, *Transplant. Proc.*, *12*:335-338 (1980).
105. W. P. Homan, M. E. French, J. W. Fabre, P. R. Millard, T. G. Denton, and P. J. Morris, *Transplant. Proc.*, *12*:287-290 (1980).
106. W. P. Homan, M. E. French, P. R. Millard and P. J. Morris, *Transplant.Proc.*, *13*:397-401 (1981).
107. W. P. Homan, M. E. French, J. W. Fabre, P. R. Millard, T. G. Denton, and P. J. Morris, *Transplantation*, *29*:262-263 (1980).
108. P. J. Tutschka, A. D. Hess, W. E. Beschorner, and G. W. Santos, *Transplantation*, *32*:203-209 (1981).
109. P. J. Tutschka, F. Pin, W. E. Beschorner, A. D. Hess, and G. W. Santos, *Transplantation*, *32*:321-325 (1981).
110. P. Jacobs, Effect of cyclosporin A on the incidence of graft-versus-host disease (GVHD) and survival of rabbits following allogeneic bone marrow transplantation, in *Experimental Hematology Today 1981* (S. J. Baum, G. D. Ledney, and A. Khan, eds.), Basel, S. Karger, 1981, pp. 87-97.
111. H. J. Deeg, R. Storb, P. L. Weiden, T. Graham, and E. D. Thomas, Cyclosporin A in marrow transplantation in the dog, in *ICN-UCLA Symposium on Molecular and Cellular Biology*, Vol. 17, *Biology of Bone Marrow Transplantation* (R. P. Gale, and C. F. Fox, eds.), New York, Academic Press, 1980, pp. 281-284.
112. H. J. Deeg, R. Storb, H. M. Shulman, P. L. Weiden, T. C. Graham, and E. D. Thomas, *Transplantation*, *33*:443-446 (1982).
113. H. J. Deeg, R. Storb, R. L. Weiden, T. Graham, K. Atkinson, and E. D. Thomas, *Transplant. Proc.*, *13*:402-440 (1981).
114. S. P. Lems and R. A. Koene, *IRCS Med. Sci.*, *7*:184 (1979).
115. S. P. Lems, P. J. A. Capel, and R. A. Koene, *Transplant. Proc.*, *12*:283-286 (1980).
116. J. F. Borel and J. Meszaros, *Transplantation*, *29*:161-162 (1980).
117. D. J. White, K. R. Rolles, T. Ottawa, and O. Turell, *Transplant. Proc.*, *12*:261-265 (1980).
118. A. J. Kostakis, D. G. J. White, and R. Y. Calne, *IRCS Med. Sci.*, *5*:243 (1988).
119. W. P. Homan, J. A. Williams, J. W. Fabre, P. R. Millard, and P. J. Morris, *Transplantation*, *31*:164-166 (1980).
120. S. W. Jamieson, N. A. Burton, C. P. Bieber, B. A. Reitz, P. E. Oyer, E. B. Stinson, and N. E. Shumway, *Lancet*, *1*:545 (1979).
121. A. B. Cosimi, C. F. Shield, C. Peters, R. C. Burton, G. Scott, and P. S. Russel, *Surg. Forum*, *30*:287-289 (1979).

122. S. L. Pennock, B. A. Reitz, C. P. Bieber, S. W. Jamieson, A. A. Raney, P. E. Oyes, and E. B. Stinson, *Transplant. Proc., 13*:390-392 (1981).
123. B. A. Reitz, C. P. Bieber, A. A. Raney, J. L. Pennock, S. W. Jamieson, P. E. Oyer, and E. B. Stinson, *Transplant. Proc., 13*:393-396 (1981).
124. J. J. Rynasiewicz, D. E. Sutherland, K. Kawahara, P. Gorecki, and J. S. Najarian, *Transplant. Proc., 12*:270-274 (1980).
125. J. F. Garvey, P. J. Morris, D. R. Finch, P. R. Millard and M. Poole, *Lancet, 1*:971-972 (1979).
126. J. F. Garvey, P. McShane, M. D. Poole, P. R. Millard, and P. J. Morris, *Transplant. Proc., 12*:266-269 (1980).
127. H. Reece-Smith, W. P. Homan, D. F. du Toit, P. McShane, and P. J. Morris, *Transplantation, 31*:442-444 (1981).
128. P. R. Bell, R. F. Wood, M. Peters, and J. R. Nash, *Transplant. Proc., 12*:291-293 (1980).
129. P. McMaster, A. Procyshyn, R. Y. Calne, R. Valdes, K. Rolles, and D. J. Smith, *Br. Med. J., 280*:444-445 (1980).
130. A. J. Norin, F. J. Veith, E. E. Emeson, K. L. Pinsker, and S. L. Kamholz, *Br. Med. Jr., 280*:444-445 (1980).
131. D. J. Coster, W. F. Shepherd, T. Chin Fook, N. S. Rice, and B. R. Jones, *Lancet, 2*:688-689 (1979).
132. D. J. Coster, W. F. Shepherd, T. Chin Fook, N. S. Rice, and B. R. Jones, *Br. J. Opthalmol., 64*:148-153 (1980).
133. D. J. Watt, T. A. Partridge, J. C. Sloper, *Transplantation, 31*:266-271 (1981).
134. A. A. Zalewski and W. K. Silvers, *J. Neurosurg., 52*:557-563 (1980).
135. A. A. Zalewski and A. K. Gulati, *Transplantation, 31*:88-89 (1981).
136. J. F. Borel, *Transplant. Proc., 13*:344-348 (1981).
137. C. Bolton and M. L. Cuzner, Modification of EAE by non-steroidal anti-inflammatory drugs, in *The Suppression of Experimental Allergic Encepholomyelitis and Multiple Sclerosis* (A. N. Davison and M. L. Cuzner, eds.), New York, Academic Press, 1980, pp. 189-197.
138. J. F. Borel, *Transplant. Clin. Immunol., 13*:3-6 (1981).
139. R. B. Nussemblatt, M. M. Rodrigues, I. Gery, W. B. Wacker, S. J. Cervario, and M. C. Salinas-Carmona, *J. Clin. Invest., 67*:1228-1231 (1981).
140. K. Thommen, *Agents Actions, 11*: (1981).
141. B. E. Bueding, J. Hawkins, and Y.-N. Cha, *Agents Actions, 11*:380-383 (1981).
142. S. Thiru, R. Y. Calne, and J. Nagington, *Transplant. Proc., 13*:359-364 (1981).
143. R. Y. Calne, K. Rolles, D. J. G. White, S. Thiru, D. B. Evans, R. Henderson, D. L. Hamilton, N. Boone, P. McMaster, O. Gibby, and R. Williams, *Transplant. Proc., 13*: 349-364 (1981).
144. T. E. Starzl, S. I. Watsuki, G. Klintmalm, G. P. Schroter, R. Weil, III, L. J. Koep, and K. A. Porter, *Transplant. Proc., 13*:281-285 (1981).
145. G. B. G. Klintmalm, S. I. Watsuki, and T. E. Starzl, *Lancet, 1*:470-471 (1980).
146. R. A. Powles, H. M. Clink, D. Spence, G. Morgenstern, S. G. Watson, P. S. Selby, M. Woods, A. Barrett, B. Jameson, J. Sloane, S. D. Lawler, H. E. M. Kay, D. Lawson, T. J. McElwain, and P. Alexander, *Lancet, 1*:327-329 (1980).
147. A. Gratwohl and B. Speck, Personal communication (1982).
148. B. Herrmann and W. Mueller, *Akt. Rheumatol., 4*:173-186 (1979).
149. W. Mueller and B. Herrmann, *N. Engl. J. Med., 301*:555 (1979).
150. G. Routhier, O. Epstein, G. Janossy, H. C. Thomas, and S. Sherlock, *Lancet, 2*: 1223-1226 (1980).

11

Tuftsin (THR-LYS-PRO-ARG)

A Stimulator of All Known Functions of Macrophage

Victor A. Najjar and Nancy J. Bump Tufts University School of Medicine, Boston, Massachusetts

I. INTRODUCTION

Tuftsin (Thr-Lys-Pro-Arg), the natural activator of macrophages and neutrophilic granulocytes has now aroused considerable interest among biologists and medical circles in the United States, Europe, Israel, and Japan. It was discovered a decade ago (1,2) as the physiological stimulator of motility, phagocytosis, and pinocytosis (2-8), both for blood neutrophils and all types of macrophages (9). It was only lately that it was recognized as a natural activator of all functions of these phagocytic cells: (a) motility, (b) phagocytosis, (c) pinocytosis (6,7,10), (d) immunogenic activity (11-13) with augmentation of the antibody response (14), (e) bactericidal activity (15,16), (f) tumoricidal activity (10,17-19) and, finally, the stimulation of the hexose monophosphate shunt (20). What this signals for research in this area is that in the investigation of general immunological stimulation, both humoral and cellular, one no longer has to resort to unphysiological compounds such as mycobacterial emulsions, endotoxins, and several synthetic compounds almost all of which at one level or another appear to be toxic. Tuftsin is now available from several commercial sources in this country and abroad.

II. THE BIOCHEMISTRY OF TUFTSIN

Tuftsin, like so many biologically active peptides, is synthesized by translation of messenger ribonucleic acid of the heavy chain of an IgG molecule, termed leukokinin, of which it is a component part.

Tuftsin is present in the Fc portion of the heavy chain (21). It is present in the C_H2 domain representing residues 289-292 in close proximity to the attachment of the carbohydrate moiety; actually five residues on the amino side of the aspartic acid-asparagisc (ASX) attachment residue.

There are two enzymes that are responsible for releasing free tuftsin from the carrier molecule leukokinin. Free tuftsin is the only form in which it is fully active and as such can stimulate the several functions of the phagocytic cells enumerated above.

Tuftsin-endocarboxypeptidase (2), an enzyme present in the spleen, is responsible for the first step in freeing tuftsin from the carrier molecule leukokinin. The splenic enzyme cleaves the carboxy end of tuftsin at the Arg-Glu bond between residues 292 and 293. Consequently, in the absence of splenic function, which results from the removal of the spleen or abrogation of its function, tuftsin remains attached to the carrier leukokinin and as such is completely inactive (22-26).

Another enzyme, leukokininase, cleaves tuftsin at the Lys-Thr bond, the amino-terminal of the tetrapeptide between residues 288 and 289. This follows the cleavage at the carboxy terminal end by the splenic enzyme. As a result of the activity of both enzymes, tuftsin is released as a free tetrapeptide which is now available for the activation of the phagocyte. Leukokininase is present on the outer surface of the cell membrane. Its active site faces outward in proximity to the binding site of leukokinin (2,6,7). These two steps can be illustrated as follows:

```
H---Ala-Lys-Thr-Lys-Pro-Arg-Glu-Gln---OH

          ↑                ↑
  [Second Cleavage      [First Cleavage
   leukokininase]        Tuftsin-endocarboxypeptidase]
```

III. THE ISOLATION OF TUFTSIN

Tuftsin was isolated from the phosphocellulose fraction IV of leukophilic human γ-globulin by digestion with leukokininase or trypsin (2-4). With the latter enzyme a short incubation was performed to liberate tuftsin, but it was insufficient to break down all sensitive bonds. This kept unwanted peptide fragments to a minimum. Large peptides were excluded on Sephadex G-10. Retarded peptides were subsequently purified on Dowex 50 (Aminex AG 50W-X4). Sequence analysis was performed with appropriate enzymes and dansyl labeling (3,4).

Synthesis of the tetrapeptide was first accomplished using the solid phase method (3,5,27). Subsequently, it was successfully prepared with conventional solution synthesis in several laboratories (28-36) and with polymeric reagents by Fridkin and his associates (28,37).

It is essential that absolute purity be attained. Several authors have stressed this point because some of the impurities are strongly inhibitory (6,10). Impurities arise readily because three of the residues involved in tuftsin synthesis are trifunctional, and protecting groups may be partially removed during the various steps, in which case, acylation of the deprotected functions may result. Furthermore, the final step in deprotection may not be complete for various reasons.

Numerous analogs of tuftsin have been synthesized for the study of the effect of structural modifications in biological activity. Fridkin and Gottlieb (38) cite a total of 67 analogs that have been reported. A look at the structure-function relationships clearly indicates that the integrity of the tetrapeptide is necessary for the full expression of biological activity. Even minor changes such as the substitution of serine for threonine (37) may lead to an 80% reduction. Other modifications produce little or no stimulation. Several analogs produce complete inhibition of the tuftsin effect (5-7,20,37-40). However, some modifications are tolerated. This was first recognized when it was found that in dogs tuftsin is Thr-Lys-Pro-Lys and represents a substitution of lysine for the carboxy-terminal arginine (2). Other exchanges between Arg and Lys do not affect activity (33). A detailed discussion of this matter has recently appeared (10,38). Thr-Lys-Pro-Pro-Arg not only was inactive but showed a strong inhibition to the stimulatory effect of tuftsin in phagocytosis and motility assays (3,5). Similarly, Lys-Pro-Arg, Ala-Lys-Pro-Arg, Ser-Lys-Pro-Arg, Thr-Glu-Pro-Arg, and tuftsinyltuftsin (Thr-Lys-Pro-Arg-Thr-Lys-Pro-Arg) also inhibit tuftsin stimulation. The first two also inhibit reduction of nitroblue tetrazolium (NBT) as well as phagocytosis stimulation (20).

IV. THE CONFORMATION OF TUFTSIN

Konopinska et al. (41), based on nuclear magnetic resonance and infrared studies, suggested that tuftsin in solution tends to form a $4 \rightarrow 1$ β-turn stabilized by hydrogen bonding which may be further stabilized by possible interaction between the carboxylate of arginine and the protonated amino group of threonine. Vicar et al. (32) at the same time suggested a similar ionic interaction with a pseudocyclic conformation. According to Fitzwater et al. (42), based on minimal energy conformation, tuftsin can exist in several low-energy conformations with a common hairpin conformation.

In contrast, my colleagues and I studied tuftsin conformation by proton and ^{13}C nuclear magnetic resonance (NMR) and found no $4 \rightarrow 1$ β-turn (43). In fact, no preferred conformation was noted. A similar conclusion was arrived at by Sekacis et al. (44) using ^{1}H- and ^{13}C-NMR studies and by Stabinsky et al. (45) by correlative structure-function studies with analogs modified at either terminal residue.

V. TUFTSIN RECEPTORS

For a study of receptor reactivity and binding, it was necessary to prepare radioactive tuftsin. Synthesis was accomplished in solution by Fridkin's group (45). This successful synthesis of [^{3}H-Arg^{4}] tuftsin was confirmed repeatedly (10,46).

It was shown that tuftsin binding to its receptors on rabbit polymorphonuclear (PMN) granulocytes is highly specific, saturable, and reversible with a K_d of 1.3×10^{-7}, which is close to the K_m of tuftsin stimulation of phagocytosis. There are about 50,000 receptors on each PMN cell (38,45). These data were reproduced with remarkable similarity with a K_d of 8.6×10^{-8} M and a receptor number of 50,000-60,000 (46,47).

Several analogs were synthesized [N-acetyl-Thr^{1}] -tuftsin, Thr-Lys-Pro, Lys-Pro-Arg, Thr-Lys-Pro-(N^g NO_2)-Arg, Thr-Lys-Pro-Homo-Arg, [O=C⊂Thr^{1}] -tuftsin (38,45). Thr-Lys-Pro-Pro-Arg, Thr-Glu-Pro-Arg, Ala-Lys-Thr-Pro-Lys-Ala-Lys, Thr-Pro-Arg-Glu-Ala_3, and Thr-Lys-Pro-Arg-Thr-Lys-Pro-Arg (tuftsinyltuftsin) were also synthesized. All show competitive binding, some of which exhibit stronger binding than exhibited by tuftsin (10). These are Lys-Pro-Arg (38) Thr-Lys-Pro-Pro-Arg, Thr-Glu-Pro-Arg, and tuftsinyltuftsin (2,10).

Receptor sites were found only on macrophages, monocytes, and PMN granulocytes. Lymphocytes were almost devoid of binding sites (45). However, others using derivatized tuftsin analog tuftsinyl-[^{125}I]-tyrosine, showed substantive binding to lymphocytes. Furthermore, binding to PMN and monocytes was found to be minimal at 22°C (48). This and the binding to lymphocytes are contrary to the results obtained with radioactive underivatized tuftsin when excellent binding was shown at 22°C (38,45). It appears that this discrepancy can be explained by the fact that the pentapeptide tuftsinyltyrosine cannot mimic the binding of the tetrapeptide tuftsin with the appropriate fidelity.

Binding studies were also performed on elicited mouse macrophages with underivatized [^{3}H-Arg^4]-tuftsin (47). The characteristics of binding were very similar to those obtained with human PMN cells and monocytes with a K_d of 5.3×10^{-8} and 72,000 receptors per cell of thioglycolate-induced mouse macrophages. Thr-Lys-Pro and [N-acetyl-Thr^1]-tuftsin showed no competitive effective while [D-Arg^4]-tuftsin bound to some extent. These binding characteristics ran parallel to the extent of phagocytic stimulation. The first two analogs are biologically inert, whereas [D-Arg^4]-tuftsin yields a small degree of phagocytic stimulation. Again, lymphocyte preparations from mouse thymus and spleen showed no binding (47,49).

Two types of phagocytic cells were further tested for receptor binding to tuftsin. A mouse mononuclear phagocyte, grown in vitro of bone marrow origin, showed phagocytic stimulation with tuftsin and a binding capacity that were threefold greater than that obtained in induced mouse peritoneal macrophage (50). Another cell line, a macrophage-type cell P388D1, also exhibited tuftsin-stimulated phagocytosis and a binding capacity comparable with that of peritoneal macrophage. It thus appears certain again that membrane receptors to tuftsin are found only on cells with phagocytic activity. The presence of receptors is, therefore, a necessary requisite for phagocytic stimulation by tuftsin. However, certain leukemic cells do not respond to tuftsin stimulation. Cells obtained from patients with acute granulocytic leukemia, which involves the polymorphonuclear series, and leukemic cells from patients with a related disorder, myelofibrosis, do not respond to phagocytic stimulation even when exposed to very high concentrations of tuftsin (24-26). Another type of leukemia that affects the monocytic series shows excellent stimulation of phagocytosis by very low levels of tuftsin (26). It is quite possible that leukemic undifferentiated PMN cells do not possess tuftsin receptors which might have been lost or possibly never acquired in this disease. By contrast, leukemic monocytes still possess tuftsin receptors. It should be pointed out, however, that the deficiency in leukemic cells may well be at a step beyond the receptor level. This remains to be determined (24-26).

VI. TUFTSIN RECEPTORS AND TUFTSIN ANTIBODY

During our studies on receptor binding of tuftsin to rabbit neutrophils and several of its analogs, we noted that some bound more tightly than tuftsin. This was reminiscent of our very early studies on antibody binding to structural or conformational varients of a hapten (51). At the time, we showed that such variants can bind more tightly than the hapten itself (52). The findings with binding of tuftsin analogs to tuftsin receptors prompted a similar study of antibody bindings to tuftsin and its analogs. The results with antibody duplicated those with the receptor to a remarkable degree.

The binding affinities were equally characteristic of receptor or antibody binding to the various oligopeptides as though both antibody and receptor were one and the same.

Thr-Lys-Pro and Ala-Lys-*Thr-Lys-Pro-Arg*-Glu-Ala$_3$ showed no measurable binding to either antibody or receptor. Ala-Lys-*Thr-Lys-Pro-Arg* showed less binding than tuftsin to both receptor molecules. However, three analogs showed stronger binding than tuftsin. The order of binding among these was the same for antibody and receptor: Thr-Lys-Pro-Arg < Thr-Glu-Pro-Arg < Thr-Lys-Pro-Pro-Arg < Thr-Lys-Pro-Arg-Thr-Lys-Pro-Arg. The unexpected similarity of binding characteristics between antibody and receptor gave rise to the notion that the receptor binding site may well display immunoglobulin characteristics. For this, we utilized goat antirabbit-IgG, purified by affinity chromatography. This was allowed to react with tuftsin receptors on rabbit peritoneal neutrophils. It was then followed by assessing the effect of [^{3}H]-tuftsin binding. For control, we also used affinity-purified anti-poly(A):poly(dT). (Both purified antibodies were gifts from David Stollar, Tufts University, School of Medicine, Boston, Mass.) In every case, treatment with antirabbit-IgG resulted in inhibition of tuftsin binding. Identical results were obtained with mouse peritoneal macrophages using affinity-purified goat antibody to mouse IgG. The number of tuftsin molecules denied access to their sites by antibody per cell and the number of radioactive antibody molecules prevented from binding by cold antibody were approximately the same. These values also correspond to the number of receptors per cell for both PMN and macrophages and indicate the IgG nature of the receptor.

VII. STIMULATION OF THE HEXOSE MONOPHOSPHATE SHUNT

It has been shown by Spirer et al. (20) and Fridkin and Gottlieb (38) that tuftsin stimulates the reduction of nitroblue tetrazolium to a considerable degree and to an extent similar to the stimulation by endotoxin. This dye reduction has been shown to result from the stimulation of the hexose monophosphate shunt (53-57). During this process hydrogen peroxide and the superoxide anion, among others, accumulate within the cell. These are presumed to be lethal to prokaryotic and eukaryotic cells. Good correlation was found between the stimulation of the shunt and phagocytic activity as measured by reduction of the tetrazolium dye (20,38). Iguchi and Nakazawa (58) also utilized the dye reduction for tuftsin stimulation.

That tuftsin stimulation of glucose oxidation during shunt activation occurs with increased release of carbon dioxide was clearly shown in Fridkin's laboratory (38,53). Analogs of tuftsin were studied for their ability to stimulate shunt activity in both human and guinea pig granulocytes. It was found that the augmentation of $^{14}CO_2$ with the various analogs followed the same relative order whether cells were in the phagocytosing or resting state. The same relative stimulation by (Thr-Lys-Pro-Arg)-tuftsin, [homoarg^4]-tuftsin, [O = C $\Diamond$ Thr^1]-tuftsin, [Arg-NH$_2$^{4}]-tuftsin, and [D-Arg^4]-tuftsin was found for both human and guinea pig cells whether resting or phagocytosing. By contrast, [Ala^1]-tuftsin and [des-Thr^1]-tuftsin, which are both inhibitors of phagocytosis as well as NBT reduction, were both inactive in glucose oxidation (20,38,53).

VIII. STIMULATION OF THE IMMUNOLOGICAL RESPONSE

Antigen activation of lymphocytes, which ultimately results in antibody production, has been shown to be macrophage dependent. The role played by the macrophages in processing the antigen is to trigger a series of events ("education of the T-lymphocyte") that is finally translated into antibody production. On this basis, Tzehoval et al. (11) were able to show that tuftsin considerably improved the capacity of the macrophage to influence the T-lymphocyte. Adherent mouse macrophages were incubated with T-dependent keyhole limpet hemocyanin, as antigen, in the presence and absence of tuftsin, or its analogs for 4 hr. After thorough washing away of the unreacted antigen, spleen cells were added to the adherent macrophages and cultured for 24 hr. The spleen lymphocytes, having presumably gotten the message from the macrophage-antigen complex, were killed by irradiation and injected into the footpad of syngeneic mice. The draining lymphnodes were removed 6 days later and their lymph cells tested for their specific response to antigen through incorporation of [^{3}H] thymidine uptake. From these studies, it was clear that tuftsin stimulates the uptake of thymidine to a considerable extent at a maximal concentration of 5 μM. Furthermore, protein and ribonucleic acid syntheses were also augmented by tuftsin (11-13).

In general, tuftsin stimulation was specific to the extent that several analogs were much less active. In addition, the correlation between immunostimulation and phagocytic stimulation was not absolute. For example, [Ala^1] tuftsin was more potent than tuftsin in this system, whereas it was not only inactive in phagocytosis assay but also inhibitory to tuftsin stimulation. Analysis of this and other analog effects with respect to activity led Feldman and Fridkin's groups to the conclusion that the dipeptide sequence Pro-Arg is essential for activity since this dipeptide showed definite stimulation of thymidine uptake. However, it lacked any stimulation of phagocytosis or shunt activation (11-13). In such an analysis, it is necessary to recall that the two assay systems are completely different. An analog, compared with tuftsin, can have a mild stimulatory effect toward a particular activity, but that effect can be much longer lasting than that of tuftsin. In that event, it would appear to be more active. What is significant is that three separate pathways may be required to activate three separate systems, namely, motility, immunostimulation, and phagocytosis. Thus, maximal stimulation of these systems has been shown to require completely different concentrations of tuftsin. Maximal stimulation of motility requires five times the concentration needed for maximal immunostimulation which, in turn, requires more than 10 times the concentration necessary for maximal stimulation of phagocytosis: 25 μM, 5 μM, 0.5 μM, respectively (6,7,10).

This type of immunostimulation, shown by the Weizmann Institute group (11), could be translated into an actual augmentation of the antibody level. This indeed proved to be the case. Florentin et al. (14) showed clearly that a different augmentation of the immunological response was obtained following injection of tuftsin into immunized mice. Tuftsin was injected at various intervals of time before immunization. There was a maximal increase of antibody forming splenic cells against injected trinitrophenyl-KLH (TNP-KLH) when the antigen was administered 5 days after tuftsin injection. Antibody response to the thymus-independent antigen TNP-lipopolysaccharide (TNP-LPS) also was increased starting 1 day after tuftsin injection. Furthermore, tuftsin also potentiated the antibody-dependent cell cytotoxic activity of spleen cells, as well as activation of the cytotoxic capability of the macrophage against mouse leukemia L1210 cells as measured in vitro.

Tuftsin has been lately shown by Bruley-Rosset et al. (59) to reverse the age-depressed tumoricidal activity of mouse peritoneal macrophages. In fact, the stimulation by tuftsin of this activity in naturally depressed macrophages of aged mice gave values higher than those obtained with macrophages from young mice. Similar results were obtained with cytolytic T-cell activity. At effector to target cell ratio of 3, 10, and 30, stimulation of age-depressed macrophages was 5- to 10-fold with tuftsin 10 μg per mouse given IP as compared with control. Again, the stimulated activity of these depressed macrophages rose to levels severalfold higher than those obtained with macrophages from young mice.

IX. ANTITUMOR EFFECT OF TUFTSIN

Antitumor activity against L1210 cells was obtained in vivo by Nishioka (17). Tuftsin injection caused a statistically significant prolongation of survival of L1210-injected mice.

Nishioka's laboratory further showed that tuftsin exerts antitumor activity on Cloudman S-91 melanoma cells (17,18,39). The injection of the tumor resulted in implantation in the lungs with readily visible pigmented colony proliferation. These could be easily counted on autopsy of the injected mouse a month after tumor injection. The administration of tuftsin three times weekly led to a marked decrease in the number of melanoma colonies as compared with controls. Tuftsin, at various doses, was injected 1-4 days after tumor administration with significant effects.

Four separate experiments were performed with doses varying from 1-1000 μg/mouse given intraperitoneally three times weekly. Melanoma cells 1×10^5 were injected intravenously. In all experiments, the tuftsin effect was dramatic. What is of special interest is that in each single experiment lower doses were more effective than the larger doses used. Again, this suggests that the inhibitory tripeptide Lys-Pro-Arg might have accumulated at the higher doses, and strengthens our suggestion that small tuftsin dosages repeatedly given would yield better results, which was highlighted by the greater effect of tuftsinyltuftsin discussed earlier (10).

Single injections at various doses were not effective. It thus appeared that multiple injection of tuftsin at a lower dosage was necessary to keep a high level of macrophage activation (17,18,39). It was also demonstrated that levels as high as 10 μg/mouse (approximately 500 μg/kg) injected on alternate days did not result in observable toxicity, nor was a dose of 24 mg/kg of rat given intravenously (2,10).

Our group used L1210 cells in order to test tuftsin and obtained mixed results. Our concern was that with the doses used the inhibitory tripeptide Lys-Pro-Arg might accumulate due to rapid aminopeptidase activity (60). Should the level of this inhibitor increase it would nullify the effect of tuftsin. To that end, we synthesized tuftsinyltuftsin (Thr-Lys-Pro-Arg-Thr-Lys-Pro-Arg) with the expectation that it would yield tuftsin in a gradual manner through the action of trypsinlike enzymes. Consequently, the inhibitor tripeptide either will not be formed at all or not accumulate if formed. Indeed, this prediction proved correct. The tuftsin dimer was very effective, and some 20-40% of mice treated with 20 μg/mouse three times weekly survived over 90 days after a challenge with 20×10^3 - 100×10^3 L1210 cells. All controls died after 10 days.

We have also studied the effect of the monomer tuftsin on B16 melanoma in C57 syngeneic mice. This was remarkably effective, albeit to a varying extent depending on the experiment. Figure 1 shows the results of an average experiment. In some experiments the intraperitoneal (IP) injections of 2-20 μg/mouse effected complete inhibition of subcutaneous melanoma implantation at 2×10^4/mouse, while in other experiments, tuftsin considerably delayed the appearance of melanoma growth (10). By contrast, the subcutaneous administration of tuftsin was not as effective.

Recently, Catane et al. (19) studied the effect of tuftsin injections three times weekly on the growth of a fibrosarcoma induced by 3-methyl-cholanthrene in C_3H mice. Tumor cells, 10^6, were injected IP into each mouse with and without injection of tuftsin, 0.2-500 μg/kg of mice. Controls showed a median survival of 21 days. Tuftsin animals, however, showed about double this survival time of 39 days. Furthermore, 20% of those mice did not develop tumors after 80 days or more of observation.

An additional parameter was also considered, namely, the dimensions of tumor growth in addition to survival. Here the fibrosarcoma was injected subcutaneously while tuftsin administration was maintained with IP injections as before. Tumor growth was then measured as a function of time. The results were less dramatic but definitely showed that tuftsin retards tumor growth. Two additional, supportive, and pertinent results were

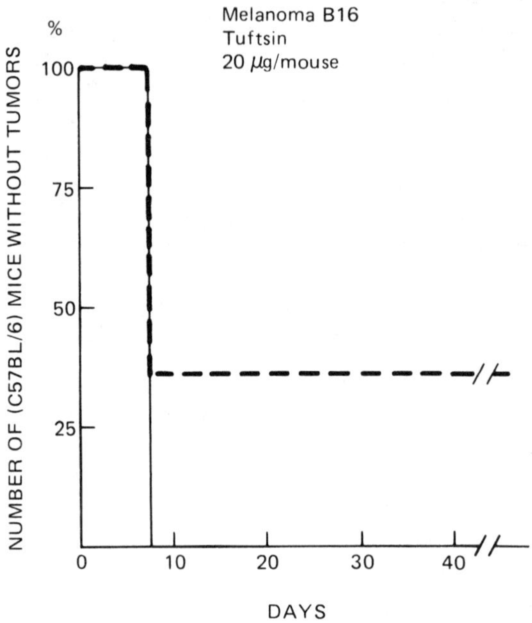

Figure 1 B16 melanoma was propagated subcutaneously in syngeneic C57BL/6 mice. For these experiments tumors weighing approximately 2-3 g were removed, cut up in slices with scissors, and teased in phosphate-buffered saline (PBS), pH 7.2 After sedementing for 10 min on ice, the supernatant was passed through several layers of gauze. Viable cells were estimated by dye exclusion, counted, and 5×10^5 cells were injected subcutaneously into each of the 4-6 week-old animals on day zero in the lower right abdominal surface. Prior to this, 20 experimental mice were injected intraperitoneally (IP) in the left lower abdomen with 1 ml of PBS containing 20 μg of tuftsin per mouse on days −7, −4, and day zero. Control mice, also 20, were injected only with PBS. All experimental and control mice subsequently received 20 μg of tuftsin or PBS IP, respectively, twice weekly, and observed daily for visible tumors. Control mice are shown in a solid line. Tuftsin-treated mice are shown in a broken line.

obtained in this study; [Ala-^{1}]-tuftsin, an inhibitor of tuftsin phagocytic effect, neither inhibited nor enhanced antitumor activity as measured by survival and tumor size (19,38).

X. ANTIBACTERIAL EFFECT OF TUFTSIN

We have discussed earlier in this chapter the stimulation by tuftsin of the hexose monophosphate shunt and the production of H_2O_2 and O^-_2. Both of these compounds are strongly bactericidal in their effect (53-57). Consequently, if tuftsin stimulates the shunt and the production of these compounds (20), then tuftsin must necessarily augment bactericidal killing. Recently, Tritsch and Niswander (61,62) showed that tuftsin indeed augments the production of O^-_2.

This aspect was tested in an exhaustive study by Martinez et al. (15,16). These authors showed increased killing by peritoneal macrophages exposed to various bacteria injected IP with and without tuftsin 10 or 20 mg/kg of body weight. Five minutes later the animals were sacrificed and the peritoneal macrophages harvested, washed, and then incubated at 37°C. At various intervals samples of the phagocytic cells were taken and assayed for live bacteria. The results show that after 15 min of incubation about 5% of the bacteria in the control were killed, whereas the experimental cells with tuftsin showed 50-70% killing for 10 and 20 mg/kg doses, respectively.

The ability of injected tuftsin to augment blood clearing of bacteria was then studied. The bacteria chosen for this study were *Listeria monocytogenes*, *Escherichia coli*, *Staphylococcus aureus*, and *Serratia marcescens*. Mice were injected intravenously with these bacteria, followed immediately by tuftsin IP at 10-20 mg/kg. Blood samples were obtained at various intervals and live bacteria assayed. Impressive reductions in circulating bacteria were observed with the four microorganisms and with both doses of tuftsin.

Similar effects of tuftsin were recorded in leukemic mice. Like normal mice, bacterial clearing was enhanced by tuftsin injection. However, the overall effect, though quite definite, was less than that obtained in normal healthy mice.

Recently, Dobrowska et al. have been studying the lethal effects of lysine containing basic peptides on several bacteria (63). Because of the structure of tuftsin it was subjected to similar tests and found remarkably effective. At 62 μg/ml of tuftsin, there was a strong and direct bactericidal effect on many bacteria, most notably the *Pneumococcus* (64).

XI. OTHER EFFECTS OF TUFTSIN AND RELATED OBSERVATIONS

A. Stimulation of Motility by Tuftsin

Early in the investigation of tuftsin activity it was shown (2-5) that in addition to the stimulation of phagocytosis, tuftsin also stimulated cellular motility of PMN blood cells in vertically held glass microtubules. The stimulation was dramatic. Whether this motility has a chemotactic component is debatable. However, if indeed chemotactic motility is, by definition, that which occurs against a concentration gradient, then there is little doubt that a gradient is formed in this experiment by simple diffusion of tuftsin from an upper tuftsin layer into a bottom cell layer devoid of tuftsin. Furthermore, in such a setup, the PMN cells consume tuftsin as these move into the upper compartment, thus sharpening the gradient. This notion was confirmed by the demonstration in Nishioka's laboratory that tuftsin is chemotactically active under classic conditions with the use of the two-well system in soft agar (18,39).

B. The Effect of Tuftsin on Cyclic Nucleotide Levels

Stabinsky et al. (65) demonstrated an increase in intracellular cyclic GMP to almost double the nonstimulated level. At the same time there was a simultaneous decrease in cyclic AMP approximately to three-quarters of control level. These two effects were exerted quite rapidly and were detectable after 4 min, reaching a maximum in 10-20 min which was maintained for 1 hr. The concentration dependence for cyclic nucleotide modulation and that for phagocytosis are similar. The implication of a cause and effect is clear and was strongly supported by the fact that the addition to the phagocytic cells of the permeable 8-bromo derivatives of cGMP and cAMP was expressed, respectively, by a stimulation and inhibition of phagocytosis.

The mechanism by which biologically active compounds augment the levels of cGMP is perhaps through the alteration of the intracellular levels of Ca^{2+} (66). It was shown by Stabinsky et al. that Ca^{2+} uptake by PMN leukocytes is not affected by tuftsin

(65). However, there is a definite enhancement of calcium efflux from cells previously loaded with $^{45}Ca^{2+}$. This activity is specific for tuftsin and is absent in analogs that are inert in phagocytic stimulation such as [Des-Thr^1]-tuftsin and [N-Acetyl-Thr^1] tuftsin. The Israeli group favors the possibility that the stimulatory activity of tuftsin on the phagocytic process is mediated through stimultaneous modulation of the levels of both cyclic nucleotides; stimulation being effected by increase in cGMP with a simultaneous decrease in cAMP. Earlier studies on cAMP levels in PMN cells by Constantopoulos and Najjar did not reveal any lowering of that nucleotide after tuftsin stimulation (67). This discrepancy may be due to technical problems inasmuch as a 20-25% decrease in cAMP level may not have been readily detected with earlier methodology.

XII. TUFTSIN AND ITS ANALOGS: RADIOIMMUNOASSAY

Our group (10,46) and Fridkin and his colleagues (28,68) developed a radioimmunoassay for tuftsin. Earlier work by Spirer et al. (28,68) established the fact that tuftsin, appropriately conjugated, is antigenic. Consequently, a bovine serum albumin (BSA)-tuftsin conjugate was prepared through p-diazoniumphenylacetyltuftsin. This was used to establish normal values through a simplified method of tuftsin extraction (28,68). Normal levels were established at 255.7 ± 10.2 ng/ml. This level was found to be much lower, 118 ± 7.9 ng/ml, in 20 patients with elective splenectomy for various diseases and 126.05 ± 10.2 ng/ml in 38 splenectomized patients with Hodgkin's disease. However, splenectomy following accidental rupture of the spleen yielded close to normal values in 50 subjects, 234 ± 10.2 ng/ml. These observations fully confirm earlier phagocytosis assays which indicated an absence of tuftsin activity in all cases of splenectomized patients, or in patients who showed extensive disease of the spleen as in severe cases of sickle cell disease, with the exception of splenectomy following traumatic rupture of the spleen (7,22-23,25,26).

Our values in general were higher with our immunoassay (10) where the hapten employed was p-NH_2-phenylacetyl Gly-Gly-Thr-Lys-Pro-Arg. This was coupled after Fridkin's methodology (28) to BSA. Our normal values vary from 350 to 500 ng/ml of serum. The highest values were obtained in two cases of tuftsin deficiency. These were approximately 10 times higher than the average normal value. Such high values were anticipated in these human mutants. However, these values are highly diagnostic of the congenital type of tuftsin deficiency. The rationale which led us to expect high values is simple. We had shown earlier that γ-globulin from patients with tuftsin deficiency yields an analog of tuftsin that is strongly inhibitory. It inhibits tuftsin stimulation of phagocytosis even at considerable excess of tuftsin. This results from a greater affinity of the receptors to the mutant peptide Thr-Glu-Pro-Arg. It is in the nature of radioimmunoassay that an analog that binds tighter than tuftsin would give very high false values for tuftsin. We have obtained values in such patients of amounts as high as 2500-3500 ng/ml.

XIII. CONGENITAL FAMILIAL TUFTSIN DEFICIENCY

Our group has identified 17 cases of deficiency comprising 8 families. There was always one parent with this deficiency. In one family, one parent and two children were tuftsin deficient (7,22-23,69). The assay was in all cases, phagocytosis. γ-Globulin from patients was digested with leukokininase or trypsin, extracted with four volumes of alcohol, and assayed. Such studies showed that these cases did not possess a stimulatory peptide. On the contrary, a mixture of patients' extracts and an extract from normal γ-globulin, even

Table 1 Clinical and Laboratory Findings in 17 Patients Studied in United States and 2 in Japan

Characteristics	Remarks
1. Respiratory infection	
Tonsillitis	Frequent, sometimes suppurative
Pharyngitis	Frequent in adults
Bronchitis	Frequent in adults and children
Broncheolitis	Severe and recurrent in children
Pneumonitis	Severe and recurrent in children, *Pneumococcus* and *Staphylococcus*
2. Skin infection	Furunculosis frequent in adults, extensive seborrheic dermatitis in children
3. Lymph nodes infection	Frequent in children, often purulent and draining
4. Blood signs	Septicemia occasionally
5. Sex frequency	Both sexes are involved
6. Tuftsin activity	Absent or markedly reduced
7. Peptide extracts from patients	Inhibitory to normal tuftsin activity
8. Reduction of nitroblue tetrazolium	Below normal values
9. γA, γM, and γG_{1-4} levels	Within normal levels
10. Polymorphonuclear leukocyte level	Low, normal, or increased
11. Complement component C5	Normal quantitatively and functionally
12. Plasma opsonic activity to yeast particles	Normal activity
13. Response to γ-globulin injection	Infection alleviated
14. Infecting organisms	*Staphlococcus aureus* coagulase positive, *Streptoccocus pneumoniae*, *Monolia albicans*

at three equivalents of the latter, always yielded a negative effect. Radioimmunoassay of two of these patients yielded the typically high values given above.

The genetics of tuftsin deficiency is not yet defined. In our 8 families, representing 17 patients, as well as in the family described in Japan (70), only 1 of the parents exhibited the disease, both chemically and by tuftsin inhibition. The affected parents were of both sexes. One possibility that might explain this type of inheritance is that the unaffected parent has a normal gene which is producing the normal extra peptide and an abnormal gene which might be a deletion producing either nothing or some nonsensical nonfunctioning protein containing neither tuftsin nor the mutant inhibitor. In that case, the patient would be a double heterozygote; that is, one of the genes is producing the mutant tuftsin, and the other is producing either nothing or the nonsense protein. Deletions are now known to account for some of the thalassemia mutants.

XIV. ACQUIRED TUFTSIN DEFICIENCY

We have discussed earlier that tuftsin is active only in the free tetrapeptide state. It appears to be inactive when derivatized unless enzymes are present to release free tuftsin from the derivatized form. As an illustration, Konopinska et al. synthesized two derivatives of tuftsin, Lys-(tuftsin) and Ala-Lys-(tuftsin). Both of these were inactive in the phagocytosis assay (71). In order to release free tuftsin from the heavy chain of carrier leukokinin, two enzymatic steps are required to cleave at both amino and carboxy terminals of tuftsin. One step is the cleavage at the carboxy terminal arginine by a splenic enzyme. In the absence of the spleen or in diseases that nullify its function, tuftsin remains attached on the heavy chain and consequently inactive. Such acquired tuftsin deficiency has been observed following elective splenectomy, in sickle cell anemia, Hodgkin lymphomas, and leukemias of the granulocytic series (7,25,26,28,68).

These results, which were obtained in two laboratories, clarify a long-held observation that removal of the spleen from animals or humans results in a high vulnerability to severe infections that are sometimes lethal (72-74).

ACKNOWLEDGMENTS

We are grateful to Dr. Barton Childs for discussion on the genetic aspects of tuftsin deficiency. Supported by NIH Grant AI09116, NSF Grant PCM-7623008, and the March of Dimes Birth Defects Foundation Grant 1-556.

REFERENCES

1. V. A. Najjar and K. Nishioka, *Nature, 228*:672 (1970).
2. V. A. Najjar, in *Advances in Enzymology 4* (A. Meister, ed.), John Wiley & Sons, Inc., New York, 1974, p. 129.
3. K. Nishioka, A. Constantopoulos, P. Satoh, and V. A. Najjar, *Biochem. Biophys. Res. Commun., 47*:172 (1972).
4. K. Nishioka, A. Constantopoulos, P. S. Satoh, W. M. Mitchell, and V. A. Najjar, *Biochim. Biophys. Acta, 310*:217 (1973).
5. K. Nishioka, P. S. Satoh, A. Constantopoulos and V. A. Najjar, *Biochim. Biophys. Acta, 310*:230 (1973).
6. V. A. Najjar, in *Advances in Experimental Medicine and Biology, Macrophages and Lymphocytes: Nature, Functions and Interaction* (M. R. Escobar and H. Friedman, eds.) Plenum Press, New York, 1980, p. 131.
7. V. A. Najjar, in *The Reticuloendothelial System*, Vol. II (A. J. Sbarra and R. R. Strauss, eds.), Plenum Press, New York, 1980, p. 45.
8. P. S. Satoh, A. Constantopoulos, K. Nishioka, and V. A. Najjar, in *Chemistry and Biology of Peptides* (J. Meinhoffer, ed.), Ann Arbor Science Publisher, Ann Arbor, Mich., 1972, p. 403.
9. A. Constantopoulos and V. A. Najjar, *Cytobios, 6*:97 (1972).
10. V. A. Najjar, M. K. Chaudhuri, D. Konopinska, B. D. Beck, P. P. Layne, and L. Linehan, in *Augmenting Agents in Cancer Therapy* (E. M. Hersh, M. A. Chirigos, and M. J. Mastrangelo, eds.), Raven Press, New York, 1981.
11. E. Tzehoval, S. Segal, Y. Stabinsky, M. Fridkin, Z. Spirer, and M. Feldman, *Proc. Natl. Acad. Sci. USA, 75*:3400 (1978).
12. E. Tzehoval, S. Segal, Y. Stabinsky, M. Fridkin, Z. Spirer, and M. Feldman, *Springer Semin. Immunopathol., 2*:205 (1979).
13. E. Tzehoval, S. Segal, Y. Stabinsky, M. Fridkin. Z. Spirer, and M. Feldman, in *Advances in Pharmacology and Therapeutics*, Vol. 4 (B. B. Vargaftig, ed.), Pergamon Press, Oxford and New York, 1979.
14. I. Florentin, M. Bruley-Rosset, N. Kiger, J. L. Imbach, F. Winternitz, and G. Mathé, *Cancer Immunol. Immunother., 5*:211 (1978).
15. J. Martinez, F. Winternitz, and J. Vindel, *Eur. J. Med. Chem.–Chim. Thera., 12*:511 (1977).

16. J. Martinez, in *These Docteur de Science Physiques*, Academie de Montepellier, Université des Sciences Techniques de Languedoc, 1976, pp. 1-144.
17. K. Nishioka, *Br. J. Cancer*, *39*:342 (1979).
18. K. Nishioka, A. A. Amoscato, and G. F. Babcock, *Life Sci.*, *28*:1081 (1981).
19. R. Catane, S. Schlanger, P. Gottlieb, J. Halpern, A. J. Treves, Z. Fuks, and M. Fridkin, Am. Soc. Clin. Oncol. Meet., Washington, D.C., 1981, p. 371.
20. Z. Spirer, V. Zakuth, A. Golander, N. Bogair, and M. Fridkin, *J. Clin. Invest.*, *55*:198 (1975).
21. G. M. Edelman, B. A. Cunningham, W. E. Gall, P. D. Gottlieb, U. Rutishauser, and M. J. Waxdal, *Proc. Natl. Acad. Sci. USA*, *63*:78 (1969).
22. V. A. Najjar, *Exp. Cell Biol.*, *46*:114 (1978).
23. V. A. Najjar, *Klin. Wochensch.*, *57*:751 (1979).
24. V. A. Najjar and J. J. Schmidt, in *Lymphokine Reports*, Vol. 1 (E. Pick, ed.), Academic Press, New York, 1980, p. 157.
25. A. Constantopoulos, V. A. Najjar, J. B. Wish, T. H. Necheles, and L. L. Stolbach, *Am. J. Dis. Child.*, *125*:663 (1973).
26. A. Constantopoulos, V. Likhite, W. H. Crosby, and V. A. Najjar, *Cancer Res.*, *33*: 1230 (1973).
27. M. K. Chaudhuri and V. A. Najjar, *Anal. Biochem.*, *95*:305 (1979).
28. Z. Spirer, V. Zakuth, N. Bogair, and M. Fridkin, *Eur. J. Immunol.*, *7*:69 (1977).
29. Y. Stabinsky, M. Fridkin, V. Zakuth, and Z. Spirer, *Int. J. Pept. Protein Res.*, *12*: 130 (1978).
30. H. Yajima, H. Ogawa, H. Watanabe, N. Fujii, M. Kurobe, and S. Miyamoto, *Chem. Pharm. Bull.*, *23*:371 (1975).
31. O. Mishimura and M. Fujino, *Chem. Pharm. Bull.*, *24*:1568 (1976).
32. J. Vicar, V. Gut, I. Frič, and K. Blaha, *Collection Czechoslov. Commun. Chem.*, *41*:3467 (1976).
33. S. Nozaki, K. Hisatsune, and I. Muramatsu, *Bull. Chem. Soc. Jap.*, *50*:422 (1977).
34. D. Konopinska, E. Nawrocka, I. Z. Siemion, S. Slopek, S. Szymaniec, and E. Klonowska, *Int. J. Peptide Protein Res.*, *9*:71 (1977).
35. Y. Stabinsky, M. Fridkin. V. Zakuth, and Z. Spirer, Israel Chem. Soc., Proc. 44th Ann. Meet., 1977.
36. M. Fridkin, Y. Stabinsky, V. Zakuth, and Z. Spirer, in *Peptides 1976* (A. Loffet, ed.), *Proceedings of the Fourteenth European Peptide Symposium*, Editions de l'Universite de Bruxelle, Belgium, 1976, p. 541.
37. M. Fridkin, Y. Stabinsky, V. Zakuth, and Z. Pirer, *Biochim. Biophys. Acta*, *496*:203 (1977).
38. M. Fridkin and P. Gottlieb, *Mol. Cell. Biochem.*, *41*:73 (1981).
39. K. Nishioka, *Mol. Cell. Biochem.*, *41*:13 (1981).
40. V. A. Najjar and A. Constantopoulos, *J. Reticuloendothel. Soc.*, *12*:197 (1972).
41. D. Konopinska, E. Nawrocka, I. Z. Siemion, S. Szymaniec, and S. Slopek, in *Peptides 1976* (A. Loffet, ed.), Editions de l'Universite de Bruxelle, Belgium, 1976, p. 535.
42. S. Fitzwater, Z. I. Hodes, and H. A. Scheraga, *Macromolecules*, *11*:805 (1978).
43. M. Blumenstein, P. P. Layne, and V. A. Najjar, *Biochemistry*, *18*:5247 (1979).
44. I. P. Sekacis, E. E. Liepins, N. I. Veretennikova, and G. I. Chipins, *Bioorg. Chim.*, *5*:1617 (1979).
45. Y. Stabinsky, P. Gottlieb, V. Zakuth, Z. Spirer, and M. Fridkin, *Biochem. Biophys. Res. Commun.*, *183*:599 (1978).
46. M. K. Chaudhuri and V. A. Najjar, *Fed. Proc.*, *40*:1737 (1981).
47. Z. Bar-Shavit, Y. Stabinsky, M. Fridkin, and R. Goldman, *J. Cell. Physiol.*, *100*:55 (1979).
48. R. M. G. Nair, B. Ponce, and H. H. Fudenberg, *Immunochemistry*, *15*:901 (1978).

49. Z. Bar-Shavit, I. Bursuker, and R. Goldman, *Mol. Cell. Biochem.*, *30*:151 (1980).
50. Y. Stabinsky, P. Gottlieb, and M. Fridkin, *Mol. Cell. Biochem.*, *30*:165 (1980).
51. V. A. Najjar and M. Griffith, *Biochem. Biophys. Res. Commun.*, *16*:472 (1964).
52. V. A. Najjar, *Phys. Rev.*, *43*:243 (1963).
53. Y. Stabinsky, *Studies on the Phagocytosis Stimulating Peptide Tuftsin*, Ph.D. thesis, The Weizmann Institute of Science, Rehovot, Israel, 1979.
54. B. N. Babior, *N. Engl. J. Med.*, *298*:659 (1978).
55. T. P. Stossel, *N. Engl. J. Med.*, *290*:717 (1974).
56. R. L. Baehner, L. A. Boxer, and J. Davis, *Blood*, *48*:309 (1976).
57. R. L. Baehner and D. G. Nathan, *N. Engl. J. Med.*, *278*:971 (1968).
58. H. Iguchi and S. Nakazawa, *Jap. J. Bacteriol.*, *31*:81 (1976).
59. M. Bruley-Rosset, T. Hercend, J. Martinez, H. Rappaport, and G. Mathé, *JNCI*, *66*: 1113 (1981).
60. R. A. Rauner, J. J. Schmidt, and V. A. Najjar, *Mol. Cell. Biochem.*, *10*:77 (1976).
61. G. L. Tritsch and P. W. Niswander, *Immunol. Commun.*,*10*(1):1-8 (1981).
62. G. L. Tritsch and P. W. Niswander, *Mol. Cell. Biochem.*, *49*:49 (1982).
63. M. Dobrowska, G. Kupryzewski, F. Muzalewski, and J. Kochanowski, *P. J. Pharmacol. Pharm.*, *28*:77 (1976).
64. F. Muzalewski, Personal communication.
65. Y. Stabinsky, Z. Bar-Shavit, Z. Fridkin, and R. Goldman, *Mol. Cell. Biochem.*, *30*:71 (1980).
66. G. Schultz, J. G. Hardman, K. Schultz, C. E. Baird, and E. W. Sutherland, *Proc. Natl. Acad. Sci. USA*, *70*:3889 (1973).
67. A. Constantopoulos and V. A. Najjar, *Nature New Biol.*, *243*:268 (1973).
68. Z. Spirer, V. Zakuth, S. Diamant, W. Mondorf, T. Stefanescu, Y. Stabinsky, and M. Fridkin, *Br. Med. J.*, *2*:1574 (1977).
69. A. Constantopoulos, V. A. Najjar, and J. W. Smith, *J. Pediatr.*, *80*:564 (1972).
70. K. Inada, N. Nemoto, A. Nishijima, S. Wada, M. Hirata, and M. Yoshida, in *Phagocytosis: Its Physiology and Pathology* (Y. Kokobun and N. Kobayashi, eds.), University Park Press, Baltimore, 1979, p. 101.
71. D. Konopinski, I. Z. Siemion, S. Szymaniec, and S. Slopek, *Pol. J. Chem.*, *53*:343 (1979).
72. W. D. Erikson, E. O. Burgert, and H. B. Lynn, *Am. J. Dis. Child.*, *116*:1 (1968).
73. H. R. Shinefield, C. R. Steinberg, and D. Kaye, *J. Exp. Med.*, *123*:777 (1966).
74. R. A. Seeler, W. Metzger, and M. A. Mufson, *Am. J. Dis. Child.*, *123*:8 (1972).

Section C

Synthetic Polymers

12
MVE-2
Development of an Immunoadjuvant for Cancer Treatment

Richard A. Carrano, John D. Iuliucci, James K. Luce, James A. Page, and Anthony R. Imondi Adria Laboratories, Inc., Columbus, Ohio

I. INTRODUCTION

Immunotherapy with biological response modifiers offers the potential of providing the medical community with safer and more effective therapy of cancer, especially when used in conjunction with cytotoxic chemotherapy or surgery to lower tumor burden. This chapter will describe some of the events that have occurred during the development of an immunomodulating agent.

In the early 1960s a preparation of maleic anhydride divinyl ether copolymer having a broad range of molecular weights from a few thousand to several hundred thousand was tested for antiviral and antitumor effects. This preparation, called divema (NSC-46015, XA124-177, or pyran copolymer), demonstrated antitumor activity or enhanced host resistance used either alone or as an adjuvant with chemotherapy or surgery in murine cancer systems (1). It also demonstrated antiviral activity and other pharmacological effects indicative of immunostimulating activity (2-16).

A clinical study of divema reported in 1978 delineated the major dose-limiting toxicity as thrombocytopenia (17). Other major side effects included leukopenia, hypotension, headaches, seizures, weakness, numbness, and transient vision loss.

Results of studies suggesting that the toxicity was associated with high molecular weight polymers led to the development of a refined method for the synthesis of copolymers with narrower molecular weight distributions designated as MVE-1 to MVE-5 (18). The antiviral and antitumor effects and toxicity of these MVE copolymers were tested in mice by Morahan et al. (19). The tumors consisted of the Lewis lung carcinoma and P815 mastocytoma and the viruses, encephalomyocarditis (EMC) virus and ATCC VR 129.

Acute toxicity increased with increasing molecular weights of the MVEs. The higher molecular weight MVE also increased the susceptibility of mice to bacterial endotoxins. The platelets were especially sensitive, with higher molecular weight MVE causing the most severe platelet depression. The content of several microsomal mixed-function oxidases (MMFO) was lowered by MVE, with the most severe effect caused by the the larger molecular weight fractions. The MMFO levels returned to normal between 7 and 14 days after treatment.

Effects on the reticuloendothelial system were also molecular weight dependent. Higher molecular weight MVE produced greater hepatosplenomegaly and decrease in thymus weight than lower molecular weight MVE. Uptake of sheep red blood cells (SRBCs) into spleen and lung was increased with MVE-3, -4, and -5.

Survival of mice who had the primary site of transplanted Lewis lung carcinoma excised at day 14 (at which time the tumor had already metastasized to the lung) was increased with increasing molecular weight MVE. Similar effects were seen in the P815 mastocytoma which metastasized primarily to the liver and spleen.

Stolfi and Martin (20) tested MVE-1 through MVE-5 against a spontaneous murine virus-induced breast cancer which is antigenic in its host of origin. At high doses, MVE-1 to MVE-4 all produced significant inhibition of tumor growth. Toxicity increased with increasing molecular weights.

Effects on blood-clotting mechanisms, leukocytes, serum glutamic pyruvic trans-aminase, and inulin clearance were more pronounced with MVE-3, -4, and -5 than with MVE-1 and -2. Based on the observation that toxicity increased with increasing molecular weight of MVE-3, -4, and -5 and evidence that MVE-1 had the least antitumor potential, it was decided to develop MVE-2 for use as an immunomodulating agent.

MVE-2 (Fig. 1) has the advantage over earlier biological response modifiers such as BCG, *Corynebacterium parvum*, and products derived from natural sources as it is a well-defined reproducible synthetic entity, with defined purity.

As synthesized, MVE-2 is an anhydride, but in solution with pH adjusted with sodium hydroxide to pH 7 it forms the sodium salt of the free acid (Fig. 2). MVE-2 has a weight average mol wt of 11,500 daltons as determined by size-exclusion chromatography and laser light scattering using polystyrene as a standard.

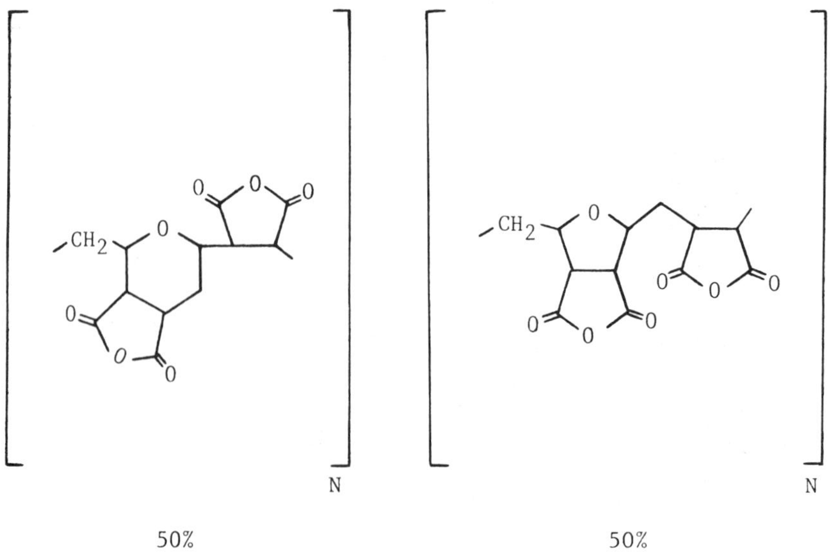

Figure 1 MVE-2: 1:2 divinyl ether-maleic anhydride cyclic copolymer.

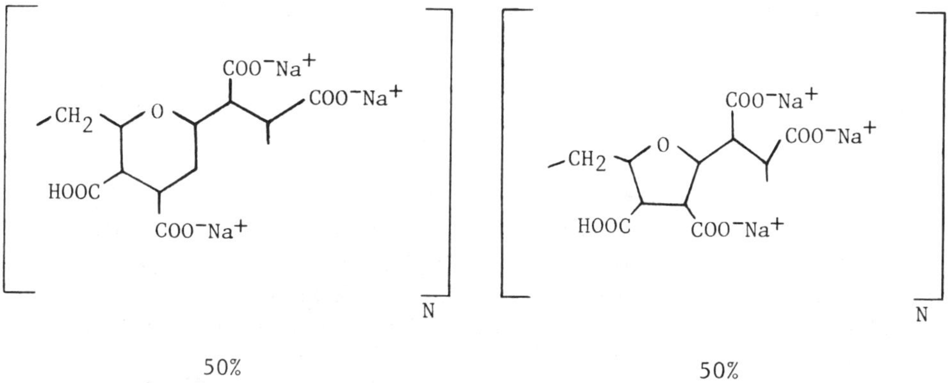

Figure 2 MVE: 1:2 divinyl ether-maleic anhydride cyclic copolymer in solution of aqueous NaOH, pH 7.0.

The action of biological response modifiers on the immune system is not fully understood. However, several studies, mostly in murine systems, have indicated certain mechanisms by which MVE-2 may be exhibiting its effects in experimental tumor systems. Figure 3 is a schematic drawing of possible immunomodulating and toxic effects of MVE-2 in mice. The next sections of this chapter will summarize some of the studies that support this speculation and further comment will be found in the discussion section.

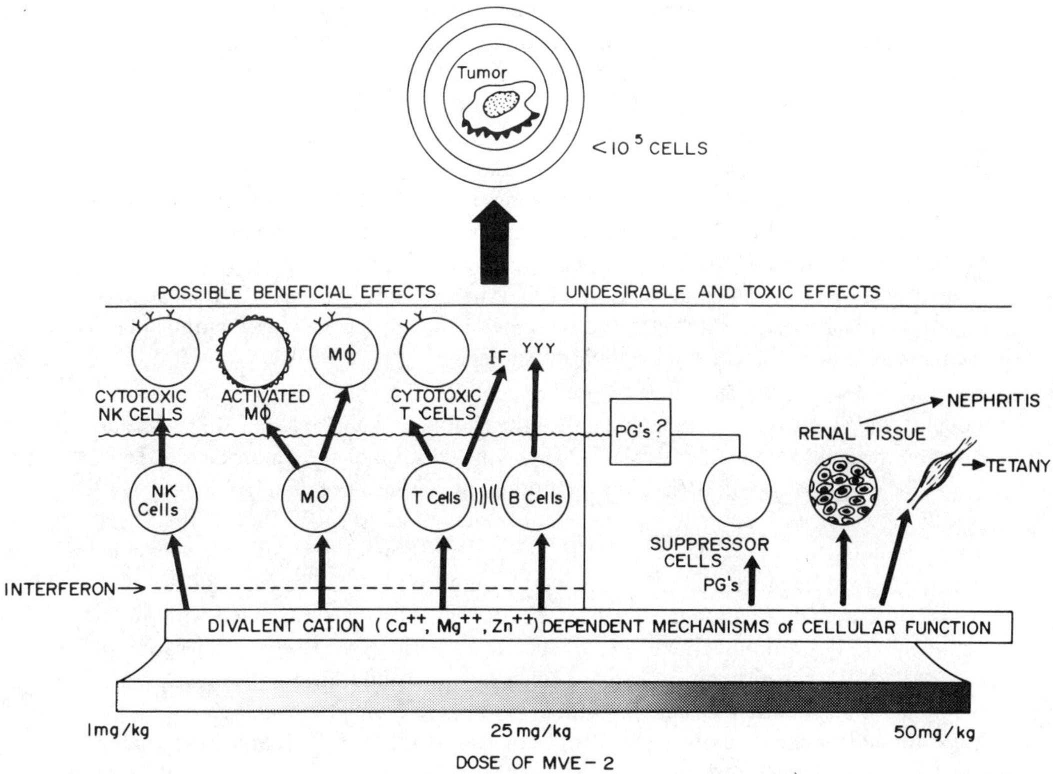

Figure 3 Possible immunomolding and toxic effects of MVE-2 in mice.

II. IMMUNOMODULATION

A. Antitumor Activity

Immunomodulators by themselves do not exhibit antitumor activity to the extent observed with chemotherapeutic agents. However, MVE-2 as a single agent was found to have antitumor activity in various animal models. Single doses of 500 mg/kg and 1000 mg/kg IP on day 0 inhibited the growth of spontaneous autochthonous breast tumors by approximately 60% in CD8F1 mice (20). Chirigos and Stylos (21) reported that MVE-2 was active against the poorly immunogenic L1210 tumor (tumor/control ratio (T/C) = 130) but not against LSTRA at doses of 20 mg/kg, IP on days 1-5. In B16 melanoma-bearing BDF_1 mice, MVE-2 resulted in a dose-related increase in median survival time (MST) at doses of 5 and 25 mg/kg IP on a -1-, +2-, +5-day schedule. T/C for the 5 and 25 mg/kg doses were 128 and 156, respectively (22).

MVE-2 was not effective against Lewis lung carcinoma, a tumor which metastasizes primarily to the lung, but did increase survival time in mice bearing P815 mastocytoma, a tumor which metastasizes to the liver and spleen (19,23). Pulmonary metastases induced by either IV (21,24) or footpad (25) inoculation of Madison 109 (M109) cells, an immunogenic tumor which is relatively resistant to chemotherapy, were inhibited by MVE-2.

MVE-2 also inhibited the growth of primary M109 lung carcinoma (26). In this model the antitumor effect of MVE-2 was dependent upon the route of administration, with the intravenous and intratumor routes being more effective than the IP route. These studies suggest that tissue distribution and, in particular, localization within or close to the tumor, is an important determinant of the antitumor activity of MVE-2.

Several studies have demonstrated antitumor efficacy of MVE-2 when used as an adjuvant in combination with chemotherapy or surgery. Thus, although MVE-2 was inactive in the LSTRA leukemia model when administered alone, it significantly enhanced the efficacy of 1,3-Bis(β-chloro-ethyl)-1-nitroso urea (BCNU) in this model (2,27). Similarly, Chirigos et al. (28) have demonstrated marked synergism between MVE-2 and cyclophosphamide in MBL2 leukemia. These findings are particularly important because a major therapeutic use for MVE-2 may be in combination with chemotherapy. Moreover, the potential for MVE-2 to be an effective adjuvant in chemotherapy may be greatly increased if it can be demonstrated that, like pyran copolymer (29), its ability to activate macrophages is not affected by some of the more widely used antineoplastic agents such as doxorubicin and cyclophosphamide.

MVE-2 was also effective when used in combination with surgery in the Lewis lung model in which the tumor was injected into the footpad. An increase in MST was obtained in those mice treated with MVE-2 following removal of the tumor-bearing leg (24).

The combination of MVE-2 with radiotherapy has also been studied in animal models; however, the results to data have not been conclusive (30). On the other hand, studies to determine the efficacy of MVE-2 in combination with a vaccine have yielded encouraging results. It has been demonstrated, for example, that a single IP dose of MVE-2 potentiated radiation-inactivated L1210 vaccine in mice inoculated with L1210 tumor cells (21). Although the degree of specificity with regard to the potentiation of vaccine by MVE-2 is not known, earlier studies by Mohr and Chirigos (9) using pyran copolymer indicated that vaccine potentiation was specific for the vaccinating cell type. It was found, for example, that mice protected against the LSTRA tumor were unable to reject L1210 leukemia. Additional studies of this type with MVE-2 would be of interest.

B. Antiviral Activity

MVE-2 at a dose of 25 mg/kg IP decreased mortality by 10% in mice infected with encephalomyocarditis virus (24) and by 60% in mice infected with herpes simplex virus 2 (23). More recently, MVE-2 was reported to protect mice against influenza virus but not against mouse hepatitis virus (32).

C. Cell Activation

The activation of peritoneal macrophages by IP administration of MVE-2 has been demonstrated in several laboratories (19,21,23,24,27,28).and is thought to be responsible, at least in part, for the antitumor effects of this drug. Target cells for MVE-2-activated macrophages included M109, MBL-2, Lewis lung carcinoma, and B_{16} melanoma. MVE-2-activated macrophages were not cytotoxic to mouse embryo fibroblasts (24). Tumoricidal and tumoristatic activity against M109, B_{16}, and L5178Y lymphoma cells have also been demonstrated with MVE-2-activated alveolar macrophages (23). In the latter study, the alveolar macrophages were activated by two doses of MVE-2 (25 mg/kg) administered IV on 2 consecutive days. In mice inoculated with M109 in the footpad, the 2-day dosing regimen at weekly intervals also resulted in a significant increased life span (ILS). These results, together with those of Chirigos et al. (28) showing an increase in M109 tumor growth in mice at a time when MVE-2 induced macrophage tumoricidal activity was decreasing, suggest that there is a relationship between the activation of macrophages and antitumor activity.

Macrophage activation has also been implicated in antibacterial activity of MVE-2. For example, IP administration of MVE-2 protected mice against mortality induced by the IP administration of *Shigella flexneri* but not against *Diplococcus pneumoniae*. The former required intracellular transport to be pathogenic, whereas the latter does not require a macrophage transport system (31).

The activation of macrophages may involve an interaction with lymphokines released by T lymphocytes (32). MVE-2 is thought to stimulate T cells in vivo since it is a potent stimulator of delayed-type hypersensitivity (21,33). Recent studies have shown that stimulation of DNA synthesis in vitro by T-cell mitogens, phytohemagglutinin (PHA) and concanavalin A (ConA), was much greater in spleen cells taken from MVE-2-treated mice than in those taken from control mice (31). However, in these studies, stimulation of DNA synthesis was also observed with lipopolysaccharide (LPS), a B-cell mitogen, suggesting that MVE-2 may have an effect on B cells. Moreover, the possibility that B cells may be involved in the activation of macrophages by MVE-2 is suggested by results of studies showing activation of macrophages by pyran copolymer in nude mice (34).

It has been suggested that MVE-2 may exert its antimetastatic activity via natural killer (NK) cell activation as well as by macrophage activation (23). Results of early studies on the effects of pyran copolymers on NK cell activity were not clear; both augmentation and suppression of NK activity following administration of pyran copolymer were reported (35,36). More recently, however, Chirigos et al. (28) and Bartocci et al. (37), using both YAC and M109 target cells, have shown that MVE-2 does stimulate NK cells. In these studies, NK activity exhibited a peak effect on day 3 postdose with diminished activity on day 6, whereas maximum macrophage activation was noted on days 3 and 6. Thus, at least two cell types, macrophages and NK cells, presumed to play an important part in tumor surveillance, have been shown to be activated by MVE-2.

Although mediation by T and/or B cells in the activation of macrophages by MVE-2 was suggested from in vivo studies, activation was also demonstrated when MVE-2 was added to normal macrophages in vitro (27), suggesting that activation of macrophages by MVE-2 may involve a direct effect.

D. Mechanism of Action

The mechanism by which MVE-2 activates macrophages remains obscure. MVE-2 has a high affinity for divalent cations, and it is possible that the ability of MVE-2 to bind or sequester these cations plays a role in its immunomodulating activity (38).

Studies by Mohr et al. (39) demonstrated that MVE-2 derepressed the DNA from isolated murine liver nuclei and that this effect was influenced by the concentration of Mg^{2+}. However, the interaction of MVE-2 with Mg^{2+} in these studies was complex and suggested that derepression and inhibition were proceeding concomitantly with Mg^{2+}, affecting both processes.

Greene and Munson (40) reported that MVE-2 inhibited wheat germ DNA-dependent RNA polymerase by a mechanism involving competition for divalent cations. In these studies, MVE-2 inhibited both chain initiation and chain elongation similar to the effects observed with ethylenediamine-tetraacetic acid (EDTA). It has also been suggested that a shift in Ca^{2+} flux is involved in the activation of macrophages by MVE-2 (41). While no direct evidence for this has been reported, the hypothesis is certainly tenable in view of the known affinity of MVE-2 for Ca^{2+} and the important role of Ca^{2+} in the activation of lymphocytes (42,43).

The broad-spectrum molecular weight pyran copolymers were reported to be interferon inducers (44); however, there have been no reports of interferon induction with MVE-2. Although the role of interferon in tumor immunology is yet to be determined, studies on the effects of MVE-2 on interferon induction may prove to be a fruitful area for research.

III. PHARMACOLOGY

A. Cardiovascular Effects

MVE-2 is synthesized as an anhydride, but in aqueous media it is converted to a polycarboxylic acid with properties of a metal chelator. The rapid intravenous administration of MVE-2 in mice caused convulsions, respiratory depression, and cardiac fibrillation (45); symptoms also associated with hypocalcemic tetany were observed upon rapid intravenous administration of EDTA (46,47).

Studies in our laboratories using anesthesized dogs (48) showed that the IV administration of MVE-2 at doses of 0.1 or 1.0 mg/kg over a 30-sec time period had no significant effects on the cardiovascular, respiratory, or autonomic nervous systems. Responses to epinephrine, acetylcholine, norepinephrine, histamine, tyramine, 1,1-dimethyl-4-phenyl piperazinium iodine (DMPP), and isoproterenol were not modified by MVE-2 (30).

In doses greater than 10 mg/kg per 30 sec, there were dose-related depressor responses, pulsus alternans, reduced myocardial contractility, ECG changes, and increased central venous pressure. These effects were reversed following intraaortic administration of $CaCl_2$. The untoward cardiovascular and respiratory effects were lessened considerably by slowing the infusion rate of MVE-2. For example, there were no effects on cardiovascular or respiratory function in the anesthetized dog when MVE-2 was infused at a rate of 0.8 mg/kg/min for up to 180 min. At doses of 1.27 mg/kg/min and 1.67 mg/kg/min, a fall in systolic blood pressure was observed within 45 min and 1.5 min, respectively. Within 3 hr, systolic blood pressure fell to 500 mmHg or respiration stopped. Thus, the magnitude of the acute cardiovascular and respiratory effects of MVE-2 are dose-dependent and rate-dependent, similar to the hypocalcemic effect induced by the IV administration of EDTA (47).

B. Pharmacokinetics

The tissue distribution of [^{14}C]MVE-2 has been studied in rats (30), dogs (49), and mice (50). [^{14}C] 2,3 Maleic anhydride was used in the synthesis to label the polymer backbone.

In the rat, a single IV bolus of 25 mg/kg was rapidly cleared from the blood. Within 4 hr, concentrations in the blood were approximately 500 ng/ml; at 24 hr, concentrations in the blood were 180 ng/ml and 26 ng/ml in males and females, respectively. Excretion of the drug was primarily via the kidney, but total excretion, urinary plus fecal, was about 20% in 48 hr in this study. Data obtained recently in our laboratory suggest that the total 24 hr urinary and fecal excretion in the rat may be about 35%.

Tissue distribution of MVE-2 was extensive, and removal from the tissues was slow (30). Significant amounts of radioactivity were found in the liver (8% of dose), carcass (11% of dose), and kidney (1% of dose) 28 days postdose. The levels of ^{14}C in the brain were practically nondetectable, representing much less than 0.1% of the dose at all time intervals. Levels of $^{14}CO_2$ in respired air were essentially nil, suggesting that the polymer was not catabolized.

In the dog, tissue distribution and elimination of MVE-2 (35 mg/kg) were studied using both rapid (10 min) and slow (180 min) infusions. Clearance from blood was rapid with a half-life of approximately 0.25 hr and 1.5 hr for the a and b phases, respectively. Tissue concentrations of MVE-2 at 24 hr postdose were generally greater in the dogs given the slow infusion. Twenty-four hour urinary excretion was about 80% of the dose following rapid infusion and about 65% following the slow infusion. Excretion in the feces, indicative of biliary excretion, was less than 1% of the dose. It was also found that approximately 10% of the dose remained in the liver for up to 20 weeks after either rapid or slow infusion of [^{14}C]MVE-2.

In view of the apparent importance of route of administration on the antitumor efficacy of MVE-2 (26), a study was conducted in mice to compare the tissue distribution of [^{14}C]MVE-2 following IV and IP administration (Table 1). Percentage of the dose in

Table 1 Tissue Distribution of [^{14}C]MVE-2 in the Mouse (% of dose/organ)

		Hours postdose			
Tissue	Route	1	4	24	72
Liver	IP	2.34 ± .98	5.07 ± .60	6.51 ± 2.41	7.02 ± 1.50
	IV	3.95 ± .37	4.37 ± .87	4.34 ± 0.74	4.58 ± 1.34
Kidney	IP	1.24 ± .91[a]	0.78 ± .29[b]	0.60 ± 0.11[a]	0.48 ± 0.23
	IV	5.02 ± .89	2.01 ± .49	0.87 ± 0.10	0.71 ± 0.11
Spleen	IP	0.18 ± .06	0.30 ± .10	0.42 ± 0.12[b]	0.33 ± 0.10
	IV	0.16 ± .06	0.18 ± .07	0.18 ± 0.03	0.18 ± 0.05
Lung	IP	0.37 ± .23[b]	0.85 ± .54[b]	0.25 ± 0.20	0.75 ± 0.65
	IV	0.13 ± .02	0.13 ± .02	0.13 ± 0.03	0.13 ± 0.04

[a]$p < 0.05$, between IV and IP. Data are mean ± SD% of dose, N = 5.
[b]$p < 0.01$ between IV and IP. Data are mean ± SD% of dose, N = 5.

the kidney during the first 24 hr postdose was significantly higher following IV administration. The amount of [^{14}C]MVE-2 in the lung was generally much higher in mice receiving the IP dose. The significance of this finding is not clear, particularly in view of the apparently greater efficacy of MVE-2 in the M109 model when given IV as compared with IP (26). However, additional studies in which tissue concentrations of MVE-2 are determined at shorter and more frequent postdose intervals may shed some light on this question.

C. Antigenicity

Studies have also been carried out in our laboratories to evaluate the antigenic potential of MVE-2 (30). In guinea pigs, doses of 1 and 100 mg/kg IP did not cause an anaphylactic response following an IV challenge 2 weeks later, but a dose of 10 mg/kg did produce a slight reaction suggesting that MVE-2 may be antigenic under certain conditions or at specific doses. MVE-2 was also administered IV to rabbits using various dosing regimens, and no anti-MVE-2 IgG was detectable by either RIA or precipitin assays. There was no induction or reaginic antibody as measured by the passive cutaneous anaphylaxis (PCA) reaction in the guinea pig.

IV. TOXICOLOGY

Several preclinical safety evaluation studies have been performed on MVE-2 using both single and repeated administration. The intravenous route has been studied to the greatest extent.

A. Acute Toxicology

Acute toxicity studies have been performed on MVE-2 in mice and rats by the oral, intraperitoneal, intramuscular, and intravenous routes of administration, and in dogs by the intravenous route (Table 2) (30).

Acute toxic and lethal effects were only observed when MVE-2 was administered by the intravenous route. The acute effects appear to be due to a hypocalcemic effect and can be circumvented by coadministration of calcium. In mice treated intravenously with

Table 2 Summary of Acute Toxicity Studies on MVE-2

Species	Method of administration	LD_{50} (mg/kg)
Mice	PO	> 1000
	IP	> 1000
	IM	> 1000
	IV (rapid)	80-100
	IV (Ca^{2+} form)	250-> 750
Rats	IV (rapid)	45-75
	IP	> 1000
	PO	> 1000
	IM	> 1000
Dogs	IV (1 ml/kg, 3 ml/min)	> 100 mg/kg

single doses of MVE-2 in which 20 or 40% of the carboxyl functions on the molecule were neutralized with Ca^{2+}, the LD_{50} values were greatly increased (Table 2) (45). Mice can also be protected from lethal intravenous doses (100 mg/kg) by prior treatment with intravenous $CaCl_2$ (51).

The acute effects of MVE-2 can also be circumvented by decreasing the rates of injection. MVE-2 at a single dose of 100 mg/kg caused death in 100% of rats treated by intravenous bolus, but was without effect when administered over a 3-hr period (52). The influence of injection rate on acute toxic events has also been demonstrated in beagles. Behavioral signs of toxicity occur with intravenous administration of MVE-2 at a dose of 25 mg/kg when given at a rate of 9 mg/kg/min, whereas the same dose produces no behavioral signs of toxicity when administered at a slower rate of 4 mg/kg/min (53).

B. Multiple Dose Toxicology

One-month intravenous toxicity studies were performed in rats and dogs (30) to support initial clinical trials of MVE-2. Rats were administered MVE-2 by rapid intravenous injection at daily dosage levels of 3, 6, and 15 mg/kg for 30 days or at a twice-weekly dose of 15 mg/kg for 4 weeks. Hematology, clinical chemistry, and urinalysis were not altered by MVE-2 treatment. Phagocytic cells of the liver, lymphatic system, and lungs were stimulated at all dosage levels. This effect was characterized by ballooning of the Kupffer cells, increased number of histiocytes in the spleen and sinus of the mesenteric lymph nodes, and increased numbers of alveolar macrophages.

Beagles were administered MVE-2 intravenously at dosage levels of 1, 5, and 20 mg/kg/day for 28 consecutive days at injection rates of 0.4, 2, and 9 mg/kg/min, respectively. Animals from each group were sacrificed at the end of the 28-day dosing period or after a 28-day recovery period. No deaths occurred at any dosage level, and only one dog in the high-dose group had a progressive loss of appetite, weight, and general health from the second week of dosing until the scheduled sacrifice at the end of the dosing period. No outstanding effects on hematology or urinalysis parameters were seen in any animal during the dosing phase of this study. However, proteinuria was seen during the recovery phase in both sexes at the higher dosage levels.

Elevated serum glutamic pyruvic transaminase (SGPT), serum alkaline phosphatase, lactate dehydrogenase (LDH), and cholesterol values were noted in the high-dose male dogs from the second week of treatment. With the exception of cholesterol, these parameters returned to normal at the end of the recovery period.

Macrophage accumulation was seen in the spleen, liver, kidneys, and regional and systemic lymph nodes of dogs at the higher dosage levels at the end of the dosing period and after the 28-day recovery period. A slight to moderate multifocal tubular degeneration was seen in the kidney cortex, with occasional necrosis of tubular epithelial cells at the end of the 28-day dosing period. After the recovery period, the renal cortical tubular degeneration was present in varying degrees in the MVE-2 treatment groups. Extensive liver damage with infiltration of large numbers of macrophages, resulting in necrosis of centrilobular hepatocytes, was seen in at least one dog in the high-dose group after the recovery period. Thus, the kidney and liver are two potential target organs of toxicity for MVE-2 in humans. The kidney is more sensitive than the liver.

Consecutive daily dosing schedules were employed in the initial preclinical toxicology studies to produce optimal conditions for identifying potential target organs of toxicity. The question whether the toxicological profile of MVE-2 is altered when the material is administered on an intermittent dosage regimen and at a much slower rate of injection was studied in dogs (53). MVE-2 was administered intravenously to male beagles at dosage levels of 25 mg/kg (500 mg/m^2) and 150 mg/kg (3000 mg/m^2) twice weekly for up to 4 weeks, with each dose being given in a constant volume of 30 ml/kg over a 3-hr infusion period (i.e., 0.14 mg/kg/min and 0.83 mg/kg/min, respectively). A group of dogs was kept under observation after the dosing phase to determine reversibility of toxic effects.

Unexpectedly, severe renal toxicity occurred at low cumulative doses which were safe in previous multiple-dose studies in which MVE-2 was administered by the more rapid intravenous injection. Elevations in BUN and serum creatinine, cholesterol, and phosphorus and decreases in serum total protein, albumin, and globulin were seen after cumulative doses of 1500 mg/m^2 had been administered. Quantitative analyses for urinary protein revealed severe proteinuria, in some cases over 300 mg/dl. Several animals subsequently developed a complete nephrotic syndrome, including generalized edema and ascites, which in some cases progressed to mortality or morbidity.

Histopathological renal changes in the infused animals included glomerular nephritis with fibrin in the glomerulus, protein casts in the tubules, tubular dilatation, the adhesion of glomerular capillaries to Bowman's capsule, and mononuclear infiltration.

Two beagles showing proteinuria were monitored during a posttreatment recovery period for reversibility of the renal lesion. One animal continued to show proteinuria for the first 2 months after being removed from treatment. Urinary protein levels appeared normal at 3 and 4 months after treatment, after which the animal was sacrificed and necropsied. Histopathological examination of the kidneys revealed that the glomeruler lesion was still present, although the severity of the lesion was reduced as compared with that seen in the dogs sacrificed at the end of the treatment period. The other animal still demonstrated moderate to severe proteinuria 12 months after the last treatment.

The studies described above suggest that the induction and/or severity of the renal lesion is related to the injection rate of MVE-2. Therefore, an intravenous infusion versus intravenous injection toxicity study on MVE-2 was performed in dogs (54). One group of dogs was administered 25 mg/kg of MVE-2 (500 mg/m^2) at an injection rate of 4 mg/kg/min. A second group of dogs was administered MVE-2 also at a dose of 25 mg/kg; however, this dose was administered as a 3-hr infusion in a constant volume of 30 ml/kg (0.14 mg/kg/min). In each case, the dose was administered twice a week for an intended 4-week period, and necropsies were scheduled for the week after the eighth and final dose.

Animals infused with MVE-2 over a 3-hr period had proteinuria within 24 hr after the first treatment which progressed to levels between 4000 and 5000 mg/dl. Changes seen in serum chemistries prior to the second dose included decreased albumin and total protein which were followed by increased BUN, creatinine, and phosphorus. One dog in the 3-hr infusion group died on the third day after receiving the fourth treatment. Fluid accumulation was first noted in the abdominal area on the last dose day. At necropsy, approximately 1 L of clear fluid was found in the peritoneal cavity.

In contrast, dogs treated with MVE-2 by intravenous injection (4 mg/kg/min) survived the duration of the study, and no proteinuria was seen until after the eighth and final dose. Relatively slight proteinuria was noted on the day after the last dose. The amount of protein appeared to peak at 3 days after this last dose (up to 1000 mg/dl) but did not reach the level seen in dogs receiving MVE-2 by infusion. On the fourth day after the last treatment, a downward trend in the protein values was observed before the animals were sacrificed. Histopathological evaluation revealed that infusion dogs have severe glomerular damage as well as severe tubular damage similar to observations made in the previous studies. However, dogs receiving MVE-2 by intravenous injection showed only occasional mild glomerular damage.

Thus, it is apparent that the rate of MVE-2 intravenous administration has a marked influence on the induction of renal pathology. While the 3-hr infusion caused proteinuria and microscopic pathology leading to death or severe nephrotic syndrome at a cumulative dose of 1500 mg/m^2, dogs treated with the IV injection tolerated the drug much better, overtly and microscopically.

The temporal aspects of the renal lesion have been studied in the dog infusion model (53). MVE-2 was administered intravenously to four groups of male beagles as a single 3-hr infusion of 500 mg/m^2. Different groups were sacrificed 4, 12, 24, and 72 hr after initiation of drug administration. An additional group similarly received two MVE-2 doses of 500-mg/m^2 3 days apart and was sacrificed 24 hr after the second treatment.

Light microscopy revealed proliferative glomerular nephritis in all MVE-2-treated groups which consisted mainly of mesangial cellular proliferative changes with increases in the amount of mesangial matrix. The proliferation was relatively mild and focal in the group administered one dose of MVE-2 and sacrificed at 4, 12, and 24 hr, and more pronounced and diffuse in the group sacrificed at 72 hr and in the group sacrificed at 24 hr after receiving a second treatment. Some cellular necrotic changes were seen in the latter two groups; however, there was no evidence of fibrin deposition signifying that no necrotizing changes were present. These light microscopic observations indicate that glomerular damage, similar to that seen in the earlier infusion studies, can be initiated by a single infusion of MVE-2 and that the severity of the renal lesion is both time and dose dependent.

Electron microscopic examination of the kidney from one of the animals sacrificed 24 hr after a single treatment revealed glomerular ultrastructural changes consisting mainly of an expanded mesangium filled with many discrete electron-dense deposits. The glomerular endothelial and epithelial cells appeared enlarged, and the podocytes showed focally fused foot processes at the sites of the dense deposits. The dense deposits resemble those seen in immune complex-mediated glomerulonephritis in human and animal kidneys.

C. Teratology

The teratogenic potential of MVE-2 was investigated in rats administered MVE-2 intravenously by slow IV administration at dosage levels of 10, 20, and 40 mg/kg/day. MVE-2 produced no teratogenic or other adverse effects on normal fetal development (55).

V. CLINICAL

Phase I clinical studies with MVE-2 took into account the toxicological effects seen in animals as well as the toxicity observed in clinical trials with Divema, a broad molecular weight pyran copolymer (17). In addition to toxicity monitoring, it was considered important in a phase I study of MVE-2 to observe patients for any immunomodulating effects in an attempt to identify a maximum immunostimulating dose consistent with tolerable toxicity. Antitumor activity in animals had been demonstrated using single doses, doses three times a week, or doses given days 1-5. Although immunomodulating agents should theoretically be more effective in animals with minimal tumor burdens, MVE-2 did demonstrate activity in animals with measurable amounts of tumor.

A. Clinical Phase I Protocols

Phase I studies were performed on patients with disseminated malignant neoplasms who, for the most part, had had extensive prior chemotherapy. The initial regimen consisted of doses given once weekly in 3-hr dextrose and water or saline infusions. The duration of infusions was subsequently shortened to 1 hr when no immediate adverse effects were noted. In an additional phase I study, patients without prior chemotherapy were treated once every 3 weeks. The initial dose administered was 25 mg/m^2. This dose was chosen to be in the nontoxic range, but consistent with the dose that had shown antitumor effects in animals. The following immunological tests were performed on patients prior to treatment days 3, 4, and 5, and then weekly: serum interferon and lysozyme levels, monocyte adherence determinations, and antibody-dependent cell-mediated cytotoxicity to chicken and human red blood cells and natural killer cell assays. Renal function, liver function, and hematological tests were also obtained. Comprehensive eye examinations were performed serially.

B. Results of Phase I Studies

Rare, transient fevers were seen that could not, however, be related to dose. Patients tolerated the medications well without any other side effects. No changes in total serum calcium were observed; however, ionized calcium was not measured.

The first reproducible toxicity seen consisted of proteinuria observed in patients who received 300 mg/m^2 or greater of MVE-2 per dose to a cumulative dose of 900-1200 mg/m^2 or greater. The protein in the urine consisted of approximately 80% albumin and 20% globulin. If MVE-2 was continued, over 1 g of protein per day was excreted, and patients developed hypoproteinemia, hypercholesterolemia, hyperlipidemia, and peripheral edema characteristic of the nephrotic syndrome. The proteinuria was reversible in from 1 week to several months, depending upon the severity. Six patients developed transient prolongation of the partial thromboplastin time (up to twice the control value). No hepatic toxicity was observed. Mild hypoalbuminemia occurred in patients who developed proteinuria. Patients did not develop mucositis, alopecia, diarrhea, or consistent fever.

Immunological function tests performed for up to 10 weeks were generally inconclusive. In two of three patients who had no prior chemotherapy and were treated every 3 weeks, increases in antibody-dependent cell-mediated cytotoxicity and natural killer cell activity occurred at doses of 400 mg/m^2. No increases were observed in serum interferon or lysozyme levels. In patients treated with extensive disease who had had considerable prior treatment, little effect on immune parameters resulted. They were not good candidates in which to evaluate immunological effects of MVE-2.

A complete response was recorded in one patient with subcutaneous melanoma metastases. Partial responses were seen in one patient each with chronic lymphocytic leukemia, melanoma, and soft tissue sarcoma. Three patients with metastatic soft tissue sarcomas, rendered disease-free by surgery or radiation therapy, have continued in complete remission 6 months to over 1 year following treatment with MVE-2.

The phase I trials had two aims:

1. To determine side effects and dose-limiting toxicity of MVE-2
2. To determine the dose and regimen that produced maximum immunostimulation

To date, neither of these objectives has been definitely accomplished. Although glomerular dysfunction appears to be the dose-limiting toxicity, dog studies and, recently, clinical trials indicate this can be lessened by shortening the duration of infusions. Several patients demonstrated increases in levels of both lymphocyte and monocyte antibody-dependent cell-mediated cytoxicity to red blood cells and NK cell activity, but no clearly defined dose-related effect on the immune system has been observed.

Pharmacokinetic studies using ^{14}C-labeled MVE-2 will be conducted in humans to determine serum levels and drug elimination rates.

Phase II trials with MVE-2 will be planned, using doses and duration of treatment found to cause minimal or no renal effects and with schedules that produced some changes in immune tests during the phase I trails. It appears inappropriate to conduct classic phase II studies, that is, in patients with advanced disease. With an immunomodulating agent, it is reasonable to conduct trials early in phase II in patients with minimal disease. This includes adjuvant therapy in patients with high risk for recurrence such as soft tissue sarcoma patients with advanced but recently excised tumor, and in combination with chemotherapy in patients with a high rate of complete response but without an expected prolonged duration of remission.

VI. DISCUSSION

Figure 3 is a schematic diagram of the possible immunomodulating and toxic effects of MVE-2 that may play a role in adjuvant antitumor therapy with MVE-2. Table 3 summarizes several points evident on this speculative scheme that have been suggested from preclinical and clinical studies with MVE-2.

In the early 1960s, an anionic polymer consisting of maleic anhydride and divinyl ether was prepared with a broad molecular weight distribution ranging from a few thousand to several hundred thousand daltons. Early work on this copolymer demonstrated that it had antitumor, antibacterial, and antiviral activity, resulting presumably from its immunomodulating ability, especially macrophage stimulation. This copolymer was tested clinically in patients with malignant tumors and was found to be quite toxic. Further clinical trials were abandoned. Antitumor studies with other similar copolymers, referred to as pyran copolymers, were often done in animals with palpable tumors where the activity was understandably rather minimal, possibly due to the inability of the immune system to eradicate a large, growing tumor.

Table 3 Summary of Important Preclinical and Clincial Findings with MVE-2

1. MVE-2 acts best when tumor burden is low. It is not particularly active as a direct cytotoxic agent.
2. MVE-2 has a high affinity for divalent cations, and it is strongly suspected that this plays a role in both its beneficial and toxic effects.
3. The main target organ of toxicity after acute rapid administration (< 10 min) is muscle tetammy leading to cardiovascular effects and finally respiratory collapse. Slow administration (> 10 min) does not appear to produce these effects.
4. The main target organ of toxicity for prolonged infusion is the kidney, leading to proteinuria and a progressive glomerular nephritis with infiltration of inflammatory cells. This effect does not occur as severely with rapid infusions (> 10 min, < 1 hr).
5. The optimal dose level and scheduling and optimal route of administration of MVE-2 necessary for optimal effect are not yet known but are under investigation.
6. MVE-2 affects many cell types including macrophages, NK, T, and B cells. The effect is most marked on macrophages and NK cells, but the effect and duration differ, depending on the cell type. Further studies need to be done to apply these differential effects to selecting the optimal dose and treatment schedule.

In 1973, the efficacy of the pyran copolymers as an adjuvant to conventional chemotherapy and other effects on the immune system was demonstrated. It was then recognized that their full potential in cancer treatment might be in patients with a small tumor burden and a competent immune system.

A process was developed to synthesize anionic polymers with the same chemical structure but with much narrower molecular weight distributions than divema and the early pyran copolymers. These new polymers were more correctly called maleic vinyl ethers (MVE). Five preparations, designated MVE-1 to MVE-5, were synthesized.

Animal tests with these preparations demonstrated that the higher molecular weights (MVE 3-5) were both more toxic and more effective as antitumor, antiviral, and immunomodulating agents than preparations with lower molecular weights (MVE 1-2).

Based on a compromise between toxicity and effectiveness it was decided to develop MVE-2 for eventual clinical trials, as it retained the basic immunomodulation effects and was less toxic. MVE-1 was less effective than MVE-2 as an immunomodulator. Characterization of MVE-2 and methods for its reproducible synthesis on a large scale were crucial steps which had to be solved early in the program.

Animal studies with MVE-2 demonstrated antitumor activity with the drugs given both IP and IV. Doses IP ranging from 5 to 1000 mg/kg inhibited tumor growth.

The IV route was found to be more effective than the IP route in some animal tumors. Antitumor effects were demonstrated at doses of 25 and 50 mg/kg (75 and 150 mg/m^2) IV. Full dose-ranging studies were not performed since doses higher than 50 mg/kg given by rapid IV injection were lethal, probably because of the calcium-chelating properties of MVE-2.

MVE-2 demonstrated antitumor efficacy when given as an adjunct to chemotherapy or surgery. Since the adjuvant use of an immunomodulating agent such as MVE-2 is the most likely circumstance in which it will be clinically effective, the results of these studies stimulated further development of the drug.

The immunomodulating effects of MVE-2 include activation of both peritoneal and alveolar macrophages. These MVE-2-activated macrophages have shown greater activity against malignant than nonmalignant cells.

Several possible mechanism of macrophage activation have been proposed. MVE-2 may stimulate T cells since it stimulates delayed-type hypersensitivity. The stimulated T cells may then release lymphokines which interact with macrophages. It may interact with B cells since it activates macrophages in nude mice. On the other hand, MVE-2 may activate macrophages directly. Its antitumor activity may be due to activation of NK (natural killer) cells. It was shown to stimulate NK cells in tests using both YAC and M109 target cells. Immunostimulation with MVE-2 has been seen at doses as low as 1 mg/kg.

Its mechanism on the subcellular level is unknown. MVE-2 has a high binding affinity for divalent cations such as Ca^{2+}, Mg^{2+}, and Zn^{2+}. The concentration of Mg^{2+} has been shown to influence the derepression of DNA from isolated murine liver nuclei. MVE-2 inhibited wheat germ DNA-dependent RNA polymerase by a mechanism involving competition for divalent cations. The activation of macrophages may be related to a shift in Ca^{2+} flux produced by MVE-2.

Animal toxicology of MVE-2 has translated to humans with remarkable accuracy. MVE-2 causes convulsions, respiratory depression, and cardiac fibrillation when given rapidly IV in mice. This is felt to be due to hypocalcemia induced by the calcium-chelating action of MVE-2. Cardiovascular alterations produced by MVE-2 are reversed by intravascular $CaCl_2$ administration or by slowing the rate of MVE-2 infusion.

Pharmacokinetic studies performed with ^{14}C-labeled MVE-2 in the rat demonstrated principally urinary excretion; however, total urinary and fecal excretion was less than 35% during the first 48 hr. Extensive tissue distribution with slow removal was demonstrated. In the dog, MVE-2 was rapidly cleared from the plasma. The 24-hr urinary excretion was about 80% following a rapid (7-10 min) infusion and 65% following a 3-hr infusion. About 10% of the dose remained in the liver 20 weeks after either a rapid or slow infusion.

The acute cardiovascular toxic effects of larger doses of MVE-2 are less if the carboxyl functions on the molecule are partially neutralized by Ca^{2+}. Prolonging the duration of the infusion permits larger doses to be given, presumably because of rapid metabolic compensation for hypocalcemia.

Chronic toxic effects in animals involve the liver and the kidneys. Repeated daily bolus doses appear to stimulate the reticuloendothelial system, manifested by ballooning of the Kupffer cells in the liver, increased number of histiocytes in the spleen and lymph nodes, and increased numbers of alveolar macrophages. Transient rises in hepatic enzymes were recorded as well as necrosis of centrilobular hepatocytes.

Repeated slow infusions in dogs produced renal glomerulonephitis manifested by proteinuria. If infusions were continued, a typical nephrotic syndrome resulted. The renal damage for the same cumulative dose was much more severe if the drug was given by prolonged (3 hr) rather than rapid (7-10 min) infusions. Histologically, kidney changes consisted of fibrin in the glomerulus, protein casts, tubular dilatation, adhesion of capillaries to Bowman's capsule, and mononuclear cell infiltration. Electron microscopy performed on renal tissue obtained 24 hr after a single dose showed an expanded mesangium with discrete electronodense deposits resembling those seen in immune complex-mediated glomerulonephritis.

Whether or not the results of animal efficacy studies performed with MVE-2 will extrapolate to humans remains to be seen. Additional preclinical studies on the mechanism of action and potential application of MVE-2 appear warranted. However, it is difficult to predict if any of these studies will clarify ultimate clinical utility. Surely, cell specificity, dose level, and dose scheduling may be very important determinants of efficacy.

Phase I clinical studies have been performed. MVE-2 initially was administered by a 3-hr infusion; later during the studies some patients received 2-hr, 1 hr, and 20- or 10-min infusions.

Patients were monitored both for toxicity and for stimulation of the immune system. No consistent immune stimulation was seen with tests that included measurement of NK activity, interferon induction, macrophage activation, PHA and PWM blastogenesis, increase in T or B cells, and antibody-dependent (ADCC) cytotoxicity to human or chicken red blood cells. At least one center reported increased monocyte maturation and increased monocyte ADCC.

The drug was given either once weekly or once every 3 weeks. Doses from 25 mg/m^2 to 300 mg/m^2 were tolerated without acute or chronic side effects or organ dysfunction. Doses 400 mg/m^2 or higher to cumulative doses of 1200 mg/m^2 or greater generally produced proteinuria. One patient manifested signs of a nephrotic syndrome when MVE-2 administration was continued after proteinuria developed. This suggests that the glomerulus is the principal target organ of toxicity in man. With doses 1200 mg/m^2 or greater infused over 2 or 3 hr, proteinuria appeared following the first dose of the drug.

Based on animal studies that showed less proteinuria with shorter duration infusions, the duration of infusion was shortened to 30, 20, or 10 min. Under these conditions, approximately twice the amount of the drug could be administered before proteinuria developed; however, as predicted in animal studies, signs of hypocalcemia developed, including perioral numbness and muscular irritability. The serum ionized, but not total, calcium fell as much as to 50% of the preinfusion level.

Tumor regression was noted in a few patients with malignant melanoma, soft tissue sarcoma, and lymphatic malignancies. Most patients in the phase I trial had far-advanced disease. While they were suitable for phase I studies in that no other known effective treatment was available, they were patients with little likelihood of responding to the modest effects expected of an immunomodulating agent. Stimulation of the immune system has rarely been shown to produce antineoplastic effects in animals bearing more than 10^5 malignant cells. The role of immunomodulating agents will probably be in circumstances in which other therapy rids the body of the bulk of the malignant cells, then host defenses, augmented by an immunomodulating agent, should be able to control the remaining small number of cancer cells. In addition, the doses used in these phase I effects in animals, as the phase I studies were primarily safety studies. Other immunomodulating agents are known to span biphasic effects between high and low doses.

Despite the lack of a clear demonstration of immunostimulation by the tests performed during the phase I study, MVE-2 remains an attractive immunomodulating agent to study. It has clearly demonstrated antitumor and antiviral activity as well as stimulation of the immune system in animals. Its dose-limiting toxicities are predictable, preventable, and reversible and are at doses well above those that produced antitumor effects in animals. It has a defined chemical composition composed of a polymer with a narrow molecular weight distribution. Various investigators may then study MVE-2 with an assurance of no significant batch-to-batch variation. This contrasts sharply with such agents as BCG and *C. parvum* which have a history of showing considerable variation in activity, depending on the source.

Clinical studies are planned for MVE-2 as surgical adjuvant in which MVE-2 should show effectiveness if it is active in humans. It is not known whether low, moderate, or high doses will be the most effective, thus a range of doses will be tested. Similarly, the most effective regimen is not known. Because it is retained in reticuloendothelial organs, widely spaced doses might be most effective. Conversely, frequent dosing to continually stimulate the immune system may produce the best antitumor effect. Ongoing preclinical studies may shed more light on the schedule most likely to succeed.

REFERENCES

1. D. S. Breslow, *Pure Appl. Chem.*, *46*:103 (1976).
2. S. J. Mohr, M. A. Chirigos, F. S. Fuhrman, and J. W. Pryor, *Cancer Res.*, *35*:3750 (1975).
3. R. M. Schultz, W. A. Woods, S. J. Mohr, and M. A. Chirigos, *Cancer Res.*, *36*:1641 (1976).
4. J. W. Pearson, M. A. Chirigos, S. D. Chaparas, and N. A. Sher, *J. Natl. Cancer. Inst.*, *35*:463 (1974).
5. P. S. Morohan, J. A. Munson, L. G. Baird, A. M. Kaplan, and W. Regelson, *Cancer Res.*, *34*:506 (1974).
6. R. M. Schultz, J. D. Papamatheukis, J. Luetzeler, and M. A. Chirigos, *Cancer Res.*, *37*:358 (1977).
7. J. Sandberg and A. Goldin, *Cancer Chemother. Rep.*, *55*:233 (1971).
8. P. S. Morahan, W. Regelson, and A. E. Munson, *Antimicrob. Agents Chemother.*, *2*:16 (1972).

9. S. J. Mohr and M. A. Chirigos, in *Control of Neoplasia by Modulation of the Immune System* (M. A. Chirigos, ed.), Raven Press, New York, 1977, pp. 421-435.
10. D. S. Breslow, *Pure Appl. Chem.*, *46*:103 (1976).
11. W. Regelson, *L'Interferon*, *6*:353 (1970).
12. W. Regelson, A. E. Munson, W. R. Wooles, W. T. R. Lawrence, and I. T. Levy, *L'Interferon*, *6*:381 (1970).
13. A. E. Munson and W. Regelson, *Proc. Soc. Exp. Biol. Med.*, *137*:553 (1971).
14. L. H. Dennis, A. Angeles, M. Baig, and B. I. Shnider, presented at *Am. Soc. Clin. Pharm. Chemother.*, May, 1969.
15. P. S. Roberts, W. Regelson, and B. Kingsbury, *J. Lab. Clin. Med.*, *2*:822 (1973).
16. Y. Shamash and B. Alexander, *Biochim. Biophys. Acta.*, *194*:449 (1969).
17. W. Regelson, B. I. Shnider, J. Colsky, K. B. Olson, J. F. Holland, C. L. Johnson, Jr., and L. H. Dennis, in *Immune Modulation and Control of Neoplasia by Adjuvant Therapy* (M. A. Chirigos, ed.), Raven Press, New York, 1978, pp. 469-490.
18. D. S. Breslow, United States Patent Office, Patent No. 3, 974, 622, patented February 26, 1974.
19. P. S. Morahan, D. W. Barnes, and A. E. Munson, *Cancer Treat. Rep.*, *62*:1797 (1978).
20. R. L. Stolfi and D. S. Martin, *Cancer Treat. Rep.*, *62*:1791 (1978).
21. M. A. Chirigos and W. A. Stylos, *Cancer Res.*, *40*:1967 (1980).
22. R. L. Wolgemuth, Unpublished observations.
23. D. W. Barnes, P. S. Morahan, S. Loveless, and A. E. Munson, *J. Pharmacol. Exp. Ther.*, *208*:392 (1979).
24. N. A. Pavlidis, R. M. Schultz, M. A. Chirigos, and J. Luetzeler, *Cancer Treat. Rep.*, *62*:1817 (1978).
25. S. E. Loveless and A. E. Munson, *Cancer Res.*, *41*:3901 (1981).
26. P. C. Klykken, B. R. Kipps, P. S. Morahan, and A. E. Munson, Submitted to *Cancer Res.*
27. J. H. Dean, M. L. Padarathsingh, and L. Keys, *Cancer Treat. Rep.*, *62*:1807 (1978).
28. M. Chirigos, V. Papademetriou, A. Bartocci, and E. Read, *Adv. Immunopharmacol.*, *Proc. Int. Conf. Immunopharmacol.*, *1*:217 (1981).
29. J. N. Stoychkov, R. M. Schultz, M. A. Chirigos, N. A. Pavlidis, and A. Goldin, *Cancer Res.*, *39*:3014 (1979).
30. R. A. Carrano, F. K. Kinoshita, A. R. Imondi, and J. D. Iuliucci, *Progr. Cancer Res. Ther.*, *16*:345 (1981).
31. A. M. Isetta, D. Trizio, M. A. Verini, and D. Jabes, Unpublished.
32. P. A. Campbell, *Bacterial Rev.*, *40*:284 (1976).
33. E. L. Read, V. Papademetrious, M. A. Chirigos, and A. Bartocci, *Fed. Proc.*, *40*:990 (1981).
34. J. D. Stinnett and J. A. Majeski, *J. Surg. Oncol.*, *14*:327 (1981).
35. P. Puccetti, A. Santoni, C. Riccardi, H. T. Holden, and R. B. Herberman, *Int. J. Cancer*, *26*:837 (1980).
36. A. Santoni, C. Riccardi, T. Barlozzari, and R. B. Herberman, *Int. J. Cancer*, *26*:837 (1980).
37. A. Bartocci, V. Papademetrious, and M. A. Chirigos, *J. Immunopharmacol.*, *2*:149 (1980).
38. R. J. Fiel, E. H. Mark, and H. I. Levine, *J. Colloid Interface Sci.*, *55*:133 (1976).
39. S. J. Mohr, J. G. Massicot, and M. A. Chirigos, *Cancer Res.*, *38*:1610 (1978).
40. R. Greene and B. Munson, *Can. J. Biochem.*, *58*:295 (1980).
41. W. Regelson, *Cancer Treat. Rep.*, *62*:1853 (1978).
42. R. G. Coffey, E. M. Hadden, and J. W. Hadden, *J. Immunol.*, *119*:1387 (1977).
43. R. Y. Tsien, T. Pozzan, and T. J. Rink, *Nature*, *295*:68 (1982).
44. T. C. Merigan, *Nature*, *214*:416 (1967).

45. V. G. Stygles, G. P. O'Hara, J. D. Iuliucci, T. L. Robbins, and A. R. Imondi, *Fed. Proc.*, *38*:847 (1979).
46. A. Popovici, C. F. Geschichter, A. Reinovsky, and M. Rubin, *Proc. Soc. Exp. Biol. Med.*, *74*:416 (1950).
47. W. G. Nayler, *J. Pharmacol. Exp. Ther.*, *137*:5 (1962).
48. E. J. Belair, Manuscript in preparation.
49. J. R. Baldwin, R. A. Carrano, and A. R. Imondi, *Fed. Proc.*, *41*:1558 (1982).
50. R. L. Wolgemuth, Manuscript in preparation.
51. V. G. Stygles, Unpublished.
52. S. W. Mann, Manuscript in preparation.
53. J. D. Iuliucci, Manuscript in preparation.
54. J. D. Iuliucci, S. W. Mann, and R. A. Carrano, *The Pharmacologist*, *24*:190 (1982).
55. J. J. Mitala, Manuscript in preparation.

13

NED 137

A Low Molecular Weight Polycarboxylate with Immunostimulatory Activity

Julia A. Teodorczyk-Injeyan, Judith A. Falk, Leonardo Makowka, Leo Filion, and Rudolf E. Falk University of Toronto, Toronto, Ontario

Frederick L. Moffat Toronto General Hospital and University of Toronto, Toronto, Ontario, Canada

I. INTRODUCTION

Therapy of neoplasia by immunostimulatory intervention began with specific active immunotherapy by the injection of autologous tumor cells performed by von Leyden and Blumenthal (1). Introduction of bacterial adjuvants to immunotherapy (2) has stimulated much interest in nonspecific active immunotherapy of cancer. Nonspecific activation of the immune system by adjuvants of bacterial origin such as Bacille Calmette-Guérin (BCG) or *Corynebacterium parvum* (*C. parvum*) may exert protective and/or therapeutic effects in experimental and clinical neoplasia (3-5). However, despite effectiveness in experimental tumor models (6-8), the clinical application of BCG and *C. parvum* is still controversial. General activation of the cellular components of the immune system frequently provides undesirable effects such as stimulation of already activated suppressor cells (9,10). Moreover, cross reactivity of bacterial adjuvants with host and/or tumor tissues has been demonstrated (11,12). Therefore, agents capable of more selective activation of cells involved directly or indirectly in the antitumor response could have a significant clinical potential. In addition to bacterial fractions, several families of polyanionic synthetic polymers have been shown to be highly active as immunomodulators and demonstrated specific host-mediated antitumor activity (13). Antitumor effects of the most widely studied polycarboxylic acid polymers have been demonstrated in a variety of experimental and clinical models (14-16), and therapeutic efficacy of these compounds has been attributed to their intrinsic biological activity. Polycarboxylatès such as pyran copolymer (divinyl ether maleic anhydride copolymer, DIVEMA, MVE) can enhance antibody production to test antigens (17,18), virus and tumor vaccines (13,19), and alter the lymphoproliferative response of B or T cells to mitogens (20,21). The cellular mechanisms of the mode of action of pyran and its related analogs are complex. The immunomodulating activity of polycarboxylates has been shown to be mediated through T and B lymphocytes (22-26) and/or through the stimulation of the reticuloendothelial system and activation of macrophages (20,21). Polycarboxylates have been frequently regarded as interferon inducers (27) but without any correlation with their antitumor activity (28).

The immunomodulating properties of synthetic polyanions derived from ethylene maleic anhydride copolymers (EMA) relate to their molecular weight (29,30). Recent studies of defined molecular weight fractions of pyran have indicated that the toxicity of EMA copolymers is associated with high molecular weight fractions and can be reduced in low molecular weight material (31). Increasing interest in the investigation of uniform low (mol wt $<$ 15,000) molecular weight polycarboxylates affecting the immune system resulted in the development of the biofunctional polymer NED 137 (Monsanto Co., St. Louis, Missouri) derived from EMA copolymers and selected after preliminary screening of over 60 analogs.

This review describes biological properties of NED 137 as an immunomodulatory agent in augmentation of the immune response to cellular and soluble antigens in vivo and in vitro in rodents. The activity of NED 137 in stimulating the immune response to weakly antigenic experimental tumors is compared with that demonstrated by conventional bacterial and synthetic adjuvants including pyran copolymer.

We report on the status of the clinical testing program using NED 137 in patients with gastrointestinal cancer, and the efficacy of this substance as an immunotherapeutic agent. Finally, we present data elucidating the mode of action of NED 137 and evaluating its potential as a polyclonal activator of the lymphoid system.

II. NED 137: STRUCTURE AND TOXICITY

NED 137 is a relatively well-defined synthetic copolymer of olefin monomers with 2-4 carbon atoms and α, β-unsaturated polycarboxylic anhydrides having 4-6 carbon atoms. The molecular weight of NED 137 and its analogs ranges from 300-1500 daltons (average 800). The optimal biological activity was achieved with copolymer ethylene and maleic anhydrides modified to contain half amide, half carboxylate salt function (Fig. 1a) and unsubstituted imide comprising 5-40% of modified function (Fig. 1b).

(a)

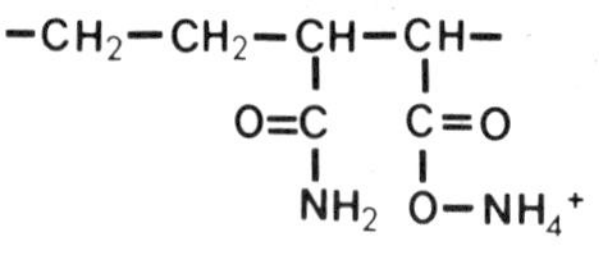

(b)

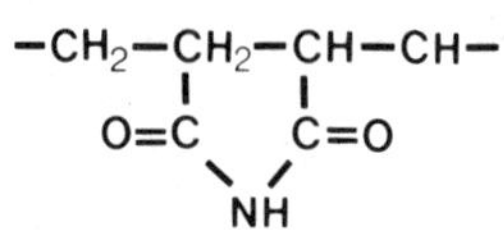

Figure 1 Structural units of NED 137. (a) Half amide, half carboxylate salt. (b) Imide group.

Acute and chronic toxicity of NED 137 has been tested and is not apparent until doses of 1000-5000 times the therapeutic dose are administered on a daily basis. At the very high doses administered on a daily basis, some anterior horn cell degeneration was observed in dogs (Paget, personal communication).

III. BIOLOGICAL ACTIVITY OF NED 137 IN EXPERIMENTAL STUDIES

A. Effect on Antibody Production In Vivo

Early experiments by Regelson and Chirigos indicated that administration of EMA copolymers could significantly increase antibody response to sheep erythrocytes (32,33). Immunostimulatory activity of pyran was frequently correlated with its antitumor effect (34,35), although enhanced tumor growth was reported in certain systems, depending on the time and route of drug administration (36,37).

The effect of NED 137 on the plaque-forming cell (PFC) response was studied in normal and T-cell-depleted Lewis (L) male strain rats, normal CBA/J, C57BL/6, and congenitally athymic BALB/c male and female mice (38,39). The rat and murine humoral responses to both T-dependent (TD) and T-independent (TI) antigents were assessed using the Jerne plaque assay (PFC) (40). Intravenous administration of antigen together with NED 137 at doses ranging from 0.01 to 32 mg/kg of body weight induced a significant increase ($p < 0.05$) in the PFC response to sheep red blood cells (SRBC) in L rats (Table 1).

The duration of the effect of NED 137 was assessed by determining the number of antibody-producing cells in animals at varying time intervals after the treatment. The increase in the number of PFCs was evident up to 8 weeks after administration of the polymer (Table 2).

These results corroborated the data on the retention of ^{14}C-labelled NED 137 in rats (41). The effect of NED 137 on the PFC response to sheep erythrocytes was then tested in thymectomized, 950 R-irradiated and bone marrow reconstituted L rats (38,41). Animals were treated with NED 137 at 30 mg/kg and immunized with SRBCs. Both oral and intraperitoneal administration of NED 137 resulted in a 3.5 fold increase in the

Table 1 Effect of NED 137 on the IgM PFC Response to Sheep Erythrocytes (SRBCs) in L Rats[a]

Intravenous dosage (mg/kg body weight)	Mean PFC/10^6 spleen cells ± SE
0	562 ± 17
0.05	620 ± 22
0.1	1021 ± 83[b]
0.5	1173 ± 72[b]
1	1257 ± 86[b]
2	1144 ± 60[b]
4	1178 ± 53[b]
8	1215 ± 78[b]
16	1138 ± 88[b]
32	1298 ± 121[b]

[a]Animals were immunized by intraperitoneal injection of SRBCs and treated with various doses of NED 137.
[b]$p < 0.05$.

Table 2 Long-Term Effect of NED 137 on the IgM PFC Response to Sheep Erythrocytes in L Rats

Day	Experimental[a]	Control
	Mean PFC/10^6 spleen cells ± SE	
7	1281 ± 86[b]	565 ± 15
14	1071 ± 57[b]	535 ± 13
21	1188 ± 81[b]	563 ± 13
28	1122 ± 46[b]	538 ± 17
56	1026 ± 76[b]	584 ± 13

[a]Animals were treated IP with NED 137 at 30 mg/kg and immunized with SRBCs 4 days before the PFC assay.
[b]$p < 0.05$.

number of PFCs in intact L rats (Table 3). A significant ($p < 0.05$) increase of the PFC response to this TD antigen was also noted in B-cell-enriched animals (Table 3).

Administration of NED 137, however, had no effect on the direct PFC response to sheep erythrocytes in adult BALB/c nude mice (39). A significant increase in number of antibody-producing cells was observed only in the polymer-treated BALB/c nu/+ control mice (Table 4). Similarly, in normal C57BL/6 and CBA/J strain mice treated with the polymer and immunized with sheep erythrocyte antigens the direct anti-SRBC PFC response was consistently significantly elevated (Table 5). The effect of NED 137 appeared to be antigen-specific since no increase in PFCs to horse red blood cells (HRBCs) was found.

Administration of NED 137 induced a significant increase in the direct PFC response to another TD antigen, DNP-dependent antigen (DA) incorporated in $Al(OH)_3^-$ (42). Anti-DNP PFC response measured using trinitrophenylated SRBCs (43) was significantly elevated after drug administration (Table 5). A threshold dose of the polymer was sufficient for the induction of the elevated response to DNP-DA. The effect of the polymer on the murine response to TI antigen was assessed in CBA/J mice injected intravenously with DNP-Ficoll and treated with varying doses of NED 137. The results presented in Table 6 demonstrate that the anti-DNP response of animals injected with NED 137 was again significantly enhanced.

The antigens which were used in the described systems had either intrinsic adjuvant properties or were administered with adjuvant. It has been shown that administration of certain antigens such as TNP-ovalbumin (OA) without adjuvant can induce B memory cells (44) and

Table 3 The Effect of NED 137 on the IgM PFC Response in T-Cell-Depleted L Rats

Treatment	Mean PFC/10^6 spleen cells ± SE
NIL	522 ± 14
NED 137, IP[a]	1425 ± 84[b]
NED 137, PO	1329 ± 106[b]
Tx, 950R, BM	55 ± 5
Tx, 950R, BM, NED 137 IP	707 ± 48

[a]NED 137 was administered at 30 mg/kg.
[b]$p < 0.05$.

Table 4 Effect of NED 137 on the IgM PFC Response to SRBC in BALB/c Nude Mice

NED 137 (mg/kg)	BALB/c[a]	PFC/spleen ± SE
0	nu/nu	2495 ± 296
15	nu/nu	1819 ± 119
0	nu/+	55,800 ± 1160
15	nu/+	118,000 ± 3622[b]

[a]Athymic (nu/nu) and normal (nu/+) BALB/c mice were immunized with sheep erythrocytes and treated with NED 137 on day zero. The anti-SRBC PFC response was measured 5 days later.
[b]$p < 0.05$

prime T lymphocytes (45). The effect of NED 137 in this adjuvant-free model was tested in C57BL/6 mice injected with TNP-OA in saline and treated with varying doses of the polymer. The results presented in Table 7 demonstrate that in NED 137-treated mice the direct PFC response was significantly higher than that of the control group. In another experiment the administration of the polymer was delayed to day 21. The direct and indirect anti-TNP PFC responses were significantly elevated in the animals which had received NED 137 (Table 7).

To determine whether NED 137 could influence the generation of T-suppressor cells, the effect of the polymer on tolerance induction to DNP-DA in $Al(OH)_3$ was investigated. C57BL/6 mice sensitized with antigen on day zero received 1 mg of DA 4 weeks later with or without NED 137 (Table 8). The administration of NED 137 significantly increased the direct and indirect anti-DNP PFC response compared with controls where tolerance had been achieved.

B. Studies In Vitro

Administration of NED 137 in vivo significantly improved the rodent humoral immune response to T-dependent and T-independent antigens. The mechanism of action of the

Table 5 Effect of NED 137 on the PFC Response to TD Antigens in Mice

Treatment NED 137 (mg/kg)	Direct PFC/spleen ± SE ($\times 10^{-3}$)	
	SRBCs[a]	DNP-DA[a]
0	57.0 ± 10.7	0.6 ± 0.02
1	20.5 ± 1.5	1.25 ± 0.14[d]
5	115.0 ± 14.3[c]	1.02 ± 0.16[d]
10	82.5 ± 1.1[c]	1.45 ± 0.11[d]
15	92.4 ± 6.8[b]	1.42 ± 0.14[d]
30	60.6 ± 5.6	1.27 ± 1.56[d]

[a]C57B1/6J mice were immunized with 0.5 ml of 1% SRBC or 1 μg of DNP-DA in $Al(OH)_3$ and treated IP with NED 137. Direct and anti-SRBC and anti-TNP PFC responses were measured on day 5.
[b]$p < 0.01$.
[c]$p < 0.05$.
[d]$p < 0.001$.

Table 6 Effect of NED 137 on the PFC Response to DNP-Ficoll[a]

Treatment, NED 137 (mg/kg)	PFC/spleen ± SE (X 10^{-3})
0	45.5 ± 3.8
1	43.0 ± 8.8
5	269.5 ± 50.5[b]
15	264.5 ± 29.0[c]
30	213.5 ± 27.0[c]
60	239.5 ± 19.5[b]

[a]CBA/J mice were immunized IV with 30 μg of DNP-Ficoll and treated IP with NED 137. The direct anti-TNP PFC response was measured 5 days later.
[b]$p < 0.001$.
[c]$p < 0.01$.

Table 7 Effect of NED 137 on the PFC Response of Mice Immunized with TNP-OA without Adjuvant

NED 137 (mg/kg)	PFC/spleen ± SE		
	Direct[a]	Direct[b]	Indirect
0	10 ± 1	120 ± 55	250 ± 55
1	390 ± 100[c]	1070 ± 195[d]	1225 ± 220[d]
5	570 ± 73[d]	995 ± 180[d]	1035 ± 133[d]
15	490 ± 65[d]	1225 ± 193[d]	1375 ± 190[d]
30	575 ± 83[d]	1490 ± 270[d]	1605 ± 260[d]

[a]C57BL/6 mice were immunized with TNP-OA (20 μg) in saline and treated with NED 137.
[b]C57BL/6 mice immunized with TNP-OA (20μg) were treated with NED 137 3 weeks later. Direct and indirect anti-TNP PFC response was measured 5 days after NED 137 administration.
[c]$p < 0.05$.
[d]$p < 0.001$.

Table 8 The Prevention of T-Cell Tolerance by NED 137

Treatment	Anti-TNP PFC/spleen ± SE	
	Direct	Indirect
Saline	2175 ± 275	2500 ± 213
NED 137	10,450 ± 1525[b]	12,500 ± 1138[b]
1 mg DA	400 ± 108	850 ± 175
1 mg DA + NED 137	4625 ± 338[b]	5975 ± 588[b]

[a]C57BL/6 mice were immunized on day zero and 28 with DNP-DA (1 μg) incorporated in AL $(OH)_3$ (1 mg). Tolerance was then induced by administration of 1 mg of DA and animals were treated IP with NED 137 at 15 mg/kg. The anti-TNP PFC response was measured on day 33.
[b]$p < 0.001$.

polymer, however, was unclear since its effects could be mediated by lymphoid cells, accessory cells, or both. We further characterized the influence of NED 137 on the antibody response in a system modulated by an adherent/phagocytic cell (46). It has been demonstrated that the in vitro PFC response of normal rat spleen cells to SRBCs is seldom, if at all, observed (47,48). Depletion of phagocytic-adherent cells from rat spleen preparations generally induces a significant increase in reactivity of lymphoid cells and permits the generation of antibody-producing cells in vitro (49).

Unfractionated spleen cells from normal L strain rats exposed to NED 137 simultaneously with antigen, that is at the time of culture initiation, demonstrated a significant increase in the number of PFCs at drug concentrations of 3.0×10^{-7} M and 2.5×10^{-6} M per culture (Fig. 2). Higher concentrations of NED 137 were less effective, although no cytotoxic effect could be detected in any of the cultures where the drug was present. In spleen cultures depleted of phagocytic adherent cells the effect of NED 137 was detectable at lower concentrations of the drug and was dose dependent (Fig. 2). The addition of NED 137 alone (without antigen) did not increase the background PFC response in rat spleen cultures with or without accessory cells. The optimal activity of NED 137 was demonstrated in cultures maintained in the presence of both the polymer and antigen throughout the entire culture period.

The effect of NED 137 on the secondary response to SRBCs was tested in lymphocyte cultures prepared from animals previously immunized with SRBCs (46). Carbonyl

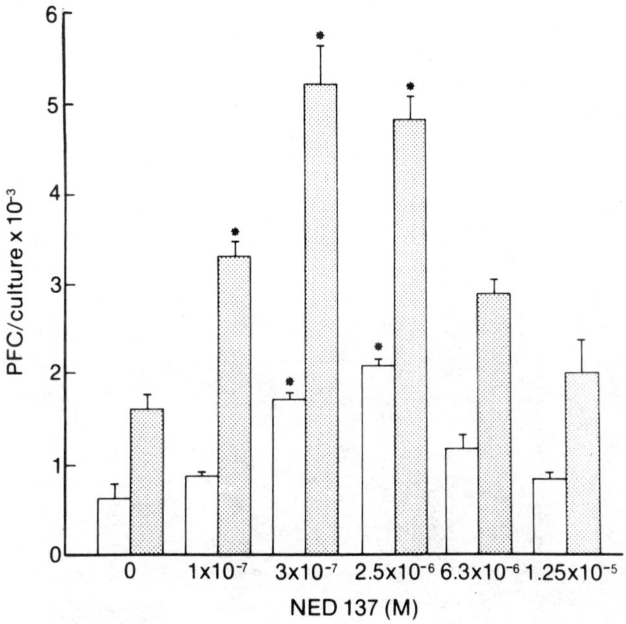

Figure 2 Effect of NED 137 on the plaque-forming cell (PFC) response of rat spleen cells to sheep erythrocytes (SRBCs) in vitro. Normal spleen lymphocytes (open bars) or carbonyl iron-treated cells (stippled bars) were cultivated in the presence of the indicated concentrations of NED 137 and SRBCs. The number of direct PFC per culture were assessed on day 5. $^*p < 0.05$. (From Ref. 46.)

iron-treated cultures were exposed to several concentrations of NED 137 in the presence or absence of SRBCs (Fig. 2). SRBC-primed spleen cells cultured in the presence of NED 137 but without antigen manifested only a moderate increase in the PFC numbers compared with the control. The greatest response was observed in secondary cultures, that is cultures rechallenged with SRBCs and incubated with increasing concentrations of NED 137 (Fig. 3).

The increase in the level of PFCs in the secondary antibody response in vitro appeared to be antigen specific. Spleen cultures prepared from animals primed with SRBCs and exposed in vitro to homologous or heterologous antigen and NED 137 demonstrated a significant increase in the secondary PFC response (Fig. 4). The polymer did not significantly enhance a relatively low primary PFC response in cultures derived from rats primed to an unrelated antigen. This may reflect sequential antigenic competition between sheep and horse erythrocytes which has been described in the rodent system (50).

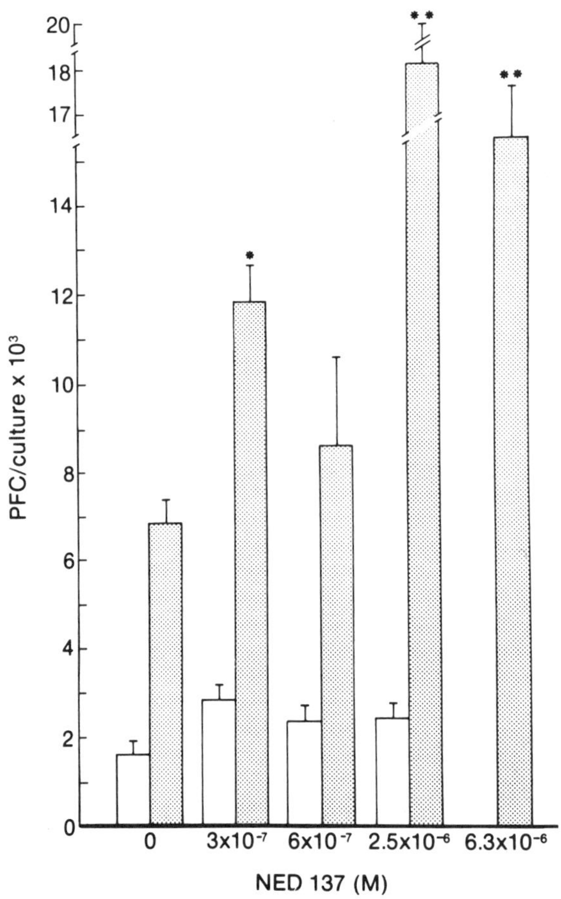

Figure 3 Effect of NED 137 on the secondary in vitro antibody response of rat spleen cells. Animals were immunized intravenously with 10^8 sheep erythrocytes and killed 5 days later. Carbonyl iron-fractionated splenocytes were cultured in the absence (open bars) or presence (stippled bars) of antigens and with the indicated concentration of the drug. $^{**}p < 0.001$; $^{*}p < 0.05$. PFC = plaque-forming cells. (From Ref. 46.)

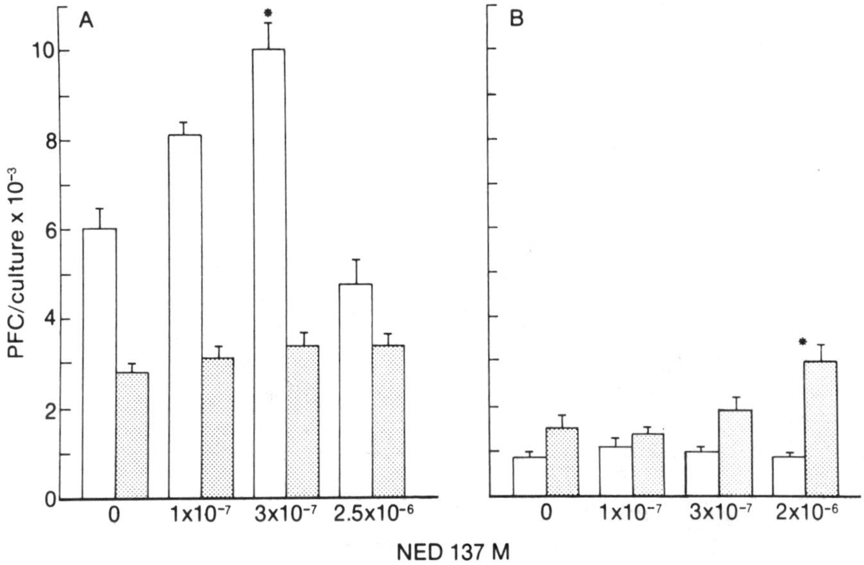

Figure 4 Specificity of the augmenting effect of NED 137 in the secondary in vitro antibody response to sheep (SRBC; open bars) and horse (HRBC; stippled bars) erythrocytes. Rats were immunized intraperitoneally with 1 ml of 10% of SRBC or HRBC and killed 2 weeks later. Carbonyl iron-fractionated spleen cultures from SRBCs (A)- or HRBCs (B)-sensitized animals were cultured in the presence of homologous or heterologous antigen with the polymer at the indicated concentrations. *$p < 0.05$. PFC = plaque-forming cells. (From Ref. 46.)

However, NED 137 did not have a significant effect on induction of the in vitro PFC response to SRBC in normal or macrophage-depleted cultures dervied from T-cell-deficient rats (Tx, 950R, BM reconstituted).

The effect of pretreatment with NED 137 in vivo on the ability of splenic cells to respond to the antigen challenge in vitro was investigated in normal and carbonyl iron-fractionated cultures from L rats pretreated with the polymer at 30 mg/kg at preselected times (46). Figure 5 illustrates PFC levels in unfractionated and carbonyl iron-treated (macrophage-depleted) cultures expressed as a percentage of their appropriate controls from spleens of untreated rats. The PFC response was completely inhibited in cultures prepared from the animals pretreated with NED 137 3-5 days before culture initiation. Plaque formation in macrophage-depleted spleen cultures was restored 1 week after NED 137 treatment but by 2 weeks later in intact (unfractionated) cultures (Fig. 5).

NED 137 did not alter the rate of DNA synthesis of rat spleen cells cultured with various concentrations of the polymer with or without conventional B- and T-lymphocyte mitogens (unpublished observations). The effect of in vivo pretreatment with the therapeutic dose (30 mg/kg) of the polymer on mitogen-induced blastogenesis of rat spleen cells was then assessed. A significant decrease in DNA synthesis was observed in cultures initiated 3-5 days after NED 137 administration and exposed to mitogenic concentrations of concanavalin A and phytohemagglutinin (Fig. 6). The mitogenic response of splenocytes to both mitogens returned to normal (control) values by 7 days after NED 137 treatment, therefore preceding the restoration of the PFC response (Fig. 5).

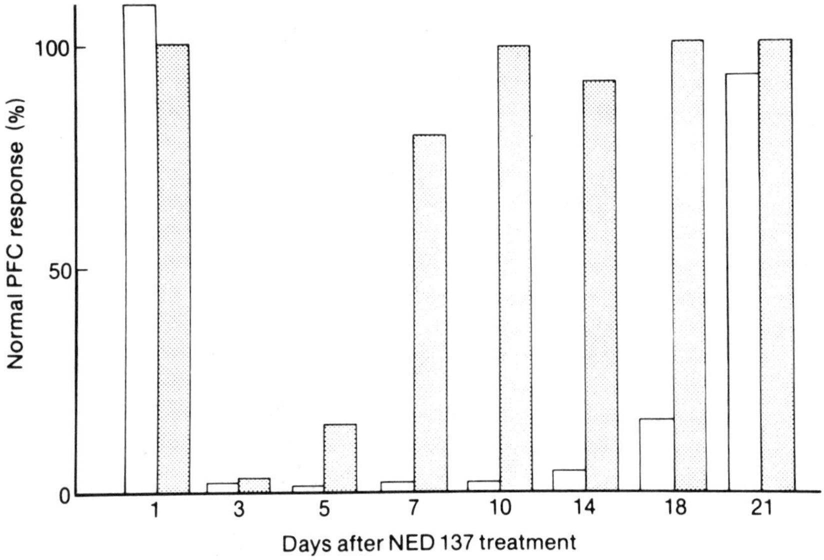

Figure 5 Effect of in vivo pretreatment with NED 137 on rat plaque-forming cell (PFC) response in vitro. Animals treated with NED 137 at 30 mg/kg body weight were killed at various time intervals after treatment. Unfractionated (open bars) or carbonyl iron-fractionated (stippled bars) splenocytes were cultured in the presence of sheep erythrocytes. The IgM-PFC response was assessed on day 5. Results are expressed as the percentage of the PFC response generated by splenocytes from normal (untreated) rats. (From Ref. 46.)

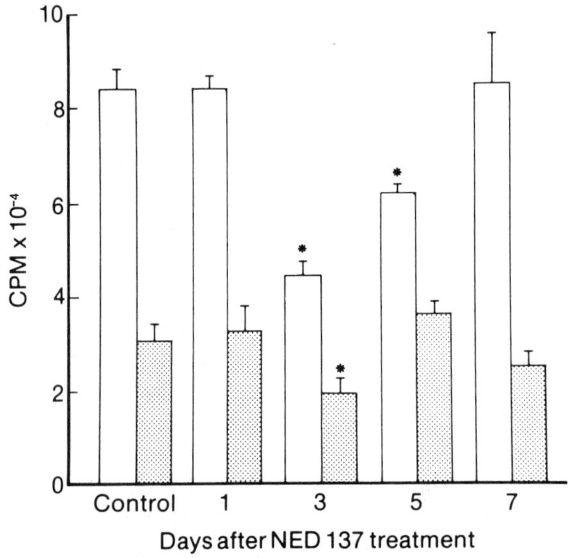

Figure 6 Blastogenic response to concanavalin A (ConA) (open bars) and phytohemagglutinin (PHA) (stippled bars) of splenocytes from rats pretreated with NED 137 1-7 days earlier. Ficoll-Hypague-isolated splenocytes were activated with either 10 μg/ml of ConA or 1% of PHA, and ^{3}H-TdR-incorporation into DNA was measured 3 days later. *$p < 0.05$. (From Ref. 46.)

C. Antitumor Activity of NED 137

The tumor used was a methylcholanthrene-induced carcinoma of the bladder syngeneic in Fischer 344 (FBCa) strain rats. This tumor grows rapidly and metastasizes 5-7 days after subcutaneous implantation of tissue fragments (200-225 mm^3). A single administration of NED 137 at a dose of 30 mg/kg body weight resulted in a 50% increase in the survival time although all experimental animals eventually died (51). Moreover, when autopsied, treated animals were found to be free of pulmonary metastases, contrary to the control rats. Therefore, the effect of the polymer was assessed after surgical excision of the primary tumor. A single administration of NED 137 (intraperitoneally or orally) at the time of excision of FBCa prevented recurrence of the local tumor for over 8 weeks and significantly decreased the incidence of distant metastases (Table 9). Repeated excision of the recurrent tumor and wound closure with syngeneic skin grafts followed by NED 137 treatment at 6 weekly intervals rendered animals tumor free at a 12-month follow-up.

When the polymer was administered at 6-week intervals after excision of the local tumor, the animals treated with multiple injections of the compound remained disease-free for over 14 months (Fig. 7). However, a single administration of NED 137 did not prevent tumor recurrence and eventual mortality, although the treatment significantly, prolonged survival of these animals compared with saline-injected controls (Fig. 7).

The antitumor effect of NED 137 in terms of affecting survival, prevention of recurrent tumor, and presence of metastases after excision of FBCa at day 7 was compared with that of standard immunostimulants such as BCG, *C. parvum*, Freund complete adjuvant (FCA), levamisole, and pyran copolymer (52). NED 137 was administered as a single dose at 30 mg/kg, and the other immune stimulants were given as described elsewhere (35,53-55). Clearly, there was a significant improvement in the survival of the NED 137-treated animals as compared with other adjuvants (Fig. 8).

Animals receiving any of the standard adjuvants survived a mean of 30-40 days, with 100% tumor recurrence and 60-90% incidence of pulmonary metastases (Table 10).

D. Mechanisms of Antitumor Effect of NED 137

Administration of NED 137 at a therapeutic dose of 30 mg/kg into tumor-bearing or tumor-sensitized animals significantly increased their ability to respond to the second challenge with the same cell-bound tumor antigen (41,56). The degree of recognition and specific destruction of radiolabeled tumor cells were assessed in vivo as described

Table 9 Effect of NED 137 on Recurrence and Metastasis of Surgically Removed FBCa[a]

Treatment	Recurrence (mean days)	Incidence of metastases
0	17 + 6	60/60
NED 137, IP	$>60^b$	$3/60^b$
NED 137, PO	$>60^b$	$9/60^b$

[a]FBCa primary tumors were excised 7 days after implantation and animals received NED 137 at a dose of 30 mg/kg intraperitoneally or orally.
[b]$p < 0.001$.

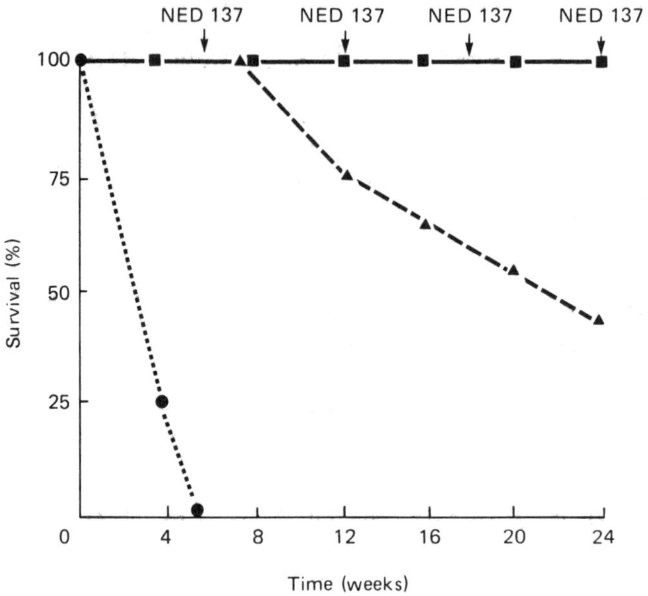

Figure 7 The effect of NED 137 on survival of F344 rats, after excision of the primary FBCa, comparing single administration with treatment every 6 weeks for 6 months. The polymer was administered intraperitoneally at 30 mg/kg on the day of excision (broken line) or at 6-week intervals following surgery (solid line). Control rats (dotted line) received a single injection of saline.

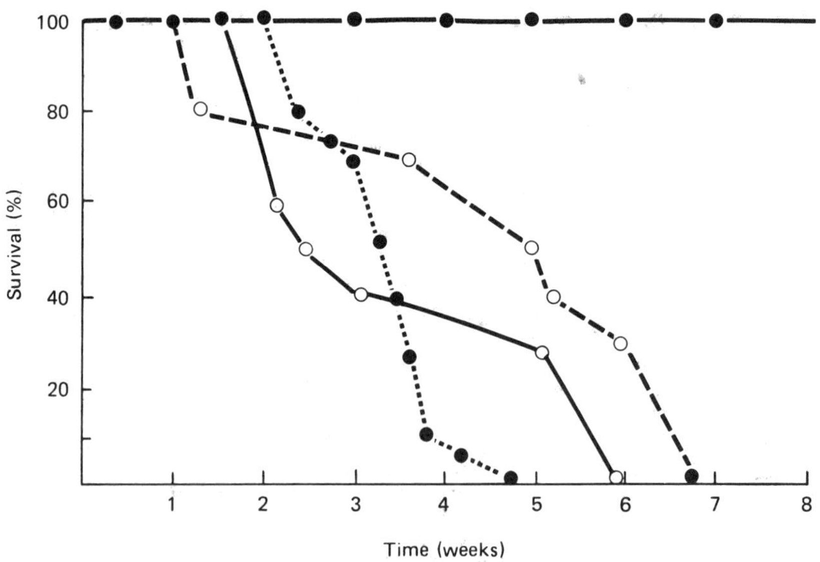

Figure 8 A comparison of the effect on survival, after FBCa excision, of NED 137 versus other adjuvants. NED 137 (solid line) was administered intraperitoneally as a single dose of 30 mg/kg; BCG (broken line) was injected once at a dose of 0.1 mg/kg and *C. parvum* (open circles, solid line) was given both intravenously and intraperitoneally at total of 1.5 mg per rat for 4 consecutive weeks. Control animals (dotted line) were left without treatment.

Table 10 Recurrence of Primary FBCa and Incidence of Metastasis after Adjuvant Treatment[a]

Adjuvant[b]	Recurrence (day ± SD)	Metastases
0	18 ± 5	10/10
BCG	21 ± 10	8/10
C. parvum	29 ± 5	6/8
Levamisole	16 ± 9	9/11
Pyran copolymer	16 ± 7	7/11
FCA	18 ± 10	11/12
NED 137	>60	0/10

[a]Surgical excision of FBCa was performed at 7 days after implantation of the tumor tissue.
[b]Rats were treated with a single (BCG, FCA, NED 137) or multiple (*C. parvum*, levamisole, pyran copolymer) dose of adjuvant on the day of tumor resection.

previously (51). Table 11 shows that F344 rats sensitized by intravenous administration of FBCa cells and treated with varying doses of NED 137 are able to eliminate ^{51}Cr-labeled sensitizing tumor cells at a significantly higher rate.

The activated component(s) and specificity of NED 137-mediated augmentation of the antitumor response were examined in cellular and serum transfer experiments (52,56) and in studies on functional activity of adherent cells after administration of the polymer (56). NED 137 did not have a direct cytotoxic effect on tumor cells in vitro (41).

Sera and spleen cells for transfer experiments were obtained from "cured" animals, which had been treated with multiple injections of NED 137 after surgical resection of

Table 11 Effect of NED 137 on Elimination of FBCa Cells in Tumor-Sensitized F344 Rats[a]

Group	NED 137 (mg/kg)	CPM/g[b]	Index of recognition[c]
1	0	6399 ± 227	1.00
2	0	6267 ± 64	0.98
3	0.05	6024 ± 97	0.94
4	0.5	4991 ± 265	0.78[d]
5	1.3	4928 ± 220	0.77[d]
6	5.0	4208 ± 268	0.66[e]
7	30.0	4359 ± 111	0.68[e]

[a]Rats in groups 2-7 were sensitized by the intravenous injection of 1×10^6 FBCa cells 10 days before assay. Group 1 was the normal (unsensitized) control. At the time of testing each animal received 1×10^6 ^{51}Cr-labeled FBCa cells intravenously.
[b]The radioactivity of weighed spleens removed 24 hr after injection of radiolabeled tumor cells was measured in a gamma counter and expressed as the mean counts per minuts (CPM) ± SD per gram of tissue.
[c]An index of antigen recognition was calculated as a ratio of CPM/g experimental group/ CPM/g control group. Therefore, a lower index reflects a greater degree of antigen recognition and destruction of the radiolabeled target cells.
[d]$p < 0.005$
[e]$p < 0.001$.

primary tumors, as described in the preceding section (Fig. 7). Cells and/or serum were then transferred to normal Fischer rats followed by the injection of ^{51}Cr-labeled FBCa cells.

We demonstrated that transfer of serum (but not spleen cells) from NED 137-treated, "cured" animals caused a 45% increase in destruction of labeled tumor cells over serum from normal animals (Fig. 9). The active component of the serum could be precipitated by 40% ammonium sulfate without deterioration of activity.

The specificity of antitumor activity induced by NED 137 was demonstrated by a comparison of the effect of active ("cured") sera on FBCa and mammary adenocarcinoma (MACa, unrelated tumor, syngeneic in Fischer 344 rats) tumor cells. As shown in Fig. 10 a significant antitumor effect of the transferred serum was demonstrated with FBCa but not with MACa cells. Figure 11 illustrates the time course of the transferred antitumor effect. The destruction of ^{51}Cr-labeled FBCa tumor cells was assessed 1-10 days after the transfer of cells or serum from "cured" rats. The specific effect of "cured" serum was time-limited. On the other hand, the activity of the spleen cells increased after 5 days and persisted up to 10 days after the transfer.

Functional activity of peritoneal exudate cells in NED 137-treated animals was tested by the assessment of phagocytosis of latex particles and enumeration of latex-containing cells. In contrast to BCG, no increase in macrophage numbers or in their phagocytic activity was observed in NED 137-treated L strain rats (Table 12).

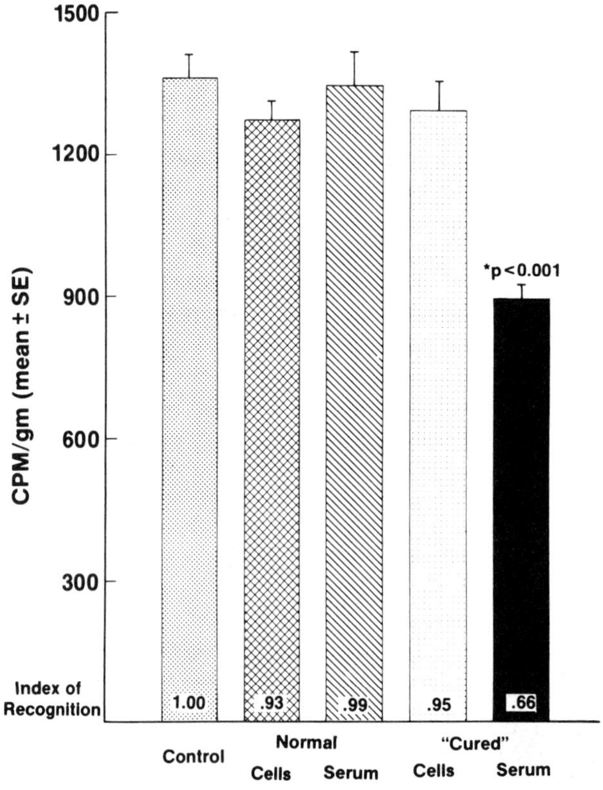

Figure 9 The effect of cell/serum transfer on the in vivo lysis of ^{51}Cr-labeled FBCa cells. Cells or serum from normal and "cured" animals were transferred to normal F344 rats, and these animals received ^{51}Cr-labeled tumor cells 10 min later.

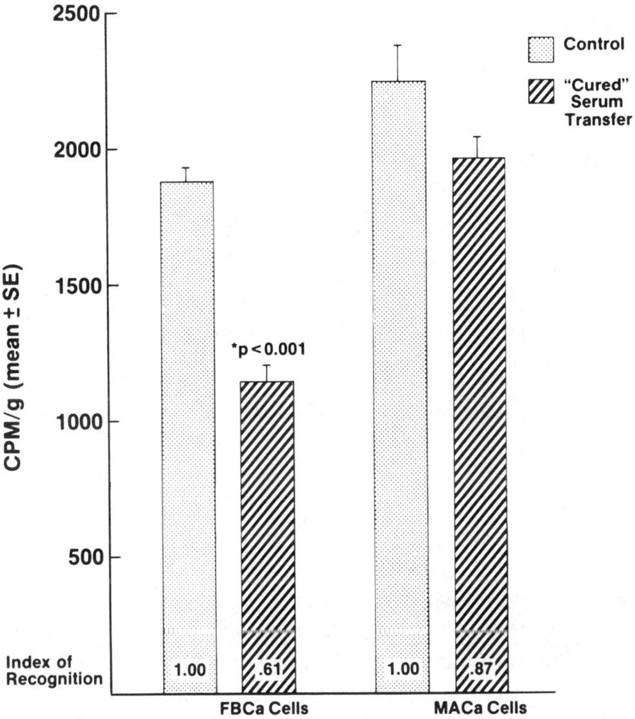

Figure 10 Specificity of FBCa "cured" serum transfer. Normal F344 rats received serum from FBCa "cured" animals and ^{51}Cr-labeled FBCa or MACa cells.

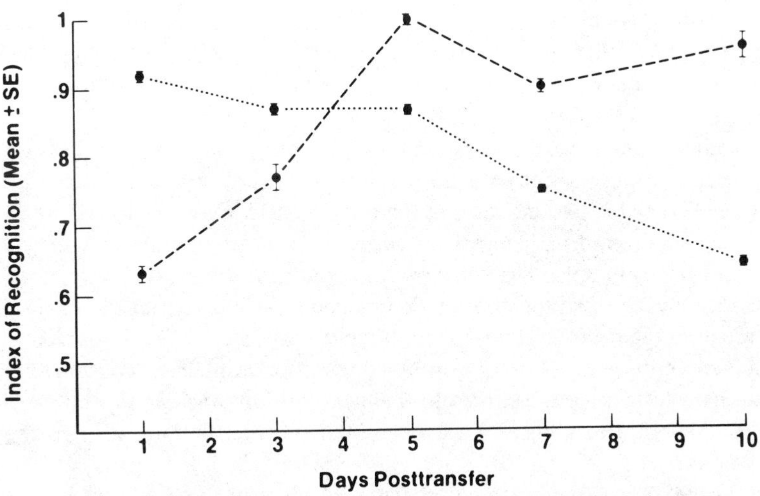

Figure 11 Assessment of in vivo cytotoxicity versus time for cell/serum transfer. Cells (dotted line) or serum (broken line) from "cured" animals were transferred to normal F344 rats, and challenge with ^{51}Cr-labeled FBCa took place on days 1, 3, 5, 7, and 10. At day 1 serum transfer produced significant cytotoxicity ($p = 0.05$), and at days 5, 7, and 10 the cell transfer produced significant cytotoxicity ($p < 0.05$).

Table 12 Effect of NED 137 on Number and Phagocytic Activity of Peritoneal Macrophages in F344 Strain Rats

	Days after treatment[b]					
	1	3	5	1	3	5
Treatment[a]	Number of recovered cells (x 10^6)[c]			Latex-containing cells (%)[c]		
0	4.6 ± 0.5	4.4 ± 1.0	5.6 ± 1.1	19.6 ± 1.4	21.8 ± 2.4	17.0 ± 1.6
NED 137, IP	5.3 ± 0.8	5.0 ± 1.1	4.2 ± 1.2	21.2 ± 1.3	20.4 ± 1.4	19.2 ± 1.9
NED 137, PO	6.2 ± 1.2	4.8 ± 0.6	4.2 ± 0.8	18.0 ± 2.5	18.9 ± 2.9	19.2 ± 1.7
BCG, IP	28.0 ± 2.8	45.4 ± 4.5	22.6 ± 2.9	67.2 ± 3.7	68.4 ± 4.2	36.2 ± 4.9

[a]NED 137 was administered to F 344 strain rats either intraperitoneally or orally at a dose of 30 mg/kg. BCG was given at a concentration of 0.1 mg/kg.
[b]Animals were sacrificed 1-5 days after the treatment, and cells were harvested from the peritoneal cavity by irrigation with RPMI 1640 tissue culture media.
[c]Expressed as mean ± SE.

IV. CLINICAL STUDIES WITH NED 137

The clinical trial of NED 137 (phases I-II) was begun in February 1979 after approval was obtained from the Human Experimentation Committee at the University of Toronto and from the Health Protection Branch of the Department of National Health and Welfare (Government of Canada). Informed consent was obtained from all participating patients. One hundred and twenty-four patients were entered into a consecutive trial, and included individuals with carcinoma of the colon, rectum, stomach, and pancreas (57,58). The results reported here were analyzed on November 14, 1980. Follow-up results to November 1982 will also be discussed.

All patients had histologically proven gastrointestinal malignancies; some had undergone resection of the primary tumor, other resections of metastases, and a number had had incomplete resection with residual disease. The remaining patients had recurrent or diffuse tumors (see Table 13). The results obtained in these patients with NED 137 are compared with 213 historical control patients with a similar spectrum of malignant disease who were treated at this center with 5-fluorouracil or BCG between 1974 and 1978.

NED 137 was administered every 6 weeks to each patient. A total of 94 individuals were treated intravenously, 5 mg/kg body weight per dose to a maximum of 250 mg, 15 received intraperitoneal NED 137, 30 mg/kg, and the remaining 15 were given the drug orally, 30 mg/kg, the lyophilized drug being dissolved in sterile water and diluted with 0.9% saline. In 75% of the cases, cytotoxic systemic or hepatic artery infusional chemotherapy was given, with NED 137 administration commencing 7-14 days after the final dose of chemotherapeutic agent(s). Systemic chemotherapy consisted of 5-fluorouracil alone, 5-fluorouracil and mitomycin-C or 5-fluorouracil with doxorubicin and mitomycin C. In patients with metastatic disease confined to the liver, 5-fluorouracil and/or mitomycin C was given by hepatic artery infusion via a percutaneous transfemoral angiographically positioned catheter.

Routine laboratory studies (complete blood count, liver function tests, serum creatinine, urea nitrogen, calcium, and urinalysis) were performed prior to NED 137 administration and at least every 6 weeks thereafter (every 1-2 weeks for those on chemotherapy). Skin testing with PPD (tuberculin), mumps antigen, *Candida* antigen, and streptokinase/steptodornase was carried out every 6 weeks. The first 30 patients underwent further immunological testing consisting of peripheral blood counts of T and B

Table 13 Patient Breakdown by Age, Sex, Site, and Extent of Disease for NED-137-Treated Group versus Historical Control Group

	NED 137				Historical Control			
Site	Primary resection	Secondary resection	Minimal residual disease	Extensive metastases	Primary resection	Secondary resection	Minimal residual disease	Extensive metastases
Pancreas	11 (9.7%)	–	1 (.87%)	10 (8.8%)	5 (2.3%)	–	–	19 (8.9%)
Stomach	–	–	9 (7.9%)	9 (7.9%)	16 (7.5%)	–	26 (12.2%)	34 (15.9%)
Colorectal	–	10 (8.8%)	12 (10.5%)	44 (38.6%)	–	–	16 (7.5%)	97 (45.5%)
Hepatocellular carcinoma	1 (.87%)	–	1 (.87%)	1 (.87%)	–	–	–	–
Gall bladder	–	–	1 (.87%)	1 (.87%)	–	–	–	–
Esophagus	1 (.87%)	–	1 (.87%)	1 (.87%)	–	–	–	–
Total	13 (11.4%)	10 (8.8%)	25 (21.9%)	66 (57.9%)	21 (9.9%)	0 –	42 (19.8%)	150 (70.3%)
Mean age (range)		56.3 years (22-76)				60 years (29-85)		
	75 males (65.8%)	+	39 females (34.2%)	= 114	134 males (63%)	+	79 females (37%)	= 213

lymphocytes and monocytes/macrophages, assessment of monocyte/macrophage activity by studies of EA rosette formation and latex phagocytosis, leukocyte migration inhibition by autologous or allogeneic tumor antigen, and measurement of the proliferative response to mitogenic lectins and specific antigen. Survival was assessed by plotting corrected survival curves for the NED 137 and historical control groups and using the log rank test for comparison of the two groups (Fig. 12) (59).

Of the 124 patients entered, 10 were excluded because of lack of compliance, diagnostic error, or transfer to another center. The remaining 114 patients, of whom 66% were male, had a median follow-up period of 44 weeks. Age ranged from 22 to 76 years (mean 56.3 years); 63% of the 213 control patients were male, with ages ranging from 29 to 85 years (mean 60 years). Disease extent for each group is shown in Table 13.

There was no measurable toxicity attributable to NED 137 in any patient, nor was toxicity of chemotherapy enhanced by the addition of NED 137. Skin testing and the immunological parameters assayed were not altered by administration of the polymer.

Figure 12 suggests that survival was improved by the use of NED 137. As of November 1980, there had been 47 deaths among patients treated with the polymer occurring in 21 of 66 with colorectal carcinoma, 7 of 22 with pancreatic carcinoma, 13 of 18 with gastric primaries, 2 of 3 with hepatomas, 2 of 3 with esophageal carcinoma, and in the 2 patients with gallbladder tumors. There were two additional perioperative deaths, one from pulmonary embolism and the other from sepsis following spinal decompression.

In patients treated with NED 137, survival of those with minimal disease was better than that of patients with extensive disease (Fig. 13). Only 9 of the 40 patients with minimal disease died, and all had proven minimal residual tumor.

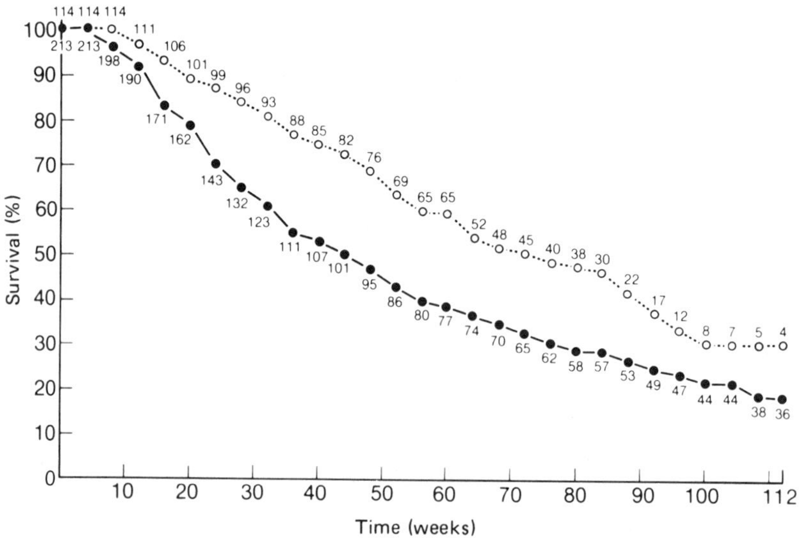

Figure 12 Total patient population (open circles) NED 137; (closed circles) historical control. Corrected survival of patients with gastrointestinal cancer, one group treated with NED 137 and the other (historical control from the same institution) treated with 5-fluorouracil alone or with BCG.

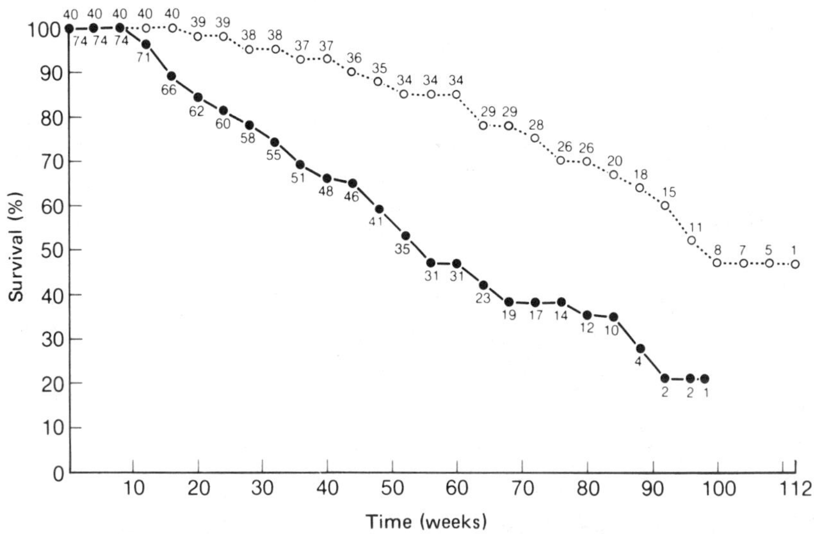

Figure 13 Extensive (open circles) versus minimal (closed circles) disease. Corrected survival of patients treated with NED 137, stratified for minimal and extensive disease.

For those patients with gastric adenocarcinoma, NED 137 did not produce improvement in survival; however, survival was enhanced in those with colorectal or pancreatic primaries (Figs. 14 and 15).

Follow-up data to November 1982 are available for 110 of the 114 patients followed to November 1980; the 4 lost patients were all male, 3 of whom had potentially resectable disease and 1, extensive disease. Of the 110 patients, 63 had extensive and 47 potentially resectable disease; 61 of those with extensive disease died, 9 of these deaths occurring

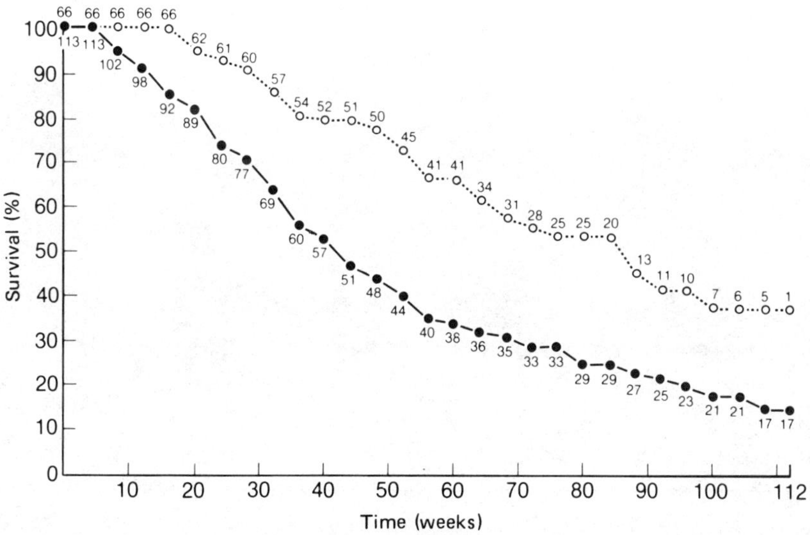

Figure 14 Corrected survival of patients with adenocarcinoma of the colon and rectum. NED 137 (open circles); historical control (closed circles).

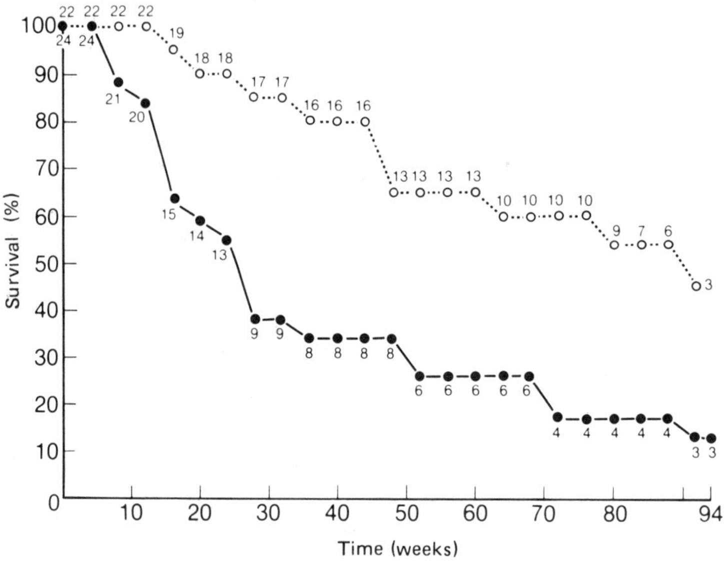

Figure 15 Corrected survival of patients with adenocarcinoma of the pancreas. NED 137 (open circles); historical control (closed circles).

after NED 137 was discontinued. Of the 29 deaths in patients with potentially resectable disease, 9 also occurred after treatment with NED 137 was stopped. Figure 16 depicts the survival curve for all 110 NED 137-treated patients followed up to November 1982, and Fig. 17, showing data collected in November 1982, confirms the improved survival seen in patients with nonextensive disease when compared with those with extensive tumors.

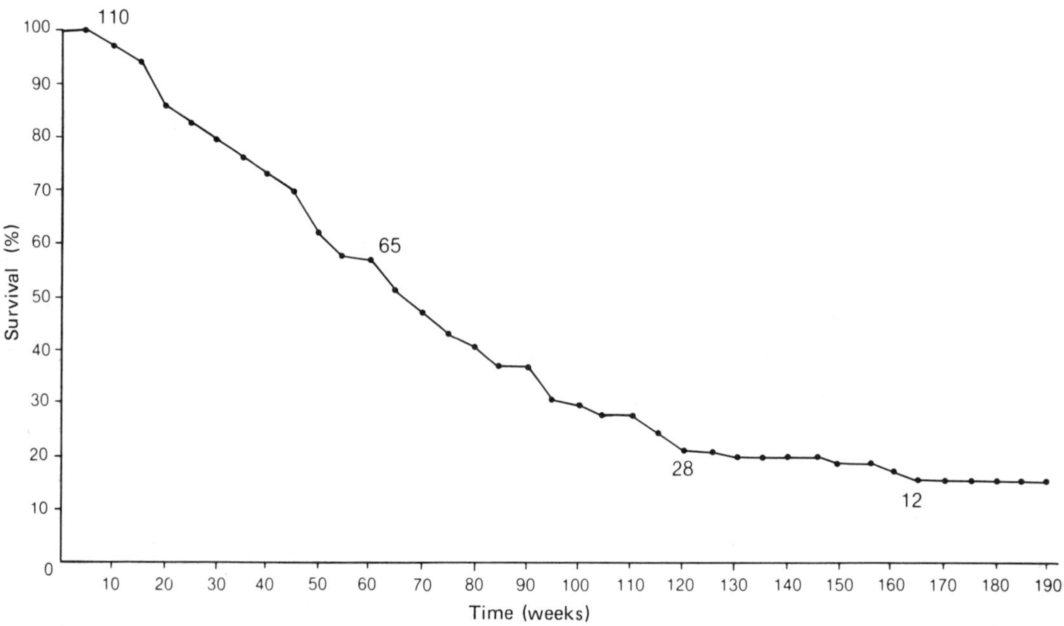

Figure 16 Corrected life-survival curve to November 1982 for 110 patients with gastrointestinal carcinoma treated with NED 137.

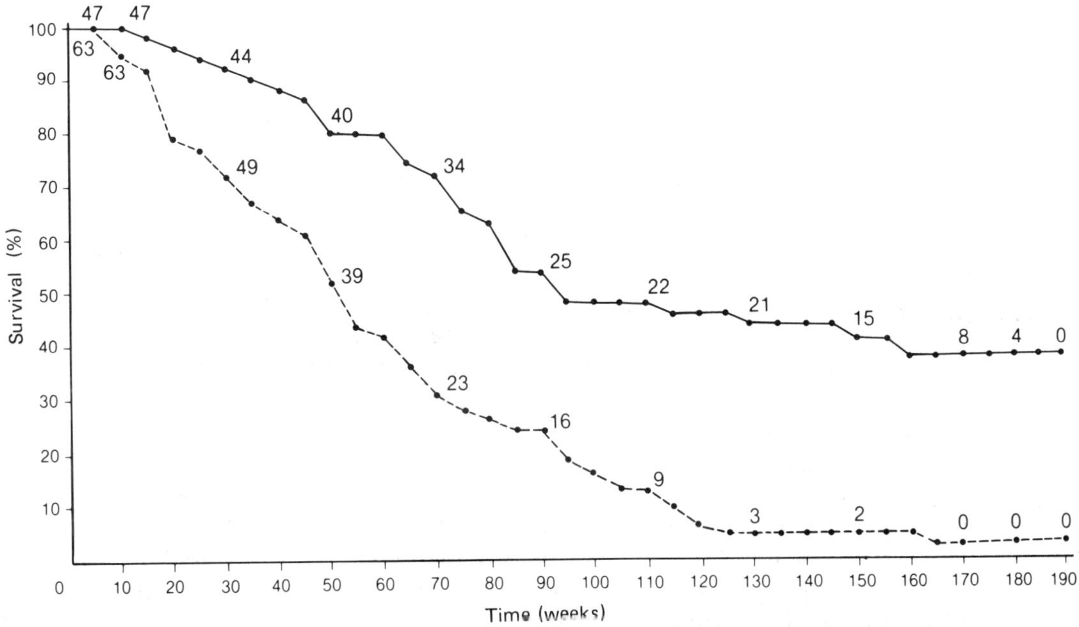

Figure 17 Corrected life-survival curve to November 1982; extensive versus minimal disease (NED-137-treated patients). Extensive, 63 patients (broken line); minimal, 47 patients (solid line).

V. DISCUSSION

The enhancement of humoral and cellular immunity through adjuvant therapy has great relevance to the treatment of neoplasia. However, synthetic immunomodulators with multiple negative charges, including polycarboxylic acids, have heterogeneous effects on the immune system with respect to the cellular site of action, specificity, and adjuvant and/or suppressive activity. Most of the commonly used immune stimulants have multiple cellular targets depending on the system under study. Elucidation of the structure-activity relationship in modulating the immune response is likely to be achieved by the application of chemically defined, small molecular weight polymers with the appropriate specificity.

We have demonstrated that one such polymer, NED 137, significantly stimulates the humoral immune response in rodents. An increased number of antibody-producing cells in the polymer-treated rats was observed even in animals with severe T-cell depletion (38). NED 137 significantly increased the IgM and IgG PFC response to TD and TI antigens in normal mice. However, it could not restore the PFC response to sheep erythrocytes in athymic (nu/nu) mice (39). The polymer increased both the primary and secondary IgM response in rat spleen cultures. Immunopotentiating activity of NED 137 was greatest in macrophage-depleted spleen cell preparations (46). The polymer did not effect or directly induce the proliferation of lymphoid cells in vitro, but PFC and mitogenic responses were markedly inhibited in cultures prepared from rats pretreated with NED 137 before culture initiation.

NED 137 had a dramatic antitumor effect and reduced the development of recurrent cancer and incidence of metastases after excision of a methylcholanthrene-induced bladder carcinoma in Fischer rats (41,51). The effect of NED 137 was clearly more significant than any of the standard bacterial or synthetic adjuvants tested. It would appear that NED 137 can stimulate the production of a specific serum factor which can be precipitated without decreasing the antitumor activity (52,56).

NED 137 was effective over a broad dose range and was not toxic at doses 100 times those with therapeutic efficacy. Moreover, the polymer had not demonstrated suppressive activity in modulating the immune response to tumor-associated antigens at any of the doses used.

The exact mechanisms of antitumor activity of NED 137 are still unclear. However, it is accepted that the B lymphocyte can play an important role in the antitumor immune response. Specific antibodies can destory malignant cells either directly in the presence of complement, or through a mechanism of antibody-dependent cellular lysis (60) and the involvement of macrophages (61,62). The use of specific monoclonal antibodies in the diagnosis and prevention of vascular dissemination of solid malignant tumors is now accepted as a postsurgical therapy (63-65).

NED 137 enhanced the differentiation of B lymphocytes to antibody-producing cells after immunization with T-dependent and T-independent antigens (39). The mechansims of enhancement of the humoral response to TD antigen could be mediated through an adjuvant effect on B or T lymphocytes and/or macrophages. Previous results obtained in our laboratory suggested that NED 137 may act as a polyclonal B-cell activator (PBA). Most PBAs induce differentiation to antibody-producing cells (66,67). NED 137 could, therefore, accentuate the B-cell response to weakly immunogenic molecules (tumor-associated antigens) by triggering appropriate clones of antibody-producing cells. It is known that polyclonal activators can directly trigger a resting B lymphocyte without the involvement of T cells or accessory cells (68,69). However, we were not able to demonstrate an increase in the antigen-independent (background) PFC response in the polymer-treated athymic (nude) mice and rat spleen cultures exposed to effective concentrations of NED 137. Furthermore, NED 137 did not induce or alter the proliferation of nylon-wool fractionated mouse, rat, or human lymphocytes. Mitogen-induced [^{3}H] thymidine incorporation was shown to be depressed at various time intervals after in vivo administration of NED 137. However, mitogen-independent (background) proliferation was similar in the polymer-treated animals and untreated controls. These observations would distinguish NED 137 from other EMA copolymers such as pyran. Pyran showed activity similar to that of NED 137 in reducing the lymphoproliferative response to mitogens following in vivo administration, but was found to be mitogeneic for B and T lymphocytes in vivo (70) and B cells in vitro (20).

Several other lines of evidence suggest that NED 137 does not act directly on the B cell. We did demonstrate that T-depleted rats were capable of generating essentially normal levels of PFCs following immunization to sheep erythrocytes (38).

Similarly, Diamantstein et al. (71) observed that certain polyanionic immunomodulators were capable of replacing T-cell function, since treatment of Tx, BM mice with these agents significantly increased anti-SRBC response. However, adult thymectomy and reconstitution with normal bone marrow cells seldom eliminates T lymphocytes completely (72). Therefore, the possibility of NED 137-mediated amplification of residual T cells cannot be ruled out. Restoration of the immune response to TD antigens in animals depleted of T lymphocytes has also been described in animals treated with single-stranded polymers of polyadenylic and polyuridylic acids [poly (A:U)] (73). Studies of Scheid et al. (74) revealed that treatment with [poly (A:U)] could render precursor cells from athymic mice Thy-1 antigen and result in development of antibody response to SRBCs. Further experiments of Cone and Johnson (75) suggested that poly (A:U) acted, indeed, at the level of thymus-derived lymphocytes. Although we did not study effects of NED 137 on expression of lymphocyte surface markers, the polymer-induced differentiation of percursors to functional T cells is unlikely, since the compound did not affect the immune response to SRBC in nude mice.

Our in vitro studies demonstrated that NED 137 stimulated primary and secondary immune response to sheep erythrocytes in a dose- and time-dependent manner. The specificity of the enhancing effect of the polymer was demonstrated in vivo and in vitro using unrelated antigen to challenge primed spleen cells. Recently, Schreier et al. (76) demonstrated that specificity resides at the level of a T-helper cell endowed with antigen-specific receptors which exerts a nonspecific, lymphokine-mediated, helper effect on B cells. Specificity of the NED 137 effect was also observed in tumor studies involving transfer experiments. These data may suggest that a lymphoid cell of T-cell lineage is affected by NED 137.

It has been suggested that adjuvant activity of an agent could be screened by its ability to abrogate tolerance to soluble proteins (77). Abrogation of tolerance by [poly (A:U)] has been attributed to a direct effect of this polyanion on T cells. Administration of NED 137 immediately after antigen, therefore at a time before T cells became tolerant (78,79), resulted in effective prevention of tolerance. In contrast, agents able to prevent tolerance induction in B lymphocytes and/or to overcome the normal requirement for carrier-specific helper T cells could be administered up to 3 days later (78,79). A significant increase in the PFC response to TI antigen such as DNP-Ficoll is insufficient evidence that the polymer selectively triggered the TI portion of the immune response to this antigen. The response to cross-reactive antigen, TNP-Ficoll, remains under the control of T cells, and anti-TNP reactivity of spleen cells is greatly reduced after the removal of T lymphocytes (80). NED 137 did not produce hepatosplenomegaly and had no effect on phagocytic activity of peritoneal macrophages. Since diverse effects of immunopotentiators on different subpopulations of macrophages have been described, we cannot entirely exclude the possibility that NED 137 could still affect accessory cells. We described the enhancing effect of the polymer in rat spleen cell cultures and observed that NED 137 demonstrated phagocytic/adherent cells (39). This may suggest that the in vitro effect of NED-137 does not result primarily from its direct interaction with splenic macrophages. On the other hand, antibody response to SRBCs was inhibited in cultures derived from rats pretreated with NED 137 3-5 days earlier (46). Since rat splenic suppressor cells have been identified as macrophages (81,82), this effect might reflect in situ activation of adherent cells, which in turn would suppress in vitro plaque formation. Such activation, however, could also result from activating signals provided by T-cell-derived soluble factors (83).

Finally it is difficult to accept that a single administration of NED 137 could lead to a long-lasting enhancement of the immune response due to more efficient processing or presentation of antigen administered at a much later date. It has been shown that primary antibody response is independent of macrophages after 24 hr (84).

The results obtained with this compound prompted a search for another of the same generic type; an immunostimulative polymeric substance produced by Pharmacia AB (Uppsala, Sweden) was introduced into a clinical phases I-II trial on June 30, 1982. To date, some 50 patients have been treated by the oral route with this compound. No toxicity has been observed, but it is too early to comment on efficacy. Immunological testing of patients in this study has been limited to skin testing; the use of the new compound has not altered patient reactivity to any of the tested antigens. Incidental observations suggest that the incidence of common viral and bacterial infections in these patients is reduced, but this has not been formally documented.

The concept of selective immune stimulation with enhanced antibody production in patients with malignant disease is an attractive one. Production of specific antibodies to tumor cell components could result in better efficacy of chemotherapy or radiotherapy. The marked reduction in metastatic potential of neoplasms seen in animal experiments and the early clinical studies is particularly noteworthy. The potential of this therapeutic modality in combination with existing treatment regimens is considerable, especially in view of the surprisingly low incidence of toxicity associated with these compounds.

REFERENCES

1. V. E. Von Leyden and F. Blumenthal, *Dtsch. Med. Wochenschr.*, *28*:637 (1902).
2. G. Mathé, J. L. Amiel, L. Schwarzenberg, M. Schneider, A. Cattan, J. R. Schumberger, M. Hayat, and F. DeVassal, *Lancet*, *1*:697 (1969).
3. R. W. Baldwin and M. V. Pimm, *Adv. Cancer Res.*, *28*:98 (1978).
4. L. Milas and M. T. Scott, *Adv. Cancer Res.*, *26*:257 (1978).
5. M. G. Hanna, Jr. and L. C. Peters, *Cancer Res.*, *38*:204 (1978).
6. L. J. Old, D. A. Clark, B. Benacerraf, and M. Goldsmith, *Ann. N. Y. Acad. Sci.*, *88*:264 (1970).
7. L. J. Old, B. Benacerraf, D. A. Clark, E. A. Carswell, and E. Stockert, *Cancer Res.*, *21*:1281 (1961).
8. B. N. Halpern, G. Biozzi, C. Stiffel, and D. Mouton, *Nature (London)*, *212*:853 (1966).
9. I. Hellström, I. D. Bernstein, *Proc. Natl. Acad. Sci., USA*, *76*:5294 (1979).
10. J. J. Mulé, T. H. Stanton, and I. Hellström, *Int. J. Cancer*, *28*:353 (1981).
11. J. Borsos and H. J. Rapp, *J. Natl. Cancer Inst.*, *51*:345 (1966).
12. C. Bucana and M. G. Hanna, *J. Natl. Cancer Inst.*, *54*:1085 (1973).
13. A. M. Kaplan, in *Anionic Polymeric Drugs* (L. G. Donaruma, R. M. Ottenbrite, and O. Vogl, eds.), John Wiley, New York, 1980.
14. R. M. Ottenbrite, W. Regelson, A. M. Kaplan, R. Carchman, P. S. Morahan, and A. E. Munson, in *Polymeric Drugs* (L. G. Donaruma and O. Vogl, eds.), Academic Press, New York, 1978.
15. R. M. Ottenbrite, in *Anionic Polymeric Drugs* (L. G. Donaruma, R. M. Ottenbrite, and O. Vogl, eds.), John Wiley, New York, 1980.
16. W. Regelson, B. I. Shnider, J. Colsky, K. B. Olson, J. F. Holland, C. L. Johnston, Jr., and L. H. Dennis, in *Immune Modulation and Control of Neoplasia by Adjuvant Therapy* (M. A. Chirigos, ed.), Raven Press, New York, 1978.
17. W. Braun, W. Regelson, Y. Yajima, and M. Ishizuka, *Proc. Soc. Exp. Biol. Med.*, *133*: 171 (1970).
18. P. S. Morahan, W. Regelson, and A. E. Munson, *Antimicrob. Ag. Chemother.*, *2*:16 (1972).
19. M. C. Breinig, A. E. Munson, and P. S. Morahan, in *Anionic Polymeric Drugs* (L. G. Donaruma, R. M. Ottenbrite, and O. Vogl, eds.), John Wiley, New York, 1980.
20. L. G. Baird and A. M. Kaplan, *Cell. Immunol.*, *20*:165 (1975).
21. L. G. Baird and A. M. Kaplan, in *Anionic Polymeric Drugs* (L. G. Donaruma, R. M. Ottenbrite and O. Vogl, eds.), John Wiley, New York, 1980.
22. B. N. Jaroslow and L. Oritiz-Oritiz, *Cell Immunol.*, *3*:123 (1972).
23. T. Hamaoka and D. H. Katz, *Cell. Immunol.*, *7*:246 (1973).
24. P. R. Narayanan and G. Sundharadas, *J. Exp. Med.*, *147*:1355 (1978).

25. T. Diamantstein, W. Vogt, H. Ruhl, and G. Bochart, *Eur. J. Immunol.*, *3*:488 (1973).
26. A. Coutinho, G. Möller, and W. Richter, *Scand. J. Immunol.*, *3*:321 (1974).
27. T. C. Merigan, *Nature*, *214*:416 (1967).
28. W. Regelson, *L'Interferon*, *6*:353 (1970).
29. W. Regelson, M. Kuhar, M. Tunis, J. E. Fields, J. H. Johnson, and E. W. Gluesenkamp, *Nature*, *186*:778 (1960).
30. W. Regelson, *Adv. Chemother.*, *3*:303 (1968).
31. D. S. Breslow, *Pure Appl. Chem.*, *46*:103 (1976).
32. P. S. Morahan, W. Regelson, and A. E. Monson, *Antimicrob. Ag. Chemother.*, *2*:16 (1972).
33. M. A. Chirigos, J. W. Pearson, and J. Pryor, *Cancer Res.*, *33*:2615 (1973).
34. W. Regelson, *Adv. Exp. Med. Biol.*, *1*:315 (1967).
35. P. S. Morahan, J. A. Munson, L. G. Baird, A. M. Kaplan, and W. Regelson, *Cancer Res.*, *34*:506 (1974).
36. A. F. Gazdar, A. D. Steinberg, G. F. Spahn, and S. Baron, *Proc. Soc. Exp. Biol. Med.*. *139*:1132 (1972).
37. G. B. Schuller, P. S. Morahan, and M. Snodgrass, *Cancer Res.*, *35*:1915 (1975).
38. R. E. Falk, N. A. Nossal, L. Makowka, L. E. Rotstein, and J. A. Falk, in *Regulation by T Cells* (D. G. Kilburn, J. G. Levy, and H. S. Teh, eds.), University of British Columbia Press, Vancouver, 1979.
39. J. A. Teodorczyk-Injeyan, L. Filion, J. A. Falk, R. E. Falk, and L. Makowka, *J. Immunopharmacol.*, *5*:147 (1983).
40. N. K. Jerne and A. A. Nordin, *Science*, *140*:405 (1963).
41. L. Makowka, R. E. Falk, N. A. Nossal, L. E. Rotstein, and J. A. Falk, in *Augmenting Agents in Cancer Therapy* (E. M. Hersh, M. A. Chirigos, and M. J. Mastrangelo, eds.), Raven Press, New York, 1981.
42. W. Y. Lee and A. H. Sehon, *J. Immunol.*, *114*:829 (1975).
43. J. R. Little and H. Eisen, *J. Exp. Med.*, *129*:247 (1969).
44. D. H. Katz, in *Lymphocyte: Differentiation, Recognition and Regulation* (F. J. Dixon and H. G. Kunkel, eds.), Academic Press, New York, 1977, p. 357.
45. D. H. Katz, in *Lymphocyte: Differentiation, Recognition and Regulation* (F. J. Dixon and H. G. Kunkel, eds.), Academic Press, New York, 1977, p. 195.
46. J. A. Teodorczyk-Injeyan, L. Makowka, R. E. Falk, and J. A. Falk, *Scand. J. Immunol.*, *15*:9 (1982).
47. J. R. F. Corvalan and J. C. Howard, *Eur. J. Immunol.*, *8*:331 (1978).
48. A. Weiss and F. W. Fitch, *J. Immunol.*, *120*:357 (1978).
49. R. Oehler, R. B. Herberman, D. A. Campbell, and J. Y. Djeu, *Cell. Immunol.*, *29*:238 (1977).
50. H. O. Besedovsky, A. Del Rey, and E. Sorkin, *Clin. Exp. Immunol.*, *37*:106 (1979).
51. R. E. Falk, L. Makowka, N. Nossal, J. A. Falk, J. E. Fields, and S. S. Asculai, *Br. J. Surg.*, *66*:861 (1979).
52. R. E. Falk, L. Makowka, N. A. Nossal, L. E. Rotstein, and J. A. Falk, *Surgery*, *88*:126 (1980).
53. V. V. Likhite, *Cancer Immunol. Immunother.*, *2*:173 (1977).
54. J. Symoens, M. Rosenthal, M. De Brabander, and G. Goldstein, *Springer Semin. Immunol. Pathol.*, *2*:49 (1979).
55. G. B. Mackaness, D. J. Auclair, and P. H. Lagrange, *J. Natl. Cancer Inst.*, *51*:1655 (1973).
56. R. E. Falk, L. Makowka, N. A. Nossal, J. A. Falk, L. E. Rotstein, J. E. Fields, and S. S. Asculai, *J. Surg. Res.*, *28*:485 (1980).
57. R. E. Falk, L. Makowka, R. Bugala, J. A. Falk, L. E. Rotstein, and U. Ambus, *Clin. Invest. Med.*, *4*:155 (1981).

58. R. E. Falk, L. Makowka, L. E. Rotstein, J. A. Falk, N. Nossal, and U. Ambus, in *Augmenting Agents in Cancer Therapy* (E. M. Hersh, M. A. Chirigos, and M. J. Mastrangelo, eds.), Raven Press, New York, 1981.
59. R. Peto, M. C. Pike, R. Armitage, N. E. Breslow, D. R. Cox, S. V. Howard, N. Mantel, K. McPherson, J. Peto, and P. G. Smith, *Br. J. Cancer*, *35*:1 (1977).
60. H. S. Shin, R. J. Johnson, G. R. Pasternak, and J. S. Economou, *Prog. Allergy*, *25*: 163 (1978).
61. R. C. Bast, R. C. Knapp, A. K. Mitchell, J. G. Thurston, R. W. Tucker, and S. F. Schlossman, *J. Immunol.*, *123*:1945 (1979).
62. S. P. Richman, V. T. Chisim, and S. G. Murphy, *Cancer Immunol. Immunother.*, *11*:233 (1981).
63. E. S. Lennox and K. Sikora, in *Monoclonal Antibodies in Clinical Medicine* (A. J. McMichael and J. W. Fabre, eds.), Academic Press, London, 1982.
64. D. G. Gilliland, L. Steplewski, R. J. Collier, K. F. Mitchell, T. H. Chang, and H. Koprowski, *Proc. Natl. Acad. Sci. USA*, *77*:4539 (1980).
65. D. C. Edwards, A. J. S. Davies, and W. C. J. Ross, in *Monoclonal Antibodies in Clinical Medicine* (A. J. McMichael and J. W. Fabre, eds.), Academic Press, London, 1982.
66. T. Kunori, O. Ringden, and E. Möller, *Scand. J. Immunol.*, *8*:451 (1978).
67. R. Dziarski, *J. Immunol.*, *125*:2478 (1980).
68. G. Möller, *Transplant. Rev.*, *23*:126 (1975).
69. E. Gronowicz and A. Coutinho, *Transplant. Rev.*, *24*:3 (1975).
70. L. G. Baird and A. M. Kaplan, in *Immune Modulation and Control of Neoplasia by Adjuvant Therapy* (M. A. Chirigos, ed.), Raven Press, New York, 1978.
71. T. Diamantstein, B. Wagner, J. L'Agestehr, I. Beyse, M. V. Oldenwald, and G. Schultz, *Eur. J. Immunol.*, *1*:302 (1971).
72. R. Roy, J. McNicoll, and F. Daguillard, *Int. Arch. Allergy Appl. Immunol.*, *52*:32 (1976).
73. R. E. Cone and A. G. Johnson, *J. Exp. Med.*, *133*:665 (1971).
74. M. P. Scheid, M. K. Hoffmann, K. Komuro, V. Hammerling, J. Abbot, E. A. Boyse, G. H. Cohen, J. A. Hooper, R. S. Schulof, and A. L. Goldstein, *J. Exp. Med.*, *138*: 1027 (1973).
75. R. E. Cone and A. G. Johnson, *Cell. Immunol.*, *3*:283 (1972).
76. M. H. Schreier, J. Andersson, W. Lernhardt, and F. Melchers, *J. Exp. Med.*, *151*:194 (1980).
77. D. W. Dresser, *Clin. Exp. Immunol.*, *3*:877 (1968).
78. Y. C. M. Kong and S. L. Capanna, *Cell. Immunol.*, *11*:488 (1974).
79. S. L. Capanna and Y. C. M. Kong, *Immunology*, *27*:647 (1974).
80. J. J. Mond, P. K. A. Mongini, V. Freckman, and W. E. Paul, *J. Immunol.*, *125*:1066 (1980).
81. H. V. Raff and D. J. Hinricks, *Cell. Immunol.*, *29*:109 (1977).
82. H. V. Raff and D. J. Hinricks, *Cell. Immunol.*, *29*:118 (1977).
83. R. N. Pantalone and R. C. Page, *Proc. Natl. Acad. Sci. USA*, *72*:209 (1975).
84. C. W. Pierce and B. Benacerraf, *Science*, *166*:1002 (1969).

Section D

Role of Immunomodulating Agents in Autoimmune and Degenerative Diseases

14

Immunomodulators in the Treatment of Selected Autoimmune Diseases

Bruce Freundlich and Robert B. Zurier University of Pennsylvania, Philadelphia, Pennsylvania

I. INTRODUCTION

A. Immune Function

The past two decades of immunology research have underscored the notion that the immune system is not composed of different cells performing isolated functions, but is instead a complex network of interacting cell subsets and associated molecules. This network is substantially intertwined with the inflammatory system which further increases the permutation of events involved in an immune response. The concept of the immune system as a network therefore has several pathophysiological implications: (a) perturbation of a discrete population of cells within this system may effect many other cells indirectly; (b) diseases characterized by abnormalities within the immune system have potential built-in complexities; (c) treatment of such diseases may therefore be complicated and results of therapy unpredictable.

This biological complexity also means that interpretation of underlying problems in autoimmune diseases (which usually exhibit both disordered immune and inflammatory responses) may be less than accurate. For example, because of the interaction of B lymphocytes and their secreted products with many other immune response cells, a primary disturbance of B-cell function may be difficult to trace to its original source. If a B-cell disturbance produced a polyclonal antibody response, as seen in systemic lupus erythematosus (SLE), emergence of antibodies directed against T-suppressor cells (T_{supp}) might evoke the theory that the polyclonal antibody response is actually a function of impaired T_{supp} (particularly if it was not known which came first, the polyclonal antibody secretion or the defective T_{supp}). A similar dilemma could arise with an increase in number or reactivity of T-inducer cells (T_{Ind}) or antigen-presenting cells (monocytes or dendritic cells). A resultant enhancement of B-cell activity which could elicit polyclonal antibody secretion might also be misinterpreted as an intrinsic B-cell abnormality.

By the time a patient with SLE or rheumatoid arthritis (RA) presents with clinical manifestations, multiple abnormalities (or simply responses) of the immune and inflammatory system are often found. Recent studies have concentrated on testing discrete aspects of these systems in an attempt to better identify primary as opposed to secondary abnormalities. This focus has followed advances in modern immunology with respect to separation of distinct T-cell subsets based upon surface antigens, and characterization of bioactive molecules produced by and/or affecting the immune response. For T cells, a basic outline of subsets as defined by monoclonal antibodies consists of inducer cells (Ly1+ in mice, OKT4+ in humans); suppressor/cytotoxic cells (Ly 2+3+ in mice, OKT5+/T8+ in humans); suppressor inducer cells (Ly 1+2+3+ in mice, not yet identified in humans as a discrete subset) (1,2). In the mouse, with the introduction of antibodies to newly defined cell surface antigens (e.g., anti-Qa), the concept of this circuitry has increased in complexity, and an entire murine contrasuppression system has been postulated (3). Some important recently discovered immune-related molecules included Interleukin 1 (IL-1), produced by activated monocytes, is a molecule which activates lymphocytes but may also affect synovial cells (4,5); Interleukin 2 (IL-2), an important growth factor for T cells, might be critical for clonal expansion during immune responses (5); interferon, a glycoprotein which protects against viral infection, may be a mediator of T-cell suppression and is an important positive modulator of NK cells (6,7); arachidonic acid metabolies [prostaglandins (PGs), leukotrienes (LTs), and thromboxanes (Txs)] are a family of fatty acid derivatives that have diverse effects on the immune system (8,9). These compounds are mentioned as they will appear in discussions to follow.

B. Autoimmunity

As knowledge of the immune system evolves, the definition of autoimmunity must likewise evolve. Two excellent reviews of this subject are available (10,11). Talal (10) views autoimmune disease as "an abnormal or excessive activity on the part of immune effector cells that induce immunologic self injury" which is "not intended to imply an etiologic mechanism." This allows us to understand autoimmunity as a final common pathway that can result from intrinsic immune system abrnormalities or an overzealous response to an offending agent such as a microorganism in which the self-defence mechanism itself produces tissue damage. Autoimmunity also is no longer synonymous with autoantibodies since it is now clear that T cells and mononuclear phagocytes also participate in immune-induced damage. Furthermore, autorecognition by immune cells (lymphocytes and mononuclear phagocytes) is a well-aceepted and necessary phenomenon for generation of immune responses specifically via immune antigens (Ia), HLA determinants, and anti-idiotypes. Lymphocytes and accessory cells communicate with each other in the context of both a receptor for antigen plus a receptor for the Ia molecule. The Ia molecule on the accessory cell corresponds to the lymphocyte Ia receptor and this specific correspondance is necessary for an immune response. Anti-idiotypes, on the other hand, are normally occurring antibodies directed at the hypervariable portion of idiotypes (antibodies against specific antigens). Anti-idiotypes provide a feedback network that helps contain the humoral response to a specific antigen (12,13). Therefore, a distinction should be made between autoimmunity and autoimmune disease.

II. DRUGS

What follows is a synopsis of current understanding of commonly used immunomodulatory drugs, with specific reference to their effect on the immune system. Our knowledge in this regard has several important limitations. Many concepts concerning mechanisms of action of these drugs are based on experiments in animals, in vitro studies, and occasional trials with normal volunteers. All of these results may be irrelevant to the patient with a deranged immune system. In addition, these studies have trailed new developments in immunology such as anti-idiotypes, dendritic cells, and lymphokines which may be relevant to drug use. Furthermore, interpretation of a particular drug effect on the autoimmune disease process may be obscured by the wide spectrum of some of these diseases (e.g., SLE), producing divergent study populations. Finally, polypharmacy including ingestion of drugs such as cimetidine, aspirin, and other nonsteroidal anti-inflammatory drugs (NSAIDs) is often overlooked as a means of immunomodulation.

A. Cytotoxic Agents

Cytotoxic agents are drugs that are generally reserved for severe manifestations of autoimmune disease (i.e., for life-threatening problems or to spare the adverse effects of long-term high-dose corticosteroids). Those used most extensively are cyclophosphamide (CTX) and azathioprine (AZA). These drugs have been used in neoplastic disease therapy for their ability to kill rapidly dividing cells by either interfering with DNA synthesis and/or cell metabolism. Since lymphocytes that have been stimulated to undergo an immune response become metabolically activated and increase their DNA turnover, they should be prime targets for cytotoxic agents. In fact this reasoning led to their initial use in autoimmune diseases. However, the actual mechanism by which they affect the immune system is complex and may encompass not only antiproliferative but also anti-inflammatory and noncytotoxic immunomodulatory effects. A major limitation in using these agents is their toxicity, which can occasionally be lethal.

1. Cyclophosphamide (CTX)

CTX is one of a group of compounds known as alkylating agents which affect cells by combining with nucleotides to form abnormal DNA molecules. Single-stranded DNA, which appears both during DNA replication and RNA transcription, is most sensitive to its effect, a phenomenon which accounts for greatest efficacy of the drug against cells in the G1 and S phases of the cell cycle, Nitrogen mustard, a highly toxic agent, was the first alkylating agent used to treat RA in the early 1950s. A less toxic drug, chlorambucil, which is used in therapy of chronic lymphocytic leukemia, was also tested in RA and continues to be employed in Europe (14). However, CTX has been the favored alkylating agent in the United States, and its effects on the immune system have been studied most carefully.

The B lymphocyte clearly appears to be directly affected by CTX. In CTX-treated mice and guinea pigs the cortical zones of lymph nodes (15) and spleen (16), which are B-cell dependent, become depleted within 2-3 days after treatment. This depletion lasts for several weeks with only a modest effect on T-cell-dependent areas. In animals given a dose of CTX, response to pokeweed mitogen (PWM), a stimulant of B cells dependent upon T-cell presence, remains depressed for more than a week, while response to phytohemagglutinin (PHA) a stimulant of T cells, returns to baseline in a few days (16). Humans receiving CTX treatment also exhibit a decreased response to PWM (17). This decrease is linked directly to B-cell function rather than T-cell regulation, as shown by cocultures of T and B cells from treated patients and normal controls (17).

CTX produces a profound lymphopenia in animals (18) and humans with various autoimmune diseases (19-21); however, there is no selective decrement of either B or T cells. Circulating immunoglobulin levels are decreased after treatment (22-24). The effect of CTX, however, on antibody secretion to specific antigens in experimental models is dependent upon the antigen used (25), dose of antigen or CTX administered (26), and most importantly the timing of drug delivery in relation to antigen delivery (26-28). A sufficiently high dose of drug, administered between 2-3 days before to 3-7 days following antigen delivery, will block antibody response to a specific test antigen. If antigen is given more than 3 days before drug or 7 days after therapy is begun, specific suppression does not occur (26). This specific lack of immune reactivity is called tolerance. Drug-induced tolerance is not permanent, and immune responsiveness returns shortly after drug is discontinued. Therefore, all antigen-responsive lymphocyte clones are not simply eliminated during induction of tolerance. B cells are particularly sensitive to drug-induced tolerance probably because regeneration of cell surface antigen specific receptors is impaired with treatment (28). There is also some evidence for enhanced antigen-specific T_{supp} activity in CTX-induced tolerance (29).

Delayed hypersensitivity (DTH) (a T-cell and monocyte-dependent response) is impaired in animals (30,31) and humans (32) when CTX is given in a time frame similar to that described for suppressing antibody response. This diminished responiveness also returns to baseline within 3-20 days after drug is discontinued. Despite an inability to initiate DTH to a new antigen, CTX-treated RA patients exhibit no change in DTH status to previously tested antigens (32). In humans, blastogenic response to T-cell-directed mitogens [PHA and concanavalin A (ConA)] are similar in CTX-treated and untreated patients (20).

The effect of CTX on response to antigen is not uniformly suppressive. Under certain conditions in fact, CTX can enhance immune responses (33-35), and tolerance may even by reversed (36). In these experiments, drug is usually given at least 3 days before antigen, and higher CTX doses are required. These findings may be due to loss of T suppression (36-38).

Other studies on T-cell-related function also show a complex picture: When donor spleen cells from CTX-treated mice are injected into F1 hybrid mice, recipients demonstrate an increased graft-versus-host (GVH) reactivity at day 6 which is suppressed at day 8, likely reflecting CTX-induced changes in spleen cell populations (39). In addition, dissociation of response to modified syngeneic spleen cells and allogenic cells is found in CTX-treated mice (40). Response to syngeneic TNP coupled cells is depressed, whereas the responses to allogeneic cells is normal. It was noted that in autoimmune diseases where syngeneic cell surfaces may be altered, depression of the self-directed immune response may potentially be beneficial.

Toxicity. Toxicity has been a major limiting factor in the use of CTX. Leukopenia is frequent but usually controllable when small doses are used and can almost always be reversed by drug withdrawal (41). Severe bacterial infections can occur, but their incidence can be minimized by maintaining the WBC count above 3000 (PMN $>$ 1500). Thrombocytopenia occurs not uncommonly, but less often than with other alkylating agents. Hemorrhagic cystitis occurs in 5-10% of cases, and often requires drug discontinuation (42). Azoospermia is a frequent problem in males, as is amenorrhea in females. Of great concern is a possible increased incidence of malignancy, particularly bladder carcinoma and possibly lymphoma (42-44). Although this point is controversial and several reviews have concluded that CTX therapy is not associated with an increased incidence of malignancy (45,46), the possibility must be factored into any treatment decision. Patients therefore deserve careful explanation of potential adverse effects before embarking on a course of CTX, especially for a nonlethal disease such as RA.

2. Azathioprine (AZA)

AZA has been widely used as an immunosuppressive agent in transplantation and a cytotoxic agent in cancer. It is a purine analog derivative of 6-mercaptopurine (6-MP) and is classified as a thiopurine (TP). AZA was synthesized in 1961, 10 years after 6-MP, in an effort to slow drug catabolism with an added imidazole group (47). This effort proved to be unfounded as in vivo conversion of AZA to 6-MP occurred within minutes (48); however, AZA is now the TP of choice because it is better absorbed (49) and may be less toxic (50). There is probably not much difference in immunosuppressive abilities of 6-MP and AZA (49,51), and they will be considered interchangeable for purpose of discussion (most studies were done with AZA). It is likely that TP works through formation of thioinosinic acid, a purine analog thought to inhibit DNA synthesis and affect cell function predominantly in the S phase of the cell cycle (52). AZA may also prolong the cell cycle (53).

As with CTX, AZA administration in man produces a lymphopenia which is nonselective for B or T cells (54,55). Short courses of TP shrink the thymus in mice, particularly the corticosteroid-sensitive cortical zone composed of more immature cells (56,57). Other lymphoid tissues are drug-sensitive, although specific cell depletion has not been defined. A 12-week course of AZA decreased numbers of plasma cells in rectal mucosa of patients with ulcerative colitis (58).

Mouse B cells are relatively resistant to the effects of AZA in vitro (59,60), particularly with respect to mitogen or T-cell-independent antigen exposure. However, in one system the number of B cells expressing surface antibodies or plaque-forming cells (PFCs) to a specific T-cell-dependent antigen sheep red blood cells (SRBCs) was markedly diminished by AZA (60). Human peripheral blood mononuclear cells showed a reduced response to PWM when cells were taken from normals and exposed to AZA (2.0 μg/ml) in vitro (61) or when AZA-treated multiple sclerosis patients were tested (62). High AZA doses (4-10 μg/ml) added to mononuclear cells in vitro, on the other hand, enhanced antibody-producing cells by PFCs and this was traced to an inhibitory effect on T_{supp} cells (61). Similar enhancement of humoral responses has been shown in animals (63,64) treated before antigen delivery.

Consistent with a suppressive effect by TP is an impaired primary antibody response in both animals (65) and humans (54,66,67). It has been demonstrated that antigen (68), drug dose (61), and timing of drug delivery are all important factors (66,69). Unlike CTX, AZA must be given with antigen within a few days after antigen administration to obtain maximum suppression of antibody response. Of interest is the observation that in both mouse and humans the IgG responses is more susceptible to inhibition than is IgM (65,67). Borel found in mice that antigen rechallenge of TP-treated animals also produced mostly an IgM response as opposed to the strong IgG response seen in untreated mice. AZA may therefore inhibit the B-cell switchover from IgM to IgG or effect a specific B-cell subpopulation. Secondary responses are affected less than primary responses by AZA and require large drug doses for inhibition (68-71). Isoagglutinin levels in treated patients are normal (54,67).

Despite evidence for AZA-induced suppression of antibody response, immunoglobulin levels in treated humans are not consistently lowered and are frequently unchanged from pretreatment levels (54,62,67), particularly short term. Some studies have found lower Ig serum levels (72,73). In one report, despite a decrease in immunoglobulin synthesis in RA patients by 4 months of AZA treatment, serum immunoglobulin levels were not consistently reduced and did not reflect the low Ig synthesis rates (72). This finding implies that an actual reduced Ig synthesis may be masked by a concomitantly reduced catabolism and that absolute amount of new antibody formation does decrease with chronic treatment.

Cell-mediated immune responses have been considered highly susceptible to AZA and led to successful use of this agent to treat several animal models thought to have T-cell-induced disease such as experimental allergic encephalomyelitis (74), autoimmune thyroiditis (75), and experimental myasthenia gravis (76). The T_{Ind} cell is probably resistant to AZA in vitro, whereas the T_{supp} cell is vulnerable, an effect which is similar to irradiation (61). Response to T-cell mitogen appears intact in treated humans (55,58) and animals (77). Mixed lymphocyte reactions (MLR) are intact in treated humans (62) but, in contrast to the response to CTX, are depressed in mice when drug is added in vitro (78,79). GVH reactions can be decreased by AZA in animals (78). This is not the case in human transplantation (80), although allograft rejection itself appears to be suppressed (81,82). This would be partially consistent with the high degree of sensitivity of cytotoxic T cells found in vitro (59).

Delayed hypersensitivity in humans is unaffected as a secondary response; however, DTH induction to new antigens is either abrogated or delayed (54,72). Timing of drug delivery once again is crucial (69,77). Effector cell (i.e., mononuclear phagocytes) impairment may partially account for the decreased response seen in animal studies (83). Early in vitro administration of AZA, but not CTX, in relation to antigen also decreased production of macrophage-inhibitor factor (MIF) (77).

Schwartz (84) showed that AZA could incude an antigen-specific tolerance but only with both large doses of antigen and drug. This tolerant state faded with time. The effect on tolerance of continuous administration of drug (as is often done to treat humans) is unknown. A further interesting effect of AZA is suppression of killer cells. Antibody-dependent cell-mediated cytotoxicity (ADCC) is reduced in mouse (85) and humans (58, 86) after AZA treatment. The effect on NK is unknown.

Toxicity. Of concern has been an increased incidence of non-Hodgkin lymphoma in renal transplant patients treated with AZA (87,88) over a short time span. While a review of the literature did note 18 cases of malignancy in 542 patients with RA taking AZA, this was not an increased incidence compared with the general population. Lymphomas are rare, and there is no good evidence yet that AZA predisposes to neoplasia in RA (45,89). A major adverse effect of AZA is severe bone marrow depression with potentially dire consequences if the drug is not discontinued immediately; discontinuation usually results in a prompt recovery. Liver toxicity with hepatic necrosis is another potential though less frequent side effect.

The complex and incompletely studied effects of CTX and AZA on the immune system make it difficult to construct a simple formulation of their mechanisms of action in autoimmune disease. Several possibilities include (a) anti-inflammatory effect which has been found for both drugs (90); (b) toxic effect on proliferating B and/or T cells that non-specifically suppresses immune responsiveness; (c) the induction of drug-induced tolerance (b and c may be the same process). This last possibility is of particular interest since autoimmune diseases represent a limited breakdown of tolerance to self-antigens. Unlike in animal immune response and drug-induced tolerance studies, the relevant disease-provoking antigen(s) in autoimmune diseases (if it exists) is unclear. This may be an antigen cross reacting with normally nonantigenic host molecules appearing intermittently (with disease exacerbation), as can be seen for example with herpes virus infections. However, by the time treatment is initiated, the immune response would be akin to a secondary response which we have seen is relatively resistant to cytotoxic agents. On the other hand, if autoimmune disease is not simply an abnormal or exaggerated response to an antigen but a more generalized (but limited) process such as breakdown of tolerance, these drugs could temporarily suppress this process by killing dividing self-directed clones, producing a limited "clonal abortion" and thereby allowing other natural suppressive mechanisms to intercede. Also, CTX and AZA are usually administered daily to humans which could sustain a re-tolerization. In summary, cytotoxic drugs have been and continue to be used empirically in the treatment of autoimmune diseases, and they do not generally produce an immunocure but more of an immunosuppression.

B. Corticosteroids (CSs)

In 1951 Dr. Philip Hench from the Mayo Clinic won the Nobel Prize for having cured RA with CSs. Within a few years it became clear that not only were steroids not a cure for RA but that serious adverse effects of these drugs demanded a reappraisal of their role in treatment. Nevertheless, CSs do have a profound effect on both inflammation and the immune system. Several excellent reviews are available (91-95). Key points will be summarized briefly.

The mechanisms whereby CSs exert their biological effects are complex. Highly specific intracellular CS receptors have been found (91,92). Although CSs may enhance some cyclic AMP (cAMP) functions, unlike other hormones they do not appear to act through this messenger (96). Instead, the CS receptor complex enters cell nuclei and modulates RNA production in either positive or negative fashion, depending on the cell (92). CSs do not appear to mediate a consistent biochemical change in different cells. As a general concept though, Baxter and Harris proposed that the actions of CSs can be conceptualized as an evolutionary mechanism to prepare for nutritional deprivation and stress with conservation of glucose producing an antianabolic and procatabolic state which spares vital organs such as heart, brain, and liver (93).

CSs have a marked anti-inflammatory effect (91,92). After CS delivery, there is a release of granulocytes (PMN) from the bone marrow (97), and an increase in their numbers in peripheral blood (98), due in part to demargination and decreased egress to sites of inflammation (99). Adherence of PMNs to surface decreases (100,101) returning to baseline within 24 hr. PMNs do not respond as well to chemotactic factors (102) and when treated with very high doses exhibit impaired phagocytosis (103). According to Fauci et al. the major anti-inflammatory effect of CSs on PMNs is decreased migration of these cells into the inflammatory site (94). Others have proposed that stabilization of lysosomal membranes may be important (104,105). There is some evidence that this can occur by restricting motion of the phospholipid acyl chains that extend into the hydrophobic regions of membranes (106) preventing regurgitation of lysosomal enzymes during particle uptake (107). High doses may be necessary for this effect, however, and its relevance in vivo is uncertain. CSs probably inhibit prostaglandin synthesis by blocking arachidonic acid release from phospholipids (108,109) through a mechanism that is distinct from NSAID.

Some effects of corticosteroids on mononuclear phagocytes (MPs) include: decreased phagocytic and bactericidal activity in vivo (110) at lower doses than are needed to inhibit PMNs, although in vitro studies on these functions have been inconsistent (111, 112); depressed DTH due to a lack of monocyte influx into skin and not to diminished number of sensitized cells (113,114); decreased MP egress to inflammatory sites (115); reduced numbers of circulating monocytes (116); inhibition of clearance of IgG-coated RBCs and platelets (117-119).

CSs given to humans intravenously cause a marked lymphopenia which peaks at 4-6 hr and returns to baseline about 24 hr. T cells are decreased out of proportion to B cells, and specifically T cells with IgM FcR (Tμ) are affected with a relative increase in T cells with IgG FcR (Tγ) (120). Since the Tγ population contains killer cells, it is not surprising that ADCC increases after CSs during the period of relative circulating Tγ increase. NK, however, which is probably mediated by the same cell, declines approximately 24 hr after administration of drug (121). The change in circulating lymphocyte composition induced by CSs is not due to a simple lympholysis as is seen in rodents (122) but represents a cellular redistribution (116,123) which, at least in the guinea pig, may be to the bone marrow (124).

After high-dose CSs, circulating B cells are relatively increased. However, serum Ig levels may be modestly decreased (125,126) and reman lowered for weeks to months after treatment, although not everyone has noted this decrease (127). Saxon et al. (128) found diminished Ig and total protein synthesis in normal volunteers taking CSs (48.5 mg/day) and in treated patients with immune thrombocytopenia. Human lymphocytes in vitro, however, exhibit enhanced Ig synthesis with addition of low CS concentrations alone (129) or in the presence of PWMs (130), compared with untreated controls. Interestingly, blastogenesis was not increased in proportion to Ig synthesis in both these experiments. In the study with PWMs when subjects were given a single dose of 400 mg hydrocortisone. (in vivo), no enhancing effect was seen when their cells were removed and studied in vitro.

Primary antibody response to various antigens does not seem to be effected by CSs (127,131) and, in fact, an enhanced response has been reported (132). Also mononuclear cell antigen sensitization is not inhibited by CSs in vitro (133). Secondary antibody responses may be normal after high doses (122) or decreased (131). CSs have been postulated to decrease generalized lymphocyte proliferation (94). Physiological concentrations of CSs, for example, markedly decrease T-cell proliferation in autologous MLR (AMLR) (134). Healthy volunteers taking as little as 10 mg of prednisone also exhibit low AMLR aftivity (135). Allogeneic MLR, however, was not affected by the same CS dose. Cytotoxic T-cell activity directed against tumor- and virus-infected targets is suppressed by CS (136,137), a finding which could explain the usefulness of CSs in halting acute transplantation rejections (80). Although the production of two lymphokines, MIF and macrophage-activating factor (MAF) is normal after CSs (94), of great theoretical interest is the recent report by Crabtree et al. (138) that inhibition of Interleukin 2 (IL-2) (or T-cell growth factor) by dexamethasone resulted in lowered antigen- or mitogen-induced T-cell proliferation. This decreased proliferation could be reversed by adding back exogenous IL-2. Therefore, an interesting possibility is that CSs can suppress clonal expansion of an immune response by effecting IL-2 production.

Toxicity. There are several regimens for administering CSs and many different preparations of varying strengths and adrenal mineralocorticoid effects. What is important to note here is that different autoimmune diseases require different dosages for different periods of time. Larger doses for longer durations have more severe untoward effects.

Doses of > 5-7 mg prednisone daily can suppress adrenal function, and dose reduction must be performed cautiously.

The adverse effects of CSs are legion, but the important ones are osteopenia with fractures, susceptibility to infections, Cushingoid features (particularly upsetting to young patients), amenorrhea, hypertension, posterior subcapsular cataracts, aseptic necrosis of bone, psychosis, hyperglycemia (occasionally requiring insulin), fluid retention, myopathy, and possibly peptic ulcers. Many of these unpleasant effects are common, and the treatment plan must balance these risks against the benefits of therapy for a particular disease. Reviews of CS therapeutic guidelines can be found in Refs. 139 and 140.

C. Antimalarials

These drugs have been used to treat SLE and RA, among other autoimmune diseases. Their mode of action remains undetermined. Primary and secondary antibody responses are not affected (141,142). Experimental data suggest that chloroquine interferes with immune complex formation (142-144). Antimalarials interact with nucleoproteins and could potentially render them less immunogenic, a finding which might be relevant to treatment of SLE (146). A few studies on mononuclear cell function indicate that antimalarials can inhibit lymphocyte responses to mitogens (145,147) and increase survival of rat skin allografts (146). Finally, these agents exhibit an anti-inflammatory effect, possibly due to their capacity to bind and stabilize lysosomal membranes. Prostaglandin antagonism and other mechanisms (148-152) can also be demonstrated for these drugs. The overriding concern when using antimalarials is potential retinal toxicity. A careful review of this subject concluded that the problem is rare if daily dosage guidelines are followed (153).

D. Prostaglandin (PG) Synthesis Inhibitors

PG production is inhibited by aspirin, NSAIDs, CSs, and antimalarials. It is becoming clear that PGs have an important role in immunoregulation, and this is not simply a suppressive effect (reviewed in Refs. 154 and 155). They can affect mitogenic response of lymphocytes, suppress NK activity, and affect antibody production. The effect of PG blockade in autoimmune diseases and their interactions with other immunomodulators in these situations is basically unknown. An indication of the uncertain importance of PG inhibition is the fact that PGE suppresses inflammation and tissue injury in several experimental animal models (156-158).

III. SYSTEMIC LUPUS ERYTHEMATOSUS (SLE)

SLE has often been referred to as a prototype autoimmune disease because of a high incidence of multiple autoantibodies with deposition of resultant immune complexes leading to tissue injury. From both clinical and immunofunctional standpoints, SLE can be characterized by the word "complex." This is probably related to the numerous immunological abnormalities in a given single patient and the heterogeneity among SLE patients as a group.

Clinically, the definition of SLE has recently been restructured by a committee of the American Rheumatism Association (ARA) to accommodate some newer serological tests and to enhance sensitivity and specificity of clinical parameters compared with the older ARA criteria (159) (see Table 1). These criteria are useful as a research tool for reporting more homogeneous patient populations.

Table 1 The 1982 Revised Criteria for Classification of Systemic Lupus Erythematosus[a]

Criterion		Definition
1. Malar rash		Fixed erythema, flat or raised, over the malar eminences, tending to spare the nasolabial folds
2. Discoid rash		Erythematous raised patches with adherent keratotic scaling and follicular plugging; atrophic scarring may occur in older lesions
3. Photosensitivity		Skin rash as a result of unusual reaction to sunlight, by patient history or physician observation
4. Oral ulcers		Oral or nasopharyngeal ulceration; usually painless, observed by a physician
5. Arthritis		Nonerosive arthritis involving two or more peripheral joints, characterized by tenderness, swelling, or effusion
6. Serositis	(a)	Pleuritis—convincing history of pleuritic pain or rub heard by a physician or evidence of pleural effusion *or*
	(b)	Pericarditis—documented by ECG or rub or evidence of pericardial effusion
7. Renal disorder	(a)	Persistent proteinuria greater than 0.5 g/day or greater than 3+ if quantitation not performed *or*
	(b)	Cellular casts—may be red cell, hemoglobin, granular, tubular, or mixed
8. Neurological disorder	(a)	Seizures—in the absence of offending drugs or known metabolic derangements (e.g., uremia, ketoacidosis, or electrolyte imbalance) *or*
	(b)	Psychosis—in the absence of offending drugs or known metabolic derangements (e.g., uremia, ketoacidosis, or electrolyte imbalance)
9. Hematological disorder	(a)	Hemolytic anemia—with reticulocytosis *or*
	(b)	Leukopenia—less than $4000/mm^3$ total on two or more occasions *or*
	(c)	Lymphopenia—less than $1500/mm^3$ on two or more occasions *or*
	(d)	Thrombocytopenia—less than $1000{,}000/mm^3$ in the absence of offending drugs
10. Immunological disorder	(a)	Positive LE cell preparation *or*
	(b)	Anti-DNA: antibody to native DNA in abnormal titer *or*
	(c)	Anti-Sm: presence of antibody to Sm nuclear antigen *or*
	(d)	False-positive serological test for syphilis known to be positive for at least 6 months and confirmed by *Treponema pallidum* immobilization or fluorescent treponemal antibody absorption test
11. Antinuclear antibody		An abnormal titer of antinuclear antibody by immunofluorescence or an equivalent assay at any point in time and in the absence of drugs known to be associated with drug induced lupus syndrome

[a]The proposed classification is based on 11 criteria. For the purpose of identifying patients in clinical studies, a person shall be said to have systemic lupus erythematosus if any 4 or more of the 11 criteria are present, serially or simultaneously, during any interval of observation.
[b]*Source*: Ref. 159.

The prevalence of SLE in the general population is about 1:2000 (160) with a female-to-male predominance of 8 or 9:1. American black females have a particularly high disease prevalence (1 in 245). SLE appears through a wide age range with a peak at about 20 years and a mean age of onset at 30 years (161). Idiopathic SLE must be distinguished from drug-induced SLE and from hypocomplementemia with a lupuslike syndrome. Some commonly used drugs that are well known to produce an SLE-like syndrome include procainamide, hydralazine, dilantin, and penicillamine (162,163). In general, lupus seen with these drugs does not involve the central nervous system (CNS) or kidneys and remits soon after drug is discontinued. However, antinuclear antibodies, arthritis, and rashes may persist for years. Both early and late complement component deficiencies (particularly C2) have been associated with an SLE syndrome that can be identified by studying family members (164). Another disease entity of note is discoid lupus which appears to be lupus confined to the skin, progressing to the systemic form in about 5% of cases (165). These conditions are mentioned for pathophysiological consideration and to keep in mind the possibility that what we call SLE the disease may actually be a syndrome (i.e., final common pathway of several different processes). This concept is reinforced by murine lupus models and immunological studies of patients. It may potentially complicate both treatment and evaluation of therapeutic trials.

The clinical manifestations of SLE are well documented in several reviews and monographs (161,166,167). Some common symptoms such as fatigue, arthritis, and pleuritis may be managed by conservative treatment, such as aspirin or other nonsteroidal anti-inflammatory drugs, and rest. However, more potent (toxic) therapy is often required, particularly when kidneys and/or the nervous system are involved. Immune thrombocytopenia, prominent vasculitis, severe skin disease, high fevers, and debilitating constitutional symptoms seem to respond best to CSs. Before discussing some specific questions of therapy, the rationale behind using immunomodulating agents will be examined in light of what is known about immune function in SLE. In this regard several murine lupus models have been useful, including the NZB/W, MRL, and BXSB strains and will be referred to below (see Refs 168 and 169 for reviews).

SLE patients often exhibit a significant lymphopenia with an absolute decrease in both B and T cells, particularly when disease is active (170,171). T cells are disproportionately low (172); this is not thought to be an artifact of surface antigen blocking by anti-lymphocyte antibodies, as similar results can be obtained with overnight preincubation of cells to allow for antibody shedding (although permanent modulation by antibody has not been ruled out).

Despite low B-cell numbers, a polyclonal hypergammaglobulinemia is common with numerous autoantibodies that vary in specificity, affinity, and quantity in different patients. It is not clear what proportion of the increased gammaglobulin is actually autoantibodies although serum anti-ds-DNA alone has been found at concentrations up to 4 mg/ml (173). Autoantibody production by SLE patients and lupus mice can be characterized as polyclonal. Anti-DNA antibodies and antinuclear antibodies are heterogeneous (174) although some cross-reacting idiotypes have been found (175,176). Autoantibodies in SLE have been found to RNA, ribosomes, single-stranded DNA, cardiolipins (accounting for biologically false-positive serology test for syphilis), platelets, RBCs, neurons, interferon, and lipomodulin, to name a few autoantigens. After in vitro DNA stimulation, lymphocytes from active SLE patients synthesize antibody to DNA, whereas lymphocytes from inactive patients do not unless they are cultured with T cells reactive with active SLE serum (176a). Lymphocytes which bind anti-DNA antibodies can also be found in stimulated lymphocytes from normal volunteers (177), although in lower numbers than SLE patients. This observation indicates that normal people have the potential to make antibodies to DNA. These clones of B cells may be inactivated or suppressed under normal circumstances. That antinuclear antibody (ANA) producing clones are ubiquitous in the general population is supported by the near 100%+ ANA reaction in patients taking the antiarrythmic drug procainamide (162). One way to shut off autoantibody production is through anti-idiotypes. Interestingly, anti-idiotypes to DNA are found in serum from inactive but not active SLE patients (178).

When lymphocytes from SLE patients are studied in vitro, spontaneous IgG synthesis is enhanced (this is not limited to autoantigens) (179-181), whereas antibody response and proliferation to PWMs are diminished (181,182). Steroid treatment tends to normalize Ig-secreting cell numbers (182). Cocultures of SLE B cells with normal T cells or their supernatants, in an attempt to see if SLE B cells respond to PWMs with normal T_{Ind} cells, have yielded conflicting data (181-184). Normal T cells do partially suppress spontaneous in vitro antibody secretion (181). It is not known therefore whether these B-cell secretory abnormalities in SLE patients are primary B-cell defects or secondary to defective T-cell regulation.

Despite high levels of spontaneous antibody production, SLE patients exhibit normal or low antibody responses to immunization with influenza vaccine (185, 186), tetanus toxoid (187,188), *Brucella* (189,190), *Rickettsieae* (189,191), and pneumococcal (192) vaccine. Depressed responses were not simply related to therapy. Interestingly in one study there was a good IgG response to immunization, while IgM response was impaired (190) to both *Brucella* and KLH antigens. Antibody titers to isohemagglutinins are normal in SLE (193), although hyperresponsiveness to rare blood-group antigens occurs (194). Hyperresponsiveness has also been noted to penicillin (195).

Of recent interest is the ability to grow B-cell colonies in vitro from human peripheral blood. In a method used by Kumagai et al. (196), enriched B cells incubated in endotoxin were grown above a layer of PHA-stimulated T cells. SLE B cells grew about twice the number of colonies as normal, although their T cells were impaired in supporting B-cell colony formation in normals.

In summary, B cells in SLE appear to be activated in that they secrete large amounts of Ig and expand in colonies faster than normal B cells. However, this activation may not include the entire B-cell repetoire since several different antigenic challenges produce normal or even depressed antibody responses. Also SLE B cells may be reponsive to T_{supp} from normals.

Analysis of T cells in SLE is evolving rapidly. In the 1970s a defect in T_{supp} was noted in both mice and humans (197-200). In the NZ mouse, early thymectomy accelerated disease (201), which was partly blocked by replacement with young but not old thymocytes (202). Increased antibody production has been documented within the first 2 weeks of life in these animals (203) and could be due to lack of immunoregulation, an intrinsically abnormal B cell, or both. This defect predates the appearance of a "natural" antithymocyte antibody (204) found in these mice which interferes with T_{supp} function.

It was reasoned that a defect in T_{supp} may help explain the polyclonal B-cell response in murine lupus and perhaps in human SLE. Therefore, treatments aimed at correcting this defect were implemented in mice. Chronic young NZ thymocyte (given before clinical autoimmune disease) injections, although preventing Coombs+ antibody production, had little effect on other autoantibodies (205,206). Thymosin (a thymic hormone) corrected NZB T-cell abnormalities in vitro (207) but had little effect on disease (208).

Soluble immune response suppressor (SIRS), a product of ConA-stimulated lymphocytes capable of suppressing B-cell secretion in vitro, significantly decreased autoimmunity and renal pathology, and increased survival when given to these mice three times per week (as ConA-induced supernatant) (209). Therefore, a basic correctable T_{supp} cell defect seemed feasible.

The issue of impaired suppression, however, is no longer so clear. Other mouse models (MRL/1pr and BXSB) show important differences from NZ mice. T-cell numbers which are low in NZ mice are normal in BXSB and increased in MRL strains (210). Thymectomy in MRL mice prevents disease expression and prolongs survival (211). Also genetically manipulated NZB/W mice that have an X-linked immunodeficiency gene (XID) (frm CBA/N mice associated with a specific B-cell subset deletion defined by lack of Ly b5+ cells) do not generate autoantibodies (except occasionally in low titer in old age) (212). Furthermore, as reviewed by Theofilopolous (210), several laboratories have questioned whether there really is a generalized T_{supp} defect in the NZ mice or if this is a dysfunction secondary to circulating immune complexes and antilymphocyte antibodies. Finally, the ConA supernatants that were called SIRS, used to treat NZ mice, are complex mixtures containing other ingredients including interferon (213) and IL-2 (214) which can influence immunoregulation so that increased T_{supp} may not have been the critical therapeutic element.

In humans a similarly complex T_{supp} story has emerged. Substantial experimental evidence has supported the view that T_{supp} is defective in active SLE. ConA-generated suppressor activity is low (198,199,215-217), and the T subset, which contains at least some suppressor function, is decreased in number during active disease (218,219). SLE serum contains antibodies to suppressor cell (OKT4$^-$) but not inducer cell (OKT8$^-$) enriched lymphocytes (220). Antibodies have also been found to ConA-activated T cells (221). Finally, in one study an increase in peripheral blood OKT4/OKT5 or T8 ("helper"/ "suppressor") ratio was particularly associated with active disease, and in an individual patient normalization of this ratio accompanied clinical improvement (222). A second study of SLE T-cell subsets, however, found an entirely different situation with a wide variety of ratios between "helper" and "suppressor" cells (223). In fact, a low "helper"/ "suppressor" ratio was found more frequently in patients with severe renal disease and thrombocytopenia, and other clinical subsets were identified based on these ratios. Further complexity may ensue with the recently discovered heterogeneity among OKT4+ and OKT8+ cells. Recent studies have also questioned the functional defect of T_{supp} in human SLE (218,224,225) and have suggested instead that T-cell inducer function of antigen-specific antibody formation may be depressed (224,226), which could explain why some immunizations in SLE patients do not evoke a good antibody response. This antigen-specific induction is likely to be a different process from more generalized antigen-nonspecific suppression which may be abnormal in SLE.

Other T-cell-related functions such as PHA and ConA proliferation are depressed in SLE patients in most studies (227-230), particularly in the presence of autologous serum (230) and with a direct relation to disease activity. Allogeneic MLRs are probably defective in SLE (228,231), which may be due to anti-T antibody (231) or diminished IL-2 production. Autologous MLR which involves an Ia-dependent T-cell proliferative reaction to autologous non-T cells is also depressed particularly in active SLE patients (232,233). DTH is diminished (228,234) which may be related to a reduced monocyte response (235).

Finally, both NK activity and ADCC are low (235a), despite frequently observed high levels of circulating IFN (235b). SLE NK/N cells may possibly be activated effector cells in vivo, killing antibody-coated cells, a theory which we are currently pursuing.

In the past two decades some progress has been made in the understanding of lupus. From the mouse models it is now apparent that diverse immune defects (as seen in each different model) can lead to a similar disease state (236). Genetic control of the composite autoimmune manifestations (e.g., antibodies to RBCs or DNA) involves multiple genes (237). Sex hormones, viral infection, thymic hormones, certain genes (1pr), and diets are modifiers of disease rather than primary elements (168). Hyperactivity of B cells, autoantibody production, and decreased IL-2 production are common demoninators in lupus mice, whereas the role of T_{supp} is controversial (168,210).

In human SLE, marked heterogeneity is also the rule. This relates to both clinical and immunological parameters. Although antinucleic acid antibodies are usually prominent, occasionally they are difficult to demonstrate (238, 239). It is also interesting that in patients with drug-induced lupus the major ANA is directed toward histones and not nucleic acids (240). As in the mouse model, a T_{supp} defect in human SLE is likely, but it is unclear whether this is a primary or secondary abnormality.

One element common to both murine and human lupus is the production of autoantibodies and resultant immune complexes. These antibodies in a sense represent a failure or breakdown of normal tolerance. In accordance with this idea is the demonstration that all three lupus mouse models, unlike normal strains, show resistance to induction of tolerance to heterologous proteins (241,242).

Although a clear picture of the immunopathogenesis of SLE is not yet available, it remains possible and necessary to design therapy in general terms. B-cell suppression, reduction of inflammation, and T_{supp} enhancement should theoretically be beneficial. One might expect CSs and cytotoxic agents to be effective since in general they decrease B-cell activity and are anti-inflammatory with a less clear effect on T_{supp}. However, the many uncontrolled variables involved in the use of these drugs and in the disease itself preclude a specific predictable response to any treatment scheme.

A. Treatment of SLE

The treatment of SLE patients has traditionally been a mixture of art and science. The great spectrum of disease manifestations, disease course, and even pathology have hampered clear interpretation of data.

To begin with, SLE patients frequently have arthralgias, arthritis, and many nonspecific aches and pains. These symptoms tend to be treated with salicylates and other nonsteroidal anti-inflammatory drugs (NSAIDs), agents which inhibit PG synthesis and can affect immune responses. In addition, functional interactions of these agents with immunomodulatory agents are largely unknown. Salicylates, which were once advocated as the main therapy of SLE (167), are now known to be not entirely benign in this disease. They have the capacity to produce gastric ulcers and prolong bleeding time in patients who are frequently on CSs, have low platelet counts, and circulating anticoagulants. SLE patients also appear to be susceptible to salicylate-induced hepatic toxicity (243) and reduction of glomerular filtration rates (244,245). Furthermore, since large doses of PGE have been shown by several groups to dramatically modify murine lupus (156), the effect of chronic administration of arachidonic acid metabolism inhibitors becomes intriguing.

Another group of commonly used potential immunomodulators in SLE is antimalarial agents (246). These drugs should be reserved for skin or mucous membrane manifestations and mild systemic involvement such as fatigue, arthralgias, and mild serositis.

In these situations they have been reported to be effective in up to 75% of cases (246). Antimalarials work very well for discoid lupus (246,247). They should not be used for acute flares of SLE or for serious internal organ involvement. Although double-blind controlled studies of antimalarial treatment of SLE have not been done, Dubois showed that five patients doing well on amodiaquin all had flares within 3 months when switched to a placebo (246). All improved within days of restarting medication. Also, Rudnicki et al. (248) studied 43 chloroquine-treated patients who developed retinal toxicity requiring drug withdrawal. Disease activity was compared for years on chloroquine with activity in matched years after drug discontinuation. There was a significant decrease in number of flares, constitutional symptoms, and skin lesions during the treatment years. However, no difference was found in specific internal organ disease, and there was no steroid-sparing effect, although this has been mentioned anecdotally (246). Of interest, although unproven, is the claim by Dubois (246) that Atabrine (Quinacrin) can be added profitably as a second antimalarial for extensive skin lesions.

1. Costicosteroids

Corticosteroids are the most commonly used immunomodulatory agents in SLE, As has been noted many times, there are no controlled clinical trials that address its efficacy in treatment or prevention of acute flares. Probably the reason for this is that CSs are in fact highly effective, often work rapidly in acute downhill situations, and physicians who have treated SLE patients would consider it unethical to withhold this therapy. In the long term, severe adverse effects of therapy are encountered. This must be balanced, however, against the greatly improved prognosis in SLE over the past 30 years which can be attributed in part to more refined use of CS (249-251).

A few general points about CS treatment can be made. Dosages must be individualized for each patient. Prior responsiveness to a particular dose may be helpful. Not all patients with SLE or all flares require CSs. Severe flares, i.e., acute CNS disease, renal deterioration, marked hematological abnormalities such as platelet count less than 10,000 severe gastrointestinal and pulmonary disease (after causes other than lupus have been ruled out) generally require acutely at least 1 mg/kg/day of prednisone. Doses are tapered in accordance with clinical response as rapidly as possible, but this often encompasses a period of months to years and is best done by physicians experienced in treating these patients. Divided doses (t.i.d.-q.i.d.) are used initially, and this is switched to a daily dose in the course of tapering. A change from divided to daily dose may provoke a relapse so that total dose should not be cut simultaneously. Moderately severe flares do not require large doses of CSs, 20-30 mg/day of prednisone often suffice. Very high-dose (1g methylprednisolone intravenously for 1-3 days) or pulse therapy seems useful for recent onset of renal insufficiency (252), and may spare the side effects associated with prolonged CS use. In other situations, pulse therapy of SLE is still experimental. Prolonged treatment with high doses of CSs ($\geqslant$1 mg/kg) as had been used for severe CNS and renal disease is more likely to result in life-threatening complications (253,254) and should be avoided. In fact, the requirement for prolonged high-dose CSs is a major indication for adding cytotoxic therapy (for possible CS sparing). The goal of CS therapy should be to control disease flares with the least morbidity from treatment itself. Some investigators therefore consider it advisable to switch to alternate-day therapy once disease activity is well controlled. As reviewed by Axelrod (140), many unwanted effects of CSs can be avoided, including hypertension, susceptibility to infections, alterations of the hypothalamic-pituitary-adrenal axis, and possibly osteoporosis. It is not known whether the dramatic effects of steroids in SLE is due to their anti-inflammatory or immunosuppressive effects or both. For further details of CS treatment the reader is referred to Refs. 140 and 255.

2. Use of Cytotoxic Agents (CTX and AZA) in SLE

A considerable amount of energy has been devoted to studying the effects of cytotoxic agents in SLE patients. Although there are many theoretical reasons why they could be useful in this disease, and results of initial uncontrolled studies bred enthusiasm for their use (256,257), the bottom line is that they exhibit only marginal, if any, benefit when compared with standard CS therapy in controled double-blind studies. This issue has been evaluated most clearly with regard to renal involvement. There are at least three reasons for examining nephritis to test these agents: first, renal disease in SLE often requires large quantities of CSs for treatment; adding a cytotoxic drug might decrease CS side effects. Second, there is precedence for these agents as immunosuppressants in renal transplantation. Third, several objective measurements can be followed in patients with lupus nephritis such as proteinuria, urine sediment, creatinine clearance, BUN, and renal histology.

In controlled studies, comparison of prednisone (Pred) treatment alone with Pred + AZA indicated zero to marginal benefit with addition of AZA in three trials (258-261) and significant benefit in two (254,262), with regard to renal function and survival. The two positive studies are flawed for different reasons. In the Downstate trial (262) seven patients that did not survive initial hospitalization (five were in the experimental group) were discarded from the data. The Cade study (254), on the other hand, used, by today's standards, extraordinarily high doses of Pred (60-100 mg/day for 6 months) in their control group, which probably accounts for the extremely high mortality (13 of 15 in 19 months) in the control Pred-alone group, and makes comparison with an AZA-alone group unjustified.

Similar studies using Pred versus Pred + CTX have yielded only marginally positive results in the CTX groups. Although a trial by Donadio et al. (263) showed no added benefit in the Pred + CTX (2 mg/kg/day, adjusted for leukopenia) group at 6 months, at 2 years (18 months after stopping CTX) renal function was similar in both groups although there were less renal flares in the CTX group. However, survival was not improved by CTX. Studies from the NIH (258,259), on the other hand, showed that addition of CTX (4 mg/kg/day for years) offered little advantage. Side effects were carefully delineated. Two patients in the CTX group developed malignancy (carcinoma in situ of cervix and bladder carcinoma). Also, a higher number of CTX-treated patients developed infections, including herpes zoster, and one-third of the females became amenorrheic.

One further attempt to use cytotoxic agents in randomized studies from the NIH combined AZA and CTX (1 mg/kg/day each) compared with intravenous boluses of CTX (0.5-1 g/m^2) every 3 months, and Pred alone (264). The rationale behind the combination therapy was the good response shown by NZB/W mice to similar therapy. The CTX boluses were given to better kill rapidly dividing activated immune cells with lower toxicity to patients. Despite encouragement from "early" results (2 years), at 3.5 years there was no statistically significant difference in renal function, despite a positive trend, in the cytotoxic-treated groups compared with Pred. All treatment groups compared with pretreatment had much lower titers of anti-DNA antibodies, higher C3 complement levels (Pred group less so), and less hematuria and proteinuria (Pred group less so). The Pred-alone group had more extrarenal disease manifestations during therapy than groups treated with cytotoxic drugs. Hahn et al. (260) had not shown a difference in AZA + Pred versus Pred in extrarenal manifestations. Previously, Ginzler et al. (265) could not show a difference between Pred versus Pred + AZA + CTX-treated patients. Currently, the NIH group is studying "vigorous treatment" for "more acute disease" with less therapy during remission (264). What they and others (254,263) have noted was a marked improvement in the prognosis of lupus nephritis compared with the 1960s and early 1970s. Better general patient management, dialysis, and more appropriate use of corticosteroids may account for this finding. Disease evolution may be another explanation. This improved prognosis with Pred and the above-cited studies must make one question the justification of using cytotoxic agents in a nonexperimental fashion. These drugs may be useful for sparing intolerable side effects of CSs and in severely ill patients not responding to CSs alone, although this has not been clearly proven. It should be noted that controlled trials of cytotoxic agents for lupus CNS, pulmonary, or hematological involvement, which can also be life-threatening complications, have not been done. In controlled studies, not all patients enjoyed a steroid-sparing effect with addition of cytotoxic drugs (260), and both cytotoxic agents and Pred alone influenced ANA, anti-DNA antibody, and serum complement similarly, with only occasional small differences (260-264).

3. Other Experimental Treatment

Plasmapheresis (PLP). (see Ref. 266 for review). Many case reports have been compiled extolling the benefits of PLP in SLE, particularly in combination with cytotoxic drugs which seem to prevent rebound of disease when PLP is discontinued. The rationale for PLP is to remove harmful circulating immune complexes and perhaps allow the mononuclear phagocyte system to more efficiently clear remaining complexes. Although anecdotal reports have been positive, double-blind studies have not yet been done.

Theoretically it is possible to remove a specific antigen or antibody from the circulation was an abosrbant column. Such a system was successfully used to remove anti-DNA antibody from rabbits (267). This concept has not yet been applied to human disease.

Levamisole. Levamisole can restore certain T-cell responses in immunodeficient animals (268,269), perhaps by enhancing monocyte-lymphocyte interactions. A preliminary report indicated that some SLE patients respond clinically to this drug (270). In a controlled study of 26 patients where levamisole was used with Pred versus Pred alone, no added benefit was found (271). The toxicity of this drug can be severe, especially at higher doseas. Granulocytopenia and gastrointestinal intolerance are limiting factors.

Frentizole. This is an immunosuppressive drug that does not affect PMN counts. Although anti-DNA antibody is decreased and longevity increased when given to NZB/W mice, neoplasms are frequent (272). A double-blind human study which indicated significant steroid sparing and reduction of joint symptoms had to be abandoned because of a high incidence of bowel ischemia/infarction and hepatotoxicity (273).

Prostaglandins (PG). Large doses of PGE_1, given to NZB/W mice prevent clinical disease and prolong survival (156). This observation was extended to the MRL mouse (158). Survival of older NZB/W mice with established autoimmune and renal disease also improved when treated with PGE_1 (157). Although mice continued to make autoantibodies, several impaired cellular immune responses were restored. The potential for use of these molecules in human SLE is currently under investigation in our laboratory.

Total Lymphoid Irradiation (TLI). This treatment, described more fully under RA, induces a brief period when antigen presentation will produce tolerance (274). It also increases survival of NZB/W mice (275). A reinduction of tolerance to autoantibodies could potentially occur.

Soluble Immunoreactive Suppressor Substance (SIRS). It is conceivable that this substance or other specific lymphokines which might suppress disease in NZB mice, could potentially be produced by cloned DNA, manufactured, and used as treatment for humans. SIRS is thought to be the same as macrophage migration-inhibition factor (MIF) (276).

Thoracic Duct Drainage. This will be discussed in the RA section. One case with severe cutaneous lupus vasculitis responded to a course of drainage (277).

IV. RHEUMATOID ARTHRITIS (RA)

Rheumatoid arthritis is a symmetrical polyarthritis that occurs at any age with peak incidence at 35-45 years of age with a 2-3:1 predominance of females (278). Etiology is unknown. That RA is an autoimmune disease is evident from the IgM anti-IgG antibody called rheumatoid factor (RF) found in greater than 80% of cases, the presence of other autoantibodies, an exuberant lymphocyte proliferation within the synovium, and a rapid response of clinical symptoms to lymphocyte depletion. Extraarticular manifestations such as lung, cardiac, and ocular involvement can occur, but RA is predominantly a disease of the joints (278,279). The literature on RA has concentrated on problems of inflammation since RA synovial fluid consists mostly of PMN cells and anti-inflammatory drugs work well as first-line therapy. However, there is increasing interest in mononuclear and synovial cell interaction in the formation of two molecules that may participate in cartilage destruction, PGE_2 and collagenase. A review by Krane (280), whose group has spearheaded this work, proposed a model whereby monocytes secrete a factor known as mononuclear cell factor (MCF; probably the same as IL-1) which acts on synovial cells to induce both collagenase and PGE. T-cell interaction with these monocytes may further modulate this reaction.

Immunohistological studies which identify large numbers of T cells in the synovium (281) and studies of thoracic duct drainage (TDD) indicate that lymphocytes are important in RA synovitis. Most patients showed an excellent response to TDD in which the thoracic duct was cannulated and 10^9-10^{10} lymphocytes were removed (282,283). When live lymphocytes were reinfused intravenously without the patient's knowledge, exacerbation of disease followed, whereas heat-killed cells produced no reaction (283). When the reinfused cells were ^{51}Cr-labeled, a small proportion could be found in synovial fluid and synovium by autoradiography. In addition, intraarticular injection of 1×10^9 live lymphocytes produced acute and persistent inflammation, whereas control dead cells caused no response (283). Early in the course of TDD peripheral blood lymphocytes transiently increase and then decrease while cellular infiltrates in synovial biopsies decrease markedly with circulating lymphocyte depletion (284). Ueo et al. therefore postulated that TDD creates a flux of cells from tissue to blood to thoracic duct, thereby leaching lymphocytes from synovium.

Inducer (OKT4, Leu 3) T cells appear to predominate in RA synovium (up to 9:1) compared with suppressor cytotoxic cells (OKT8, Leu 2a) (284,285). Many of these T cells may be Ia+ and are considered "activated" (286,287). Unlike normals, peripheral blood of RA patients often contain 5-30% Ia+ T cells (287-290). Circulating T-cell subsets are either in normal proportions (287,291) or have decreased OKT8+ cells (290,292).

One interesting Ia+ cell in synovium, particularly of RA patients, is a large cell with elongated projections (293). This dendritic cell has several characteristics of a unique nonmonocyte antigen-presenting cell described in peripheral blood (294). If these are indeed the same cell, an exciting possibility is that in synovium the dendritic cell presents antigen to OKT4 cells which proliferate and either directly or indirectly stimulate local monocytes to secrete IL-1, which can in turn act upon synovial cells to release factors that degrade cartilage. A good strategy to treat RA might therefore be to modulate the T inducer, the dendritic cell, the synovial cell, the monocytes, or combinations of these.

The role of RF is unknown and mysterious. IgM anti-IgG RF predominates in the sera but correlates only roughly with disease and is absent in approximately 20% of patients (294a). Serum IgG RF (most is found in synovial fluid) correlates best with rheumatoid vasculitis which can be a severe leukocytoclastic vasculitis that requires aggressive therapeutic intervention (295). These RF do bind complement and could contribute to joint damage.

A. Treatment

It has been tacitly assumed that anti-inflammatory drugs work in RA because of their effects on inflammation via inhibition of PG production, influence on migration patterns of inflammatory cells, and effects on chemotaxis and phagocytosis. As noted above, however, CSs and NSAIDs can affect the immune system, and the anti-inflammatory action may only represent part of their effect in RA. For example, T-cell retrafficking out of the circulation after steroid administration could have an effect on synovial T cells similar to that of TDD.

There are four goals in treating RA: (a) to relieve systemic manifestations (e.g., fatigue, fever); (b) to reduce joint inflammation; (c) prevent deformities; (d) prevent erosions and joint destruction. The first two goals are often accomplished by therapy with aspirin or other NSAIDs. Prevention of joint deformity usually is dependent upon physical measures and general control of disease process. It is the prevention of erosions and joint destruction that make RA a particularly difficult therapeutic challenge.

It is clear that no medicine used to treat RA, after the NSAID alone is both highly effective and without significant toxicity. It is also not known whether NSAIDs affect the natural history of RA. Historical controls from the literature cannot be compared as early studies often contain many uncontrolled factors such as variable diagnostic criteria for RA. The initial enthusiasm for CS was dampened by lack of significant advantage over aspirin in 1-3 year follow-up in two large prospective controlled British studies (296,297). Also, despite maintenance of functional status in these patients, radiographic deterioration occurred (298,299), and steroid-treated patients often developed severe drug-induced side effects (298). Nevertheless, small doses in short courses are occasionally useful in active young patients while waiting for other slow-acting therapy (such as hydroxychloroquine, penicillamine, or gold) to take effect. Despite an encouraging report on high-dose pulse therapy (300), a double-blind crossover trial with placebo showed symptomatic improvement in the treated group but no inhibition of radiological progression (301). This therapy is still experimental and, although there were few side effects in the above study, sudden deaths have been reported (252).

Even the efficacy of gold therapy, a time-honored treatment for RA, must be called into question. Lipsky and Ziff have shown that gold is capable of inhibiting antigen- or mitogen-induced responses by human lymphocytes, and this is likely related to the antigen-presenting cell (302). Since gold is found in synovial cells in treated individuals (303), it could play a role in suppression of local antigen presentation. Gold may also decrease macrophage phagocytosis (304) and chemotaxis of monocytes (305). Gold-treated patients can mount an appropriate antibody response to vaccine (305), although effects on Ig metabolism and RF are controversial (306-310). Unfortunately, after more than 20 years of study, there is still controversy as to whether gold is effective treatment for moderate to severe RA (311-318). The early short-term double-blind trial of 5 months of gold treatment by the Empire Research Council (312) is suspect in that during the 13-month follow-up period after gold was stopped, relatively little deterioration in both gold and control groups was observed. This finding is contrary to common experience and may indicate that patients were taking other medications. There was a strong and persistent response in the placebo group, a finding also noted by others (315). X-ray changes were similar in both groups, even after a second gold course (313). In other words, joint disease progressed despite gold. During the next decade claims were made for the capacity of gold treatment to halt erosive disease (311,318). However, these studies either included small numbers of patients and/or had problems with control-group comparability. Other studies have not found gold beneficial (314,315,317). In addition, a major problem with gold has been toxicity, which can include occasional life-threatening cytopenias, glomerulonephritis, severe skin eruptions, and other complications (319,320).

Antimalarials, which may be as efficacious as gold (321,322) are probably considerably more benign if used carefully. Retinal damage is dose dependent so recommended doses must not be exceeded. More than 6 months of therapy is needed to show statistical differences from controls with regard to joint function and subjective patient improvement (322-326). However, inhibition of x-ray progression has not yet been demonstrated convincingly.

Another drug that has been considered in the same line of defense as gold and antimalarials is the copper chelator penicillamine (PN). PN has no anti-inflammatory effects (327), but can inhibit mononuclear cell response to mitogens (328,330). and reduces titers of RF (331-333). Under certain conditions it can act as a polyclonal B-cell activator (334), which may relate to PN's ability to occasionally initiate several different autoimmune diseases such as SLE, myasthenia gravis, polymyositis, and Goodpasture's syndrome (335). Interestingly these side effects are not exclusive to treatment of RA but are also found in PN-treated patients with Wilson's disease, which is a genetic derangement of copper metabolism with an intact immune system. Results of three separate large controlled studies indicate that PN is useful therapy for RA, although its mechanism of action is unknown (331,333,336). One study showed statistically less erosion in the PN-treated group (333). Lower doses produce less toxicity, although adverse reactions can be a limiting factor in up to 30% of cases (335,336).

Cytotoxic drugs may be considered when all other agents fail to control severe disease. CTX used in patients who had failed gold and other milder therapy worked well in four of five trials (337-340). The trial in which no response was observed (341) used relatively low doses (<1 mg/kg). The other studies gave at least 1.5 mg/kg/day. In the carefully controlled study by Currey et al. (338), CTX was compared with AZA and gold. Both cytotoxic-treated groups had less radiographic deterioration than patients on gold. Furthermore, the cytotoxic agents, but not gold, provided a steroid-sparing effect. Unfortunately there was no comparison with placebo. Several doubled-blind studies, however, have shown beneficial effects of AZA (321,342-345) compared with placebo. RF and Ig tended to decrease with longer therapy. The limiting factor of cytotoxic therapy for RA, a nonlethal disease, continues to be potentially severe side effects as previously discussed. In one of the above CTX studies a patient died from infection that might have been related to drug-induced leukopenia (340). Therefore, these agents should probably be reserved for severe resistant cases or experimental trials.

B. Experimental Approaches

1. Combination Therapy

A recent study using combined therapy of CTX, AZA, and hydroxychloroquine in low doses achieved good to excellent responses in most refractory patients tested (346). There were a large number of side effects, but these were mostly reversible.

2. Total Lymphoid Irradiation (TLI)

Based on animal studies in which TLI induced a relative augmentation of nonspecific T suppression and tolerance (347,348), and successful treatment of Hodgkin disease (348), two groups of patients with severe RA were treated with different regimens which produced somewhat different results. Lymphopenias with high T_{supp}/T_{Ind} (Leu 2/Leu 3) ratios and decreased mitogen and antigen-specific responsiveness in vitro were described. RF titers did not change, but ANA, circulating immune complexes, and antibodies to collagen actually increased despite clinical improvement in most patients, further indicating the secondary importance of some of the common humoral abnormalities in RA. In the Stanford study (349), responding patients obtained relief for at least 1 year, while in the Harvard study (350) patients experienced recurrence of disease within a year of treatment concomitant with return to normal of peripheral lymphocyte counts and other immunological measurements.

3. Plasmapheresis

In one uncontrolled study (351) six of eight patients on gold or PN that received 11 weeks of plasmapheresis went into remission for an average of 4 months. RF decreased even in nonresponders. However, in a trial by Rothwell (352), using a control group receiving physiotherapy and bedrest similar to the experimental group, no advantage of plasmapheresis was observed (this was without even using the more appropriate control of sham-pheresis).

Lymphaphoresis (LP) via peripheral access could potentially function similarly to TDD. One study showed a good clinical response in four of four patients (353). Patients were on other medications and did not exhibit rebound of symptoms when LP was stopped. This procedure may be useful in the future, especially when it becomes feasible to remove specific lymphocyte subsets such as OKT4+ cells via monoclonal antibodies.

3. Levamisole (reviewed in Ref. 354)

Several double-blind studies using relatively high doses have shown benefit in treated groups. At low, less toxic doses (150 mg/week) however, data suggest a lack of efficacy (355).

V. VASCULITIS

It is hoped this final section will impart a note of optimism to the treatment of autoimmune diseases with immunomodulators. The outcomes of three separate vasculitidies [polyarteritis nodosa (PAN), Wegener's granulomatosis, and giant cell arteritis (GCA)] have all been altered dramatically by these agents. Until a few years ago PAN and Wegener's were almost uniformly fatal, while untreated GCA not uncommonly resulted in blindness. New treatment, although basically empirical, has been highly effective in decreasing morbidity and mortality in all three diseases.

A. Polyarteritis Nodosa (PAN)

PAN is a necrotizing vasculitis characteristically of medium-sized muscular arteries that produces a multisystem disorder with an untreated 5-year survival of 13% or less (356, 357). Males are affected three to four times more than females, often after the fourth decade, although the age range is wide (358). Circulating immune complexes (CICs) are likely to play an important role in pathogenesis (359,360). Vascular pathology closely resembles the serum sickness produced in animals by intravenous injections of CIC (361). Hepatitis B antigen has been recovered from about 30% of CIC, and several underlying antigenic exposures have been implicated in PAN (357,358). RF is positive in 40% of patients (titer $\geqslant$ 1:160) with lowered CH50 in 47%. Cryoglobulins occur in 25%, and ANA are generally not present (357).

Excellent results of treatment are obtained with high initial doses of steroids plus cyclophosphamide (362-365) even in advanced cases (364). A retrospective study (363) showed 5-year survivals of 53% with CS treatment alone, 80% with CSs and CTX, and 12% untreated. It is not yet clear whether all patients with a diagnosis of PAN should be on CSs and CTX agents or CSs alone. Patients without kidney involvement or hypertension may not need cytotoxic drugs, at least not immediately (366). However, of possible importance with long-term survival of PAN patients, is that late causes of death not uncommonly are due to myocardial infarction or cerebral vascular accidents in the absence of active vasculitis (363,366a). These events may be steroid-related and may provide a rationale for employing the potential steroid-sparing effects of CTX in all cases.

B. Wegener's Granulomatosis

This necrotizing granulomatous vasculitis of unknown etiology affects people over 40 years of age, uniformly strikes the lungs, and is fatal if untreated with a mean survival time of 9 months (351,367-369). Upper respiratory and renal involvement are common, and skin and neuromusculoskeletal systems can be involved.

Pathology reveals a necrotizing vasculitis with granulomas (370). A polyclonal increase in IgA and IgM is not uncommonly seen (41,367) and IC-like material can be seen in some kidneys (371), although IC have not been found in the lungs (372). Mononuclear cell numbers and response to mitogens are normal (372). RF is positive in at least 50% of cases (357,372). CTX-treated patients experience lymphocytopenia and reduction in Ig levels with maintained normal response to mitogens (368,373). CTX has been found to be the most effective drug for treatment of Wegener's, and should be started with CS. Long-term remissions with this therapy can be achieved in over 90% of cases (41,373). TP may not work as well as CTX (41,372) in induction of remission but may be useful as maintenance therapy in patients who cannot tolerate CTX (41).

Few immunological studies have been done on these diseases, probably because they are uncommon and because potent therapy is generally started almost immediately.

C. Giant Cell Arteritis (GCA) (Temporal Arteritis)

This disease usually afflicts people over 50 years of age and in its classic presentation produces a boring-type headache with tender temporal arteries, constitutional symptoms, and a high erythrocyte sedimentation rate (ESR). There is a strong association with polymyalgia rheumatica (357,375,376). Temporal artery histology reveals vessel wall infiltration by PMN and mononuclear cells, with varying numbers of giant cells. Left untreated, sudden blindness secondary to arteritis may occur, usually a few months after symptoms have begun (377).

In GCA Ig and RF have been noted in temporal artery biopsies (378,379), and serum IgG is often elevated (380). An observation of proliferation by lymphocytes exposed in vitro to arterial smooth muscle cells (381) has not been confirmed (382,383). Steroid use has greatly decreased the dreaded ocular complications of this disease, and in fact in a recent report (384) of 90 cases with 3-10-year follow-up, no severe eye lesions were found and normal life expectancy was observed. Although 1 year of treatment is occasionally sufficient, many patients require several years as relapses can occur (384, 385). Alternate-day steroid therapy, although useful for maintenance (386), should not be used initially (387).

VI. CONCLUSION

In summary, our ability to manipulate the immune system and control autoimmune diseases is proportional to our knowledge of normal immunology. Since the enormous complexities and subtleties of the normal immune system are becoming more apparent, it is not surprising that early attempts to treat autoimmune disease should be mostly empirical. Despite this, patients with several previously fatal diseases have benefited from such therapy. Nevertheless, as our knowledge of the immune system and autoimmunity expands, more specific, less toxic treatment for these diseases can be anticipated.

REFERENCES

1. E. Reinherz and S. F. Schlossman, *N. Engl. J. Med., 305*:370 (1980).
2. H. Cantor and R. K. Gershorn, *Fed. Proc., 38*:2058 (1979).
3. R. K. Gershorn, D. D. Eardley, S. Duram, D. R. Green, *J. Exp. Med.*
4. F. H. Bach, B. J. Alter, S. Sollidy, D. C. Zoschke, and M. Janis, *Cell Immunol., 1*:219 (1970).
5. K. A. Smith and F. W. Ruscetti, *Adv. Immunol., 31*:137 (1981).
6. S. Baron, F. Dianzani, and G. J. STanton (eds.), *Tex. Rep. Biol. Med., 41*: (1981-1982).
7. G. Trinchieri, D. Santoli, D. Granato, and B. Perussià, *Fed. Proc., 40*:2705 (1981).
8. M. E. Goldyne and J. D. Stobo, *R. C. Crit. Rev. Immunol., II*:189 (1981).
9. J. S. Goodwin and D. R. Webb, *Clin. Immunol. Immunopathol., 15*:106 (1980).
10. N. Talal, in *Basic and Clinical Immunology* (H. H. Fudenberg, et al., eds.), Los Altos, Calif., 1980, p. 220.
11. A. N. Theofilopoulos and F. J. Dixon, *Am. J. Pathol., 108*:21 (1982).
12. N. K. Jerne, *Ann. Immunol., 125*:373 (1974).
13. E. S. Golub, *Cell, 22*:641 (1980).
14. B. Amor and C. Mery, *Clin, Rheum. Dis., 6*:567 (1980).
15. J. L. Turk and L. W. Poulter, *Clin. Exp. Immunol., 10*:285 (1972).
16. G. D. Stockman, L. R. Heim, M. A. South, and J. J. Trentin, *J. Immunol., 110*:277 (1973).
17. T. R. Cupps, C. E. Lynn, and A. S. Fauci, *J. Immunol., 128*:2453 (1982).
18. A. Winkelstein, *Blood, 50*:81 (1977).
19. P. J. Clements, D. T. Yu, J. Levy, H. E. Paulus, and E. V. Barnett, *Arthritis Rheum., 17*:347 (1974).
20. D. A. Horwitz, *Arthritis Rheum., 17*:363 (1974).
21. A. S. Fauci, D. C. Dale, and S. M. Wolfe, *Arthirits Rheum., 17*:355 (1978).

22. A. S. Fauci, S. M. Wolff, and J. S. Johnson, *N. Engl. J. Med.*, *285*:1493 (1971).
23. F. P. Alepa, N. J. Zvaifler, and A. J. Sliwinski, *Arthritis Rheum.*, *13*:754 (1970).
24. Cooperating Clinics Committee of the American Rheumatism Association, *N. Engl. J. Med.*, *283*:883 (1970).
25. D. Parker and J. L. Turk, *Immunology*, *34*:115 (1978).
26. A. C. Aisenberg, *J. Exp. Med.*, *125*:33 (1967).
27. G. W. Santos and A. H. Owen, *Nature*, *209*:622 (1966).
28. J. G. Howard and F. L. Shand, *Immunol. Rev.*, *43*:43 (1979).
29. I. A. Ramshaw, P. A. Bretscher, and C. R. Paush, *Eur. J. Immunol.*, *7*:180 (1977).
30. H. C. Maguire and H. I. Maibach, *J. Invest. Derm.*, *37*:427 (1961).
31. J. L. Turk, *Int. Arch. Allergy*, *24*:191 (1964).
32. A. S. Townes, J. M. Sowa, and L. E. Shulman, *Arthritis Rheum.*, *19*:563 (1976).
33. J. L. Turk and D. Parker, *J. Immunopharmacol.*, *1*:127 (1979).
34. H. C. Stevenson and A. S. Fauci, *Immunology*, *39*:391 (1980).
35. T. Diamenstein, E. Willinger, and J. Reinan, *J. Exp. Med.*, *150*:1571 (1979).
36. L. Polak and J. L. Turk, *Nature*, *249*:654 (1974).
37. L. Polak, H. Geleick, and J. L. Turk, *Immunology*, *28*:939 (1975).
38. M. Rollinghoff, A. Starzinski-Powitz, K. Pfizenmaier, and H. Wagner, *J. Exp. Med.*, *145*:455 (1977).
39. R. H. Wander and H. R. Hilgard, *J. Immunol.*, *126*:901 (1981).
40. M. Hurme, *J. Exp. Med.*, *149*:290 (1979).
41. A. S. Fauci, B. F. Maynes, P. Katz, and S. M. Wolff, *Ann. Int. Med.*, *98*:76 (1983).
42. P. H. Plotz, J. H. Klippel, J. L. Decker, D. Grauman, B. Wolff, B. C. Brown, and G. Rutt, *Ann. Int. Med.*, *91*:221 (1979).
43. S. J. Farber, R. P. Sheon, A. B. Kirsner, and R. I. Finkel, *Arthritis Rheum.*, *22*:608 (1979).
44. R. L. Wall and K. P. Clausen, *N. Engl. J. Med.*, *293*:271 (1975).
45. B. L. Hazelman, *Ann. Rheum. Dis.*, *415*:12 (1982).
46. A. B. Kirsner, S. J. Farber, R. P. Sheon, and R. I. Finkel, *Ann. Rheum. Dis.*, *415*:32 (1982).
47. G. B. Elion, S. Callahan, S. Bieber, G. H. Hitchings, and R. W. Rundles, *Cancer Chemother. Rep.*, *14*:93 (1961).
48. G. B. Elion, *Fed. Proc.*, *26*:898 (1967).
49. F. Spreafico, M. G. Donelli, A. Bossi, V. Vecchi, S. Standen, and S. Garattini, *Transplantation*, *16*:269 (1973).
50. J. F. Bach, in *The Mode of Action of Immunosuppressive Agents*, North-Holland, Amsterdam, 1975, p. 93.
51. A. Winkelstein, *J. Immunopharmacol.*, *1*:429 (1979).
52. A. Winkelstein, C. G. Craddock, and J. S. Lawrence, *J. Reticuloendo. Soc.*, *9*:307 (1971).
53. R. Van Furth, A. E. Gassmann, and M. Diesselhoff-Den Dulk, *J. Exp. Med.*, *141*:531 (1975).
54. R. H. Levin, M. Landy, and E. Frei, *N. Engl. J. Med.*, *271*:16 (1964).
55. D. T. Yu, P. J. Clements, J. B. Peter, J. Levy, H. E. Paulus, and E. V. Barnett, *Arthritis Rheum.*, *17*:37 (1974).
56. M. D. Berenbaum, *Immunology*, *36*:355 (1979).
57. L. W. Poulter, N. J. Bradley, and J. L. Turk, *Immunology*, *26*:777 (1974).
58. A. C. Campbell, J. M. Skinner, P. Hersey, P. Roberts-Thompson, I. C. M. MacLennan, and S. C. Truelove, *Clin. Exp. Immunol.*, *16*:521 (1974).
59. M. Rollinghoff, J. Schrader, and H. Wagner, *Clin. Exp. Immunol.*, *15*:261 (1973).
60. P. Galanaud, M. Crevon, and J. Dormont, *Clin. Exp. Immunol.*, *22*:139 (1975).
61. A. Dimitriu and A. S. Fauci, *J. Immunol.*, *121*:2335 (1978).

62. N. I. Abdou, B. Zweiman, and S. R. Casella, *Clin. Exp. Immunol.*, *13*:55 (1973).
63. D. Chanmougan and R. S. Schwartz, *J. Exp. Med.*, *124*:363 (1966).
64. E. M. Uyeki, *Biochem. Pharmacol.*, *16*:53 (1967).
65. Y. Borel, M. Fauconnet, and P. A. Miescher, *J. Exp. Med.*, *122*:263 (1965).
66. E. M. Hersh, P. P. Carbone, V. G. Wong, and E. J. Freireich, *Cancer Res.*, *25*:997 (1965).
67. M. A. Swanson and R. S. Schwartz, *N. Engl. J. Med.*, *277*:163 (1967).
68. G. B. Elion, *Transplant. Proc.*, *9*:975 (1977).
69. Y. Borel, M. Fauconnet, and P. A. Miescher, *Int. Arch. Allergy*, *33*:583 (1968).
70. E. LaPlante, R. M. Condie, and R. A. Good, *J. Lab. Clin. Med.*, *59*:542 (1962).
71. A. Winkelstein, *J. Clin. Invest.*, *56*:1587 (1975).
72. J. Levy, E. V. Barnett, N. S. MacDonald, J. R. Klinenberg, and C. M. Pearson, *J. Clin. Invest.*, *51*:2233 (1972).
73. M. B. Urowitz, D. A. Gordon, H. T. Smythe, P. Waldemar, and O. A. Metro, *Arthritis Rheum.*, *16*:411 (1973).
74. L. W. Hoyer, R. A. Good, R. M. Condie, *J. Exp. Med.*, *116*:311 (1962).
75. H. L. Spiegelberg and P. A. Miescher, *J. Exp. Med.*, *118*:869 (1963).
76. R. Tarrab-Hazdai, O. Abramsky and S. Fuchs, *J. Immunol.*, *119*:792 (1977).
77. A. Winkelstein, *J. Clin. Invest.*, *52*:2293 (1973).
78. R. S. Smith, C. Teminelli, C. T. Kipilman, and Y. Smith, *J. Immunopharmacol.*, *3*:133 (1981).
79. M. A. Bach and J. F. Bach, *Clin. Exp. Immunol.*, *11*:89 (1972).
80. D. W. Scott and D. B. Amos, in *Immunological Diseases* (M. Samte, ed.), Little Brown & Co., 1978.
81. R. Schwartz and W. Dameshek, *J. Clin. Invest.*, *39*:952 (1960).
82. J. E. Murray, A. G. R. Sheil, R. Moseley, P. Knight, J. D. McGavic, and G. J. Dammin, *Ann. Surg.*, *160*:449 (1964).
83. S. M. Phillips and B. Zweiman, *J. Exp. Med.*, *137*:1494 (1973).
84. R. S. Schwartz, in *Immunosuppressive Drug Therapy in Human Transplantation* (F. T. Rapaport and J. Dausset, eds.), Grune & Stratton, New York, 1965, p. 440.
85. E. C. Purves, *Clin. Exp. Immunol.*, *22*:348 (1975).
86. A. C. Campbell, J. M. Skinner, I. C. M. MacLennan, P. Hersey, and C. A. Waller, *Clin. Exp. Immunol.*, *24*:249 (1976).
87. R. Hoover and J. F. Frauneni, *Lancet*, *ii*:55 (1973).
88. L. J. Kinlen, A. G. Sheil, J. Peto, R. Doll, *Br. Med. J.*, *ii*:1461 (1979).
89. J. K. Whisnant and J. Pelkey, *Ann. Rheum. Dis.*, *415*:44 (1982).
90. E. R. Hurd, *Arthritis Rheum.*, *16*:84 (1973).
91. R. B. Zurier and G. Weismann, *Med. Clin. North Am.*, *57*:1295 (1973).
92. B. E. Thompson and M. E. Lippman, *Metabolism*, *23*:159 (1974).
93. J. D. Baxter and A. W. Harris, *Transp. Proc.*, *7*:55 (1975).
94. A. S. Fauci, D. C. Dale, and J. E. Balow, *Ann. Int. Med.*, *84*:304 (1976).
95. A. S. Fauci, *J. Immunopharmacol.*, *1*:1 (1979).
96. J. D. Baxter and P. H. Forsham, *Am. J. Med.*, *53*:573 (1972).
97. D. C. Dale, A. S. Fauci, D. Guerry, IV, and S. M. Wolff, *J. Clin. Invest.*, *56*:803 (1975).
98. J. W. Athens, D. P. Haab, S. O. Raab, A. M. Mauer, H. Ashenbucher, G. E. Cartwright, and M. M. Wintrobe, *J. Clin. Invest.*, *40*:989 (1961).
99. W. P. Peters, J. F. Holland, H. Senn, W. Rhomberg, and T. Baneriff, *N. Engl. J. Med.*, *282*:342 (1972).
100. R. R. MacGregor, P. J. Spagnuolo, and A. L. Lentnek, *N. Engl. J. Med.*, *291*:642 (1974).
101. D. H. Perez, R. P. Kimberley, H. B. Kaplan, H. Edelson, R. D. Inman, and I. M. Goldstein, *Arthritis Rheum.*, *24*:641 (1981).

102. P. A. Ward, *J. Exp. Med., 124*:209 (1966).
103. J. R. Clarke, R. F. Gagnon, F. M. Gotch, M. R. Heyworth, I. C. M. MacLennan, S. C. Truelove, and C. A. Waller, *Clin. Exp. Immunol., 28*:292 (1977).
104. G. Weissmann and L. Thomas, *J. Clin. Invest., 42*:661 (1963).
105. I. M. Goldstein, *Transp. Proc., 7*:21 (1975).
106. L. H. Libertini, A. S. Waggoner, P. C. Jost, and O. H. Griffith, *Proc. Natl. Acad. Science USA, 64*:13 (1969).
107. G. Weissmann, R. B. Zurier, P. Spieler, and I. M. Goldstein, *J. Exp. Med., 134*:1495 (1971).
108. G. P. Lewis and P. J. Piper, *Nature, 254*:308 (1975).
109. F. Kantrowitz, D. R. Robinson, M. B. McGuire, and L. Levine, *Nature, 258*:737 (1975).
110. J. J. Rinehart, S. P. Balcerzak, A. L. Sagone, and A. F. LoBuglio, *J. Clin. Invest., 54*:1337 (1974).
111. E. Wiener, Y. Marmary, and Z. Curelaru, *Lab. Invest., 26*:220 (1972).
112. T. L. vanZwet, J. Thompson, and R. vanFurth, *Infect. Immun., 12*:699 (1975).
113. M. M. Cummins and P. C. Hudgins, *J. Immunol., 69*:331 (1952).
114. P. W. Seebohm, M. M. Tremaine, and W. S. Jeter, *J. Immunol., 73*:44 (1954).
115. J. Thompson and R. van Furth, *J. Exp. Med., 131*:429 (1970).
116. A. S. Fauci and D. C. Dale, *J. Clin. Invest., 53*:240 (1974).
117. J. P. Atkinson and M. M. Frank, *Blood, 44*:629 (1974).
118. A. D. Schreiber, J. Parsons, P. McDermott, and R. A. Cooper, *J. Clin. Invest., 56*:1189 (1975).
119. R. I. Handin and T. P. Stossel, *Blood, 51*:771 (1978).
120. B. F. Haynes and A. S. Fauci, *J. Clin. Invest., 61*:703 (1978).
121. J. E. Parrillo and A. S. Fauci, *Scand. J. Immunol., 8*:99 (1978).
122. T. F. Dougherty, *Ann. NY Acad. Sci., 56*:748 (1953).
123. A. S. Fauci and D. C. Dale, *Blood, 46*:235 (1975).
124. A. S. Fauci, *Immunology, 28*:669 (1975).
125. W. T. Butler and R. D. Rossen, *J. Clin. Invest., 52*:2629 (1973).
126. G. A. Settipane, R. K. Pudupakkam, and J. H. McGowan, *J. Allergy Clin. Immunol., 62*:162 (1978).
127. P. T. Fan, D. T. Yu, P. J. Clements, *J. Lab. Clin. Med., 91*:625 (1978).
128. A. Saxon, R. Stevens, S. J. Raner, *J. Clin. Invest., 62*:922 (1978).
129. J. Grayson, N. J. Dooley, I. R. Koski, and R. M. Blaese, *J. Clin. Invest., 68*:1539 (1981).
130. A. S. Fauci, K. R. Pratt, and G. Whalen, *J. Immunol., 119*:598 (1977).
131. W. T. Butler, *Transplant. Proc., 7*:49 (1975).
132. M. Tuchinda, R. W. Newcomb, and B. L. DeVald, *Int. Arch. Allergy, 42*:533 (1972).
133. L. Stavy, I. R. Cohen, and M. Feldman, *Transplantation, 17*:173 (1974).
134. D. N. Ilfeld, R. S. Krakauer, and R. M. Blaese, *J. Immunol., 119*:428 (1977).
135. B. H. Hahn, R. P. MacDermott, S. B. Jacobs, L. S. Pletscher, and M. G. Beale, *J. Immunol., 124*:2812 (1980).
136. G. Fernandes, E. J. Yunis, and R. A. Good, *Clin. Immunol. Immunopathol., 4*:304 (1975).
137. Y. H. Thong, S. A. Hensen, M. N. Vincent, N. Rola-Pleszczynski, J. B. Walser, and J. A. Bellanti, *Clin. Immunol. Immunopathol., 3*:363 (1975).
138. G. R. Crabtree, S. Gillis, K. A. Smith, and A. Munch, *Arthritis Rheum., 22*:1246 (1979).
139. E. K. Garber, P. T. Fan, and R. Bluestone, *Sem. Arthritis Rheum., 11*:231 (1981).
140. L. Axelrod, in *Textbook of Rheumatology* (W. N. Kelley, eds.), W. B. Saunders, Philadelphia, 1981, p. 822.

141. G. M. Kalmanson and L. B. Guze, *J. Lab. Clin. Med.*, *65*:484 (1965).
142. T. R. Neblett, *Arch. Dermatol.*, *92*:720 (1965).
143. D. Stollar and I. Levine, *Arthritis Rheum.*, *5*:660 (1962).
144. D. Stollar and I. Levine, *Arch. Biochem. Biophys.*, *101*:885 (1963).
145. D. Hurvitz and K. Hirschorn, *N. Engl. J. Med.*, *273*:23 (1965).
146. W. S. Logan, *Prog. Dermatol.*, *14*:1 (1980).
147. W. A. Panayi, *Ann. Rheum. Dis.*, *32*:316 (1973).
148. J. Knox and A. C. Griffin, *Arch. Dermatol.*, *81*:570 (1960).
149. F. A. Gaudener and G. H. Cleich, *Proc. Soc. Exp. Biol. Med.*, *157*:129 (1978).
150. M. S. Manko and D. E. Horrobin, *Lancet*, *ii*:1115 (1976).
151. W. M. Sams, Jr., *Mayo Clin. Proc.*, *42*:300 (1967).
152. G. Weissmann, *Fed. Proc.*, *23*:1038 (1964).
153. A. H. Mackenzie and A. L. Scherbel, *Clin. Rheum. Dis.*, *6*:545 (1980).
154. C. J. Meade and J. Mertin, *Adv. Lipid Res.*, *18*:127 (1981).
155. R. B. Zurier, *Arthritis Rheum.*, *25*:802 (1982).
156. R. B. Zurier, D. M. Sayadoff, S. B. Torrey, and N. T. Rothfield, *Arthritis Rheum.*, *20*:723 (1977).
157. K. A. Krakauer, S. B. Torrey and R. B. Zurier, *Clin. Immunol. Immunopathol.*, *11*:256 (1978).
158. V. E. Kelley and J. B. Roths, *J. Immunol.*, *129*:923 (1982).
159. E. M. Tan, A. S. Cohen, J. F. Fies, *Arthritis Rheum.*, *25*:1271 (1982).
160. W. J. Fessel, *Arch. Intern. Med.*, *134*:1027 (1974).
161. N. Rothfield, in *Textbook of Rheumatology* (W. N. Kelley, et al., eds.), W. B. Saunders Co,, Philadelphia, 1981, p. 1106.
162. A. Weinstein, *Prog. Clin. Immunol.*, *4*:1 (1980).
163. C. E. Harmon and J. P. Portanova, *Clin. Rheum. Dis.*, *8*:121 (1982).
164. P. H. Schur, *Arthritis Rheum.*, *25*:788 (1982).
165. N. F. Rothfield, in *Dermatology in General Medicine*, 2nd ed. (E. Fitzpatrick, ed.), McGraw-Hill Book Co., New York, 1979.
166. E. Dubois, *Lupus Erythematosus: A Review of the Current Status of Discoid and Systemic Lupus Erythematosus*, 2nd ed., Los Angeles, University of Southern California Press, 1976.
167. M. W. Ropes, *Systemic Lupus Erythematosus*, Cambridge, Mass., Harvard University Press, 1976.
168. A. D. Steinberg, E. S. Raveche, C. A. Laskin, M. L. Miller and R. T. Steinberg, *Arthritis Rheum.*, *25*:734 (1982).
169. D. R. Milich and M. E. Gershwin, *Sem. Arthritis Rheum.*, *10*:111 (1980).
170. R. L. Williams and A. D. Bankhurst, *Arthritis Rheum.*, *21*:5202 (1978).
171. E. S. Raveche and A. D. Steinberg, *Sem. Hematol.*, *16*:344 (1979).
172. S. J. Rivero, L. Llorente, E. D'iaz-Jouanen, *Arthritis Rheum.*, *20*:1169 (1977).
173. A. D. Steinberg, H. B. Kaltreider, P. J. Staples, *Ann. Intern. Med.*, *75*:165 (1971).
174. M. Fishbach, J. Rabbie, and N. Talal, *J. Clin. Invest.*, *68*:1036 (1981).
175. C. Andrzejewski, J. Rauch, E. Lafer, D. Stollar, and R. S. Schwartz, *126*:226 (1981).
176. T. N. Marion, A. R. Lawton, J. F. Kearney, and D. E. Brites, *J. Immunol.*, *128*:668 (1982).
176a. M. Kiyotaki, T. Togushi, T. Abe, T. Takeuchi, C. Morimoto, and M. Homma, *Clin. Immunol. Immunopathol.*, *21*:237 (1981).
177. A. D. Bankhurst and R. C. Williams, *J. Clin. Invest.*, *56*:1378 (1975).
178. N. I. Abdou, H. Wall, H. B. Lindsley, F. J. Halsey, and T. Suzuki, *J. Clin. Invest.*, *67*:1297 (1981).
179. H. E. Jasin and M. Ziff, *Arthritis Rheum.*, *18*:219 (1975).

180. C. Morimoto, T. Abet, M. Hara, *Scand. J. Immunol.*, *6*:575 (1977).
181. K. Okudaira, K. Taninoto, T. Nahamura, and Y. Horiuchi, *Clin. Immun. Immunopathol.*, *16*:267 (1980).
182. W. W. Ginsburg, F. D. Finkelman, and P. E. Lipsky, *Clin. Exp. Immunol.*, *35*:76 (1979).
183. A. M. Bobrove, and P. Miller, *Arthritis Rheum.*, *20*:1326 (1977).
184. K. M. Nies and J. S. Louie, *Arthritis Rheum.*, *21*:51 (1978).
185. G. W. Williams, A. D. Steinberg, J. L. Reinerstein, L. W. Klassen, J. L. Derber, and R. Dolin, *Ann. Int. Med.*, *88*:729 (1978).
186. R. Brodman, R. Gilfillan, D. Glass, and P. Schur, *Ann. Int. Med.*, *88*:735 (1978).
187. I. Sarkang, *Arch. Dermatol.*, *84*:372 (1961).
188. T. Abe and M. Hornman, *Acta Rheum. Scand.*, *17*:35 (1971).
189. L. E. Mieselas, S. B. Zingale, S. L. Less, R. Richman, and M. Siegal, *J. Clin. Invest.*, *40*:1872 (1961).
190. J. Baum and M. Ziff, *J. Clin. Invest.*, *48*:758 (1969).
191. S. L. Lee, L. E. Miesalas, S. B. Zinagle, and R. Richman, *J. Clin. Invest.* (Abst.), *39*:1005 (1960).
192. M. P. Jarrett, *Arthritis Rheum.*, *23*:1287 (1980).
193. L. H. Muschel, *Proc. Soc. Exp. Biol. Med.*, *106*:622 (1961).
194. S. B. Zingale, A. J. C. Sanchez, J. A. Andrada, *Arthritis Rheum.*, *6*:581 (1963).
195. R. J. Muelling, T. Bevin, R. F. Samson, E. P. Jenevein, and J. D. Guillory, *Am. J. Clin. Pathol.*, *29*:503 (1958).
196. S. Kumagai, B. Sredni, S. House, A. D. Steinberg, and I. Green, *J. Immunol.*, *128*: 258 (1982).
197. N. I. Abdou, A. Sagawa, E. Pascual, *Clin. Immunol. Immunopathol.*, *6*:192 (1976).
198. B. Bresnihan and H. E. Jasin, *J. Clin. Invest.*, *59*:106 (1977).
199. T. Sakane, A. D. Steinberg, and I. Green, *Arthritis Rheum.*, *21*:657 (1978).
200. A. D. Steinberg, *Arthritis Rheum.*, *17*:11 (1974).
201. B. J. Helyer and J. B. Howie, *Lancet*, *2*:1026 (1963).
202. A. D. Steinberg, I. W. Law, and N. Talal, *Arthritis Rheum.*, *13*:369 (1970).
203. N. Talal and A. D. Steinberg, *Curr. Top. Microbiol. Immunol.*, *64*:79 (1978).
204. M. C. Gelfand, L. M. Parker, and A. D. Steinberg, *J. Immunol.*, *113*:1 (1974).
205. J. G. Knight and D. D. Adams, *J. Clin. Lab. Immunol.*, *1*:151 (1978).
206. A. A. Hoffman and R. J. Harbeck, *Arthritis Rheum.*, *22*:412 (1979).
207. M. J. Dauphinee, A. Talal, A. L. Goldstein, *Proc. Natl. Acad. Sci. USA*, *71*:2637 (1975).
208. A. D. Steinberg, M. E. Gershwin, N. L. Gerber, in *Immune Depression and Cancer* (G. W. Sisfind, C. L. Christian, S. D. Litwin, eds.), Grune and Stratton, New York, 1975, p. 42.
209. R. S. Krakauer, T. A. Waldmann and W. Strober, *J. Exp. Med.*, *144*:662 (1976).
210. A. N. Theofilopoulos, *Arthritis Rheum.*, *25*:726 (1982).
211. A. D. Steinberg, J. B. Roths, E. D. Murphy, R. T. Steinberg, and E. S. Raveche, *J. Immunol.*, *125*:871 (1980).
212. B. J. Steinberg, P. A. Smathers, K. Fredeikson, and A. D. Steinberg, *J. Clin. Invest.*, *70*:587 (1982).
213. A. S. Kodish, F. A. Tansey, G. S. Yu, A. T. Doyle, and B. R. Bloom, *J. Exp. Med.*, *151*:627 (1980).
214. S. Gillis, K. A. Smith, and J. D. Watson, *J. Immunol.*, *125*:1954 (1980).
215. A. S. Fauci, A. D. Steinberg, B. F. Haynes, and G. Whalen, *J. Immunol.*, *121*:1473 (1978).
216. R. S. Krakauer, J. D. Clough, S. Frank, and J. T. Sundeen, *J. Clin. Immunol. Immunopathol.*, *14*:327 (1979).

217. C. Morimoto, T. Abe, and M. Homma, *Clin. Immunol. Immunopathol., 13*:161 (1979).
218. A. Moretta, M. C. Mingari, E. Santoli, P. Perlmann, and L. Morretta, *Scand. J. Immunol., 10*:223 (1979).
219. M. E. Hamilton and J. B. Winfield, *Arthritis Rheum., 22*:1 (1979).
220. C. Morimoto, E. L. Reinherz, T. Abe, G. Hornna, and S. F. Schlossman, *Clin. Immunol. Immunopathol., 16*:474 (1980).
221. M. Honda, T. Sakane, A. D. Steinberg, H. Kotoni, T. Tsunematsu, K. Moriyama, and M. Fukase, *J. Clin. Invest., 69*:940 (1982).
222. C. Morimoto, E. L. Reinherz, S. F. Schlossman, P. H. Schur, J. A. Mills, and A. D. Steinberg, *J. Clin. Invest., 66*:1171 (1980).
223. J. S. Smolen, T. M. Chused, W. M. Leiserson, J. P. Reeves, D. Alling, and A. D. Steinberg, *Am. J. Med., 72*:783 (1982).
224. J. F. Delfraissy, P. Segond, P. Galanoud, P. Wallon, P. Massais, and J. Dormont, *J. Clin. Invest., 66*:141 (1980).
225. Z. Nakamura, T. Asano, K. Yano, and T. Ofuji, *Clin, Immunol. Immunopathol., 24*:72 (1982).
226. A. B. Gottlieb, R. G. Lahita, N. Chiorazzi, and H. G. Kunkel, *J. Clin. Invest., 63*:885 (1979).
227. N. Suciu-Foca, J. A. Buda, T. Theim, *Clin. Exp. Immunol., 18*:295 (1974).
228. J. G. Paty, C. W. Sienknecht, A. S. Townes, A. S. Hanissian, J. B. Miller, and A. T. Masi, *Am. J. Med., 59*:769 (1975).
229. W. Glinski, M. E. Gershwin, D. R. Budman, and A. D. Steinberg, *Clin. Exp. Immunol., 26*:228 (1976).
230. D. A. Bell, *Clin. Immunol. Immunopathol., 9*:301 (1978).
231. P. Wernet and H. G. Kunkel, *J. Exp. Med., 138*:1021 (1973).
232. T. Sakane, A. D. Steinberg, and I. Green, *Proc.Natl. Acad. Sci. USA, 75*:3464 (1978).
233. M. Kuntz, J. B. Innes, and M. Weksler, *J. Clin. Invest., 63*:151 (1979).
234. D. A. Horwitz, M. A. Garrett, and A. H. Craig, *Clin. Exp. Immunol., 27*:100 (1977).
235. F. C. Passero and A. R. Myers, *J. Rheumatol., 8*:62 (1981).
235a. T. Hoffman, *Arthritis Rheum., 23*:30 (1980).
235b. J. J. Hooks, H. M. Moutsopolous, and S. A. Geis, *N. Engl. J. Med., 301*:5 (1979).
236. F. J. Dixon, *Arthritis Rheum., 25*:721 (1982).
237. E. S. Raveche, E. A. Novotny, C. T. Hansen, J. H. Tjio, and A. D. Steinberg, *J. Exp. Med., 153*:1187 (1981).
238. M. E. Reichlin, *Arthritis Rheum., 24*:767 (1982).
239. P. J. Maddison, *Clin. Rheum. Dis., 8*:105 (1982).
240. E. M. Tan and J. P. Portanova, *Arthritis Rheum., 24*:1064 (1981).
241. C. A. Laskin, J. D. Taurog, P. A. Smathers, and A. D. Steinberg, *J. Immunol., 1278*: 1743 (1981).
242. A. N. Theofilopoulous and F. J. Dixon, *Immunol. Rev., 55*:179 (1981).
243. W. E. Seaman and P. H. Plotz, *Arthritis Rheum., 19*:155 (1976).
244. R. P. Kimberley, *Lancet, ii*:553 (1978).
245. R. P. Kimberley, *N. Engl. J. Med., 296*:418 (1978).
246. E. Dubois, *Sem. Arthritis Rheum., 8*:33 (1978).
247. R. K. Winkleman, C. F. Merwin, and L. T. Brunsting, *Ann. Int. Med., 55*:772 (1961).
248. R. D. Rudnicki, G. E. Gresham, and N. F. Rothfield, *J. Rheumatol., 2*:323 (1975).
249. J. D. Urman and N. F. Rothfield, *JAMA, 238*:2272 (1977).
250. D. A. Albert, N. M. Hadler, and M. W. Ropes, *Arthritis Rheum., 22*:945 (1979).
251. E. M. Ginzler, H. S. Diamond, and M. Weiner, *Arthritis Rheum., 253*:601 (1982).
252. R. P. Kimberly, *Clin. Rheum. Dis., 8*:261 (1982).

253. J. S. Sergent, M. D. Lockshin, M. S. Klempner, and B. A. Lipsky, *Am. J. Med.*, *58*:644 (1975).
254. R. Cade, G. Spooner, E. Schlein, and M. Pickering, *Nephron*, *10*:37 (1973).
255. A. D. Steinberg, in *Textbook of Rheumatology* (W. N. Kelley, eds.), W. B. Saunders Co., Philadelphia, 1981, p. 1133.
256. D. S. Baldwin and G. R. Gallo, *Clin. Rheum Dis.*, *1*:639 (1975).
257. E. M. Ginzler, A. J. Bollet, and E. A. Friedman, *Ann. Rev. Med.*, *31*:463 (1980).
258. J. L. Decker, J. H. Klippel, P. H. Plotz, and A. D. Steinberg, *Ann. Int. Med.*, *83*:606 (1975).
259. J. L. Decker, A. D. Steinberg, J. L. Reinersten, P. H. Plotz, J. E. Balow, and J. H. Klippel, *Ann. Int. Med.*, *91*:587 (1979).
260. B. H. Hahn, O. S. Kantor, and C. K. Osterland, *Ann. Int. Med.*, *83*:697 (1975).
261. J. V. Donadio, K. E. Holley, R. D. Wagoner, R. H. Ferguson, and F. C. McDuffie, *Ann. Int. Med.*, *77*:829 (1972).
262. M. Sztejnbok, A. Stewart, H. Diamond, and D. Kaplan, *Arthritis Rheum.*, *14*:639 (1971).
263. J. V. Donadio, K. H. Holley, R. H. Ferguson, and D. M. Ilstrup, *N. Engl. J. Med.*, *299*:1151 (1978).
264. H. J. Dinant, J. L. Decker, J. H. Klippel, J. E. Balow, P. H. Plotz, and A. D. Steinberg, *Ann. Int. Med.*, *96*:728 (1982).
265. E. M. Ginzler, H. Diamond, M. Guttadauria, and D. Kaplan, *Arthritis Rheum.*, *19*:639 (1977).
266. J. V. Jones, *Clin. Rheum. Dis.*, *8*:243 (1982).
267. D. S. Terman, D. Petty, R. Harbeck, R. I. Carr, and G. Buffaloe, *Clin. Immunol. Immunopathol.*, *8*:90 (1977).
268. G. Renoux, *Pharmacol. Ther.*, *2A*:397 (1978).
269. D. Sampson and A. Liu, *Cancer Res.*, *36*:952 (1976).
270. B. L. Gordon and R. Yanagihara, *Ann. Allergy*, *39*:227 (1977).
271. T. Hadidi, J. L. Decker, L. El-Nagdy, and M. Sany, *Arthritis Rheum.*, *24*:60 (1981).
272. S. E. Walker, M. Soloky, and B. Schnitzer, *Arthritis Rheum.*, *25*:1291 (1982).
273. N. U. Bang, *Arthritis Rheum.*, *23*:1388 (1980).
274. B. L. Kotzen and S. Strober, *J. Exp. Med.*, *150*:371 (1979).
275. S. Slavin, *Proc. Natl. Acad. Sci. USA*, *76*:5274 (1979).
276. R. J. Warrington, P. J. Sauder, S. L. Oliver, J. W. Rutherford, and J. A. Wilkins, *J. Immunol.*, *130*:237 (1983).
277. K. E. Nyman, R. Bangert, H. Machleder, and H. E. Paulus, *Arthritis Rheum.*, *20*:1129 (1977).
278. R. C. Williams, in *Arthritis and Allied Conditions* (D. J. McCarty, ed.), Lea and Febiger, Philadelphia, 1979.
279. J. W. Hollingsworth and R. J. Saykaly, *Med. Clin. N. Am.*, *61*:217 (1977).
280. S. M. Krane, *Ann. Rheum. Dis.*, *40*:433 (1981).
281. W. L. Norton and M. Ziff, *Arthritis Rheum.*, *9*:589 (1966).
282. H. E. Paulus, H. I. Machleder, S. Levine, T. Y. Yu, and N. S. MacDonald, *Arthritis Rheum.*, *20*:1249 (1977).
283. T. Ueo, S. Tanaka, T. Yoshinori, H. Ogawa, and T. Sakurani, *Arthritis Rheum.*, *22*:1405 (1979).
284. G. Janossy, O. Duke, L. W. Poulter, G. S. Panayi, M. Bofill, and G. Goldstein, *Lancet*, *ii*:839 (1981).
285. L. Klareskog, V. Forsum, A. Wigien, and H. Wigzell, *Scand. J. Immunol.*, *15*:01 (1982).
286. O. Duke. G. S. Panayi, G. Janossy, and W. Poulter, *Clin. Exp. Immunol.*, *49*:22 (1982).

287. G. R. Burmester, D. T. Yu, A. Irani, H. Kunkel, and R. J. Winchester, *Arthritis Rheum.*, *24*:1370 (1981).
288. D. T. Yu, R. J. Winchester, S. M. Fu, A. Gibofsky, H. S. Ko, and H. G. Kunkel, *J. Exp. Med.*, *151*:91 (1980).
289. O. Forre, J. H. Dobloug, and J. B. Natvig, *Scand. J. Immunol.*, *15*:227 (1982).
290. R. I. Fox, S. Fong, N. Sabhorval, S. A. Carstens, P. C. Kung, and J. H. Vaughan, *J. Immunol.*, *128*:351 (1982).
291. O. Forre, J. Thoen, J. H. Dobloug, T. Egeland, T. K. Kvien, O. J. Mellbye, and J. B. Natvig, *Scand. J. Immunol.*, *15*:221 (1982).
292. E. M. Veys, P. Hermanns, J. Schinder, P. C. Kung, G. Goldstein, J. Symoens, and J. V. Wauwe, *J. Rheumatol.*, *9*:25 (1982).
293. R. J. Winchester and G. R. Burmester, *Scand. J. Immunol.*, *14*:439 (1981).
294. W. C. VanVoorhis, L. S. Hair, R. M. Steinman, and G. Kaplan, *J. Exp. Med.*, *155*: 1172 (1982).
294a. S. A. Paget and A. Gibofsky, *Am. J. Med.*, *67*:961 (1979).
295. D. G. Scott, P. A. Bacon and C. R. Tribe, *Medicine*, *60*:961 (1979).
296. H. Cohen, E. G. L. Bywaters, and W. S. Copeman, *Br. Med. J.*, *ii*:122 (1955).
297. E. G. L. Bywaters, W. S. Copeman, and J. R. Duthie, *Ann. Rheum. Dis.*, *16*:277 (1957).
298. C. A. Bernstein and R. H. Freyberg, *Ann. Int. Med.*, *54*:938 (1961).
299. D. Glass, M. L. Snaith, A. S. Russel, *Lancet*, *ii*:334 (1971).
300. P. T. Fan, D. Y. Yu, P. J. Clements, S. Fowlston, J. Eisman, and R. Bluestone, *J. Lab. Clin. Med.*, *91*:625 (1978).
301. M. R. Leibling, E. Lieb, McLaughlin, K. Bloka, *Ann. Int. Med.*, *94*:21 (1981).
302. P. E. Lipsky and M. Ziff, *J. Clin. Invest.*, *59*:455 (1977).
303. W. L. Norton, D. C. Lewis, and M. Ziff, *Arthritis Rheum.*, *11*:436 (1968).
304. J. D. Jessop, B. Vernon-Roberts, and J. Harris, *Ann. Rheum. Dis.*, *32*:294 (1973).
305. P. K. Ho, A. L. Young, and G. L. Southhard, *Arthritis Rheum.*, *21*:133 (1978).
306. J. S. Strong, B. A. Bartholomew, and C. J. Smyth, *Ann. Rheum. Dis.*, *32*:233 (1973).
307. H. T. Mouridsen, D. Baerentsen, N. Rossing, and K. B. Jensen, *Arthritis Rheum.*, *17*:391 (1974).
308. N. L. Gottlieb, I. M. Kiem, N. S. Penneys, and D. R. Schultz, *J. Lab. Clin. Med.*, *86*:962 (1975).
309. A. Lorber, T. Simon, J. Leeb, A. Peter, and S. Wilcox, *Arthritis Rheum.*, *21*:785 (1978).
310. R. Srinivasan, B. L. Miller, and H. E. Paulus, *Arthritis Rheum.*, *22*:105 (1979).
311. J. W. Sigler, G. B. Bluhm, H. Duncan, J. T. Sharp, D. C. Ensign, and W. R. McCrum, *Ann. Int. Med.*, *80*:21 (1974).
312. Empire Rheumatism Council, *Ann. Rheum. Dis.*, *19*:95 (1960).
313. Empire Rheumatism Council, *Ann. Rheum. Dis.*, *20*:315 (1961).
314. The Cooperative Clinics Committee of the ARA, *Arthritis Rheum.*, *16*:353 (1973).
315. A. Cats, *Agents Actions*, *6*:355 (1976).
316. N. O. Rothermich, V. K. Philips, W. Beigen, and M. H. Thomas, *Arthritis Rheum.*, *19*:1321 (1976).
317. N. D. Rothermich, *Arthritis Rheum.*, *22*:423 (1979).
318. J. T. Sharp, M. D. Lidsky, and J. Duffy, *Arthritis Rheum.*, *25*:540 (1982).
319. N. L. Gottlieb, *Bull. Rheum. Dis.*, *27*:912 (1977).
320. W. F. Kean, and T. P. Anastassiades, *Arthritis Rheum.*, *22*:495 (1979).
321. I. L. Dwosh, H. B. Stein, M. B. Urowitz, H. A. Smythe, *Arthritis Rheum.*, *20*:685 (1977).

322. A. B. Kirsner, R. P. Sheon, R. I. Finkel, and S. J. Farber, *Arthritis Rheum.*, *22*(Abst.): 630 (1979).
323. A. Freedman and V. L. Steinberg, *Ann. Rheum. Dis.*, *19*:243 (1960).
324. A. J. Popert, K. A. Meijers, and J. Sharp, *Ann. Rheum. Dis.*, *20*:18 (1961).
325. D. Mainland and M. I. Sutcliffe, *Bull. Rheum. Dis.*, *12*:287 (1962).
326. L. E. Bartholomew and I. F. Duff, *Arthritis Rheum.*, *6*:356 (1963).
327. I. A. Jaffe, *Clin. Rheum. Dis.*, *6*:633 (1980).
328. P. Lipsky and M. Ziff, *J. Immunol.*, *120*:1006 (1978).
329. G. Room, L. Roffe, and R. N. Maini, *Scand. J. Rheum.*, *28S*:47 (1979).
330. L. Binderup, E. Bramm, and E. Arrigoni-Martelli, *Scand. J. Immunol.*, *11*:23 (1980).
331. Multicenter Trial Group, *Lancet*, *1*:275 (1973).
332. A. T. Day, J. R. Golding, P. N. Lee, and A. D. Butterworth, *Br. Med. J.*, *1*:180 (1974).
333. Y. Shiokowa, Y. Horiuchi, M. Homma, and T. Kageyama, *Arthritis Rheum.*, *20*: 1464 (1977).
334. M. G. Goodman and W. O. Weigle, *Cell. Immunol.*, *65*:337 (1981).
335. H. B. Stein, A. C. Patterson, R. C. Offer, C. J. Atkins, *Ann. Int. Med.*, *92*:24 (1980).
336. A. J. Dixon, J. Davies, T. L. Dormandy, E. B. Hamilton, *Ann. Rheum. Dis.*, *34*:416 (1975).
337. Cooperating Clinics of the ARA, *N. Engl. J. Med.*, *283*:883 (1970).
338. H. L. Currey, J. Harris, R. M. Mason, J. Woodland, *Br. Med. J.*, *3*:763 (1974).
339. A. S. Townes, J. M. Sowa, and L. E. Shulman, *Arthritis Rheum.*, *19*:563 (1976).
340. H. J. Williams, J. C. Reading, J. R. Ward, and W. M. O'Brien, *Arthritis Rheum.*, *23*:521 (1980).
341. M. D. Lidsky, J. T. Sharp, and S. Billings, *Arthritis Rheum.*, *16*:148 (1973).
342. M. Mason, H. L. Currey, C. G. Barnes, J. F. Dunne, *Br. Med. J.*, *1*:420 (1969).
343. M. B. Urowitz, D. A. Gordon, H. A. Smythe, W. Pruzanski, and M. A. Ogryzlo, *Arthritis Rheum.*, *16*:411 (1973).
344. F. Hunter, M. B. Urowitz, D. A. Gordon, *Arthritis Rheum.*, *18*:15 (1975).
345. R. Cade, G. Stein, M. Pickering, E. Schlein, and G. Spooner, *South. Med. J.*, *69*:388 (1976).
346. D. J. McCarty and G. F. Carrera, *JAMA*, *248*:1718 (1982).
347. S. Strober, S. Slavin, M. Gottlieb, *Immunol. Rev.*, *46*:87 (1979).
348. H. S. Kaplan, *Hodgkins Disease*, 2nd ed., Harvard University Press, Cambridge, Mass., 1980, p. 366.
349. B. L. Kotzin, S. Strober, E. G. Engleman, A. Calin, *N. Engl. J. Med.*, *305*:969 (1981).
350. D. E. Trentham, J. A. Belli, R. J. Anderson, and J. A. Buckley, *N. Engl. J. Med.*, *305*:976 (1981).
351. D. J. Wallace, D. Goldfinger, R. Gatti, C. Lowe, *Arthritis Rheum.*, *22*:703 (1979).
352. R. S. Rothwell, P. Davis, P. A. Gordon, M. K. Dasgupta, *Arthritis Rheum.*, *23*:785 (1980).
353. J. Karsh, D. G. Wright, J. H. Klippel, J. L. Decker, *Arthritis Rheum.*, *22*:1055 (1979).
354. Twenty-fourth Rheumatism Review, *Arthritis Rheum.*, *24*:285 (1981).
355. R. S. Pinals, F. Robertson, and W. J. Blechman, *J. Rheumatol.*, *8*:949 (1981).
356. P. P. Frohnert, and S. G. Sheps, *Amer. J. Med.*, *43*:8 (1967).
357. T. R. Cupps, and A. S. Fauci, *The Vasculidities*, W. B. Saunders, Philadelphia, 1981.
358. L. Vertzman, *Clin. Rheum. Dis.*, *6*:297 (1980).
359. C. L. Christian and J. S. Sergent, *Am. J. Med.*, *61*:385 (1976).
360. E. S. Lieb, H. Hibrawi, D. Chia, and R. G. Blaker, *J. Rheumatol.*, *8*:258 (1981).

361. G. C. Cochrane, and D. Kofler, *Adv. Immunol.*, *16*:185 (1973).
362. A. S. Fauci, P. Katz, B. F. Haynes, and S. M. Wolff, *N. Engl. J. Med.*, *301*:235 (1979).
363. E. S. Lieb, C. Restivo, H. E. Paulus, *Am. J. Med.*, *67*:941 (1979).
364. A. S. Fauci, Doppman, and S. M. Woff, *Am. J. Med.*, *64*:890 (1978).
365. B. Pirofsky, and E. J. Bardona, *Med. Clin. N. Am.*, *61*:419 (1977).
366. B. Zweiman, *N. Engl. J. Med.*, *301*:266 (1979).
366a. R. D. Cohen, D. L. Conn, and D. M. Ilstrup, *Mayo Clin. Proc.*, *55*:146 (1980).
367. A. S. Fauci and S. M. Wolff, *Medicine*, *52*:535 (1973).
368. S. M.Wolff, S. M. Fauci, and R. G. Horn, *Ann. Int. Med.*, *81*:513 (1974).
369. J. A. Hoekstra and A. S. Fauci, *Clin. Rheum. Dis.*, *6*:373 (1980).
370. M. J. Saldana, A. S. Patchefsky, H. I. Israel, and G W. Atkinson, *Human Pathol.*, *89*:391 (1977).
371. R. G. Horn, A. S. Fauci, A. S. Rosenthal, and S. M. Wolff, *Am. J. Pathol.*, *74*:423 (1974).
372. H. L. Israel, A. S. Patchefsky, and M. J. Saldana, *Ann. Int. Med.*, *87*:691 (1977).
373. A. S. Fauci, D. C. Dale, and S. M. Wolff, *Arthritis Rheum.*, *17*:355 (1974).
374. M. J. Reza, L. Dornfeld, L. S. Goldberg, R. Bluestone, and C. M. Pearson, *Arthritis Rheum.*, *18*:501 (1975).
375. C. R. Hamilton, W. M. Shelley, P. A. Tumulty, *Medicine*, *50*:1 (1971).
376. K. A. Huston, G. G. Hunder, J. T. Lie, R. H. Kennedy, and L. R. Elvelback, *Ann. Int. Med.*, *88*:162 (1978).
377. H. P. Wagener and R. W. Hollenhorst, *Am. J. Opthamol.*, *45*:617 (1958).
378. G. C. Liang, P. A. Simpkin, and M. Mannik, *Ann. Int. Med.*, *81*:19 (1974).
379. E. Waller, O. Tonder, and E. Milde, *Acta Pathol. Microbiol. Scand.*, *84*:55 (1976).
380. B. Malmvall, B. Bengtsson, B. Kayser, L. Nilsson, and K. Alestiz, *JAMA*, *236*:1876 (1976).
381. B. Hazelman, I. C. MacLennan, and M. Esiri, *Ann. Rheum. Dis.*, *34*:122 (1975).
382. C. C. Papaioannou, G. G. Hunder, and F. C. McDuffie, *Arthritis Rheum.*, *22*:740 (1979).
383. R. G. Jones, J. R. Park, B. I. Hazelman, M. Ward, and A. Y. Bulgen, *J. Rheumatol.*, *7*:6 (1980).
384. B. A. Bengtsson and B. E. Malmvall, *Acta. Med. Scand.*, *209*:337 (1981).
385. D. G. Beevers, J. E. Harpur, and K. A. Turk, *J. Chronic. Dis.*, *26*:571 (1973).
386. B. A. Bengtsson and B. E. Malmvall, *Acta. Med. Scand.*, *209*:347 (1981).
387. G. G. Hunder, S. G. Sheps, G. L. Allen, and J. W. Joyce, *Ann. Int. Med.*, *82*:613 (1975).

15

Tumor and Metastatic Disease

Gerald J. Elfenbein The J. H. Miller Health Center, University of Florida, Gainesville, Florida

I. PERSPECTIVE

The concept of "natural immunity" modulating the growth of malignant neoplasms has been around at least since the turn of the century, as expressed by Amedee Borrel. Paul Ehrlich suspected that "cellular forces" were predominant in host reactions against carcinoma. He firmly believed that manipulation of the immune system in animals with experimental tumors could result in protection of the animal against the ravaging effects of the neoplasm and that the results of these experiments could be translated into therapy for humans with malignant disease (1). These thoughts supported by early experiments gave birth to the fields of tumor immunology and immunotherapy.

Generations of investigators have grappled with the problem of immune-mediated destruction of malignant cells in animal models. Understanding the mechanism of immune destruction of neoplastic cells was the specific aim, but manipulation of the immune response for more effective immune destruction of cancer was the ultimate goal. The first step needed was a definition of the specific antigenic determinant(s) on the malignant cell toward which the immune response was directed. It was, in fact, this need that resulted in the development of inbred strains of laboratory animals, now about half a century ago, that permitted investigators to design experiments enquiring into the responses of the immune system to tumor-associated antigens, or tumor-specific transplantation antigens rather than tissue-specific or histocompatibility antigens (2,3).

Much has been learned since about the heterogeneity of the immune system and the multiplicity of mechanisms by which the immune system interacts with foreign antigens. Much has also been learned about the multiplicity of mechanisms by which the immune system inhibits tumor growth by killing malignant cells. It has been stated that tumor immunity per se is not a distinct entity unto itself with different mechanisms of effector functions, but just another example of how the immune system interacts with foreign antigens (4). As with microbial immunity, tumor immunity deals with antigens on viable, proliferating cells bearing foreign antigens which have the potential to multiply and overwhelm the host resulting, ultimately, in death of the host.

This monograph describes the fruits of the efforts of many investigators whose research has been directed to augmenting or modulating the immune response either to enhance tumor immunity, thereby making it more effective, or to restore immunological balance that is disturbed in autoimmune disorders. The purpose of this chapter is to describe the component parts and framework of tumor immunity, to point out where immunomodulating agents may be effective in enhancing tumor immunity, and to put these concepts into the perspective of medical management of the cancer patient. No attempt will be made to describe clinical trials of immunomodulating agents in patients with cancer. Colleagues contributing to this monograph have adequately described clinical trials, where relevant, of the particular agents in which they are interested. Principles of clinical trials to illustrate theoretical considerations will be presented when appropriate.

II. CONCEPTS OF CANCER IMMUNOBIOLOGY

Although cancer is a term used to refer to a disease process that has the characteristics of (a) unrestrained proliferation of abnormal cells, (b) ability to invade adjacent, often vital, structures, and (c) potential to spread to distant organs via vascular structures, it is well known that cancer is not a single disease but many diseases. Different types of cancers have different patterns of behavior and different clinical coureses in patients. Most nonlymphohematopoietic malignancies are characterized by (a) the typical primary lesion, often called the *tumor*, although some neoplasms may be multifocal in origin (e.g., bronchogenic carcinoma and breast carcinoma) and (b) the secondary lesions at sites distant to the primary lesion, the *metastases.*

This proclivity of malignancies to grow locally into tumors and to spread by blood vessels and lymphatic channels, to seed distant tissues, and to grow at distant sites into metastatic lesions was the fundamental reason for the choice of the title of this chapter. Until recently, however, from the point of view of the immune system this division into tumors and metastases was artificial as the cells in the secondary metastases are clonal progeny of the original malignant transformed cells, just as the cells in the primary tumor are clonal progeny. Furthermore, since cancer is a clonal disease, the cells would be expected to express the same tumor-related antigens (see Sect. IV), whether in the primary or secondary lesion. Differences in the immune response to tumor and to metastastes may exist but should be explicable by local rather than systemic factors. For instance, differences in blood vasculature and differences in tumor oxygen tension may be the explanation for differences in immune responses. Examples of these circumstances are the blood-brain barrier, across which there is a poor pentration of immunocytes, and poor function of antibody-producing cell machinery under conditions of anaerobic metabolsim (5). If it were not for these possible local differences, immune responses to malignant cells in the primary tumors and secondary metastatic lesions would be expected to be identical.

In light of recent data accumulated from experimental malignancies in animal models, this concept may be in need of revision. Specifically, there is a transplantable murine melanoma line which has the potential to metastasize from a primary implantation site to the lungs and to the brain. Cells that have metastasized to the brain on subsequent passage "prefer" to metastasize to the brain, while cells that have metastasized to the lungs on subsequent passage "prefer" to metastasize to the lungs (6). These findings suggest that metastases are not random events and that subclones of the melanoma with different tumor-related surface antigens, which may explain differential tumor immune responses directed toward the primary lesion and toward secondary lesions, and differential responses may even be noted from one secondary lesion to another because of organ of residence.

Returning to the notion that cancer is not just one disease but many diseases, cancers have for a long time been classified histologically, cytologically, and by organ of origin. By these classifcation schemes, well over 100 different cancers are known to exist. Furthermore, cancer may etiologically be related to a variety of factors. Best known in humans are environmental factors such as cigarette smoking and asbestosis in lung cancer (7,8). Well known in animal models are genetic predispositions for and viral causes of specified types of cancer. In animals, chemical carcinogens, such as methylcholanthrene, can induce tumors of the same histological appearance at injection sites in different animals, but cells from these tumors may have entirely different (i.e., unique) surface antigens (2,3). The point is that cancers are quite heterogeneous by morphological appearance, by organ of origin, and by surface antigens. It is altogether reasonable to suspect that cancers may be essentially infinitely variable. If this concept were true, even in a limited variability sense, it would preclude development of a vaccine (see Sec. VIII) with "cancer cell surface antigens" to prevent cancer by immunizing patients with "cancer antigens." On the other hand, it is altogether possible to utilize autochthonous cancer cell surface antigens to produce a vaccine which may boost the tumor immune response in an inidividual patient.

One further concept to develop concerning the variability in cancer immunobiology is the dependence of expression of tumor-related antigens on cell cycle. The cells of tumors are not all in the same stage of the cell cycle; some are synthesizing DNA (S phase), some are undergoing mitosis (M phase), some are in phases between these two phases (G_1 and G_2), and some are not in cell cycle at all (G_0). In normal tissues surface antigenic expression may be dependent upon cell cycle stage (9). There is no reason to believe this cannot be true for cancer cells as well. The implication of this concept is that any single-point-in-time immunotherapy such as passive transfer of antibodies (monoclonal or polyclonal) to specific tumor-related antigens (see Sec. VIII) may fail to be totally effective since many cancer cells may not bear the specific target antigen because of their stage of cell cycle and, therefore, not be destroyed by the antibodies (augmented by complement or linked with toxins).

III. PRINCIPLES OF CANCER PATIENT MANAGEMENT

In order to understand the role of immunomodulating agents in the therapy of cancer more clearly, one must understand some of the current principles of clinical management of patients with cancer. The diagnosis of cancer is made by obtaining a tissue specimen from a suspicious mass for pathological examination. Once the diagnosis of cancer is made, the clinician must assess the extent of the disease and estimate if the cancer may be approached with "curative" therapeutic intent or should be treated with "palliative" intent. This decision is made utilizing the histological type of cancer, stage of the disease, and knowledge of the clinical behavior of this type of malignancy.

Until recently, the primary therapeutic modalities for curative intent were those in which the primary lesion (and any local extension of the disease) could be encompassed in a limited anatomic field so that either the disease could be extirpated surgically or the field could be "sterilized" by radiation therapy. This approach is still quite effective for many solid tumors. Recently, for many lymphohematopoietic malignancies and some solid tumors (following surgical resection of primary lesions and regional nodes which are involved with disease) curative intent may be achieved with combination chemotherapy alone or with added radiation therapy (10-12).

The main principles to be derived from these clinical approaches to cancer are: (a) more complete understanding of the biological behavior of cancers have enabled oncologists to devise more effective therapy; (b) aggressive therapy is required to achieve the goal of therapeutic intent; and (c) multimodal therapy is often the best approach for many malignancies.

When the disease is of a histological type, or at an advanced stage, or has a biological behavior that currently makes it incurable, the oncologist approaches the patient with palliative intent. This simply implies that clinicians will use all therapeutic modalities (surgery, radiation and/or chemotherapy) available to them to control the malignant disease (induce a remission or delay progression) to prolong the productive life of the cancer patient. It is in patients with incurable disease that new chemotherapeutic combinations and new modality combinations are utilized in an attempt to improve survival and, perhaps, produce cures. It is also in patients with incurable disease that new therapeutic modalities such as hyperthermia and immunotherapy are tried. There are many forms of immunotherapy that have been tried, some of which have had palliative effects.

To date only one form of immunotherapy (see Sec. VIII) has actually been curative in the clinical management of malignancy. Specifically, the graft-versus-leukemia effect after allogeneic bone marrow transplantation for acute leukemia, suspected from animal models, has been quite adequately documented in humans to improve the cure rate produced by the intensive combination chemoradiotherapy used to eradicate malignant cells and prepare the recipient to accept the marrow graft from the donor (13). Although this circumstance currently has a rather restricted spectrum of clinical applications and although no immunomodulating agent was used in this form of immunotherapy, it is important to bear in mind the principle that these observations demonstrate: immunotherapy under appropriate circumstances may be effective in producing "cures" of malignant disease in humans. With advances in knowledge of tumor immunity and with improvements in immunomodulating agents, it is altogether reasonable to believe that immunotherapy may, in the future, be a modality used with curative intent for many malignancies.

IV. CONCEPTS IN TUMOR IMMUNOLOGY

There is little doubt that immune responses to tumor cells occur in humans as well as in animals models of malignant disease. As alluded to in the Perspective (Sec. I), tumor immunology does not represent a new scientific discipline but rather another circumstance in which the immune system must act upon foreign antigens, this time on malignant cells. In this section fundamental concepts of tumor immunology will be discussed. In a subsequent section the biological role of tumor immunity will be discussed.

The fundamental assumptions of tumor immunology are: (a) that tumor-related foreign antigens (i.e., neoantigens) exist on the surfaces of cancer cells and (b) that these neoantigens are sufficiently immunogenic to elicit an immune response. These neoantigens may be of two general types: (a) tumor-specific transplantation antigens (TSTAs) (i.e., antigens which are unique to the particular neoplasm) or (b) tumor-associated antigens (TAAs) (i.e., antigens frequently found on tumor cells and infrequently found on normal cells from the same lineage, including oncofetal antigens and differentiation antigens). Also, it may be expected that tumor cells bear other antigenic systems on their surfaces, for example, (a) tissue- or organ-specific antigens and (b) histocompatibility antigens. Table 1 summarizes the classification of TSTAs, TAAs, and other antigens found on the surface of tumor cells.

As is generally true in immunology, tumor immunity is antigen specific. This implies that immunity is acquired upon exposure to specific TSTAs or TAAs, that clonal expansion of immunocytes capable of recognizing and/or dealing with the antigen occurs, and that memory for the specific TSTA or TAA develops such that a later challenge with the same tumor will elicit a secondary immune response. Furthermore, challenge with a different tumor with other TSTAs or TAAs will not elicit a secondary response. In other words, the *protective immunity* which may develop after exposure to a tumor cell is *not broad* against all cancer cells *but limited* to specific TSTAs or TAAs. No antigen common to all cancer cells and not present on normal cells has yet been identified. This situation is no different from what is commonly understood to be true in microbial immunity.

The biological characteristics of cancer cells (and microbial agents) of viability and proliferative capacity (as described above) provide an extra challenge to the immune system over that presented by foreign antigens such as toxins or transplantation antigens. This challenge is related to a time factor. While the primary immune response is being stimulated and clonal expansion and development of immune effector cell populations is taking place (see Sec. V), the cancer cells are proliferating without restraint. By the time reactive effector cells are sufficiently expanded in numbers that the immune response is prepared to make a concerted attack on the tumor, the tumor may have a sufficient competitive edge in cell numbers to withstand the immunological attack with minimal losses in cell number, to exhaust the immune response, and to continue to grow

Table 1 Classification of Tumor-Related Cell Surface Antigens

I. Tumor-specific transplantation antigens (TSTAs)
   A. Unique to particular tumor
      Example: carcinogen (e.g., methylcholanthrene-induced TSTA)
   B. Inducer-specific antigen but not part of inducer itself
      Example: oncogenic viral (e.g., polyoma) induced TSTA

II. Tumor-associated antigens (TAAs)
   A. Oncofetal or maturation regression antigens
      Example: carcinoembryonal antigen
   B. Differentiation antigens
      Example: idiotypic determinant of surface immunoglobulin molecule on malignant B-cell clone

III. Other cell surface antigens
   A. Organ- or tissue-specific antigens
      Example: T-cell determinant on malignant T-cell clone
   B. Histocompatibility antigens
      Example: HLA-DR(Ia) on malignant B-cell clone

without apparently being affected at all by the immune response. This circumstance, amply supported by animal model experimental data, has led to the concept of limited capacity of tumor immunity to cope with tumor (i.e., tumor immunity is only likely to be effective when the tumor cell burden is minimal). Bearing this concept in mind, clinicians have been planning for years planning therapeutic strategies to minimize tumor burden, often by multimodal therapeutic approaches (i.e., surgery, radiation, and/or cytotoxic drugs) prior to initiating trials with immunotherapy (see Sec. IX).

V. MACHINERY OF TUMOR IMMUNITY

How is tumor immunity effected? What are the factors and cell populations which participate in tumor cell immune responses? Again, as alluded to above, the immune response to tumor cells qualitatively differs from the immune response to transplanted cells and to microbial agents only by the antigens (TSTAs or TAAs) to which the immune response is directed. The teleological goal of the immune response is protection (survival) of the host against invasion (neoplasia) by cells bearing foreign antigens. It is not the purpose of this chapter to discuss the entire immune system in its comprehensive response to foreign antigens or to discuss all the mechanisms by which individual factors or cell populations eliminate foreign cells from the host. The purpose is to describe the component parts of tumor immunity and the framework within which the parts work.

Figure 1 summarizes what is currently understood about the component parts and their framework for cytolysis of malignant cells by the immune system. Both cellular immune and humoral immune responses may be involved in the cytolysis of any particular malignant cell clone. The antigen(s) to which the immune response is (are) directed are TSTAs and/or TAAs. All known subsets of cells in the immune system may be acting on any particular malignant cell clone. It is not necessarily true that all cell populations and factors participate in the cytolysis of all types of malignant cells.

T-helper (T_h) cells recognize the neoantigens, proliferate, and cooperate with B cells with receptors (surface immunoglobulin) for TSTAs and/or TAAs for the production of specific antibody molecules and with T-killer (T_k) cells with receptors for TSTAs and/or TAAs for expansion into a specific, tumor cell cytotoxic, effector cell pool. T_h also cooperate with other T-effector cells such as lymphokine-producing $T(T_l)$ cells, which produce cytotoxins, macrophage migration-inhibition factor, tumor necrosis factor, interferon, and macrophage-activating factor (MAF), to name just a few lymphokines. These lymphokines may act directly upon tumor cells (e.g., cytotoxins or tumor necrosis factor) (14), or indirectly by activating nonspecific effector cell populations (e.g., MAF-activating macrophages and interferon-augmenting natural killer (NK) cells). It is suspected that some of the progeny of the expanded clone of TSTA/TAA-reactive T_h cells become memory $T(T_m)$ cells. T-suppressor (T_s) cells modulate immune responses; in particular T_s regulate the generation of T_k and production of antibody by B cells. Antibody molecules may be directly toxic with the assistance of the complement cascade and the terminal lytic components or indirectly by binding to tumor cells by the Fab (antigen reactive) end of the immunoglobulin molecule, leaving the Fc end of the immunoglobulin molecule free for nonspecific killer (K) cells to bind to and then lyse the tumor cell.

Much attention has been devoted above to the concept of tumor immunity being antigen specific. And this concept is true for the vast majority of cell populations participating in the tumor immune response. However, there are recently obtained data demonstrating that there are at least two subpopulations of cells participating in the immune

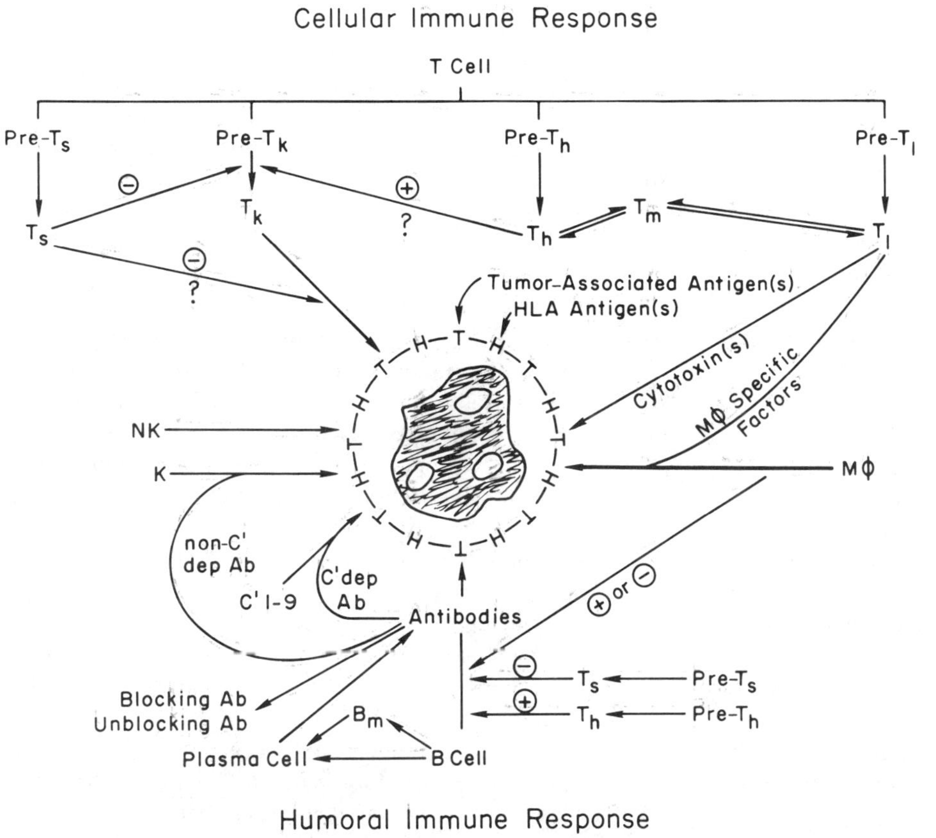

Figure 1 Cytolysis of malignant cells: This schematic diagram presents all the currently known interactions between immunocytes and tumor cells and among immunocytes for tumor lysis. Tumor cells bear HLA (H) antigens and tumor (T) associated antigens as targets for recognition and cytolytic attack. The cellular immune response involves helper $T(T_h)$, killer $T(T_k)$, suppressor $T(T_s)$, memory $T(T_m)$, and lymphokine-producing $T(T_l)$ cells. The humoral immune response involves antigen-responsive B, memory $B(B_m)$ and antibody (Ab) producing plasma cells. The interactions (⊕ signifies facilitation and ⊖ signifies inhibition) of macrophages (MΦ) with B cells are noted as are the interactions of T cells and lymphokines with MΦ and with B cells. The involvement of antibody with complement (C′ deb Ab) and with killer (K) cells (non-C′ deb Ab) for tumor lysis is shown. The participation of nonimmune natural killer (NK) cells is also represented. Production of blocking and unblocking antibodies of tumor enhancement is indicated. Details of this machinery of tumor immunity are given in the text. This schematic is a consolidation of the results of many studies. It is not necessarily true that all of the lytic mechanisms presented are operative for all types of malignant cells.

response capable of killing tumor cells that function without antigen specificity. These two populations have been named above—NK cells (15) and macrophages (16). Both of these cell types are ultimately derived from lymphohematopoietic stem cells in the bone marrow. Macrophages are well known to be derived from lymphohematopoietic stem cells in the bone marrow via the monocytic cell line (17). NK cells are apparently derived from lymphopoietic cells. At the writing of this chapter, it is not clear whether NK cells belong to the T-cell lineage or not. Experiments do show that NK cells may be generated under appropriate circumstances from thymocytes (18). Two observations made above are worth restating: macrophages become cytyolytic after activation with MAF (19) and interferon augments NK-cell activity (20). Thus, cytolytic cell populations which act antigen nonspecifically are activated or augmented by the products (lymphokines) of T cells stimulated during antigen-specific interactions, in other words, products from antigen-specific reactions effecting antigen-nonspecific cell populations.

Understanding the cell populations involved with and the mechanisms of cytolysis of malignant cells has been a major area of research that is still ongoing. Although this field is exceptionally important, a review of this field is beyond the scope of this chapter. One notion worthy of consideration because of its theoretical importance, as well as because of recently obtained data, is the concept of tumor cell cytostasis. One important function of tumor immunity may be inhibition of proliferation of neoplastic cells. This will not result in eradication of tumor cells directly, but may prevent progression of tumor growth in terms of cell numbers allowing the immune response to continue its clonal expansion until cytotoxic effector cells are present in quantitatively sufficient numbers to eradicate the neoplastic clone. Cytostasis of tumor cells may be just as important as cytostatic antibodies which prevent microbial proliferation and allow phagocytic cells and the immune reponse to cope with invading microbes. Current research suggests a cytostatic role, as well as a cytotoxic role, for macrophages (21).

VI. BIOLOGICAL RELEVANCE OF TUMOR IMMUNITY

The ability of the immune system to respond to TSTAs and TAAs is no longer subject to question. What is subject to question is the biological role of tumor immunity, especially in light of the clinical observations that most malignancies, if left untreated, ultimately overwhelm the host and prove fatal. That tumor immunity may have an important biological role in humans stems from observations, in a small proportion of cancer patients, that primary and even metastatic lesions may spontaneously shrink in size (regress) leaving the patient free of disease.

Two possible productive roles for tumor immunity that may result in protection of the host are (a) tumor surveillance and (b) tumor lysis. Much has been written about the concept of tumor surveillance. In fact, immune surveillance for neoantigens with rapid destruction of small clones of cells bearing neoantigens has been said to be, teleologically speaking, one of the major reasons why the immune system has evolved in so complex a fashion in mammals. Much data have been presented that support and contradict the concept of tumor surveillance (22). It is not the purpose of this section to review these pros and cons; however, two pertinent comments are in order. First, there is a definite increased incidence in selected types of malignancies in all clinical settings of immune insufficiency such as after renal transplantation, with immunodeficiency syndromes, and during senescence. And second, if there really is such a role for the immune system as tumor surveillance, NK cells and macrophages are likely to be the cell populations which execute the function because they do not require sensitization in order to lyse tumor cells.

The second productive role for tumor immunity stated above is tumor lysis. It has become apparent over the years that patients with tumors that have a heavy lymphocytic infiltrate have a better prognosis than those who do not (23). Furthermore, as mentioned above, spontaneous regressions of primary and metastatic lesions have been observed clinically in such diseases as melanoma and hypernephroma. And last, animal models clearly show that immunity to tumor cells can be induced and be protected against subsequent challenge with viable tumor cells. Thus, there is no doubt that under appropriate circumstance tumor immunity may be protective and lyse established, growing neoplasms.

Unfortunately, clinical observations tend to negate both of these roles as being of major biological significance because cancer is a relatively high-incidence disease (approximately 3250 new cases per 100,000 population in the United States per year) and spontaneous regressions are relatively rare events ($<1\%$ of patients with cancer have been documented to have spontaneous regressions). In defense of the biological significance of tumor surveillance and tumor lysis, it must be acknowledged that there is no method for quantitating how many nascent tumors were destroyed by NK cells and macrophages nor how many clinically measurable but undiagnosed tumors spontaneously regressed due to tumor lysis mediated by the immune system. Only prospective studies with highly sensitive methods for detecting cancer at the cellular level can resolve this dilemma. These types of studies are not likely to be performed in the near future.

Two possible counterproductive roles for tumor immunity that result in harm to the host are (a) immunostimulation of tumor growth and (b) enhancement of tumor growth—which on the surface sound very similar but really are quite different. The concept of immunostimulation of tumor growth by the host's immune response is derived from experiments in animal models of malignant disease in which transplantable tumor cells mixed with lymphoid cells prior to inoculation into the recipient animal resulted in growth of larger tumor nodules than when tumor cells alone were inoculated. In other words, a weak immune response may actually stimulate tumor growth (22). This, if true in humans, would be clearly maladaptive and pervert the attempt of the immune system to survey against nascent neoplasms and lyse neoplasms that have escaped surveillance and have grown into tumors.

The second counterproductive role for tumor immunity stated above was enhancement of tumor growth. Much research has been devoted to elucidating the mechanisms whereby tumor growth is enhanced by the immune response of the host (24). Passive transfer experiments in animal models have shown that factors exist in the serum which prevent the cytolytic arm of the immune response from killing tumor cells. In vitro correlates of these experiments have confirmed these observations and have developed the concepts of "blocking" factors (25). Blocking factors appear to be specific antibodies or antibody-neoantigen complexes which interfere with immune cell-mediated tumor lysis functions, because of their peculiar biochemical properties, either at the level of the tumor cell or at the level of the immunocyte. Enhancement may also be effected by any mechanism which prevents clonal expansion of immunoreactive cells to TSTAs/TAAs. This may be accomplished by inhibition of macrophage antigen presentation or by excessive function of suppressor cells. The mechanisms involved in immune enhancement of tumor growth are summarized in Table 2. Needless to say, enhancement is also clearly maladaptive to tumor lysis of growing malignant lesions.

There is yet a third maladaptive pattern of behavior of the immune response that may be an example of bypassing tumor immunity. In specific animal models of malignant disease, where different numbers of transplantable tumor cells were inoculated into different animals, there was a surprising biphasic pattern for tumor lesion growth. At high doses, tumors developed and apparently overwhelmed host resistance. At moderate doses, tumors failed to develop, presumably indicating that the immune response was sufficient to cope with the foreign antigenic challenge. These observations were not surprising. However, at low doses of inoculated tumor cells, tumor cell proliferation was not inhibited

Table 2 Immune Mechanisms of Enhancement of Tumor Growth

I.	Afferent block: Antigen (TSTA/TAA) is prevented from sensitizing specific immunocytes, perhaps related to inhibition of the antigen-processing function of macrophages.
II.	Efferent block: Antibody, produced by the immune response (to TSTAs/TAAs), covers sites on tumor cells which are targets for cell-mediated tumor lysis.
III.	Central block: Antibody or antigen-antibody complexes (involving TSTAs/TAAs) are present in the circulation and bind to immune effector cells, thereby neutralizing their ability to bind to tumor cells and to cause lysis.
IV.	Suppression: Excessive function of suppressor cells (antigen specific or nonspecific) prevent recognition of or effector function of immunocytes reactive with TSTAs/TAAs.

and lesions developed, suggesting that the inoculum size was either (a) below the threshold for immune recognition or (b) that, at this inoculum size, antigen processing was inhibited or suppressor cells developed quickly and turned off clonal expansion of TSTA/TAA immunoreactive cells. The experimental observations were said to represent a "sneaking through" or "escape phenomenon" from immune recognition (22). If the low inoculum size was below the threshold for recognition, the immune response would be "innocent," despite its failure to lyse the tumor. On the other hand, if one of the mechanisms of enhancement were responsible, the immune response would be "guilty."

The actual biological relevance of all of these roles of tumor immunity is not clearly understood in humans or even in animal models of malignant disease. However, it is important to make note of all of the potential roles and to try to formulate an algorithm which integrates the behavior of tumor cells and the immune system and predicts tumor growth patterns. Such an algorithm is shown in Fig. 2.

VII. MECHANISMS OF TUMOR SELF-DEFENSE

To this point it has been assumed that tumor cells overcome the host simply because of their unrestrained proliferation that exceeds the ability of the host to lyse tumor cells in a quantitative sense. This need not necessarily be true: tumor cells may be more "wily" than formerly suspected. It has been clearly shown that tumor cells may become resistant to chemotherapeutic agents (such as methotrexate) by a variety of biochemical mechanisms (26) and that tumors may transform from one histological subtype to another that is more virulent [such as the blast crisis of chronic myelogenous leukemia (27) and conversion of poorly differentiated lymphomas into histiocytic lymphomas (28)]. There is no reasons a priori to discount the notion that tumor cells may be able to develop resistant to immune attack. This would result in a qualitative change in host-tumor relationship. Undoubtedly, the development of such resistance stems from the inherent biological variablility of tumor cells and forces which tend to select a subclone with better survival potential in the host (i.e., a process much like natural selection during evolution).

The ability of tumor cells to proliferate, invade, and disseminate and to escape immune attack because of peculiar vasculature properties (e.g., sanctuary sites for tumors in the central nervous system and the testicles) has already been adequately discussed. The remainder of this discussion will be devoted to mechanisms by which tumor cells may protect themselves against attack by the immune system.

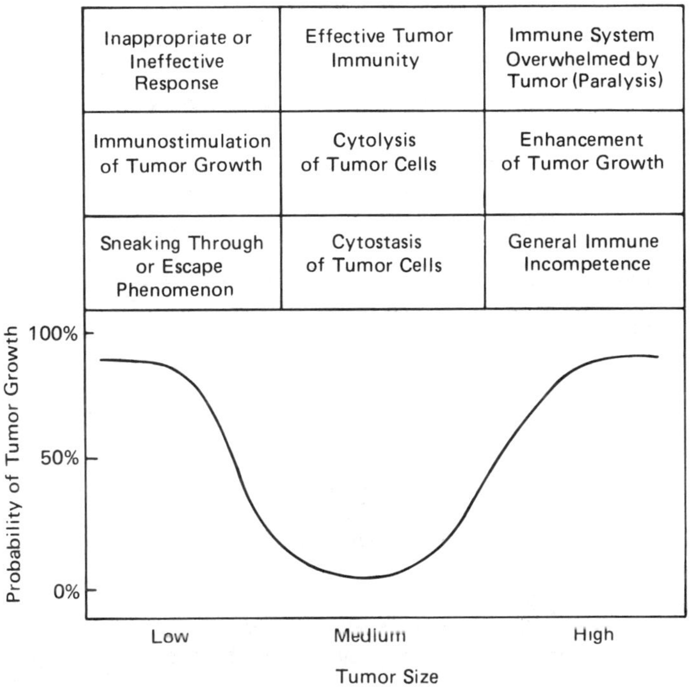

Figure 2 Tumor immunity effectiveness profile: This schematic diagram attempt to put into perspective the net result of the interactions of tumor cells with the machinery of tumor immunity in terms of tumor growth. The idealized curve is clearly biphasic with tumor immunity ineffective (for different reasons) at the two ends of the scale of tumor size and effective in the middle of the scale. Details of the rationale for the shape of this curve are given in the text. These concepts are based, in large part, upon animal models of malignant disease. Their precise role in human malignancies remains to be clarified.

Tumor cells may protect themselves against tumor immunity by two basic mechanisms: (a) prevention of immune recognition and (b) prevention of immune destruction. Prevention of immune recognition may be achieved by (a) inhibition of antigen processing (29), (b) induction of suppressor mechanisms, and (c) reduced TSTA/TAA immunogenicity due to biochemical modification of membrane-bound molecules. Examples of these mechanisms are given in Table 3. The first two mechanisms resemble two of the four mechanisms of immune enhancement of tumor growth (see Table 2), suggesting that immune enhancement may, in fact, be tumor-induced perversion of immune responses (away from protection of the host) to serve the needs of the tumor itself.

Prevention of immune destruction may be achieved (a) at the level of tumor cell surface antigens by shedding of neoantigens, cell cycle dependence of neoantigens, and modulation of neoantigens; (b) at the level of the tumor cell membrance (where transport mechanisms are often altered in tumor cells that develop cytotoxic drug resistance); and (c) by induction of general depression of host immunity or immune paralysis specific to TSTAs/TAAs. Examples of these mechanisms are given in Table 3. The shedding of neoantigens into the surrounding milieu creates a density gradient of neoantigen about the malignant cell and may induce central blockade of the immune response by competing

Table 3 Mechanisms of Tumor Self-Defense Against Immune Attack

- I. Prevention of immune recognition
  - A. Inhibition of antigen processing
    Example: elaboration of substance which inhibits a macrophage migration into tumor
  - B. Induction of suppressor mechanisms
    Example: antigen-specific or nonspecific suppressor cell inhibition of expansion of TSTA/TAA immunoreactive clones
  - C. Reduced immunogenicity
    Example: some spontaneous neoplasms in animals stimulate the immune system very weakly, if at all
- II. Prevention of immune destruction
  - A. At the level of cell surface antigens
    1. Shedding neoantigens [to induce efferent or central blockage of immune response (see Table 2)]
    2. Cell-cycle dependence of neoantigen expression (implying not all cells are subject to lysis at the same time)
    3. Modulation of neoantigens (removing antigens from cell surface induced by antibody, for instance)
  - B. At the level of the tumor cell membrane
    Example: complement resistance preventing cell lysis despite binding of complement-fixing antibody and terminal complement components
  - C. Induction of depression of host immunity
    1. General depression of immune responsiveness (as manifested by impaired reactivity to other antigens)
    2. Immune paralysis (overwhelming antigen-specific immune response to TSTAs/TAAs)

with tumor cells to occupy receptor sites on immune effector cells. Generalized immune depression and antigen-specific immune paralysis may be produced by activation of suppressor mechanisms. Again, the similarity of tumor self-defense mechanisms and immune enhancement becomes evident (see Table 2). Any tumor cells which survive immune attack may retain the ability to proliferate, a biological property of cancer cells which, in essence, negates the effect of immune attack.

As suggested above, tumor cells may be more wily than was formerly suspected. If they can biochemically alter, or immunologically modulate their TSTAs/TAAs or become resistant to autologous complement (30), they may genuinely be able to resist humoral-mediated immune attack, by, for instance, passive antibody administration (see Sec. VIII). When devising immunotherapeutic strategies, the biological variability and ability of tumor cells to adapt to their environment (just like invading microbes) must be borne in mind.

VIII. PRINCIPLES OF IMMUNOTHERAPY

The purpose of this section is threefold: (a) to develop a classification scheme for cancer immunotherapy and identify the context in which immunomodulating agents fit, (b) to define where in tumor immunity immunotherapy may be effective, and (c) to describe nonimmune system side effects which may be beneficial to the host. Toxic side effects which may damage the host are an ever-present threat of any therapeutic agent;

they have adequately been discussed by colleagues contributing to this monograph and will not be discussed here. However, one point relevant to toxicities should be stressed: no therapeutic trial with any immunotherapeutic agent should be undertaken without some estimation of the risk/benefit ratio for the patient participating in the study. The ultimate goal of any agent is selective damage to the disease process (in this case "cure" of cancer), with preservation of the host as completely intact and functional as possible.

As complete a classification scheme for cancer immunotherapy as is currently possible is presented in Tables 4 and 5. Immunotherapy may be viewed as either neoantigen specific (Table 4) or neoantigen nonspecific (Table 5). Antigen-specific immunotherapy may be either actively or passively administered, the distinction referring to the participation of the host's endogenous immune response to neoantigens. The two basic types of active, antigen-specific immunotherapy are (a) immunization with suitably prepared neoantigen/tumor cell vaccines and (b) infusion of host immunocytes reactive with TSTAs/TAAs into sites where their access had been previously restricted.

Passive, antigen-specific immunotherapy involves (a) the infusion of antibodies (monoclonal or polyclonal) utilizing endogenous complement or linked with toxic

Table 4 Classification Scheme for Cancer Antigen-Specific Immunotherapy

I. Active immunotherapy
  A. Immunization with tumor cell/neoantigen vaccine
    1. Tumor cells/neoantigens alone or with adjuvants such as BCG vaccine, MER[a], *C. parvum*
    2. Autochthonous or allogeneic cells of same histology
    3. Cells rendered nonviable by irradiation or drugs
    4. Cells with or without modification of surface antigens by formalin or neuraminidase
  B. Infusion of autologous lymphocytes reactive to tumor cells/neoantigens
    1. Directly into tumor bed
    2. After stimulation in vitro with tumor cells/neoantigens
    3. Derived from excised tumor tissue, clonally expanded in vitro with the lymphokine T-cell growth factor (interleukin 2)

II. Passive immunotherapy
  A. Infusion of antibodies to tumor cells/neoantigens
    1. Polyclonal: homologous or heterologous
    2. Monoclonal: homologous or heterologous
  B. Infusion of antibodies linked with
    1. Radioisotopes
    2. Cytotoxic drugs
    3. Toxins such as ricin or diphtheria toxin
  C. Infusion of allogeneic lymphocytes
    1. Allogeneic effect
    2. Graft-versus-tumor-effect of bone marrow transplantation
  D. Infusion of factors from immune allogeneic lymphocytes
    1. Transfer factor
    2. Immune RNA
  E. Passage of plasma over protein A columns to remove neoantigen-antibody complexes

[a]Methanol-extracted residue of BCG.

Table 5 Classification Scheme for Cancer Antigen-Nonspecific Immunotherapy

I. Direct immunotherapy
   A. Intralesional injections of immunomodulators such as BCG or MER
   B. Superficial painting of lesions with cytotoxic drugs such as 5-flurouracil or sensitizers such as dinitrochlorobenzene
   C. Intracavitary instillation of immunomodulators such as *C. parvum* or BCG

II. Indirect immunotherapy
   A. Developmental hormones for the immune system such as thymosin, thymopoietin, or thymique facteur serique
   B. Immunomodulators of populations of lymphocytes or macrophages
      1. Bacteria such as BCG or *C. parvum*
      2. Bacterial products such as MER or *C. parvum* extracts
      3. Defined organic chemicals such as diethyldithiocarbonate, isoprinosone, or tilorone
      4. Antihelminithic drugs such as levamisole or thiazolobenzimidazoles
      5. Cytotoxic drugs such as cyclophosphamide
      6. Synthetic polymers such as pyrancopolymer, MVE-2, NED 137, or lipoidal amines
      7. Suppressor agents such as tuftsin, indomethacin, or cimetidine
   C. Immune system products that influence immunocytes or tumor cells directly
      1. Lymphokines such as interferon or macrophage-activating factor
      2. Monokines such as lymphocyte-activating factor
      3. Tumor necrosis factor

moieties (radioisotopes, cytotoxic drugs, or toxins) to lyse tumor cells; (b) the infusion of allogeneic lymphoid cells to stimulate host immune effector responses or, after bone marrow transplantation, to produce a direct graft-versus-tumor effect; (c) the infusion of substances produced by immune lymphoid cells which may educate host immunocytes to participate in effector responses; or (d) the removal of neoantigen-antibody complexes by extracorporeal passage of plasma over protein-A columns, which may overcome efferent or central blockade mechanisms of tumor enhancement (see Table 4).

Antigen-nonspecific immunotherapy may be either directly applied to malignant lesions to induce tumor lysis or indirectly effective by modulating host immune effector responses systemically. The principle of direct, antigen-nonspecific immunotherapy is to induce a vigorous inflammatory response in situ in a malignant lesion which will then stimulate a vigorous neoantigen specific host immune response. Three types of direct immunotherapy are mentioned in Table 5.

The goal of indirect, antigen-nonspecific immunotherapy, on the other hand, is the modulation of host immune repsonses to TSTAs/TAAs by systemic administration, such that increased effector activity may be generated and focused at the sites of tumor and metastatic disease. Three basic types of indirect, antigen-nonspecific immunotherapies are (a) developmental hormones whose mechanism of action is stimulation of maturation of precursor cells into antigen-committed effector cells; (b) natural or synthetic chemical immunomodulators which stimulate one or more populations of lymphocytes and/or macrophages or which depress the activity of suppressor cells to result in a net improvement in tumor lysis; and (c) mediators produced by the immune system which modulate effector cell populations or act directly upon tumor cells. Details of examples are given in Table 5.

From this comprehensive classification scheme for cancer immunotherapy, it is obvious that immunomodulating agents represent but one of the possible modes of immunotherapy. It must be clearly understood that the other modes primarily represent biological methods of immunotherapy, whereas immunomodulators represent the pharmacological methods of immunotherapy. Each has great potential. The strong points of the pharmacological approach to immunotherapy are: (a) minor chemical modifications of chemical compounds may drastically and beneficially alter the therapeutic index (toxic-dose-to-therapeutic-dose ratio); (b) high purity of agent may be achieved by chemical synthesis; and (c) agent may be produced reliably from lot to lot.

There are, utlimately, only two goals of immunotherapy, whether antigen specific or nonspecific, active or passive, direct or indirect. The first is enhancement or augmentation of weak, ineffective tumor responses to produce strong, effective tumor responses. Whether the cause of the weak responses is reduced immunogenicity of the neoantigens or poor clonal expansion of effector cells or other mechanisms, the result of effective immunotherapy is improved effector function, quantitatively. The second is restoration of depressed tumor responses that would otherwise be effective by either removing suppression or accelerating maturation of immunocytes to replenish depleted effector cell pools. The result is also improved effector function, qualitatively as well as quantitatively.

Aside from immunomodulating effects relevant to TSTAs/TAAs, immunomodulating agents may have other important side effects beneficial to the host. For instance, immunomodulators may either stimulate myelopoiesis or cause increased peripheral blood leukocyte counts by demargination, which allows the oncologist to deliver more chemotherapy (31). The net effect is increased kill of tumor cells (see Sec. IX). Furthermore, immunomodulators because of their essential antigen nonspecificity will also, if effective, enhance the host's immune responses to invading microbes, in particular, opportunistic infectious agents, by the same mechanisms cited above. The effects on both myeloid cells and the general immune system result in increased resistance to infection, one of the major causes of morbidity and mortality in cancer patients.

IX. STRATEGY OF IMMUNOTHERAPY

In order to understand the role of immunotherapy in the overall management of patients with malignancy, the kinetics of tumor cell proliferation and cytoreduction must be more fully appreciated. Tumor cell proliferation may effectively counterbalance and even negate cytoreduction efforts. The ultimate clinical outcome for any patient depends on the net change in tumor cell number produced by cytoreduction acting upon proliferating tumor cells. These kinetic considerations become more complicated by the superimposition of tumor cell resistance to the specific cytoreductive agent or modality (drug or radiation). A model system for understanding the kinetics of tumor cell proliferation and cytoreduction was developed by Skipper and colleagues (32,33). Figure 3 shows the Skipper "hypothesis" adapted to the circumstances under discussion in this chapter. The basic coneepts of the Skipper hypothesis are that (a) tumor cells proliferate in log phase in most hosts (tumor lesion doubling times for changes in size are often discussed clinically) and (b) tumor lysis occurs in fractions with each cytoreductive event (90% reduction in mass represents 1 $\log_{10}$ kill, 99% represents lysis of 2 logs, 99.9% 3 logs, etc.). As clinical disease is usually detectable when tumor size is measured in grams to kilograms (10^9-10^{12} cells) and as cytoreductive events rarely produce more than 2-4 logs to kill, it is obvious that multiple cytoreductive events are necessary to cure a host of cancer (see Fig. 3).

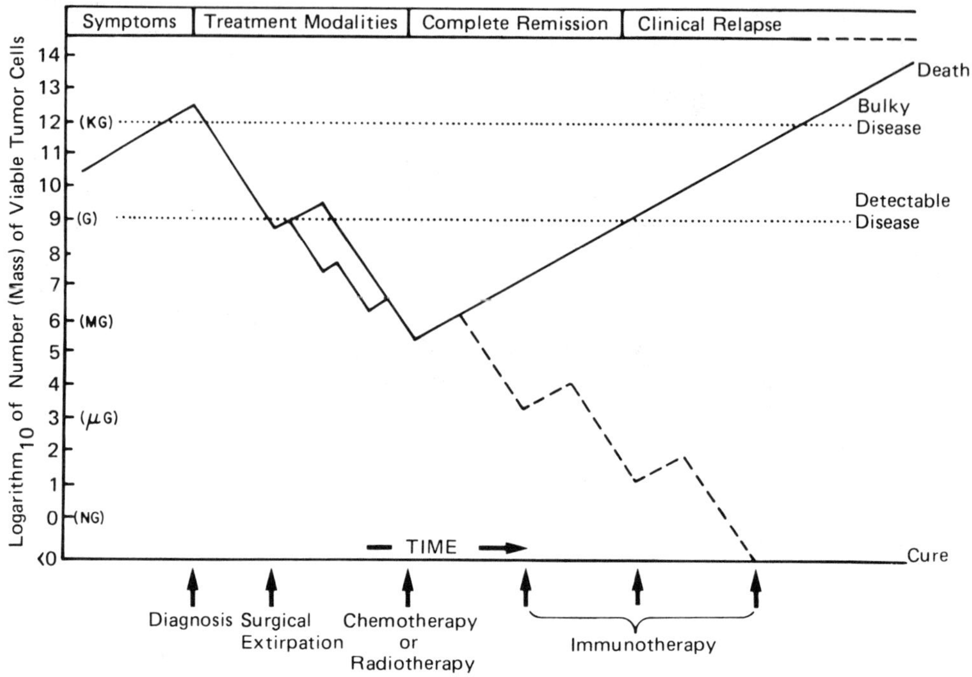

Figure 3 Kinetics of tumor cell proliferation and cytoreduction. This schematic diagram portrays tumor cell number (mass) as a function of time balancing the proliferative capability of tumor cells against the expected cytolytic effects of cytoreductive therapy. Most therapeutic modalities can reduce tumor cell numbers by 2-4 logs_{10}. Clinically detectable disease may be absent, but the patient may still have up to 10^9 viable tumor cells in situ. Without continued cytoreductive therapy, this number of tumor cells will proliferate and overwhelm the patient. In the absence of development of resistance, continued cytoreduction may ultimately eradicate the last malignant cell ($10^{<0}$). Immunotherapy may play this role as is depicted in this diagram. Death or cure hangs in the balance. Details of these concepts are given in the text.

In fact, because of development of tumor resistance or toxicity to the host of a given modality, these kinetic concepts usually imply the need for combined therapeutic modalities, often employed sequentially, to achieve a cure. Where does immunotherapy fit into this conceptual framework of tumor cell kinetics?

In therapeutic planning for patients with cancer, a strategy is developed with first, second, and third (if necessary) treatment modalities set in chronological order. Ordinarily, first treatment is surgical extirpation or radiation therapy for most solid tumors, but occasionally is chemotherapy for some solid tumors. Usually, chemotherapy or radiotherapy is first treatment for lymphohematopoietic malignancies. Obviously, second treatment depends on first treatment and usually involves radiation therapy or chemotherapy but may involve surgery as well. The ultimate goal of the strategy is the reduction of the number of tumor cells with proliferative potential until the last malignant cell is eradicated; failure to achieve the goal results in a poor outcome (see Fig. 3). As discussed above, tumor immunity is likely to be more effective when tumor cell burden is minimal (see Sec. IV). The appropriate role for tumor immunotherapy, according to current thinking in terms of cancer therapy strategy, is to be a third or second treatment, when tumor burden has been clinically minimized. The goal of immunotherapy is to enhance tumor immunity to "mop up" or lyse residual tumor cells after surgery, radiation therapy, and/or chemotherapy.

Immunotherapy, depending upon which type is employed, may have more than one beneficial effect as stated above (see Sec. VIII). All nonimmunotherapeutic modalities for cancer (surgery, radiotherapy, and chemotherapy) have been shown to be immunodepressive to one degree or another. Immunotherapy may not only restore and augment tumor immune responses depressed by other therapeutic modalities but also enhance general immunity to help protect the host against invading microbial agents. Additionally, unlike surgery, radiation therapy, and chemotherapy, immunotherapy may not behave mechanistically as a discrete cytoreductive event (as depicted in Fig. 3). If tumor immunity is continuously active against tumor cells, such time-nondiscrete behavior may be expected to magnify the ability of tumor immunity to kill the remaining 7-9 logs of tumor cells and "cure" the host of cancer.

Last, the current position of tumor immunotherapy as third among treatment modalities for human malignancy is, in part, dictated by principles of tumor immunity and, in part, by empiric results of previous clinical trials of immunotherapy, which, in general, have not been very rewarding to date. Animal models have clearly shown the protective role of tumor immunity but rarely have animal models evaluated the efficacy of tumor immunity or immunotherapy after treatment of experimental malignancies with radiotherapy and/or chemotherapy. Translating animal models into clinical trials is, therefore, not a simple matter. Moving tumor immunotherapy up to a second or first treatment in the strategy of cancer therapy will depend on clearcut good results from well-designed clinical trials more than upon observations of efficacy in animal model systems. This is, perhaps, as it should be.

X. SUMMATION

To close this chapter a summation of observations and principles has been chosen rather than a listing of definitive conclusions as the precise role of immunomodulating agents remains incompletely clarified at this point in time. The goal of the efforts of biologists studying the effects of immunomodulators in animal models of malignant disease and of clinicians delivering immunotherapy to patients with malignancy is "cure" of cancer, a ravaging disease. The potential of tumor immunotherapy as a major therapeutic modality in cancer treatment strategy has not yet been fully achieved. Development of new or refinement of old agents or methods, improvement of animal models to reflect more accurately clinical malignant disease, and better-designed clinical trials are absolute imperatives for tumor immunotherapy to achieve its full potential.

What has been attempted by this chapter is an exposition of tumor immunity and the role of immunomodulating agents in tumor and metastatic disease. This has been done in the context of cancer cell biology, clinical cancer management, and overall strategy for cancer therapy. The ultimate role of tumor immunotherapy in the clinical management of patients with malignancy rests upon the fundamental assumptions and principles of tumor immunity and immunotherapy which simply restated are (a) *tumor immunity exists* and has a degree of *effectiveness in vivo* that is *usually insufficient* to eliminate clinically detectable malignancies; and (b) *stimulation* of tumor immunity directly or indirectly, neoantigen specifically or nonspecifically, *will improve effectiveness in vivo*, but this is most likely to occur *when* the *tumor burden* is *minimal.*

REFERENCES

1. F. Himmelweit (ed.), *The Collected Papers of Paul Erhlich,* Pergamon Press, New York, 1957, p. 561.
2. R. T. Prehn and J. M. Main, *J. Natl. Cancer Inst., 18*:769 (1957).
3. G. Klein, H. D. Sjögren, E. Klein, and K. E. Hellström, *Cancer Res., 20*:1561 (1960).
4. I. Green and E. M. Shevach, in *Mechanisms of Cell-Mediated Immunity* (R. T. Mc Cluskey, ed.), John Wiley and Sons, New York, 1974, pp. 221-225.
5. H. M. Ravlin, personal communication.
6. I. R. Hart and I. J. Fidler, *Cancer Res., 40*:2281 (1980).
7. G. Berry, M. L. Newhouse, and M. Turok, *Lancet, 2*:476 (1972).
8. R. A. Bordow and A. M. Lilienfeld, in *The Health Consequences of Smoking: Cancer* (J. Luoto and D. R. Shopland, eds.), U.S. Government Printing Office, Washington, D.C., 1982, pp. 13-169.
9. T. Uchiyama, D. L. Nelson, T. A. Fleisher, and T. A. Waldmann, *J. Immunol., 126*:1398 (1981).
10. D. J. Straus, J. Myers, S. Passe, C. W. Young, L. Z. Nisce, B. J. Lee, B. Koziner, Z. Arlin, S. Kempin, T. Gee, and B. D. Clackson, *Cancer, 46*:233 (1980).
11. L. H. Einhorn and J. P. Donohue, *Ann. Int. Med., 87*:293 (1977).
12. W. Zuelzer, *Johns Hopkins Med. J., 142*:115 (1978).
13. P. L. Weiden, K. M. Sullivan, N. Flournoy, R. Storb, E. D. Thomas, and the Seattle Transplant Team, *N. Engl. J. Med., 304*:1529 (1981).
14. M. R. Ruff and G. E. Gifford, in *Lymphokines*, vol. 2 (E. Pick, ed.), Academic Press, New York, 1981, pp. 235-272.
15. R. B. Herberman and H. T. Holden, *J. Natl. Cancer Inst., 62*:441 (1979).
16. D. O. Adams and R. Snyderman, *J. Natl. Cancer Inst., 62*:1341 (1979).
17. R. P. Gale, R. S. Sparkes, and D. W. Golde, *Science, 201*:937 (1978).
18. M. Torten, N. Seidel, and S. H. Golub, personal communication.
19. J. R. David and H. G. Remold, in *Immunobiology of the Macrophage* (D. S. Nelson, ed.), Academic Press, New York, 1976, pp. 401-426.
20. I. Kimber and M. Moore, *Scand. J. Immunol., 13*:375 (1981).
21. B. M. Eggen, *Acta Path. Microbiol. Scand. (Sect. C), 89*:85 (1981).
22. R. T. Prehn, *Transplant Rev., 28*:34 (1976).
23. T. H. M. Stewart, D. Lassen, and A. F. Crook, *Can. Med. Assoc. J., 101*:191 (1969).
24. G. D. Snell, H. J. Winn, J. H. Stimpfling, and S. J. Parker, *J. Exp. Med., 112*:293 (1960).
25. I. Hellström and V. E. Hellström, *Int. J. Cancer, 4*5587 (1969).
26. V. T. DeVita, Jr., in *Cancer: Principles and Practice of Oncology* (V. T. DeVita, Jr., S. Hellman, and S. A. Rosenberg, eds.), J. P. Lippincott, Philadelphia, 1982, p. 140.
27. S. Shin-ichi and A. A. Sandberg, *Cancer, 41*:153 (1978).
28. S. M. Hubbard, B. A. Chabner, V. T. DeVita, R. Simon, C. W. Berard, R. B. Jones, A. J. Garvin, G. P. Canellos, C. K. Osborne, and R. C. Young, *Blood, 59*:258 (1982).
29. R. Synderman and M. C. Pike, *Science, 192*:370 (1976).
30. S. H. Ohanian and S. I. Schlager, in *Critical Reviews of Immunology*, vol. 1 (M. A. Atassi, ed.), CRC Press, Boca Raton, Fla., 1981, pp. 165-209.
31. M. H. Cohen, P. B. Chretien, D. C. Ihde, B. F. Fossieck, Jr., R. Makuch, P. A. Bunn, A. V. Johnston, S. E. Shackney, M. J. Matthews, S. D. Lipson, D. E. Kenady, J. J. Snyder, and J. D. Minna, *J. Am. Med. Assoc., 241*:1813 (1979).
32. H. E. Skipper, F. M. Schabel, Jr., and W. S. Wilcox, *Cancer Chemother. Rep., 35*:3 (1964).
33. H. E. Skipper and S. Perry, *Cancer Res., 30*:1883 (1970).

Part II

Effect of Chemical Agents on Biological Secretions and Mechanisms of Immune Modulation

Introduction

Michael A. Chirigos National Cancer Institute–Frederick Cancer Research Facility, Bethesda, Maryland

Recent advances in cellular and humoral immunology have been due in part to the results obtained from investigations conducted with chemical or biological agents which stimulate and/or augment specific cellular components of the immune system. The response elicited by these agents have been defined by various terms (e.g., immunomodulating, immuno-augmenting, immunostimulating, and immunorestorative). Recent studies indicate that many of these agents (often referred to as biological response modifiers) elicit responses of specific cell types (e.g., thymosin fraction V inducing maturation of pre-T-cells; interferon augmenting natural killer cells and macrophages; MVE-2, interferon, and poly ICLC causing the induction and secretion of colony-stimulating factor and prostaglandins by macrophages). Many of these agents have been investigated for their capacity to elicit a tumor reductive effect in various animal and human tumors. In many cases the selection of dose and regimen of treatment was empirical. With the acquisition of more information concerning the mechanism(s) by which these agents modify the immune response has come the indication that such agents exert a bimodal effect and that the philsophy that "if a little is good, then more should be better" does not apply.

Although major strides have been made in containing—and in some cases curing—various cancers with chemotherapy, there is still limitations which prevent more progress from being made, including insufficient selectivity for the target tumors and toxicity to normal tissues. Current evidence indicates that alteration of the tumor-host-relationship through modulation of the immune system by biological response modifiers is therapeutically beneficial when they are used alone or in combination with other therapeutic modalities. Immunointervention by these agents thus offers a unique approach based on either selective action on the cellular components of the immune system, such as augmenting effector cell responses (natural killer, macrophage, or cytotoxic T cells), or their ability to reconstitute bone marrow through their capacity to elicit the production and secretion of colony-stimulating factor.

The purpose of Part II is to provide a critical review of the experience gained in studies elucidating the mechanism(s) by which selected agents are expressing an immune effector cell response. The contributors of the chapters discuss over 30 different chemical and biologic agents concerning: their action on specific effector cells (natural killer, macrophage, cytotoxic T cells, and B cells), on various target tumor cells, and on bacteria; the elicitation of T-cell subsets; the induction and secretion of soluble products (colony-stimulating factor, prostaglandin, and interferon); and the interaction of prostaglandins and colony-stimulating factor in feedback inhibition mechanisms. Comprehensive and updated reviews are presented on the more investigative agents (muramyldipeptide, levamisole, lentinan) and new agents (NPT15392 and imuthiol). Both preclinical and clinical studies are presented describing the therapeutic response attained with various biological response modifying agents and the specific effector cells regulated by these agents.

This part will be informative and of interest to immunologists, immunopharmacologists, and experimental and clinical oncologists.

Section A

Concepts of Immunomodulation

16
Immunomodulating Agents

P. Reizenstein Karolinska Hospital and Institute, Stockholm, Sweden, and Institut de Cancérologie et d'Immunogénétique, Villejuif, France

Georges Mathé Service Des Maladies Sanguines et Tumorales and Institut de Cancérologie et d'Immunogénétique, Villejuif, France

I. INTRODUCTION

In 1908, in a lecture in Holland about cancer research, Paul Ehrlich suggested the existence of protective devices (immunological, antibody-dependent cellular forces) causing aberrant cell clones to remain latent for decades rather than to develop into cancer (1). The theory of immune surveillance, including both recognition of and defense against tumors, has since then been elaborated by Burnet and others (2), and their theory is one of the reasons why modulators of the immunological and biological response receive some attention now.

II. THE BIOLOGICAL RESPONSE TO TUMORS

A. Nonspecific Response

Every clinician has noticed the biological response, both to cancer and to chronic inflammatory disease (e.g., pulmonary tuberculosis), in the form of weight loss and anemia. These visible symptoms are only the top of an iceberg, which has less visible signs of hyperfibrinogenemia with high erythrocyte sedimentation and hypercoagulability, leukocytosis and activation of macrophages, activation of nonspecific cytotoxic cells, nutritional immunity, and a series of humoral reactions. These involve, among other things, the mediators of inflammation and cytokines such as interferon, tumor-necrotizing factor, lymphotoxin (3), or colony-stimulating activity. Tumor-necrotizing factor is a glycoprotein with a mol wt of 70,000, probably released by macrophages, toxic in vitro for human and murine cell lines, but not for mouse embryo cells. Altogether this complex, well-regulated, and poorly understood system (Fig. 1) can be interpreted as a defense reaction against infections or tumors and their complications, such as bleeding

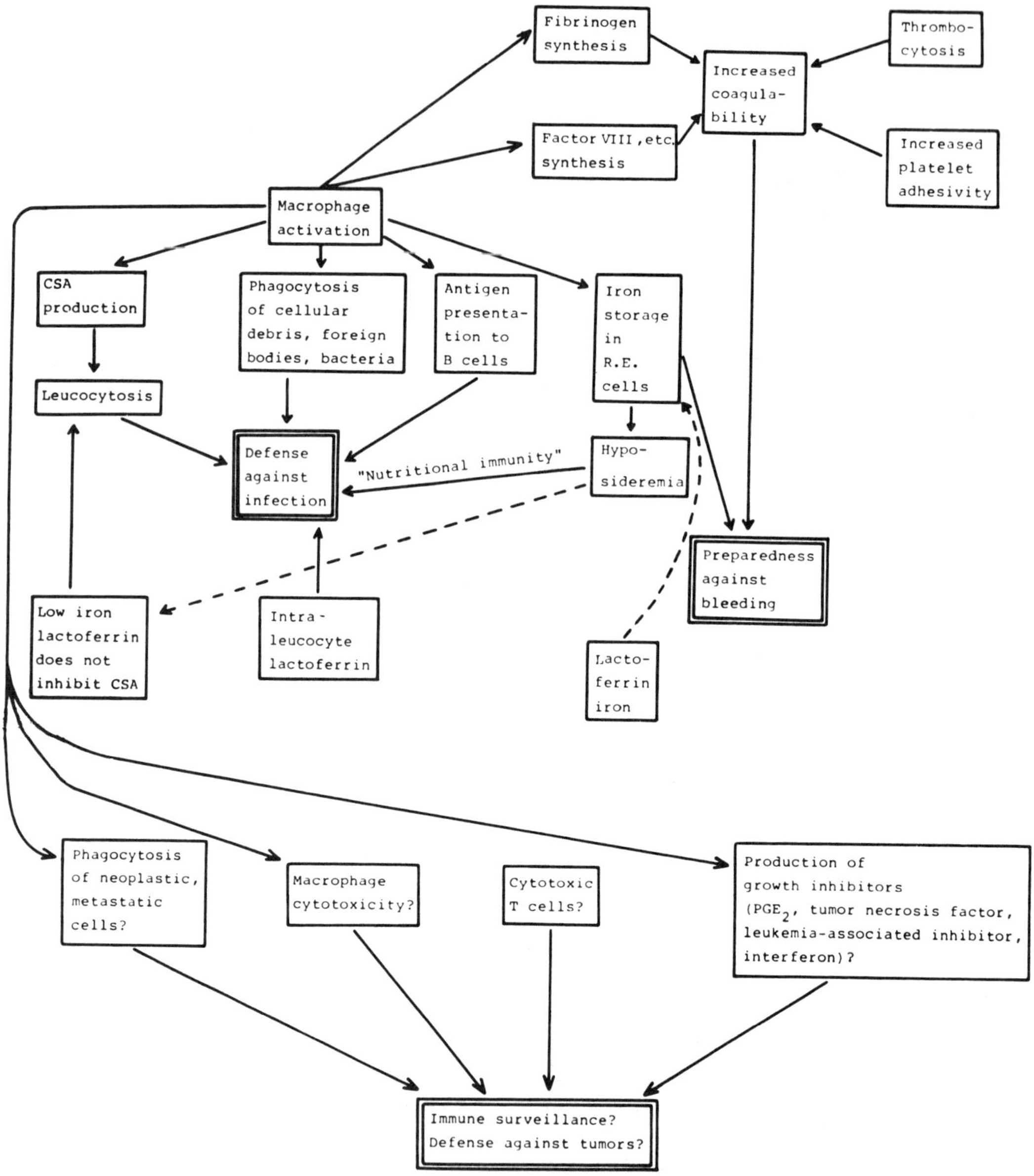

Figure 1 The nonspecific biological response to disease may well constitute a defense against infections, perhaps tumors, and bleeding. (After Ref. 4.)

It is conceivable that macrophages play a relatively central role in this defense reaction (Fig. 2) since they produce tumor-necrotizing factor, fibrinogen, prostaglandins, colony-stimulating activity, and interferon. In addition, they take up lactoferrin, which regulates serum iron and thus nutritional immunity (Fig. 1).

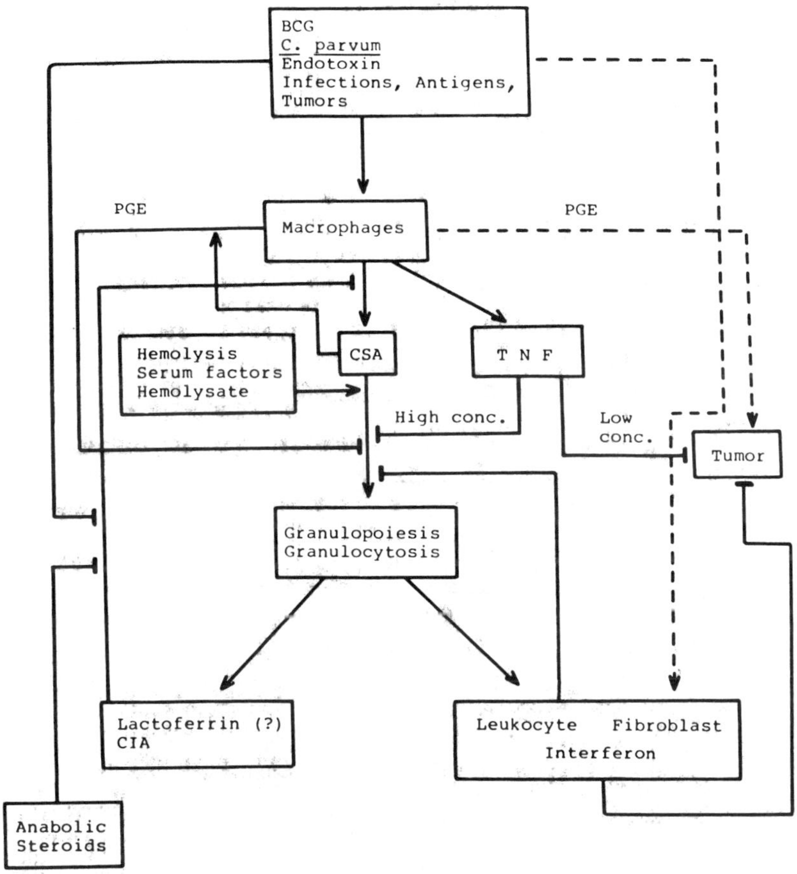

Figure 2 Macrophages activated by some immunomodulators as well as by disease itself may play a central role in the biological response to disease. Arrows indicate stimulation; bars indicate inhibition. (After Ref. 4.)

This nonspecific biological response is being treated separately (4) and will not be further dealt with here. However, there is no doubt that a nonspecific biological response to tumors, infections, and trauma exists. Biological response modifiers are drugs which can modulate this response.

B. Specific Biological Response and Immune Surveillance of Tumors in Man

Fundamentals of humoral and cellular immunity (Fig. 3) and of the occurrence of tumor-specific cell surface antigens in transplantable, experimental tumors are well known (Table 1; see, for instance, Ref. 5). The difficulties to demonstrate such antigens in all but a few spontaneous human tumors (6), and the possible therapeutic benefits which can be obtained in certain subgroups of patients and certain tumors (Table 2) from nonspecific immunotherapy with Bacillus Calmette-Guérin (BCG), or specific treatment with tumor cells are reviewed separately (7,8). The 386 references of these two reviews are not repeated here.

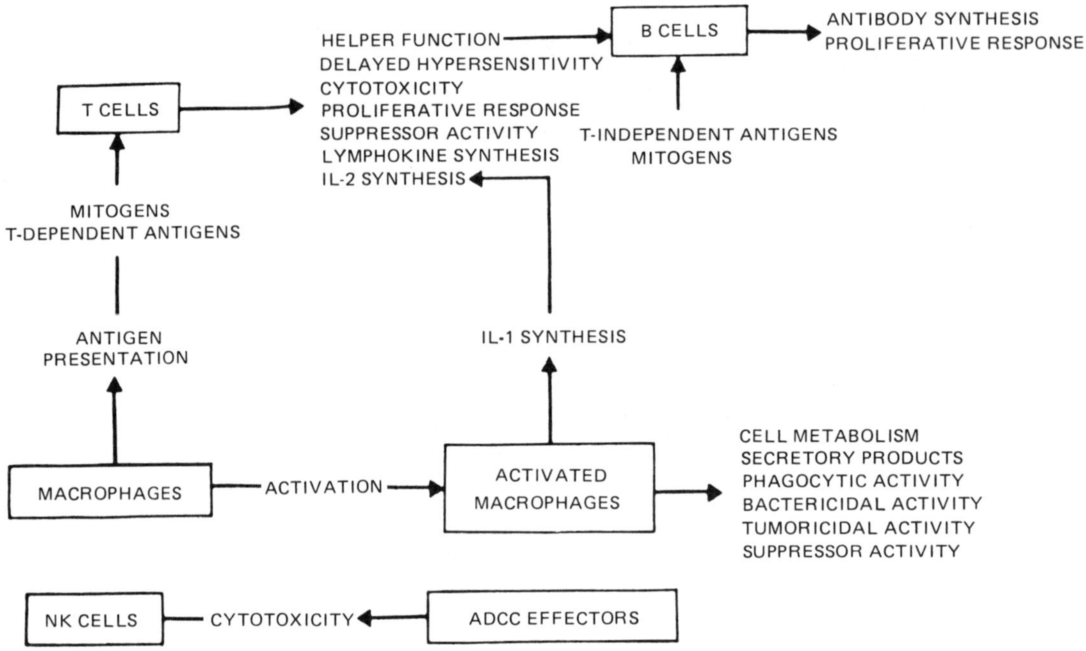

Figure 3 Brief review of interaction between T cells, B cells, macrophages, NK (natural killer) cells. ADCC: antibody-dependent cell-mediated cytotoxicity. (After Florentin, unpublished).

Table 1 Monoclonal Antibodies against Human Tumor-Associated and Oncofetal Antigens

Tumor	Probably cross reacting with
Melanoma	Astrocytoma Fetal cells Some carcinomas[a]
Colorectal carcinoma	Cirrhosis, colitis, and gastric carcinoma sera
Neuroblastoma	Fetal brain
Glioma	Melanoma
Mammary carcinoma	Other carcinomas
Acute lymphatic leukemia	Non-Hodgkin lymphoma, chronic lymphatic leukemia, proliferating T-cells, fetal kidney cells

[a]Several antibodies

Table 2 Subgroups of Patients and the Response to Nonspecific Adjuvant Immunotherapy

Diagnosis	Patient group with a significant effect	Patient group with nonsignificant effect
Acute myelogneous leukemia	A group with 35% remissions	A group with 65% remissions
Non-Hodgkin lymphoma	Young, or stage I, or women, or in initial phase of the disease	Old, or stages II-IV, or men, or in the relapse phase
Bronchial carcinoma	Non-small cell carcinoma or blood groups A, B, AB, Rh+	Small cell carcinoma, or blood groups O, Rh−
Acute lymphatic leukemia	First patients treated 1962 patients who had, without neuroprophylaxis, survived over 2 years and who frequently had HLA BW 17 and AW 33, approximately, remission frequency 80%, some patients induced with prednisone alone	First patients treated 1972 patients who had survived, with neuroprophylaxis, 0.2-0.3 years, remission frequency 93% all patients given combination chemotherapy
Gastric cancer	Stage III	Stages I and II

III. MODULATORS OF THE IMMUNE RESPONSE

Table 3 attempts to list the various drug modulating the immune responses, some of which will be discussed below.

A. BCG

In young, healthy mice, BCG, the best studied of the immunomodulators, can under certain dose and time conditions activate the phosphatase activity and the cytostatic effect of macrophages, potentiate antibody responses and antibody-dependent cell-mediated cytotoxicity, and induce nonspecific suppressor cells (9-13). BCG also stimulates the secretory activity of thymic epithelium (14,15). It may increase the lymphocyte number in the spleen and reduce that in mesenteric lymphnodes (13).

Tumors, notably lymphomas, are common in aged, immunodeficient mice. After 20 months, all nontreated mice are dead (Fig. 3). BCG treatment can increase the number of survivors (Fig. 4).

Work is in progress in the laboratories of Chedid (16) and Friedman (28) to identify the immunomodulating structures of various bacteria. Particularly lipoproteins, lipopolysaccharides, mycolic acids, and certain peptides are of interest, since they seem able to stimulate cytotoxic activity and peroxydase-positive macrophages in animals (17).

B. Levamisole

In the aged mice, levamisole treatment activates macrophages and restores the delayed-type hypersensitivity reaction and the antibody response to T-cell-dependent antigens. It prevents the appearance of suppressor cells (18), in this respect acting antagonistically

Table 3 Different Categories of Immunomodulators

I. Biological origin

1. Microorganisms

Bacterial preparations
Bacillus Calmette-Guérin (BCG)
Corynebacterium parvum
Brucella abortus
Pseudomonas aeruginosa
Bordetella pertussis
Nocardia

Extracts of microorganisms

Chemically unidentified
Picibanil (*Streptococcus pyogenes*)
ERB (*L. monocytogenes*, *S. typhimurium*)
MER (BCG)
BRU-Pel (*B. abortus*)

Chemically identified (isolated from bacteria)
WSA (dissacharide bound to a peptidoglycan, *M. smegmatis*)
Biostim (glycoprotein, *K. pneumoniae*)
Trehalose-dimycolate (*M. tuberculosis*)
Peptidoglycans (gram-negative bacteria)
Lipopolysaccharide (*E. coli*, *S. typhimurium*)
Muramyl-dipeptide[a] (*M. smegmatis*) and analogs[a]

Chemically identified (isolated from fungi)
Krestin (protein bound to a polysaccharide, Coriolus versicolor)
Glucan (β-1-3- polyglucose, *Saccharomyces cerevisiae*)
Lentinan (β-1-3 polyglucose, *Lentinus edodes*)
Cyclomunine (Cyclohexa peptide, *Fusarium equiseti*)
Bestatin[a] ([2S,3R-amino-2-hydroxy-4-phenylbutanoyl]-L-leucine, *Streptomyces olivoreticuli*)

2. Products of the immune system

Thymic hormones
Thymosine
Thymopoietine
FTS (facteur thymique sérique)[a]

Lymphokines
Lymphokines, nonpurified
Interferon
Interleukine 2

Others
Tuftsine[a] (a tetrapeptide which forms a part of the IgG heavy chain)

3. Natural compounds or their analogs

Vitamin A and its derivatives[a] (retinoids)
Vitamin E
Lysolecithenes
Lynesterol

Table 3 (continued)

II. Synthetic compounds
1. Sulfur-containing compounds
Levamisole
Diethyldithiocarbamate
Cimetidine
2. Compounds with a nucleotide
Polynucleotide (poly A:U, poly I:C)
Isoprinosine (an inosin compound)
NTP 15392 (analog of hypoxanthine)
3. Various
Azimexon (cyanoaziridine)
Therafectine (a glucofuranose derivative)
Tilorone (polymer of pyran)
Indomethacine

[a]Compounds which have now been synthesized.
Source: After I. Florentin, unpublished data.

to cyclosporin (28), and, like BCG, prolongs the mouse life span. In young healthy mice, levamisole is inactive (10,11,18).

C. Glucan

Glucan, β-1-3 polyglucose from yeast, is a classic macrophage stimulator in animals, but there are few reports in humans.

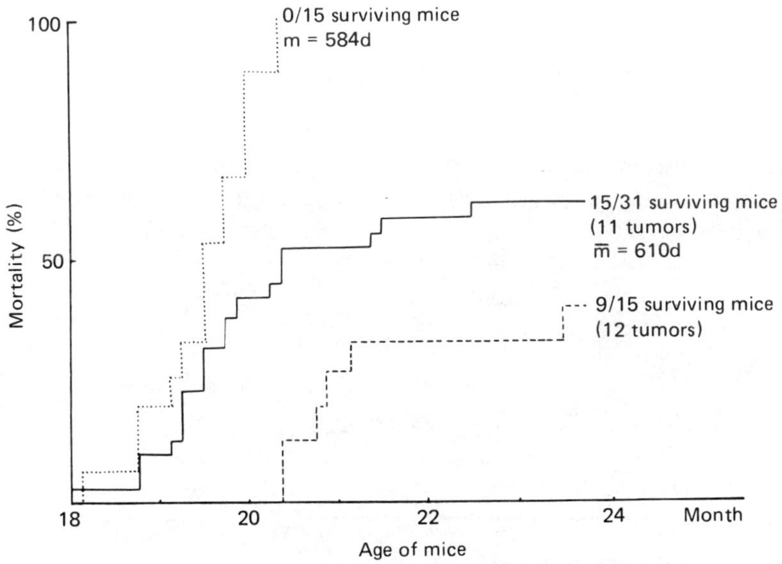

Figure 4 Age-related mortality of mice either untreated (. . . .) or treated repeatedly with BCG (——) or levamisole (- - -). The surviving mice were killed at 24 months of age and the number of mice bearing spontaneous tumors as recorded. (After Ref 18.)

D. Bestatin

Bestatin, a Japanese actinomycetes extract, may stimulate B-cell responses in small and T-cell responses in large doses (18). The latter also reduce the incidence of spontaneous tumors in old mice significantly (19; Fig. 5).

E. Azimexon

Azimexon, an aziridine derivative (BM 12531), stimulates the cytostatic activity of macrophages but not that of antibody-dependent T cells, and also stimulates antibody responses (20) and helper T-cells (21).

F. Tuftsin, Muramyl Dipeptide, and NTP 15392

Active peptides like muramyl dipeptide and the physiological basic tetrapeptide tuftsin can, like BCG, in certain doses stimulate the cytostatic activity of macrophages in vitro, both in healthy young and in immunosuppressed old mice (Fig. 6). Under certain conditions they can also stimulate the antibody response to a thymus-dependent antigen (20,22,23).

NTP 15392 (9-erythro-2-dehydroxy,3-nonyl hypoxanthine) increases mainly the natural and the T-cell mediated cytotoxicity, but it has varying effects on the lymphocyte proliferative response and the antibody-dependent cytotoxicity (24).

G. Retinoids

Synthetic vitamin A derivative are of interest because they can prevent chemical carcinogenesis in animals and possibly in humans, if they are smokers (25). They have a certain effect on the peritoneal macrophage cytotoxic effect and, in aged mice, on NK activity (Fig. 7) (26).

H. Hormones

Neither the well-known immunomodulating effects on adrenal hormones or the less well-known ones of gonadal and thyroid hormones fall within the scope of this review.

Even the thymic factors, hormones secreted by the epithelial cells in the thymus, are now so many that it becomes difficult to include them in this review. Some of the factors are mentioned in earlier reviews (27,28). The 12 different thermostable peptides of Goldstein are also not reviewed here.

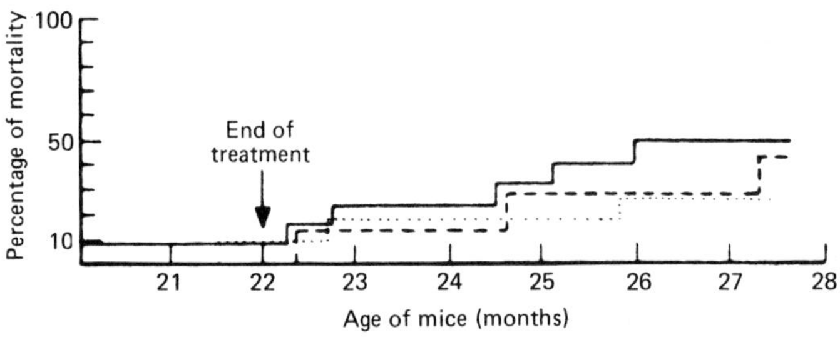

Figure 5 Percentage mortality related to aging in mice either untreated (solid line) or treated repeatedly with bestatin at the doses of 10 μg (dashed line) or 100 μg (dotted line). (After Ref. 19.)

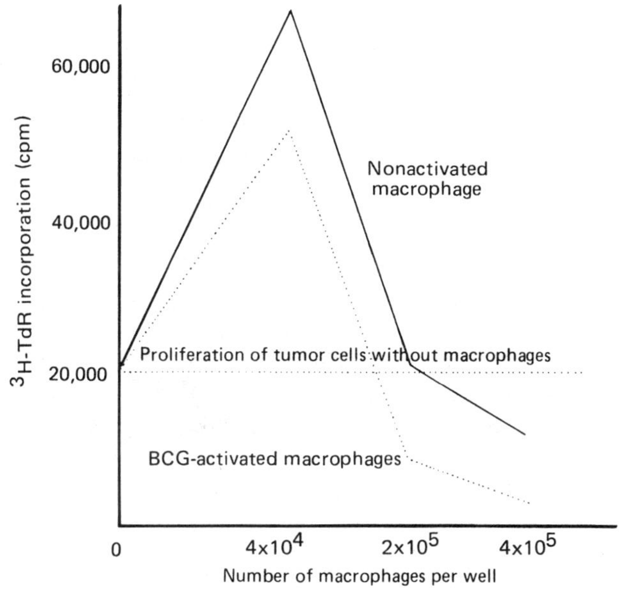

Figure 6 Proliferation of tumor cells (P815) measured by tritiated thymidine incorporation in the absence (. . . .) or in the presence of normal (——) or BCG activated (- - - -) macrophages in relation to their concentration.(After Ref. 23.)

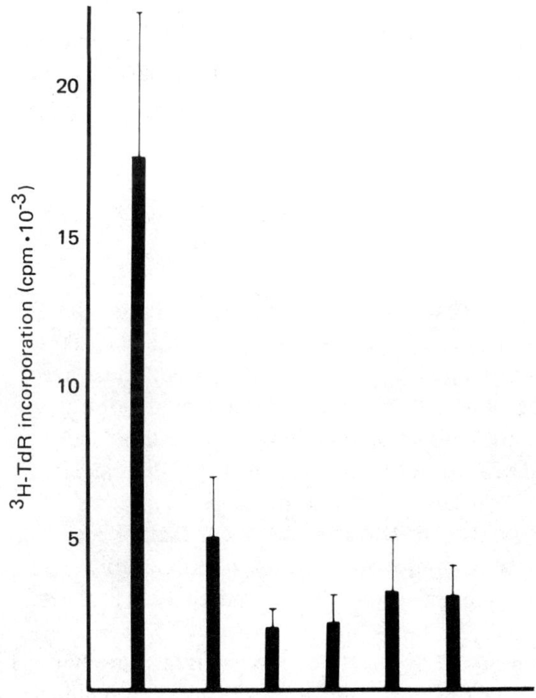

Figure 7 Macrophage activation in 2-month-old mice treated with retinoids (Ro 10-9359) at various days. (After Ref. 26.)

Several relatively impure thymus extracts are on the market and Davies and Ogier (28) have shown that they increase the percentages of E rosettes in patients with lymphomas and leukemia. Several of them increase the E-rosette expression of T cells. Thymosin has been reported to restore the antibody responses to T-dependent antigens (21). In France, the group of Bach and Dardenne (29) isolated a zinc-dependent factor, facteur thymique sérique (FTS), for which human T cells have specific receptors, and which can also induce sheep red cell receptors. Preliminary studies indicate an effect on T-helper cells in IgA-deficient children, leading to IgA production.

I. Cyclosporin

Cyclosporin, isolated from a fungus, has antimalarial, antischistostomal, and T-suppressor cell stimulating, or possible T-helper-inhibiting activity. It is not cytostatic and has no marrow toxicity. The T-suppressor cells seem to arrest B cells in the G_0 or G_1 phase, so that IgM, IgG, and IgE production is inhibited (28,30).

J. Cytostatics

The general immunosuppressive activity of many cytostatics given in doses sufficient to cause bone marrow aplasia is well known, nonspecific, and easy to understand. This effect is used in preparing patients for and protecting patients after transplantation.

Of greater theoretical interest is the apparently specific effect of low doses of certain cytostatics on T-suppressor cells. In animals, Orbach-Arbouys et al. (31) and Dray (28) have shown that low-dose methotrexate and cyclophosphamide, respectively, eliminate T-suppressor cells specifically. In humans, an increased lymphocyte mitogen response has been found in patients with acute myeloid leukemia in complete remission given low-dose maintenance treatment, mainly with antimetabolites (32).

K. Cytokines

There are a few reports and an increasing interest in studies of lymphotoxins (3). The major interest at the present time is in interferon, which stimulates both NK cells (33) and lymphokine production (34), but also has a cytostatic activity (35). Which of the two mechanisms is responsible for the clinical effects described below is difficult to say. Since there is only sometimes a correlation between the NK activity and the clinical effect, a nonimmunomodulatory mechanism cannot be ruled out (36-38). On the other hand, the interferon activity seems to be stimulated by certain immunomodulators (39). It is clear that interferon has a certain clinical effect on lymphoma, IgG (but not IgA) myeloma, acute lymphatic leukemia, and chronic lymphatic leukemia (36). In myeloma it seems less efficient than conventional cytostatic treatment (40); 0 of 18 patients reduced their M component by 50%, and only 3 of 18 patients reduced their M component by 25% (37), which is really a poor response. Interferon is not necessarily less toxic than cytostatics. Treatment has to be interrupted because of toxicity in 3 of 18 patients (37,41,42).

Of particular interest is the intrathecal use of interferon in meningeal acute lymphatic leukemia. However, it was efficient only in 1 of 6 patients (43). The interferon inducer poly: IC gave remissions in 5 of 15 acute lymphatic leukemias (44).

In metastatic, chemotherapy-resistant cancer, a complete clinical response was found in 1 of 9 breast cancers, 1 of 16 prostatic cancers, and 1 of 6 melanomas. Partial remissions were seen in about half the patients (45).

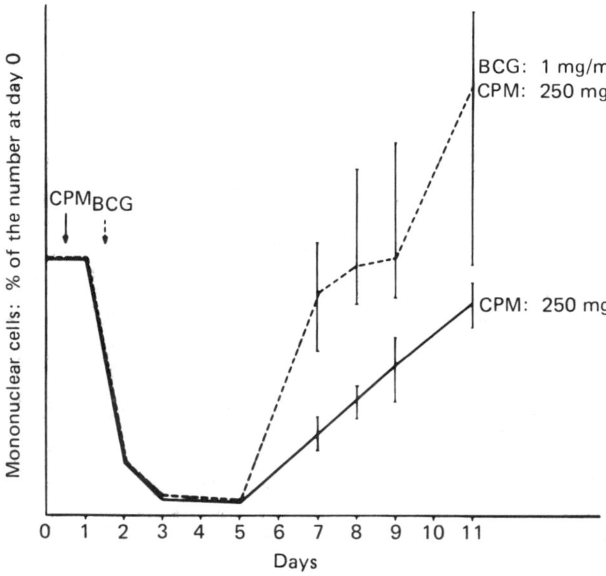

Figure 8 The restoration of blood lymphocyte number after cyclophosphamide aplasia is faster when BCG is administered 1 day after cytostatics. (After Ref. 21.)

L. Possible Effects on the Nonimmunological Biological Response

As shown in Figs. 1 and 2, BCG and conceivably other immunomodulators could in theory affect nonimmunological parts of the immune response, such as for instance the secretion of colony-stimulating activity or other poietins. In fact, such an effect has been demonstrated in a small but statistically significant number of patients (46). The finding of rapid hematological restoration after BCG (Fig. 8) supports this finding. It is conceivable that even a synthetic immunomodulator like azimexon has similar effects. It induces leukocytosis and restores leukopenia in rats (21). It is even possible that tumor-necrotizing factor secretion may be augmented by immunomodulators. Carswell et al. (47) found this in mice given first BCG, then LPS.

IV. CLINICAL RELEVANCE OF IMMUNOMODULATORS

A. Nonneoplastic Diseases

A decrease of T-suppressor cell activity appears to be a frequent pathogenetic factor in rheumatoid arthritis and other autoimmune and collagen diseases. The literature is reviewed elsewhere (4). It is possible that this is caused by suppressor cell autoantibodies (21,48). It is obviously just as logical to use a suppressor cell inducer as to use a B-cell suppressor in such diseases, and the first experiments with cyclosporin will be of interest. Levamisole has already been tried in rheumatoid arthritis (49).

B. Tumors

Chemotherapy, like radiotherapy following first-order kinetics, very rarely kills the last tumor cell. In animals and humans there are indications that 10 tumor cells suffice to cause a relapse. One of us (21,50) has suggested that, where chemotherapy does cure, it does so because of immune rejection of the last tumor cells. One of the problems is to show that we are dealing with immune rejection, as other, nonspecific rejection mechanisms are also possible.

The numerous immunomodulators and the beginning knowledge of their mechanism of action certain inspire great hope that, in the future, we shall be able to modulate the complex immune system in a direction desired. We can stimulate or suppress the antibody response to T-dependent and T-independent antigens. We can modulate the cytotoxic effects of T cells, antibody-dependent or not, of NK cells, and of macrophages. The problem is that we really do not know where we want to go. Is the fact that cancer patients normally have a suppressed mitogen response by T cells enough to make us try to restore it? Is the fact that T-suppressor cells suppress this response, as well as that of B cells, enough to try to destroy suppressors? Maybe they have a tumor cytotoxic effect at the same.time. In fact, the probable destruction of T suppressors with the relatively low-dose chemotherapy maintenance in acute myeloid leukemia is not associated with very good survival. This is better if BCG is given at the same time and the lymphocyte mitogen response thus kept low (32).

The establishment of correlations between tumor prognosis and certain immunological functions is not enough to guide us, since we do not know which is the chicken and which is the egg. Even if we had studies showing that, for instance, patients in whom we succeeded to stimulate the macrophages did better than the others, this would not be enough. The two effects can simply have a common cause. We really need the very difficult direct identification of the effect of one or several of the parts of the biological response directly on the tumor. And what is worse, we need this in humans.

V. SUMMARY

There are indications, of varying strength, that different immunomodifiers affect different parts of the immune system. A primarily depressed T-cell function seems to be restored by levamisole. Even a nondepressed T-cell response seems to be stimulated by high-dose bestatin. The E-rosette receptor expression seems to be stimulated by thymic extracts and factors such as FTS.

The appearance and/or function of suppressor T cells seems to be inhibited by levamisole (in immunosuppressed animals only) and low-dose cytostatics, but stimulated by cyclosporin and BCG. T-cell-mediated cytotoxicity may be stimulated by azimexon.

The B-cell function seems to be stimulated by low-dose bestatin, and possible also azimexon and thymosin (via helper T cells?).

Certain macrophage functions, for instance the helper function, production of colony-stimulating activity, and cytotoxicity, seem to be stimulated by azimexon, BCG, retinoids, and active peptides like tuftsin, muramyl dipeptide, and NTP 15392.

The NK-cell function seems to be stimulated by interferon, BCG, NTP 15392, and (in immunosuppressed animals) by retinoids.

The biological response to tumors consists not only of a specific humoral or cellular immunological response but also of a nonspecific biological response including hyperfibrinogenemia with a high erythrocyte sedimentation rate and hypercoagulability, leukocytosis, lactoferrin production, and activation of macrophages and nonspecific cytotoxic cells; nutritional immunity, and a series of humoral reactions involving the mediators of inflammation and cytokines such as interferon, tumor necrotizing-factors and lymphotoxins.

Some of the immunomodulators discussed seem to prolong life in patients with leukemia and lymphomas (BCG and levamisole) or to prevent tumors in old mice (BCG, levamisole, bestatin), but it is not known whether they act via specific, immunological mechanisms or via nonspecific cell-mediated cytotoxicity, or via other parts of the biological response, for instance cytokine or poietin secretion (BCG, azimexon). If their effect can be identified, biological response modifiers may come to represent an important new family of drugs.

REFERENCES

1. J. H. Humphrey, *Immunol. Today*, *2*:V (1981).
2. F. M. Burnet, *Prog. Exp. Tumor*, *13*:1 (1970).
3. A. Khan, E. S. Martin, K. Webb, D. Weldon, N. O. Hill, J. Duvall, and J. M. Hill, *Proc. Soc. Exp. Biol. Med.*, *169*:291 (1982).
4. P. Reizenstein, *The Biological Response to Tumors. I. The Hematologic Stress Syndrome*, Praeger, New York, 1983.
5. H. Yamaguchi, T. Moriuchi, M. Hosokawa, and H. Kobayashi, *Cancer Immunol. Immunother.*, *12*:119 (1982).
6. L. Olsson, G. Mathé, and P. Reizenstein, in *Anticancer Chemotherapy*, Vol. III (K. Karrer, G. Mathé, and N. Periti, eds.), G. Thieme, Stuttgart, in press.
7. J. P. Brown, R. M. Hewick, I. Hellström, K. E. Hellström, R. F. Doolittle and W. J. Dreyer, *Nature*, *296*:171 (1982).
8. P. Reizenstein, L. Olsson, and G. Mathé, in *Immunobiology of Transplantation Cancer and Pregnancy* (P. F. Ray, ed.), Pergamon, New York, 1984.
9. M. Bruley-Rosset, I. Florentin, and G. Mathé, in *Fourth Annual Conference, International Society for Experimental Hematology, Yugoslavia, Sept. 21-25,ç 1975*, Abstract No. 122, p. 54.
10. M. Bruley-Rosset, I. Florentin, A-M. Khalil, and G. Mathé, *Int. Archs. Allergy Appl. Immunol.*, *51*:594 (1976).
11. M. Bruley-Rosset, I. Florentin, N. Kiger, M. Davigny, and G. Mathé, *Cancer Treat Rep.*, *62*:1641 (1978).
12. I. Florentin, R. Huchet, M. Bruley-Rosset, O. Halle-Pannenko, and G. Mathé, *Cancer Immunol. Immunother.*, *1*:31 (1976).
13. I. Florentin, N. Kiger, M. Bruley-Rosset, J. Schulz, and G. Mathé, in *Human Lymphocyte Differentiation: Its Application to Cancer*, INSERM Symposium no. 8 (B. Serrou and C. Rosenfeld, eds.), Elsevier/North-Holland Biomedical Press, Amsterdam, 1978, p. 299.
14. A. Khalil, H. Rappaport, D. Dantchev, I. Florentin, and C. Bourut, *Biomedicine*, *25*:396 (1976).
15. A. Khalil, H. Rappaport, I. Florentin, M. Bennoun, M. Davigny, and G. Mathé, *Biomedicine*, *30*:200 (1979).
16. L. Chedid, paper presented at a *Symposium on Immunomodulators, Hôpital Necker, Paris, Nov. 19, 1981* (in French).
17. S. Orbach-Arbouys, J-P. Tenu, and J-P. Petit, *Int. Archs. Allergy Appl. Immun.*, in press.
18. M. Bruley-Rosset, I. Florentin, N. Kiger, J. Schulz, and G. Mathé, in *Cancer Chemo- and Immunopharmacology. 2. Immunopharmacology, Relations and General Problems* (G. Mathé and F. M. Muggia, eds.), *Rec. Res. Cancer Res.*, vol. 75, Springer Verlag, Heidelberg, New York, 1980, p. 139.
19. M. Bruley-Rosset, I. Florentin, N. Kiger, J. Schulz, and G. Mathé, *Immunology*, *38*: 75 (1979).
20. I. Florentin, J. Schulz, M. Bruley-Rosset, N. Kiger, J. Martinez, and G. Mathé, in *Cancer Chemo- and Immunopharmacology. 2. Immunopharmacology, Relations*

and General Problems (G. Mathé and F. M. Muggia, eds.), *Rec. Res. Cancer Res.*, vol. 75, Springer Verlag, Heidelberg, New York, 1980.

21. G. Mathé, L. Olsson, I. Florentin, N. Kiger, M. Bruley-Rosset, S. Orbach-Arbouys, and J. Schulz, in *Neoplasm Immunity: Experimental and Clinical* (R. G. Crispen, ed.), Elsevier/North-Holland, Amsterdam, 1980, p. 521.
22. I. Florentin, M. Bruley-Rosset, N. Kiger, J-L. Imbach, F. Winternitz, and G. Mathé, *Cancer Immunol. Immunother.*, *5*:211 (1978).
23. M. Bruley-Rosset, I. Florentin, and G. Mathé, *Molec. Cell Biochem.*, *41*:113 (1981).
24. I. Florentin, E. Taylor, M. Davigny, G. Mathé, and J. W. Hadden, *Int. J. Immunopharmacol.*, *4*:225 (1982).
25. J. Gouveia, G. Mathé, T. Hercend, F. Gros, G. Lemaigre, G. Santelli, J-P. Homasson, J-P. Gaillard, M. Angebault, J-P. Bonniot, A. Ledente, J. Marsac, R. Parrot, and S. Pretet, *Lancet*, *2*:710 (1982).
26. T. Hercend, M. Bruley-Rosset, I. Florentin, and G. Mathé, in *Retinoids* (C. E. Orfanos, eds.), Springer Verlag, Heidelberg, New York, 1981, p. 21.
27. L. Kesztyüs, *Ther. Hung.*, *29*:113 (1981).
28. P. Reizenstein, in the *Supplementary Treatments of Cancer*, San Rocco Symposium, 1982, *Clin. Immunol. Immunopathol.*, *26*:432 (1983).
29. J-F. Bach and M. Dardenne, paper presented at *Symposium on Immunomodulators, Hôpital Necker, Paris, 19 Nov. 1981* (in French).
30. A. Borel, paper presented at *Symposium on Immunomodulators, Hôpital Necker, Paris, 19 Nov. 1981* (in French).
31. S. Orbach-Arbouys, B. M. Castes, and M. Berardet, in *Experimental Hematology Today*, Springer Verlag, Heidelberg, New York, 1977, p. 127.
32. P. Reizenstein, C. Ogier, and A-M. Sjögren, in *Cancer Chemo- and Immunopharmacology. 2. Immunopharmacology, Relations, and General Problems* (G. Mathé and F. M. Muggia, eds.), *Rec. Res. Cancer Res.*, vol. 75, Springer Verlag, Heidelberg, New York, 1980, p. 29.
33. A. Goutner, J-L. Misset, and G. Mathé, *Antiviral Res.* (special abstracts issue): 19 p. 29
34. H. Blomgren and S. Einhorn, *Antiviral Res.* (special abstracts issue): 19 (1981).
35. N. Giannoulis, E. Osby, G. G. Hatzisotiriou, and P. Reizenstein, in *Mediterranean Cancer Conference, Cairo, Nov. 5-8, 1980*, abstract no. 80, p. 56.
36. J-L. Misset, G. Mathé, J. Gastiaburu, A. Goutner, T. Dorval, J. Gouveia, M. Hayat, C. Jasmin, L. Schwarzenberg, D. Machover, P. Ribaud, and F. De Vassal, *Anticancer Res.*, *2*:67 (1982).
37. J-L. Misset, G. Mathé, J. Gastiaburu, A. Goutner, T. Dorval, J. Gouveia, M. Hayat, C. Jasmin, L. Schwarzenberg, D. Machover, P. Ribaud, F. De Vassal, and J. S. Horoszewick, *Anticancer Res.*, *2*:63 (1982).
38. J-L. Misset, G. Mathé, J. Gastiaburu, A. Goutner, T. Dorval, J.Gouveia, L. Schwarzenberg, D. Machover, P. Ribaud, and F. De Vassal, *Biomedicine*, *36*:112 (1982).
39. M. Bruley-Rosset and I. Florentin, *Antiviral Res.* (special abstracts issue): 1981, p. 68.
40. B. Lönnqvist, A. Aahre, M. Björkholm, G. Brenning, L. Engstedt, G. Gahrton, G. Hölm, B. Johansson, R. Lerner, H. Mellstedt, B. Nordenskiöld, A. Killander, A-M. Stalfelt, B. Simonsson, H. Strander, B. Ternstedt, and B. Wadman, in *12th International Congress of Chemotherapy, Florence, Italy, July 19-24, 1981*, abstract no. 1261.
41. G. Mathé, A. Goutner, J. Gastiaburu, F. De Vassal and J-L. Misset, in *The Biology Interferon System* (E. De Maeyer, G. Gallasso, and H. Schellekens, eds.), Elsevier/North-Holland Biomedical Press, Amsterdam, 1981, p. 437

42. J-L. Misset, G. Mathé, J. Gastiaburu, A. Goutner, T. Dorval, J. Gouveia, M. Hayat, C. Jasmin, L. Schwarzenberg, D. Machover, P. Ribaud, F. De Vassal, and J. S. Horoszewicz, *Biomedicine*, *36*:55 (1982).
43. J-L. Misset and G. Mathé, *N. Engl. J. Med.*, *304*:1544, (1981).
44. G. Mathé, J-L. Amiel, L. Schwarzenberg, M. Schneider, M. Hayat, F. De Vassal, C. Jasmin, C. Rosenfeld, M. Sakouhi, and J. Choay, *Rev. Eur. Etudes Clin, Biol.*, *XV*:671 (1970).
45. R. Medenica, G. Emödi, and P. A. Miescher, in *12th International Congress of Chemotherapy, Florence, Italy, July 19-24, 1981*, abstract no. 1265.
46. P. Reizenstein, B. Andersson, and M. Beran, in *Adjuvant Therapies of Cancer* (G. Mathé, G. Bonadonna, and S. Salmon, eds.), *Rec. Res. Cancer Res.*, vol. 80, Springer Verlag, Heidelberg, New York, 1982, p. 64.
47. E. A. Carswell, L. J. Old, and R. L. Kassel, *Proc. Natl. Acad. Sci. USA*, *72*:3666 (1975).
48. A. J. Strelkauskas, V. Schauf, and B. S. Wilson, *J. Immunol.*, *120*:1278 (1978).
49. L. Hodinka, K. Merétey, Z. Zahumenszky, and S. Bozsoky, *Ther. Hung.*, *29*:162 (1981).
50. G. Mathé, L. Olsson, I. Florentin, N. Kiger, S. Orbach-Arbouys, and J. I. Schulz, in *Adjuvant Therapies and Markers of Post-Surgical Minimal Residual Disease. I. Markers and General Problems of Cancer Adjuvant Therapies*, (G. Bonadonna, G. Mathé, and S. E. Salmon, eds.), *Rec. Res. Cancer Res.*, vol. 67, Springer Verlag, Heidelberg, New York, 1979, p. 132
51. C. Canon, C. Ogier, P. Reizenstein, A. Goutner, F. de Vassal, and G. Mathé, *Biomed. Pharmakother.*, *37*:90 (1983).

17

Modulation of Human Lymphocytotoxicity by Biological Response Modifiers

Michael Micksche, Michel Colot, and Atsushi Uchida* Institute for Applied and Experimental Oncology, University of Vienna, Vienna, Austria

I. INTRODUCTION

Natural killer (NK) activity initially has been defined as an immediate lymphocyte reactivity occurring without presensitization against tumor cells and is detectable in the peripheral blood of both tumor-bearing hosts and normal individuals (1-3). Recently, this lymphocyte population has been characterized by morphology, surface marker studies, and also by in vitro culture (4-6). These cells designated large granular lymphocytes (LGLs) appear to be involved in important effector mechanisms against tumor- and virus-infected cells in vitro (7,8). Recent evidence in rodents suggests that NK cells are also able to control primary tumor development and formation of metastases in vivo (9,10). However, the biological significance of human NK cells is not yet fully established. There is evidence that NK activity is reduced in patients with advanced malignant disease (11-13), and that changes of this activity are correlated with the prognosis of the disease (14). Furthermore, low or no NK activity has been demonstrated in tumor-infiltrating lymphocytes (15,16), tumor-draining lymphnodes (17), and also in malignant effusions (18,19), indicating that an impairment of this primary defense mechanism allows tumor development and progression of the disease.

There is some knowledge on factors and cells which may be responsible for negative regulation of NK activity in humans. Prostaglandins and suppressor cells can inhibit the effector phase, the development or maintenace of NK activity in vitro and, possibly, in vivo (20-22).

*Current affiliation: Christie Hospital and Holt Radium Institute, Manchester, England.

Recent clinical studies with biological response modifiers (BRMs) have demonstrated that blood NK-cell activity of cancer patients can be augmented even in advanced stages of the disease (23).

The most pronounced increase of NK killing has been observed in patients receiving therapy with human interferon (IFN) (24), documenting that IFN is an important regulatory factor for NK activity as has been demonstrated by in vitro studies (25). However, no correlation between the augmentation of NK activity and the final clinical outcome of the patients has been found, indicating that further studies will be required.

II. MODULATION OF NK ACTIVITY IN VITRO

A. Motility of NK Cells

Recent investigations have demonstrated that the mechanism leading to target cell lysis includes several steps: target cell binding (conjugate formation), the lethal hit stage, and, furthermore, recycling to kill another target cell (26,27). All these events can be detected by a combination of the conventional cytotoxicity assay and the single cell assay (28), the latter detecting conjugate formation and also cells killed by single effectors, thus allowing estimation of the recycling capacity of NK cells (27,28). Nevertheless, prebinding events (i.e., the effector target cell recognition phase, which includes according to our studies an important motility step) cannot be detected by these assays.

There have been observations that LGLs are highly motile cells which can rapidly change their shape, form contacts with target cells, detach, and again make conjugates (recycling) (29). So far, conjugate formation has been mainly observed in the single cell assay which includes a centrifugal step by which effector cells are forced to make contacts with the targets, missing the motility step.

Cell motility can be investigated by a variety of methods, and we have adapted the agarose microdroplet assay (30) for studying the motility behavior of purified LGLs and compared this with a small lymphocyte population (31). For this assay, lymphocytes, that is, LGL-enriched (LGL+) and LGL-depleted (LGL–) fractions after Percoll separation were suspended in agarose at a concentration of 1×10^5 ml at 37°C. Two microliters of this suspension were then transferred to wells of migration plates. After solidification, droplets were overlayered with medium, with or without K 562 targets, covered with coverslips, and incubated at 37°C. After the respective time intervals, the number of migrated cells was determined under an inverted microscope or migration areas were determined by planimetry (Colot et al., in preparation).

With this method we have documented that fetal calf serum (FCS) in the surrounding medium acts as chemoattractant for LGLs as well as for small lymphocytes; the latter cell population has been found to have a four times enhanced motility in the presence of FCS (Fig. 1).

Addition of K562 targets to the medium leads to a decrease of LGL– motility, whereas LGL+ showed active cell recognition followed by directed movement towards the target, conjugate formation, and subsequent target cell lysis, as demonstrated by time-lapse cinematography.

We have further evidence that microfilament function and energy are required for NK motility. This function seems to be necessary for effector target cell contact, recycling, and subsequent target cell killing. Inhibitors such as cytochalasin B and dinitrophenol (DNP) block LGL motility and also NK killing as they also inhibit contact formation.

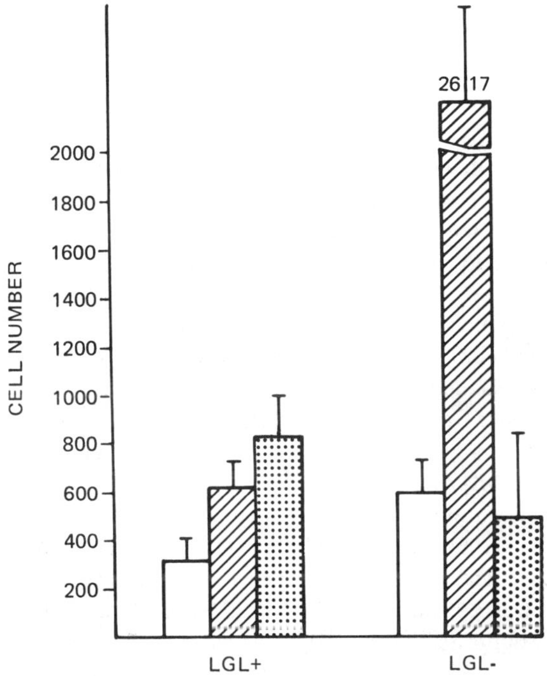

Figure 1 Motility of LGL and small lymphocytes: Motility of LGL (+) and LGL (-) fractions was investigated in agarose microdroplet assay, in presence of medium ▭ FCS ▨, and K 562 target cells ▒. Significant increase in number of LGL (+) in the presence of K 562 cells ($p < 0.01$) within the counting area.

One can conclude that LGL motility is important for the optimal NK killing and, therefore, the study of agents enhancing or inhibiting this phenomenon might be of great interest, especially in the light of BRMs applied in cancer therapy.

B. Suppression of NK-Cell Activity

Several mechanisms are involved in the in vitro and in vivo regulations of NK activity leading to its augmentation or suppression. Known regulators include cellular mechanisms such as suppressor cells (20) and humoral factors, such as IFN and Interleukin 2 (Il-2), known for their capacity of maintaining or augmenting NK activity, whereas prostaglandins of E type have been found to suppress and, under certain conditions to augment NK killing (32-34).

We have stated that patients with malignant pleural effusions have low or no NK-cell activity against K 562 cells in the effusion lymphocytes, whereas NK-cell activity can be demonstrated in the peripheral blood of the same patient (35). Moreover, we demonstrated that the Sephadex G-10 and serum-coated plastic dish adherent fraction, representing monocytes and macrophages, can suppress blood NK activity of normal donors and cancer patients. Nonmalignant pleural effusions do not contain suppressor cells and represent appreciable levels of NK activity (19).

Furthermore, we have observed that patients with malignant tumors including breast, head, and neck cancers have depressed NK activity in the postoperative period (up to 14 days) with a normal lymphocyte proliferative response (36). When these breast cancer patients were monitored before and after surgery, it was found that this depression was not present before surgery (Fig. 2). For detection of mechanisms involved in this postoperative suppression of NK killing, blood mononuclear cells were depleted by adherence (plastic dish and G-10); removal of monocytes did not cause any enhancement of NK-cell activity (Fig. 3).

When monocyte-depleted fractions were cultured for 24 hr at 37° C, a significant increase in NK activity occurred (Fig. 3). These results suggest that the peripheral blood of postoperative cancer patients contains potentially cytotoxic cells which are functionally suppressed by monocytes, and are able to recover their lytic function after removal of monocytes and culture for 24 hr.

Addition of blood monocytes of postoperative cancer patients to monocyte-depleted lymphocytes of normal donors and culture at 37°C for 24 hr resulted in a suppression of NK activity (Fig. 4). Thus, we concluded that blood monocytes obtained from postoperative cancer patients are suppressive for autologous and allogeneic (adherent cell depleted) NK-cell activity. In normal donors and preoperative breast cancer patients, we were unable to detect suppressor cells for NK-cell activity.

The possibility that suppressor substances are excreted in medium by suppressor monocytes was further examined. Culture supernatants (24 hr) of lymphocytes with or without addition of suppressor monocytes and also patients' serum (postoperative) were incubated with lymphocytes for 24 hr, washed, and tested for NK activity. None of the culture supernatants and patients' sera suppressed NK activity, whereas postoperative monocytes did. Furthermore, the presence of indomethacin failed to abrogate monocyte-mediated suppression of NK-cell activity (Fig. 5).

From these studies we concluded that suppressor-to-effector-cell contact is necessary to mediate suppression. Although monocytes were able to suppress NK-cell activity, they failed to inhibit lymphocyte mitogenic response.

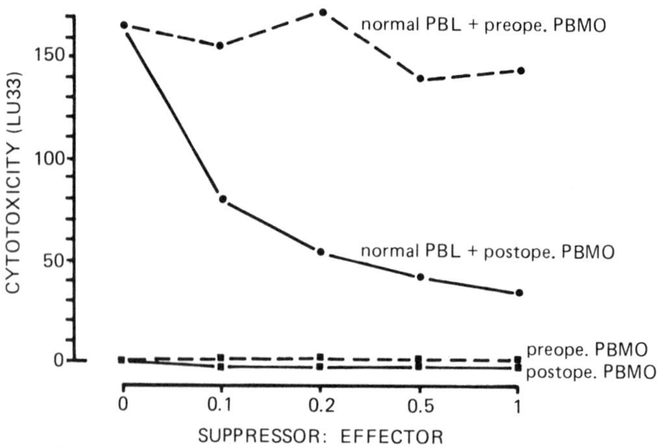

Figure 2 Suppression of NK-cell activity by monocytes: Monocytes obtained from peripheral blood of preoperative (preope. PBMo) and postoperative (postope PBMo) were mixed with normal-donor lymphocytes at different suppressor-to-effector-cell ratios and incubated at 37°C for 20 hr. Significant suppression ($p < 0.05$) of NK-cell activity by postoperative monocytes.

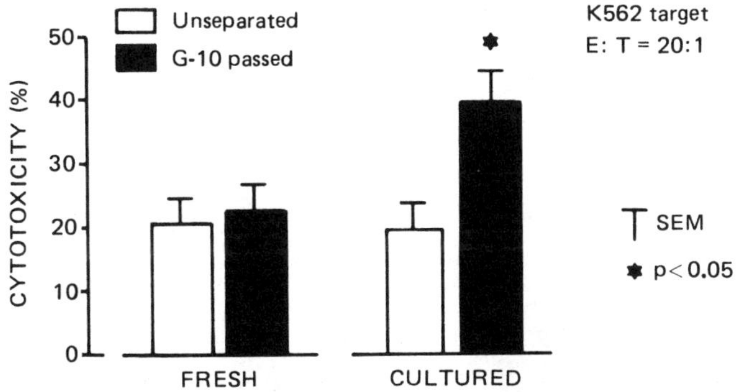

Figure 3 Adherent cell depletion influence on NK activity: Peripheral blood mononuclear cells (PBMNC) of postoperative patients were tested for cytotoxicity with or without depletion of plastic dish and Sephadex G-10 adherent cells, immediately or after culture for 24 hr at 37°C. Significant increase ($p < 0.05$) of NK-cell activity in monocyte-depletion fraction after 24 hr culture.

In order to further evaluate the mechanisms of monocyte-mediated suppression of NK-cell activity, the influence of IFN was investigated. Normal blood lymphocytes were cultured for 24 hr alone or with suppressor monocytes, either in the presence or absence of IFN. Presence of suppressor monocytes reduced the levels of NK activity, and no augmentation by IFN was observed (Table 1), suggesting that postoperative monocytes inhibit both the development and maintenance of NK-cell activity in response to IFN.

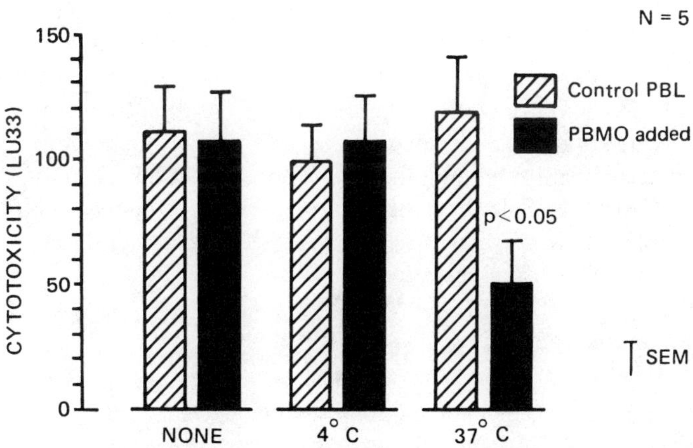

Figure 4 Influence of culture condition on NK suppression: PBMNC of normal donors were incubated, with or without preculture at +4°C or 37°C, with monocytes of postoperative cancer patients (PBMo) for 24 hr. Significant suppression ($p < 0.05$) of NK-cell activity when preculture is performed at 37°C.

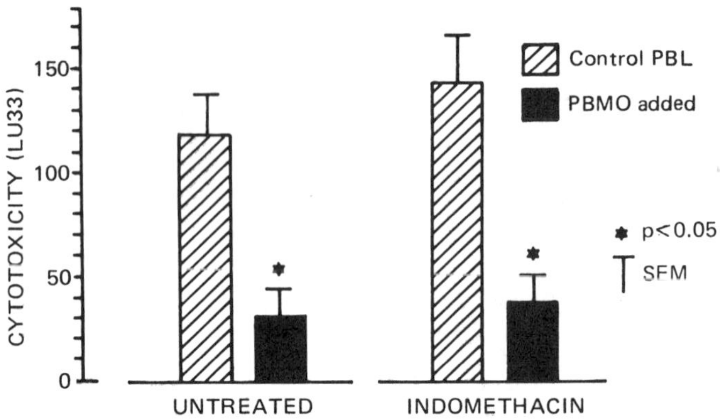

Figure 5 Effect of indomethacin on NK suppression: PBMo of postoperative were cultured, with or without addition of indomethacin (10^{-6}M), with normal-donor lymphocytes. No influence of indomethacin treatment on suppressor cell activity.

The possibility that a secretory process mediates suppression of NK killing was further investigated; postoperative monocytes, with or without pretreatment with monensin (10 μg/ml for 1 hr), were added to normal-donor lymphocytes (Table 2). Monensin treatment of suppressor monocytes abrogated the development of suppression of NK-cell activity.

From these studies one might postulate that modulation of these suppressor cells by BRMs in vivo could subsequently lead to a benefit for cancer patients.

C. Modulation of NK-Cell Activity by BRMs In Vitro

BRMs are, by definition, agents of biological and synthetic origin which are able to modulate host response and, by this, initiate or increase cellular effector mechanisms against tumor cells (37). As natural cell-mediated immunity has been recognized as one important defense mechanism, it seems to be important to know the effect of several widely used and recently developed BRMs on NK-cell activity of cancer patients. Augmentation of human NK-cell activity by BRMs after in vitro incubation may be a useful parameter to screen for agents which may be applied for immunotherapy of human cancer.

Our in vitro studies with BRMs include three different preparations of human IFN, the IFN inducers poly A:U and poly I:C, furthermore two synthetic agents, Azimexon and NPT 15392, and also the streptococcal preparation OK-432.

Table 1 Suppression of Spontaneous and IFN-Induced[a] NK Activity by Postoperative Monocytes (Mϕ)

	NK activity (LU 33) normal-donor lymphocytes		
	Fresh	Cultured	Cultured + IFN
No addition	89	95	200
Mϕ addition	86	25[b]	32[b]

[a]IFN: 100 IU/ml, 20 hr.
[b]$p < 0.05$.

Table 2 Effect on Monensin on Monocyte (Mϕ) Suppressor Activity[a]

PBL	Cytotoxicity (LU 33)	Suppression (%)
PBL	110	–
PBL + Mϕ	43[b]	61[b]
PBL + Mϕ (monensin)	96	13

[a]Treatment of monocytes with 10 μg/ml (1 hr) monensin.
[b]$p < 0.05$.

1. IFN Preparations

Studies were performed with human leukocyte IFN (Immunoloski Zavod, Zagreb, Yugoslavia), lymphoblast IFN (Namalvin, Denmark), and fibroblast IFN (Fiblaferon, Rentschler-Flow Lab., Federal Republic of Germany). Lymphocytes were incubated with 1000 IU/IFN up to 20 hr. For IFN induction *Staphylococcus aureus* protein A (SPA; Protein A, Pharmacia, Uppsala, Sweden) was added to lymphocytes in a concentration of 50 μg/ml and incubated for the same time. After intensive washing, lymphocytes were tested in a 4 hr- ^{51}Cr-release assay using K 562 targets. All IFN preparations tested significantly augmented NK activity of peripheral blood lymphocytes. This augmentation was also observed in patients with advanced malignant disease and low NK activity (Table 3).

Furthermore, SPA augmentation of NK killing was a consistent finding, suggesting that even in advanced stages endogenous IFN production can be induced and, by this, NK–cell activity augmented.

2. Poly A:U, Poly I:C

Polycyclic nucleotides are known to be potent IFN inducers, and animal studies have demonstrated that NK activity can be augmented by in vitro and in vivo application (38). Poly A:U and poly I:C (both purchased from Boehringer Mannheim, Mannheim, Federal Republic of Germany), were reconstituted with medium immediately before use. Replicates of patients' lymphocytes were incubated overnight with different concentrations (10-100 μg/ml) of the respective nucleotide and also for control with IFN-α. After intensive washing NK-cell activity was measured in the cytotoxicity assay.

None of the concentrations of poly A:U tested, in the chosen incubation period, significantly changed NK activity. A representative experiment (Fig. 6) shows that IFN-α and also poly I:C significantly augment NK killing, whereas the same concentration of poly A:U (i.e., 50 μg/ml) was without effect on NK-cell activity).

Table 3 In Vitro Effects of IFN on NK-Cell Activity[a]

	Cytotoxicity (LU/10^7)			
Experiment	Medium	IFN-α	IFN-β	SpA
A	57	100	105	245
B	36	123	152	193
C	21	85	83	100
D	41	117	127	170

[a]Lymphocytes were incubated alone, or with IFN-α, IFN-β (1000 U/ml), or SPA (50 bg/ml) for 20 hr at 37°C.

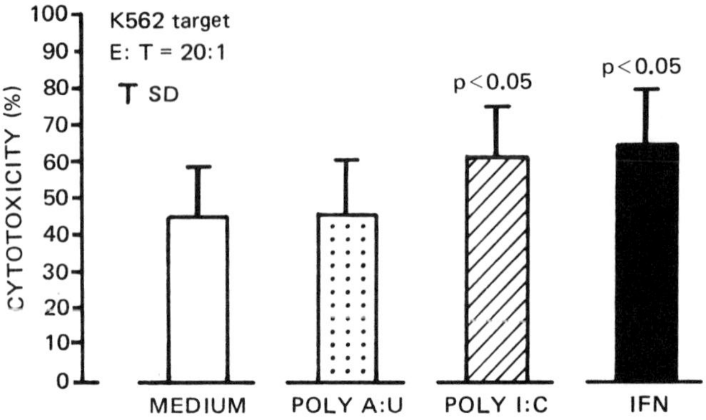

Figure 6 Effect of poly A:U, poly I:C, and IFN in vitro on NK activity: Significant augmentation of NK activity by poly I:C and IFN; poly A:U has no effect.

3. Azimexon

Two cyanoaziridine derivatives have been recently developed by Bicker: Imexon-4-imino-1, 3-diazobicyclo(3,1,0)-hexan-2-on and Azimexon-2-[2-cyanaziridinyl-(1)]-2-[2-carbamoyl aziridinyl-(1)] propane (39,40). Both preparations have been considered to be potent immunomodulating agents (41,42). As there exists evidence that Azimexon is augmenting NK-cell activity in mice after intravenous and/or intraperitoneal injection (43), we performed in vitro studies in order to evaluate the effect of Azimexon on human NK-cell killing.

Lymphocytes of patients and normal donors were incubated for 1, 4, and 24 hr at 37°C with doses of 0.2-100 μg/ml of Azimexon, intensively washed, and tested in the cytotoxicity assay. Significant inhibition of NK killing was observed at doses of 2-100 μg/ml at a preincubation time of 24 hr; 1- and 4-hr incubation did not enhance or suppress. A representative experiment is shown in Fig. 7. Removal of adherent cells before preincubation has no effect on the suppression at 24 hr suggesting that monocytes are not involved in the observed inhibition of NK killing. As viability of lymphocytes was

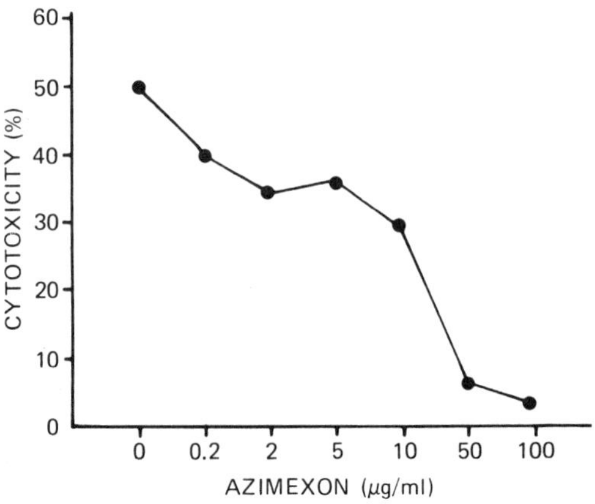

Figure 7 Effect of Azimexon in vitro on NK activity: Significant inhibition of NK-cell activity by addition of Azimexon to PBMNC (24 hr preincubation), $p < 0.005$ (E:T = 40:1).

unchanged after incubation with Azimexon, one may assume that this agent has a direct effect on the effector phase. Induction of suppressor T cells by Azimexon in vivo has been described already (43), and this is presently investigated in the in vitro system.

4. NPT 15392

NPT 15392, 9-erythro-(2-hydroxy, 3-nonyl)-hypoxanthie), is a recent development of Newport Pharmaceutical International Inc. (Newport Beach, California) and Sloan-Kettering Institute for Cancer Research (New York). Several in vitro studies indicate that NPT 15 392 is modulating a variety of T lymphocyte and macrophage reactions (44). Controversial results exist with regard to the effect of this agent on human and mouse NK-cell activity (45,46). Peripheral blood lymphocytes were incubated with NPT 15392. (kindly provided by Newport Pharm. Inc.) at concentrations of 0.001-10 μg/ml for 20 hr, washed, and tested for NK-cell activity. In none of the experiments performed with healthy donors and cancer patients' (with low or high NK activity) lymphocytes, was NPT 15392 found to enhance NK-cell activity (data not shown).

5. OK-432

The pharmaceutical preparation of a low virulent Su strain of *Streptococcus pyogenes*, OK-432 (supplied by Chugai Co., Tokyo, Japan), has been intensively investigated for its potential immunomodulating properties (47-49). We have described the augmentation of NK-cell activity of peripheral blood lymphocytes of normal donors and also cancer patients against both NK-sensitive and resistant human targets by OK-432 treatment in vitro (50). Enhancement of NK-cell activity was evident after a 4-hr treatment, with a maximum between 16 and 24 hr. Augmentation by this preparation required active cell metabolism, RNA, and protein, but no DNA synthesis. We were unable to demonstrate any augmenting factor in the supernatant of OK-432-treated lymphocytes and, furthermore, anti-IFN antibodies, directed against IFN-α and -β (kindly provided by Dr. Cantell) did not inhibit the boosting effect of OK-432. Supernatants also did not show any antiviral activity, suggesting again that IFN-α is not involved in the augmentation of NK killing (50). Thus, other mechanisms seem to be responsible for the modulation of NK killing by OK-432.

We have observed that blood of postoperative patients contains adherent cells that can suppress the maintenance and development of NK activity (36). To know whether OK-432 can modulate activity of suppressor cells, blood lymphocytes were incubated in the presence or absence of adherent suppressor cells (with or without OK-432) at 37°C for 20 hr. OK-432 treatment of monocytes resulted in an abrogation of suppressor activity (Table 4), whereas untreated adherent cells inhibited spontaneous NK activity.

Table 4 In Vitro Reduction of NK-Suppressor Activity by OK 432[a]

PBL	Cytotoxicity (LU 33)	Suppression (%)
PBL	102	–
PBL + Mϕ	39[b]	62[b]
PBL + Mϕ -(OK 432)	126	-25

[a]Monocytes were treated with 50 μg/ml OK 432 for 20 hr [Mϕ-(OK 432)].
[b]$p < 0.05$.

The mechanism of desuppression by OK-432 is not yet clear, but we suggest that macrophages and monocytes can be activated by OK-432 and by this losing their suppressor activity. Our results give evidence that OK-432 not only augments NK-cell activity but also reduced NK-suppressor activity in vitro. Recent studies in patients with OK-432 seem to confirm these in vitro findings.

III. MODULATION OF NK ACTIVITY IN VIVO

The basic findings concerning the in vivo modulation of NK activity by BRMs was the observation that IFN can boost the NK activity in mice. This phenomenon was detected with nonpurified as well as with homogenous purified IFN preparations, and also with IFN inducers (38). Additional studies in animals demonstrated that injections of agents such as poly A:U, poly I:C (38), Bacillus Calmette-Guérin (BCG) (51,52), *Corynebacterium parvum* (53), pyran copolymer (54), and so on, can significantly augment NK activity. It was assumed and recently demonstrated that endogenous IFN induction by these agents was responsible for this observed augmentation. Studies with human lymphocytes demonstrated that in vitro incubation of these effector cells with IFN increases their cytolytic activity (24). Application of IFN to healthy volunteers and cancer patients was found to be associated with an increase of blood NK activity (25). This activity reaches, after an initial drop, a maximum at 24 hr after IFN application. Augmented NK levels can be maintained by continuous therapy (25).

Clinical studies recently performed in patients with cancer have given evidence that other BRMs such as retinoids (55), *C. parvum* (56), lentinan (57), and NPT 15392 (58) can augment NK-cell activity in peripheral blood.

We have investigated the effect of therapy with IFN, poly A:U, vitamin A, NPT 15392, and OK-432 on NK-cell activity in patients with malignant disease.

A. IFN Therapy

Several clinical trials have already documented that therapy with IFN-α, with IFN-β, independent of the purity of the preparations, and with recombinant IFN, results in an augmentation of NK activity of peripheral blood lymphocytes.

We have used IFN therapy in nine patients with malignant disease in an advanced stage whom we considered unresponsive to conventional therapy, and we have monitored these patients for the influence of therapy on NK activity.

IFN-α (Namalvin) was administered peritumorally with a single dose of 0.5×10^6 IU, three times a week for 2 weeks, to a patients with multiple skin metastases of breast cancer. A second patient with multiple lung metastases (soft tissue sarcoma) received daily an IM injection of IFN-α (Namalvin) in a dose of 4×10^6 IU for 12 days. Seven more patients were treated with IFN-β (Virogen, Bern) with an initial dose of 1×10^6 IU given IV and on the subsequent 4 days 4×10^6 IU daily. This regimen was repeated after a therapy-free interval. One of these patients received this scheme four times over a period of 4 months and another five times over 6 months.

NK activity was significantly increased by day 2 in all patients receiving IFN-α This augmentation was preceded by an initial drop of activity 2-4 hr after the initial injection. After this, levels remained elevated in the patient with local therapy, whereas IM therapy resulted in a decrease to pretreatment levels after 12 days. All patients receiving IFN-β, with the exception of one of them, showed an increase in NK activity during the first treatment course (Table 5). One patients who received IFN for five

Table 5 NK Activity in Patients Receiving IFN-β Therapy[a]

Patient no.	Days of treatment 0	1	2	3	4
3	50	56	68	NT[b]	NT
4	26	26	NT	NT	13
5	6	45	63	55	33
6	11	40	31	46	33
7	4	9	24	18	34
8	33	51	21	12	30
9	9	15	41	36	NT

[a]Percent specific cytotoxicity (E:T = 40:1).
[b]NT

cycles had continuously augmented NK activity. Nevertheless, an augmentation of NK activity was not correlated with the clinical response in all patients.

B. Poly A:U Therapy

Adjuvant immunotherapy with poly A:U was investigated in a randomized trial with 300 patients with operable breast cancer who had been treated by surgery with or without radiotherapy (59). IV injection of 30 mg poly A:U per week (for 6 weeks) resulted in a significant increase in overall survival times in comparison with the control group. Furthermore, this effect was also noticed in node-positive patients (i.e., significant increase in relapse-free interval and survival time) (59).

The mechanism of action of poly A:U on immune function in humans is not yet elucidated. In one study, paradoxical immunological effects have been described (60). No data concerning the effect of poly A:U therapy on NK activity in patients are available to date, although an augmenting effect has been described in animal studies (38). For this reason, and according to the clinical benefit obtained by this therapy, we investigated the effect of poly A:U therapy on NK activity and on serum IFN levels in patients with advanced cancer.

Initially, eight patients received 20 mg poly A:U IM. No side effects were detected in these patients. Determination of serum IFN levels (before and 2, 4, 8, 12, and 24 hr after injection) did not show endogenous induction of IFN (61).

Three patients then received 30 mg poly A:U IV. In none of them could significant augmentation of NK activity in comparison with untreated patients be detected up to 24 hr after drug application and, furthermore, no significant levels of antiviral activity were detected in patients' serum at the time intervals investigated. These studies might indicate that mechanisms other than IFN induction and augmentation of NK activity seem to be responsible for the observed clinical benefit in breast cancer.

C. NPT 15392 Therapy

Therapy with this agent was investigated within a cooperative trial with the EORTC tumor immunology project group. The purpose of this study was to evaluate the effect of two fixed doses of NPT: 0.4 mg and 0.7 mg, given four times within 10 days by oral route, on several immune parameters including NK activity.

In this study, we have included 10 patients with diagnosis of malignant melanoma (n = 5) and gastrointestinal cancers (n = 5). All patients had previous surgery and have refused or not been eligible for chemo- or radiotherapy. Therapy was well tolerated by all patients. NK activity was found augmented in 6 of 10 patients, without relationship to the doses applied. Augmentation was observed mainly by day 4; after this time, NK activity returned to pretreatment levels in all patients, despite continuation of therapy until day 10. A kinetic study of NK activity of one patient is shown in Fig. 8.

The main finding from this study was that NPT therapy was able to augment NK activity, especially in those patients who had low pretreatment levels, whereas in patients with reactivity in the normal range no change of NK-killing activity has been observed. Further studies will be required in order to clarify the mechanisms involved in augmentation of NK activity and to find out the doses suitable for maintenance of high NK activity.

D. OK-432 Therapy

Clinical studies with OK-432 have documented that this agent is a potent immunomodulator with anticancer activity even in cases of advanced malignant disease (62). Immunological changes after OK-432 therapy in cancer patients include enhancement of lymphoproliferative response to mitogens and antigens, reduction of suppressor cells, and increase of skin test reactivity (63,64).

In a phase I study in patients with advanced cancer, we have investigated toxicity and immunopharmacology of OK-432 applied in either a single dose or repeatedly by various routes. Fever was the side effect always observed after the IV route occurring only rarely after IM or ID injection (65). One single dose of OK-432, 1 KE (Klinische Einheit, equaling 0.1 mg dried streptococci), could augment significantly blood NK activity with a maximum on day 3. IV and ID routes were more effective than IM application for boosting NK activity.

According to these studies and also some clinical benefits observed, we extended our clinical investigations with OK-432 in patients who received OK-432 for a longer period of time. Therapy results in patients with metastastic malignant melanoma might be considered beneficial, as objective tumor remissions have been achieved by OK-432 treatment (65). Another therapy study with OK-432 was performed in patients with

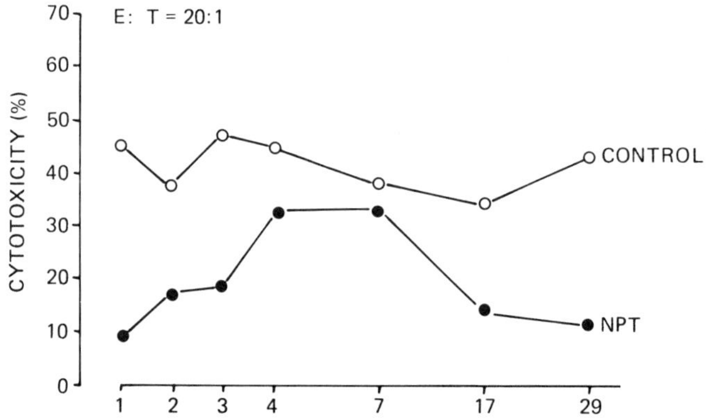

Figure 8 Influence of NPT therapy on NK activity: Significant augmentation of NK activity in a patient receiving NPT therapy (days 4 and 7, $p < 0.05$) in comparison with pretreatment level (day 1).

operated gastric cancer: patients were randomized to receive (a) no further therapy, (b) chemotherapy, and (c) immunochemotherapy including OK-432 (applied IM in a dose of 2 KE once a week for 5 weeks) before chemotherapy (66).

In patients with malignant melanoma we have not attempted to investigate the effect of OK-432 therapy on blood activity. In patients with gastric cancer a significant increase in blood NK activity was observed after IM therapy with OK-432, whereas untreated patients did not show this augmentation at the time (66).

Another therapy study with OK-432 was performed in patients with malignant pleural effusions with diagnosis of breast or lung cancer. Twelve patients received IP injections of OK-432 (10 KE/week) after drainage of all fluid. NK activity was determined in peripheral blood and in pleural effusion obtained on days 0 and 7, immediately before injection of OK-432. In untreated patients, effusion lymphocytes had, as reported previously (19), low or no NK activity, whereas blood NK activity was depressed in 9 of 12 patients, but always higher than the activity in their effusions.

Seven days after OK-432 injection, NK activity in pleural effusions was significantly enhanced in seven patients; two patients were still lacking NK activity, whereas in two other patients no fluid could be obtained due to complete disappearance of exudate after therapy. Monitoring of blood NK activity before and on day 7 of therapy did not reveal any significant changes, suggesting that the main effect of OK-432 therapy is a local one in the pleural cavity.

In order to evaluate the effect of OK-432 therapy on suppressor activity of adherent cells from pleural effusions, effusion-derived suppressor cells were tested with normal donors' lymphocytes in vitro on days 0 and 7 for presence of NK-suppressor activity. Adherent effusion cells obtained from OK-432-treated patients were no longer suppressive on day 7 (Table 6), whereas in untreated pleural effusions this activity was still demonstrable.

Beside this effect of intrapleural OK-432 therapy on local immune reactions (i.e., augmentation of NK-cell activity and abrogation of suppressor activity of adherent cells), a clinical benefit of this therapy has been observed also. Two patients had complete and seven partial remissions, as judged by the amount of fluid which could be drawn within the observation period. Furthermore, there seems to exist a correlation between clinical response and the augmentation of NK activity in pleural fluid, as all patients who were considered responders also showed this increase in reactivity, whereas nonresponders continuously had no pleural NK activity.

Table 6 Reduction of NK-Suppressor Cell Activity after Intrapleural Administration of OK-432

PEAC added[a]	Cytotoxicity (LU 33)
Ly	105
Ly + untreated PEAC	37
Ly + OK-432-treated PEAC	121

[a]Pleural exudate adherent cells (PEAC) obtained from untreated and OK-432-treated patients were incubated with normal donor peripheral blood lymphocytes (Ly).

IV. CONCLUSION

We have demonstrated that motility of NK cells is important for NK killing. Simultaneous investigations of LGL motility, using the agarose microdroplet assay, and LGL killing, using cytotoxicity assay, and of the influence of cytochalasin B and DNP on both these activities revealed that agents that inhibit motility also inhibit target cell killing. So far, little attention has been paid to the initial recognition and motility phase within the killing event by NK cells. Present attempts, therefore, should be directed at identifying agents which can modulate NK motility and thus increase killing efficacy.

Modulation of NK-cell activity by BRMs might also interfere with regulatory cells such as monocytes, macrophages, and T lymphocytes which have been reported to act as suppressor of NK activity (21,35,36). We have given evidence that treatment of adherent suppressor cells, as present in malignant pleural effusions and peripheral blood of post-operative patients, with OK-432 abrogates NK suppression and, by this, restores NK activity. This desuppression has been observed first in vitro and recently also in vivo, as patients with malignant pleural effusions who were treated intrapleurally with OK-432 developed activated pleural NK activity together with a reduction of suppressor cell activity. Furthermore, patients' clinical response was correlated with the development of significant levels of NK killing in pleural effusions. Beside this local effect of OK-432 therapy, we have found that IV or ID application of this agent significantly augments blood NK activity. From in vitro studies, also showing augmentation of NK activity by OK-432, we have evidence that IFN-α is not involved in this agumentation (50). Investigations of other researchers have pointed to a possible role of IFN-γ and/or Interleukin 2 (Il-2) in this OK-432-induced augmentation of NK killing (67).

Using different preparations of IFN, we were able to demonstrate that NK activity can be augmented in vitro in all patients so far investigated, independent of the clinical stage of malignant disease and of the level of spontaneous NK activity. These observations differ from those of other authors (68) who have demonstrated that the NK defect cannot be corrected in vitro with IFN in all patients. These discrepancies might be due to differences in IFN preparations, in methodology, and finally in the patient population investigated. Our in vitro results were confirmed by our clinical studies with IFN; in all patients except one, IFN therapy was accompanied by a significant increase in blood NK activity. Studies with IFN inducers revealed that poly A:U has neither in vitro nor in vivo an augmenting effect on NK activity, whereas poly I:C is active both in vitro and in vivo (unpublished observation).

NPT 15 392 was found ineffective in vitro, whereas in the clinical study, a significant augmentation of NK activity could be demonstrated, especially in patients with low pre-treatment levels.

Another observation was the suppression of NK killing in vitro by preincubation of patients' lymphocytes with the synthetic agent Azimexon. This seems to be controversial to in vivo studies in animals (43) and also cancer patients (69), as therapy with Azimexon was found to significantly augment NK killing. According to our studies, neither monocytes nor soluble factors are involved in this suppressed NK activity. One possibility of suppressor T cells being involved, as already demonstrated in animals receiving high doses of Azimexon (43), is presently investigated.

From all these studies with BRMs both in vivo and in vitro, showing augmentation of suppression or no change of NK activity, one achieves more insight into the mechanism of action of the different agents, and this may finally help to establish dose regimens for more successful therapy with BRMs in cancer patients.

ACKNOWLEDGMENTS

The cooperation of Dr. O. Kokron (L. Boltzmann Institute for Clinical Oncology, Hospital Lainz, Vienna), Prof. Dr. K. Moser, Dr. R. Lenzhofer, Dr. H. Rainer (Clinic for Chemotherapy, University of Vienna), Dr. E. M. Kokoschka (Dept. of Dermatology, University of Vienna), and Dr. H. Höcker (Blood Transfusion Center, General Hospital, Vienna) is gratefully acknowledged by the authors.

REFERENCES

1. M. E. Nunn and R. B. Herberman, *JNCI*, *62*:765 (1979)
2. R. Kissling and O. Haller, *Contemp. Top. Immunobiol.*, *8*:171 (1978).
3. R. B. Herberman, J. Y. Djeu, H. D. Kay, J. R. Ortaldo, C. Riccardi, G. D. Bonnard, H. T. Holden, R. Fagnani, and A. Santoni, *Immunol. Rev.*, *44*:43 (1979).
4. T. Timonen and E. Sausela, *J. Immunol. Meth.*, *36*:285 (1980).
5. J. R. Ortaldo, S. O. Sharron, T. Timonen, and R. B. Herberman, *J. Immunol.*, *127*: 2401 (1981).
6. G. Dennert, G. Yoheeswaran, and G. Yamagata, *J. Exp. Med.*, *153*:545 (1981).
7. T. Timonen, J. R. Ortaldo, and R. B. Herberman, *J. Exp. Med.*, *153*:545 (1981).
8. M. O. de Landazuri, M. Lopez-Botet, T. Timonen, J. R. Ortaldo, and R. B. Herberman, *J. Immunol.*, *127*:1274 (1981).
9. M. Kasai, J. C. Leclerc, L. McVay-Boudreau, T. W. Shen, and H. Cantor, *J. Exp. Med.*, *149*:1260 (1979).
10. N. Hanna, *Cancer Metastasis Rev.*, *1*:45 (1982).
11. S. Cunningham-Rundles, D. A. Filippa, D. W. Braun, Jr., P. Antonelli, and H. Ashikari, *JNCI*, *67/3*:585 (1981).
12. K. P. DeBoer, D. P. Braun, and J. E. Harris, *Clin. Immunol. Immunopathol.*, *23*:133 (1982).
13. N. Saijo, E. Shimizu, N. Irimajiri, K. Mimura, T. Takizawa, and N. Niitani, *J. Cancer Res. Clin. Oncol.*, *102*:195 (1982).
14. P. Hersey, A. Edwards, and W. H. McCarthy, *Int. J. Cancer*, *25*:187 (1980).
15. B. M. Vose, R. Vankey, S. Argov, and E. Klein, *Eur. J. Immunol.*, *7*:753 (1977).
16. B. M. Vose, *Int. J. Cancer*, *30*:135 (1982).
17. O. Eremin, R. R. A. Coombs, D. Plumb, and J. Ashby, *Int. J. Cancer*, *21*:42 (1978).
18. A. Mantovani, P. Allavena, C. Sessa, G. Bolis, and C. Mangioni, *Int. J. Cancer*, *25*:573 (1980).
19. A. Uchida and M. Micksche, *Cancer Immunol. Immunother.*, *11*:131 (1981).
20. G. Cudkowicz and P. S. Hochman, in *Developmental Immunology* (G. W. Siskind, S. D. Litwin, and M. E. Wechsler, eds.), Grune & Stratton, New York, 1979.
21. J. Tarkkanen and K. Saksela, *Scand. J. Immunol.*
22. M. J. Droller, M. U. Schneider, and P. Perlman, *Cell Immunol.*, *39*:165 (1978).
23. E. M. Hersh, J. Gutterman, G. Mavligit, and S. Murphy, in *Advances in Immunopharmacology* (J. Hadden, L. Chedid, P. Mullen, and F. Spreafico, eds.), Pergamon Press, New York, 1981.
24. S. Einhort, H. Blomgren, and H. Strander, *Int. J. Cancer*, *22*:405 (1978).
25. S. Einhorn, in *Natural Cell-Mediated Immunity against Tumors* (R. B. Herberman, ed.), Academic Press, New York, 1980.
26. P. Rubin, H. F. Pross, and J. C. Roder, *J. Immunol.*, *128/6*:2553 (1982).
27. O. Carpén, I. Virtanen, and E. Saksela, *Cell. Immunol.*, *58*:97 (1981).
28. M. Ullberg and M. Jondal, *J. Exp. Med.*, *153*:615 (1981).
29. E. Saksela and T. Timonen, in *Natural Cell-Mediated Immunity against Tumors* (R. B. Herbeman, ed.), Academic Press, New York, 1980.

30. J. L. McCoy, J. H. Dean, and R. B. Herberman, in *In Vitro Methods in Cell-Mediated and Tumor Immunity* (B. R. Bloom and J. R. David, eds.), Academic Press, New York, 1976.
31. A. Uchida, M. Colot, and Mi. Micksche, *Proc. Am. Assoc. Cancer Res.*, *23*:268 (1982).
32. I. Heron, M. Hokland, A. Møller-Larsen, and K. Berg, *Cell. Immunol.*, *42*:183 (1979).
33. C. S. Henney, K. Kuribayashi, D. E. Kern, and S. Gillis, *Nature*, *291*:335 (1981).
34. A. D. Bankhurst, *J. Clin. Lab. Immunol.*, *7*:85 (1982).
35. A. Uchida and M. Micksche, *Cancer Immunol. Immunother.*, *11*:255 (1981).
36. A. Uchida, R. Kolb, and M. Micksche, *JNCI*, *68*:735 (1982).
37. St. M. Mikulski, M. A. Chirigos, and F. M. Muggia, *Adv. Pharmacol. Chemother.*, *15*:263 (1978).
38. J. Y. Djeu, J. A. Heinbaugh, I. Gresser, H. T. Holden, and R. B. Herberman, *J. Immunol.*, *122*:175 (1979).
39. U. Bicker, in *Immune Modulation and Control of Neoplasia by Adjuvant Therapy*, Progress in Cancer Res. Ther. (M. A. Chirigos, ed.), Karger Press, Basel, 1978.
40. U. Bicker, *Cancer Treat. Rep.*, *62*:1987 (1978).
41. M. Micksche, P. Sagaster, E. M. Kokoschka, O. Kokron, and U, Bicker, in *Immunotherapy of Human Cancer* (W. A. Terry and St. A. Rosenberg, eds.), Elsevier/North Holland, New York, 1982.
42. M. Colot, M. Micksche, and U. Bicker, *Cancer Immunol. Immunother.*, *6*:175 (1979).
43. I. Florentin, M. Bruley-Rosset, J. Schulz, M. Davigny, N. Kiger, and G. Mathé, in *Advances in Immunopharmacology* (J. Hadden, L. Chedid, P. Mullen, and F. Spreafico, eds.), Pergamon Press, Oxford, 1981.
44. A. Goutner, L. Schwarzenberg, and G. Mathé, in *Immunotherapy of Human Cancer* (W. A. Terry and St. A. Rosenberg, eds.), Elsevier/North Holland, New York, 1982.
44. J. W. Hadden, E. M. Hadden, T. Spira, and Giner-Sorolla, *Int. J. Immunopharmacol.*, *4*:225 (1982).
45. I. Florentin, E. Taylor, M. Davigny, G. Mathé, and J. W. Hadden, *Int. J. Immunopharmacol.*, *4*:225 (1982).
46. A. Goutner, *Int. J. Immunopharmacol.*, *2*:197 (1980).
47. K. Oshimi, S. Kano, F. Takaku, and U. Kokumura, *JNCI*, *65*:1265 (1980).
48. A. Uchida,and T. Hoshino, *Cancer*, *45*:476 (1980).
49. T. Murayama, S. Natsuume-Sakai, K. Ryoyama, and S. Koshimura, *Cancer Immunol. Immunother.*, *12*:141 (1982).
50. A. Uchida and M. Micksche, *Int. J. Immunopharmacol.*, *3*:365 (1981).
51. S. A. Wolfe, D. E. Tracey, and C. S. Henney, *Nature*, *262*:585 (1976).
52. M. R. Potter and M. R. Moore, *Immunology*, *39*:427 (1980).
53. E. Ojo, O. Haller, and H. Wigzell, *Scand. J. Immunol.*, *8*:215 (1978).
54. A. Santoni, P. Pucetti, C. Riccardi, R. B. Herberman, and E. Bonmasser, *Int. J. Cancer*, *24*:656 (1979).
55. D. Cupissol, F. Favier, A. Rey, B. Longhi, C. Favier, and B. Serrou, in *Natural Cell-Mediated Immunity*, vol. II (R. B. Herberman, ed.), Academic Press, New York, 1982.
56. P. Hokland and J. Ellegard, in *Natural Cell-Mediated Immunity*, vol. II (R. B. Herberman, ed.), Academic Press, New York, 1982.
57. T. Aoki, H. Miyakoshi, Y. Horikawa, A. Shibata, and Y. Aoyagi, in *Natural Cell-Mediated Immunity* (R. B. Herberman, ed.), Academic Press, New York, 1982.
58. J. Wybran, B. Serrou, D. Belpomme, J. Boneterre, A. Desplaces, R. Favre, T. Ginsberg, J. M. Lang, G. Mayer, D. T. McKenzie, M. Micksche, D. C. Petit, G. Renoux, C.

C. Rosenfeld, M. Schneider, L. N. Simon, and L. Tojas, in *Current Concepts of Tumor Immunology and Cancer Immunomodulation* (B. Serrou, C. Rosenfeld, and J. Daniels, eds.), Elsevier/North Holland, New York, 1982.

59. L. Lacour, A. Spira, J. -Y. Petit, D. Sarrazin, J. Viguier, F. Lacour, M. Michelson, G. Delage, and G. Contesso, *Lancet*, :161 (1980).
60. H. J. Wanebo, M. Kemeny, C. M. Pinsky, Y. Hishaut, and H. F. Oettgen, *Ann. N. Y. Acad. Sci.*, *277*:288 (1976).
61. R. Lenzhofer, W. Graninger, A. Uchida, and M. Micksche, in *Current Chemotherapy and Immunotherapy* (P. Periti and G. G. Grassi, eds.), Am. Soc. Microbiol., 1982.
62. M. Yasue, M. Murakami, N. Hakazato, T. Suchi, and K. Ota, *Cancer Chemother. Pharmacol.*, *7*:5 (1981).
63. A. Uchida and T. Hoshino, *Cancer*, *45*:476 (1980).
64. A. Uchida and T. Hoshino, *Int. J. Cancer*, *26*:401 (1980).
65. M. Micksche, E. M. Kokoschka, R. Jakesz, Th. Luger, K. Moser, H. Rainer, P. Sagaster, A. Spitzy, and A. Uchida, in *Immunotherapy of Human Cancer* (W. A. Terry and St. A. Rosenberg, eds.), Elsevier/North Holland, New York, 1982.
66. M. Micksche, E. M. Kokoschka, Th. Luger, H. Rainer, C. Dittrich, K. Moser, R. Jakesz, A. Fritsch, M. Al-Hashimi, S. Yamagata, T. Hoshino, M. Colot, and A. Uchida, in *Human Cancer Immunology*, vol. III (B. Serrou and C. Rosenfeld, eds.), Elsevier Biomedical Press, 1982.
67. S. Matsurbara, F. Suzuki, and N. Ishida, *Cancer Immunol. Immunother.*, *6*:41 (1979).
68. A. S. Kadish, A. T. Doyle, E. H. Steinhauer, and N. A. Ghossein, *J. Immunol.*, *127/5*:1817 (1981).
69. A. Goutner, L. Schwarzenberg, and G. Mathé, in *Immunotherapy of Human Cancer* (W. A. Terry and St. A. Rosenberg, eds.), Elsevier/North Holland, New York, 1982.

Section B

Effects of Immunomodifiers on Thymus Lymphocytes

18
Levamisole

Willem K. Amery and Christian Hörig Janssen Pharmaceutica N.V. Research Laboratories, Beerse, Belgium

I. INTRODUCTION

Levamisole, the levoisomer of tetramisole, was first stereospecifically synthesized in 1966 and first became available as an anthelmintic for human use in 1968. The racemic compound tetramisole was already available as a dewormer in humans 2 years earlier. Le vamisole hydrochloride is a stable, white crystalline powder with a mol wt of 240.75. It is very soluble in water and aqueous acidic solutions, and soluble in polar solvents. In neutral buffer solutions and particularly in alkaline solutions, the solubility drops and hydrolysis takes place, yielding the poorly water-soluble racemate of 3-oxo-3(2-mercaptoethyl)-5-phenyl imidazoline (OMPI) which is in some studies considered the active principle or, at least, an active metabolite. The dextroisomer, dexamisole, is generally pharmacologically less active and in some tests completely inactive .

The first evidence of immunotropic properties of levamisole was obtained by Renoux and Renoux (1) in 1971, who observed in *Brucella*-vaccinated mice an increased immunity against *Brucella* infection after levamisole medication.

This observation must be considered a particularly lucky strike, because it marked the start of modern immunopharmacology. In this model, levamisole did not appear to act as a chemotherapeutic agent, but it enhanced the host-mediated defense capacity.

During about 10 years following the publication by Renoux and Renoux, an increasing number of studies has been performed which indicated the practical usefulness of levamisole in diseases where a reduced immunocompetence of the host may be suspected, and one tried to find an explanation of this activity, particularly by studying the cell-mediated immune mechanisms and by studying experimental cancer models. The growing number of results stimulated reviews (2-6) and monographs on specific subjects connected with levamisole, for example, rheumatism (7-9) and cancer (10-14), as well as symposia on the different aspects of the drug (15-19). The aim of the present review is to update the view on levamisole by means of a representative selection of publications from 1978 (4) until mid-1981.

II. PRECLINICAL INVESTIGATIONS

A. Pharmacology

Leaving aside its anthelmintic activity, other well-documented pharmacological properties of levamisole have mainly been observed at near to toxic or toxic dose levels. In vitro studies indicate a stimulation of parasympathetic and sympathetic ganglia, the latter effect being accompanied with inhibition of norepinephrine reuptake, which might be a pharmacological correlate to some antidepressive, positive inotropic and chronotropic as well as convulsant properties at high doses in vivo. Some investigators mention particularly the cholinomimetic properties of the drug, which might be of direct importance for the immunomodulating potential, because cholinergic activity results in an increased cell proliferation (20,21). It must be always kept in mind that the drug has no direct effect on bacteria, viruses, and fungi and that it is devoid of any cytotoxicity to normal and tumor cells (5). Within the context of its clinical use, levamisole is given to ameliorate the deficient host response: it has no direct effect on pathogens or degenerated cells.

B. Pharmacokinetics

Levamisole is rapidly absorbed from the gastrointestinal tract after oral administration and reaches peak plasma levels within 1-4 hr as indicated in cattle, calves, pigs, dogs, rats (22), and humans (23). The unchanged drug shows an elimination half-life of about 4 hr in humans. The major part is extensively metabolized in the liver and only about 5% of the unchanged drug was found in urine and feces. The elimination in humans is virtually complete after 48 hr. A comparison of in vitro and in vivo pharmacodynamics leads to the conclusion that the immunotherapeutic activity is not only due to the parent drug (21), since the immunological effect clearly survives the presence of analytically detectable quantities of the drug in blood and tissue. A triggering minimum effective concentration seems to be required for this immunological effect (24). More details on pharmacokinetics and metabolism were given in earlier summaries (4,7,25).

C. Toxicology

Toxicological data have been extensively reviewed in previous summaries (4,5,26). Main facts to retain are the very low acute oral toxicity in mice, rats, and rabbits and the absence of any sign of pathology after median and long-term treatment of rats and dogs with low and median doses. The high 20-mg/kg dose produced a hemolytic anemia in beagles after 2 months of treatment which is a species-specific hypersensitivity reaction. Carcinogenicity tests in rats and mice showed negative results. Reproduction studies in rats and rabbits demonstrated the absence of any teratogenic potential, and toxic signs were a consequence of maternal toxicity at high dose levels. Therefore, levamisole is a toxicologically safe compound, particularly if the 2.5-mg/kg/day schedule once or twice weekly or up to three times biweekly is followed.

D. Mechanism of Action

Several mechanisms of action have been proposed, but it is not clear at present which one is the most important.

Levamisole induces increased cyclic GMP (cGMP) levels in the immunocytes. Such an effect promotes proliferative and secretory functions and receptor reactivity in general, and of effector cells in particular. The imidazole ring seems to be one of the active moieties of the drug, responsible for the functional increase of peripheral T lymphocytes and macrophages, at least in the in vitro experiments. The thiol group is the other moiety which, however, appears only after hydrolysis of levamisole. Thiols, as many other antioxidants, have a great importance for the cellular redox potential. Another aspect is the indirect thymomimetic activity of the molecule which is mediated by a serum factor that does not depend on the presence of a functioning thymus (4). Finally, there is some preliminary evidence of calcium influx stimulation by levamisole and/or its metabolites into leukocytes, or of altered intracellular calcium distribution. Because of the well-known connection between calcium and the intracellular cyclic nucleotides, this effect could be a link to the mechanism of action (11). Therefore, it is all but sure that the levamisole effects would be monolithic. Moreover, different mechanisms may be operative, depending upon whether an experiment is performed in vitro or in vivo, and in a normal or a pathological system, respectively.

These introductory remarks concerning the relative uncertainty of the mechanism of action are not contradictory to the fact that many recent detail observations are available.

Cyclic nucleotide induction has been used for the explanation of the activation mechanism of human lymphocytes in a phytohemagglutinin (PHA)-induced proliferation experiment, in the lymphokine-induced macrophage proliferation, and the increased *Listeria*-killing activity (27). Human neutrophils show a nonsignificant enhancement of chemotaxis, probably as a result of cGMP increase (28), and the involvement of cyclic nucleotides in vitro is likely, because phosphodiesterase inhibitors (e.g., theophylline or adenosine) inhibit T-cell functions, whose effect is antagonized by levamisole or thymosin pentapeptide (TP5) (29). Another aspect in that field is the increase of adenosine deaminase by levamisole or TP5. The enzyme is defective in some cases of immunodeficiency (30). The contribution of cyclic nucleotides under in vivo conditions is less clear. In a noninfective inflammation model (acetic acid-induced pleurisy in rats), levamisole had a bidirectional action depending upon the concentration of the drug, and the effect showed time-dependent oscillations. Therefore, an inhibition of the thromboxane or prostaglandin synthetase systems was concluded which modulates the cyclic nucleotide synthesis (31). An interaction with these synthetases is also assumed by other authors. Mouse peritoneal cells showed in vitro after levamisole incubation a sharply decreased prostaglandin synthesis which was associated with a macrophage activation (32). Because the aggregation of human peripheral platelets is inhibited by levamisole in vitro, which is accompanied with a decreased oxygen consumption, cyclooxygenase inhibition might explain the prostaglandin synthesis suppression (33). Other authors explain the platelet aggregation by thromboxane synthetase inhibition (34). Free radicals and peroxides are inevitable products of metabolic cell functions and, at the same time, incompatible with life. For this reason, all organisms have developed certain protection and elimination systems which scavange and decompose these products. Antioxidants are very important in this process. Levamisole and its metabolites were tested in different systems to demonstrate the relation between immunomodulating and antioxidant properties. Levamisole was found to possess a purely antioxidant effect, whereas its decomposition product (OMPI) showed a biphasic profile: low concentrations are prooxidant, higher concentrations inhibit the peroxidation by formation of sulfhydryl metabolites, as indicated in a rat liver microsome system (35). Addition of peroxidase in the presence of H_2O_2 and iodide to peripheral human neutrophil suspensions inhibits random motility and chemotaxis. Levamisole and OMPI restore cell functions by inhibition of peroxide formation (36,37). Levamisole shares with other antioxidants the ability to stimulate the DNA synthesis which might be a key function (38). These biochemical processes proceed without additional energy requirements. The stimulation of glycolysis and an increased cell metabolism are not necessarily prerequisites of an increased neutrophil motility. Levamisole has no influence upon glycolysis, whereas ascorbic acid acts as a promoter, and both drugs improve neutrophil motility (39).

The protection of rats against carbon tetrachloride-induced liver damage by levamisole is ascribed to antioxidant effects (40). There is good evidence that the metabolite OMPI is mainly responsible for antioxidant cell protection. It is formed by catalytic hydrolysis in the presence of the ubiquitary ketoaldehyde methylglyoxal (41). An experiment with rat liver microsomes showed the transformation of levamisole into a sulfhydryl intermediate. A relation between antioxidant and immunological properties has not been found (42). In human embryonal fibroblast culture, OMPI was much more effective against autooxidative necrosis by glutathione depletion than levamisole (43). Another indicator of the importance of the levamisole metabolite is the increased E-rosette formation (ERF) in presence of viable lymphoid cells which form active metabolites with a free sulfhydryl group (44). Comparable results were obtained in a phagocytosis experiment in the presence of levamisole and nitrotetrazolium blue (NTB). Levamisole itself did not reduce the dye, but with increasing phagocytosis a parallel increased dye reduction was observed (45). Finally, the efficacy of diethyldithiocarbamate as an immunomodulator may support this assumption (20).

From these observations it can be concluded that the antioxidant effect of levamisole or its metabolite may indeed be a key effect because it increases the threshold of self-limitation of defense cell metabolism. This threshold is a natural block to prevent the accumulation of peroxides and free radicals, but can be detrimental in cases where a maximum defense activity is crucial.

III. IMMUNOMODULATION BY LEVAMISOLE

The influence of levamisole upon the immune system of normal and compromised hosts has been studied for 10 years, giving rise to an extensive series of papers describing detailed or summarized experimental or clinical results. It remains, however, a difficult and speculative task to extract common features concerning the mechanism of action, particularly since one is mainly dealing with the complex feedback mechanism of host defense processes in the living organism. Instructive reviews containing proposals for a mechanism of action are available (4,5,7,20,21,46). They can be summarized as follows.

Levamisole is able to restore to normal in vivo and in vitro the major functions of effector cells involved in cell-mediated host defense. Most pronounced effects are reached in hosts with subnormal T-lymphocyte or phagocyte functions. Adequate immune response usually remains unchanged, although some minor changes are possible. T lymphocytes show restoration of spontaneous and mitogen- or antigen-induced cell proliferation, active and total ERF capacity, lymphokine production, suppressor activity, and antibody plaque cell formation. The phagocyte function of polymorphonuclear cells, monocytes, and macrophages is normalized, including random migration, chemotaxis, antibody and complement receptor activity, adherence, phagocytosis, NTB reduction, and peroxidase activity. Levamisole does not directly influence B cells. There is, however, an influence of T cells upon B-cell activity, and one may observe a secondary effect on B cells. The effect in vivo can be a result of an enhanced maturation of circulating T cells and granulocytes. Another aspect is the induction of a serum factor which has thymopoietinlike properties but can be formed in athymic mice (4). Since the publication of the latter review, many experimental results have been published which confirm many of the older results and try to explain the different aspects of immunomodulation in vitro and in vivo.

A. General Investigations

1. In Vitro Experiments

In contrast to most of the clinical studies where a fixed dosage schedule was established, experimental and particularly in vitro studies still use very different drug concentrations. Therefore, the results must always be seen in the light of the experimental setup. Kalmár et al. (47) were able to exclude an influence of levamisole upon the ERF activity of normal human lymphocytes. They ascribed this observation to the functional state and activity of the T cells in their system. Hazama et al. (48). confirmed these findings, including the PHA blastogenesis, but detected an enhanced colony formation. Normal lymphocytes cannot be stimulated by levamisole to release a leukocyte-inhibitory factor, and the simultaneous presence of PHA even results in a suppression of this factor (49). Since a wide range of interactions between B and T lymphocytes and neutrophils may occur, the sometimes divergent experimental results must be interpreted bearing this confounding factor in mind. Levamisole does not directly act upon B cells. Helper T cells, however, act upon the B-cell population and enhance their immunoglobulin production (50). This is not the only effect, because an activation of suppressor T cells might inhibit the mitosis of B cells (51). Incoherent results are also attributable to the multiple influences upon T-cell subpopulations. Although a normal T-cell population cannot develop supranormal properties, some subpopulations can show different reactions. Even when the ERF reaction of the total population remains unchanged, the Tγ population may develop suppressor activity which is reflected after some days by a depressed B-cell population (52). In healthy organisms, levamisole may stimulate the physiologically inactive T_0 cells to form immunocompetent cells, which leads to the assumption of a constant total population with varying activities of the subpopulations (53). Monocytes from the umbilical blood of newborn infants have a lower phagocytic activity than cells from adults. Incubation of such cells in a levamisole solution matures the monocytes to the normal phagocytosis level (54). In a system of normal cells, levamisole may enhance the interaction between lymphocytes and monocytes, resulting in an increased proliferation of T cells (55). Increased ERF of lymphocytes from healthy volunteers taking a single dose of 150 mg levamisole is paralleled by an acidic phosphatase increase. Both effects may be explained by lysosome activation (56).

Physiological factors in health and disease may disturb the normal equilibrium. Histamine at moderate concentrations inhibits the PHA stimulation of lymphocytes, a reaction which is antagonized by levamisole (57). If serum from patients with Hodgkin disease or systemic lupus is added to normal lymphocytes, the ERF reaction becomes defective. Concomitant or previous addition of levamisole normalizes the reaction (58).

In conclusion, levamisole can shift the proportions within a healthy T-lymphocyte population, and this may secondarily influence B cells and their immunoglobulin production. Some proliferative action is possible. Finally, effects of physiological substances or pathogenic factors upon normal T cells can be antagonized.

The interaction with neutrophils is also complex. Lymphocyte stimulation may result in an increased lymphokine production which inhibits the leukocyte migration (59). However, depending upon the system, the opposite may also occur (49). Moreover, levamisole stimulates neutrophil motility and postphagocytic hexose monophosphate shunt activity, if the drug is applied under in vivo conditions (60).

The increased killing capacity of levamisole-treated granulocytes was indicated in a bactericidal assay (61). Levamisole-stimulated mononuclear leukocytes produce detectable amounts of interferon which might be responsible for virus-killing properties (62). Another noncellular reaction is the levamisole-induced increase in serum complement levels in vivo which might be important in cancer patients (63).

If in vitro experiments with lymphocytes of donors affected by various diseases are performed, the potential of levamisole becomes more clear. Lymphocytes from psoriatic patients can be stimulated to differentiate into more responsive T cells by pretreatment with levamisole or TPS (64).

Using lymphocytes from cancer patients, levamisole and TP5 block the induction of suppressor cells by concanavalin A (ConA) and restore the auto-rosette cell-forming activity which is a result of a modulation of helper and suppressor cells (65). Lymphocytes from tuberculosis patients who received a single dose of levamisole showed a normalized purified protein derivative (PPD)-induced lymphocyte transformation in those cases where the tuberculin skin test was previously negative (66). If the lymphocyte donors suffer from pancytopenia/aplasia, levamisole increases the number of T-lymphocyte colony-forming cells, which is subnormal in this disease as a consequence of monocyte dysfunction (67). The effect of levamisole is dependent on the stage of maturation of the lymphocytes. Azathioprine in vitro is able to inhibit the mitogen-induced blast formation. If the donor received levamisole treatment or the drug is added in vitro, this effect can be antagonized. Lymphocytes from umbilical blood are resistant to the levamisole effect, and their blast formation remains inhibited by azathioprine (68). Since the differences in lymphocyte reactivity to levamisole in healthy and diseased conditions might be receptor-mediated, trypsinized lymphocytes with damaged ERF receptors were investigated. Levamisole restored the ERF reaction and, hence, a stimulation of the protein and receptor synthesis, respectively, may be assumed (69). Although treatment of neutrophils from donors with recurrent infections in vitro resulted in increased chemotaxis and motility, oral therapy had no influence upon granulocytes (70). This indicates the difference between in vitro and in vivo results in the same subjects. Neutrophils from surgical patients without recall skin test antigen response showed an increased chemotaxis after in vitro addition of levamisole (71,72).

Although a secondary influence of levamisole upon immunoglobulin production cannot be excluded, neither treatment of allergic patients (73) nor addition of levamisole in vitro to lymphocytes of allergic or atopic patients resulted in consistent changes (73,74).

In conclusion, in vitro levamisole acts mainly toward a normalization of lymphocytes and neutrophils of ill donors. This effect, however, does not always have a clinical correlate.

2. Ex Vivo Experiments

The influence of levamisole on the immune mechanisms has been studied in various test systems. An experiment with lymphocytes from normal and *Mycobacterium bovis*-sensitized cattle demonstrated that levamisole increases the PPD blastogenesis in lymphocytes from sensitized animals only (75). Mouse macrophages harvested from subcutaneous coverslips fail to express an IgG surface receptor activity. Incubation with levamisole restores the Fc-receptor activity as indicated by ingestion of IgG-covered erythrocytes (76). Although levamisole has no influence upon chemotaxis of normal guinea pig macrophages, cells from casein-injected animals showed a clear stimulation by the drug. In vitro addition of *Rickettsia* or Bacillus Calmette-Guérin (BCG) cell walls to macrophages, followed by levamisole incubation, resulted in a stimulation of poorly reacting cells while highly reactive ones were tempered, which is another evidence of the immunomodulating rather than potentiating effect (77).

Another experiment which underlines the importance of the initial situation for the outcome is the addition of levamisole and/or inflammatory exudate to mouse macrophages. Normal cells remained unaffected while increased or decreased DNA synthesis rates were observed after addition of levamisole and the exudate, depending upon the time of addition (78). The problem of responders and nonresponders was studied by means of an in vitro model. Using lymphocytes and granulocytes from healthy human donors, different levamisole-binding capacities were found for specific lymphocyte subpopulations of the various subjects, which indicates differences in binding capacity and response (79). If mouse thymocytes were exposed to ConA alone or in combination with levamisole, the drug enhanced the cell proliferation as reflected by shortened cell cycles and an increased number of proliferating cells (80). Similar results were obtained in a comparison between levamisole and antioxidants: the DNA synthesis was enhanced whereas the RNA and protein synthesis remained unchanged in both groups. From that, the in vitro immunomodulation might be explained by an antioxidant effect (38). The addition of mercaptoethanol or cysteamine to the same system resulted in a proliferation inhibition, whereas penicillamine, glutathione, and cysteine had no effect (81). If OMPI was used in place of levamisole, the cell proliferation was even more enhanced than after levamisole, but mercaptoethanol acted again as a suppressant. From this experiment it has been concluded that levamisole is probably transformed into OMPI because the combination of this compound with mercaptoethanol acts as an antimitotic by affecting the microtubules (82). Similarly, as in human mononuclear leukocytes (62), an induction of interferon production in mouse spleen cells was found, particularly if an age-related drop had taken place (83).

3. In Vivo Experiments in Healthy Models

Sheep red blood cell injection into mice results in an antibody response reaction. This antibody-forming cell response can be potentiated by concomitant doses of 0.5 and 2.5 mg/kg levamisole, whereas 5 mg/kg has a suppressive effect. Drug administration was ineffective 1 day after sensitization or after administration to a spleen-cell sheep-erythrocyte system of nonsensitized mice (84). The injection of high doses of levamisole (2 or 20 mg/kg) to mice resulted immediately in a strongly decreased phagocytosis of ^{198}Au particles which is explained (85), as in another experiment (86), by the saturation of specific sites at the cell surface, responsible for the ingestive activity.

If guinea pigs are sensitized to levamisole by means of intradermal injections, an increased T-cell proliferation is observed. It has therefore been proposed that the immunomodulating activity would be due to a strongly sensitizing effect (87), but results from other authors classify this conclusion as less relevant. Rather, it may point to an immunological mechanism behind certain clinical side effects. The conclusion from observations under in vitro conditions using healthy animal preparations and from in vivo studies in healthy organisms has been drawn by Renoux et al. (88). The complex relationship between host, antigen, and immunopotentiator makes clear-cut relations impossible, particularly because genetic factors acting on the drug metabolism, enzyme activation, and T-cell function are involved.

4. In Vivo Experiments in Abnormal Models

The importance of health and disease for the response of a system to levamisole has already been appreciated in a former survey (4). Although the response of healthy mice to oxazolone sensitization remained unaffected by levamisole, the inhibition of this reaction by methotrexate was reversed (89). If levamisole was given during the BCG sensitization of rats, no immunomodulating effect was seen. If, however, the drug was given during the BCG challenge, an increased hypersensitivity was observed (90). Similarly, *Bordetella*-sensitized rats which were implanted with a *Bordetella*-containing sponge showed a much higher leukocyte migration after levamisole than nonsensitized animals. A stimulation of cell-mediated immune response in diseased but not in healthy conditions is concluded (91). The influence of immune dysregulation was shown by a mouse macrophage model from tumor-bearing mice. In vivo treatment as well as in vitro experiments showed an improvement of the phagocytic, cytostatic, and mitogenic responses of the macrophages after levamisole (92). Lymphocytes from rats with dimethylbenzanthracene-induced tumors regained their immunological potential after low-dose oral treatment, whereas higher doses had an immunosuppressive effect (93). If levamisole was given orally to mice 3 days after an IP peptone injection, the drug stimulated the catabolism of the antigen, whereas the phagocytosis remained unchanged after in vitro addition (94). Azocasein-induced amyloidosis in mice did not react when 1.8 mg of levamisole was injected per animal shortly after disease provocation. In this model, the high levamisole dose acted probably as an immunosuppressant (95). In a rat arthritis model where levamisole was locally applied by a sponge, responder rats, which were selected by a dextran edema test, reacted by a much higher leukocyte motility improvement than nonresponders or even normal controls (96). There are also other triggers than natural and artificial disease which can influence the immune response. Aged mice showed a restored ERF reaction after in vivo treatment, whereas in vitro addition to T cells remained ineffective. The importance of drug metabolism as an activation step is derived from this experiment (97). Zinc deprivation of rats results in a lowered mitogen response of their lymphocytes. Levamisole restores the reactivity, probably by a maturing effect upon immature T cells or differentiation of null cells. Normal lymphocytes are nonreactive (98). Malnourishment of rats results in a delayed cutaneous hypersensitivity and reduced ERF reaction. Levamisole normalized both reactions (99).

Another model is the graft-versus-host reaction after transplantation. Skin grafts in rabbits reacted differently to levamisole: the survival of the transplant was prolonged in normal animals, probably as a result of a stimulation of suppressor T cells, whereas the survival was shortened in burned rabbits because of a stimulation of cell-mediated immunity (100). Rats which were injected with a heterologous lymph node suspension showed an enhanced rejection if levamisole was given at days 5-7 after injection. Levamisole pretreatment of the injected lymphocytes in vitro was ineffective. The results are explained by an enhanced DNA synthesis and activation of immature cells in this system (101). The absence of an enhanced rejection of male skin transplants by female BALB/c mice under levamisole treatment might be understood as an expression of the immunomodulating properties of the drug, whereas some bacterial extracts yield an enhanced rejection and, therefore, are immunostimulators (102).

The modulation of the course and intensity of specific immune reactions as well as nonspecifically induced inflammatory responses by levamisole follows a similar pattern as the reaction to the thymus factor X. Therefore, a typically thymus hormonelike activity has been concluded not only from comparison of results but also from parallel experiments (103). In nude mice, a frequently used thymus-defective mouse model, levamisole produces an increased lymphoid population of the dysgenetic thymus, and this effect is similar to and even stronger than that of TP5 (104). The induction of Thy-1^+ cells from pre-T cells in nude mice was demonstrated by the depression of sd-DNA antibodies, while thymus-dependent antibodies were not affected. This probably means for this model a higher susceptibility of suppressor cells if compared with helper cells (105). Although levamisole produced some normalization in thymus-defective mice, the drug is unable to induce interferon production in these animals whereas normal controls show a clear increase (106). A comparison between nude mice and normal ones showed after levamisole and thymosin treatment an increased white blood count in both groups, but an elevation of colony-forming units in the defective ones only. This increase is explained by an increased stem cell activity which mobilizes dormant mesenchymal cell reserves, whereas in normal mice a depressionlike effect is observed as a result of a dilution by a greater population of mature cells (107).

In conclusion, levamisole yields a much stronger reaction in diseased than in healthy organisms. The choice of the dose range is very important, because high doses might be immunosuppressive. Thymus defects (e.g., in nude mice) are compensated for by levamisole, and, finally, the effect of levamisole is in many instances similar to that of thymopoietin. A clear answer to the question of whether or not levamisole or its metabolite(s) (e.g., OMPI) are (is) more important for the pharmacological activity, cannot be given by these results.

5. Clinical Implications: Treatment of Noninfectious, Noninflammatory Immune Defect Diseases

Levamisole was tested in some conditions which are frequently associated with an IgE excess (e.g., atopic dermatitis, bronchial asthma, or Buckley syndrome). For atopic dermatitis as a target symptom, the treatment was clinically and immunologically useless (108, 109). In patients with elevated IgE levels as a target symptom, levamisole produced within 8 weeks a reduction of the IgE levels in all patients. This was ascribed to a stimulation of the suppressor T lymphocytes resulting in a concomitant clinical improvement in 13 of 16 patients (110). In one Buckley syndrome child, the neutrophil chemotaxis was normalized in vitro, the IgE remained unchanged, but some clinical benefit was reported (111).

In tumor patients with a pathologically suppressed IgE level as a result of chemo- or radiotherapeutic measures, a 4-week levamisole treatment with two consecutive treatment days per week produced a highly significant increase in the IgE levels, probably as a result of T-lymphocyte maturation and B-lymphocyte stimulation (112).

Some injuries (e.g., burns or surgical interventions), as well as the physiological process of aging, result in a decreased response of the cellular immunity. In patients with burns, a normal levamisole regimen given for 3-5 weeks resulted in an improved course of the healing, less bacterial infections, a higher survival rate, and a reduction of the distance between the accident and skin grafting (113,144). The number of ERF cells was concomitantly normalized (113).

Postoperative immunodepression was reversed, and the response of lymphocytes to PHA stimulation increased in surgical patients with postoperative immunological anergy (115). Further, skin tests and neutrophil chemotaxis were improved, which resulted in a trend to less septic complications (116). Levamisole treatment of aged patients without malignancies for 3-6 months resulted in a restored skin test reactivity and an improved serum complement C3, C4, and factor-B levels which indicate a host-mediated immune response (118).

Finally, some noninfectious, noninflammatory diseases with poor treatment chances were included in levamisole trials. In six patients with sarcoidosis, levamisole increased the skin hypersensitivity reaction in three of them without any change in the clinical picture (119). In patients with fibrotic lesions of tuberculous origin without a positive tuberculin reaction, levamisole produced a positive skin reaction and increased the ERF reaction (120).

Levamisole treatment resulted in a clinical improvement in one child with cyclical neutropenia, while cessation provoked a deterioration, although neutrophil and monocyte counts remained unchanged (121). These results indicate the potential usefulness of levamisole in conditions with a clearly detectable immune defect. Whether or not the treatment has implications for the clinical picture remains a question of experience, because in some cases the improved immune situation was not associated with the expected clinical improvement.

B. Activity in Chronic Inflammatory Diseases

1. Inflammation Models and Anti-Inflammatory Mechanism

Since chronic inflammatory diseases can be defined as dysregulations of the immune system (i.e., an imbalance of cellular and humoral immune mechanisms), levamisole has been tried as a new therapeutic concept of the same category as penicillamine and gold compounds. In vivo and in vitro experiments are still ongoing to circumscribe the mode of action, and consequently, the position of the drug.

In the coverslip technique with healthy mice, levamisole yields an increased cell coverage and potentiates in adjuvant-arthritic rats the secondary arthritic lesions. These observations are explained by a stimulation of the macrophages (122). In the oxazolone-induced cutaneous basophil hypersensitivity reaction of mice, levamisole at very high doses (100 mg/kg) given before sensitization shows a suppression of the challenge reaction similar to penicillamine but different from cytostatics (123). Comparable results were obtained with picryl chloride-delayed hypersensitivity if levamisole doses of 50 mg/kg were given to mice before sensitization (124). These models indicate the dose dependence of levamisole effects but are without further implication to the practice. The immunosuppressive action of high concentrations of levamisole is supported by in vitro studies with skin of newborn rats. The drug inhibits the formation of soluble and insoluble collagen as indicated by the incorporation of [^{14}C] proline (125). A common biochemical property of levamisole, penicillamine, and gold thiomalate is to increase the sulfhydryl group reactivity in rheumatoid arthritis patients' serum as indicated by the thiol reagent 5,5'-dithiobis-2-nitrobenzoic acid. Levamisole shows this effect after oral treatment only; in vitro addition to the reaction mixture is ineffective. This indicates the possible involvement of thiol groups in the antirheumatic activity of levamisole as well as the importance of the formation of reactive metabolites (126). Some experimental results indicate the involvement of prostaglandins in the mechanism of action. Since levamisole and, similarly, penicillamine selectively release dihomo-γ-linolenic acid in tissue preparations from the stores, and this acid constitutes a precursor of prostaglandin E_1 (PGE_1) and controls autoimmune diseases, and since PGE_1 activates T lymphocytes and inhibits B lymphocytes, a prostaglandin mechanism cannot be excluded (127).

Immunological defects which are connected with systemic lupus erythematosus models poorly respond to levamisole. In female mice with a lupuslike syndrome, 25 mg/kg which was used in order to suppress helper cells and to increase the suppressor effect, reduced the antinuclear antibody titer but accelerated the nephritis (128). In another experiment using 2 mg/kg in mice, the survival was increased and the antinuclear antibody titer reduced; however, the renal involvement was unchanged (129). A dose of 20 mg/kg once weekly in New Zealand mice protected against anti-DNA antibodies, proteinuria, and lupus nephritis, but did not prevent the formation of antinuclear antibodies (130). The low reactivity of the lupus syndrome is also reflected by the in vitro resistance of mononuclear cells from SLE patients against the stimulation of the suppressor cell function by levamisole, which resembles the behavior of mononuclear cells from healthy persons (131). The result of levamisole treatment in autoimmune thyroiditis of mice depends on the timing, similar to the delayed hypersensitivity reactions to oxazolone (123) and picryl chloride (124): if the drug is given before the challenge, the thyroid infiltration and Tg-antibody formation are suppressed. Treatment after the challenge results in a slight increase. This underlines the role of cytotoxic T cells in the pathogenesis of experimental autoimmune thyroiditis (132).

Although the experimentally used inflammatory reactions are heterogeneous, which makes the divergent observations complementary rather than contradictory, two important features can be extracted: the importance of dosage and timing of the levamisole treatment for the therapeutic outcome and the resistance of some immune defects, such as lupus.

2. Clinical Implications: Treatment of Chronic Inflammatory Disease

Chronic rheumatoid arthritis has been successfully treated with levamisole as reported in summaries (4,7-9) and indicated by some recent reports (133-140). The efficacy was comparable to penicillamine (141) although the incidence of side effects was somewhat higher in one study (142). Attempts have been made to correlate experimental and clinical results. Although levamisole treatment resulted in an increased immediate and long-term phagocytic activity, there was no correlation with the clinical improvement (143).

Ceruloplasmin and IgG levels dropped under the therapy and simultaneous clinical improvement was reported (144). Furthermore, an improvement of the PHA-mitogen response of T cells, suppression of the B-cell function, and reduction of immunoglobulin and autoantibody levels were correlated with clinical improvement (145). The PHA-mitogen response seems to indicate whether patients are responders or nonresponders: after an 8-week treatment good responders show a more enhanced blast formation than nonresponders (146). In rheumatoid arthritis patients a T-cell subclass with receptor for the F_c portion of IgG was found to be increased as well as the helper T-cell immunoglobulin production. Levamisole treatment corrected both parameters (147). Isolated monocytes from rheumatoid arthritis patients demonstrated in an in vitro experiment the immunorestoring activity of levamisole. Cells from therapeutic responders showed an improved killer activity, if [^{51}Cr] labelled K562 erythroleukemia cells served as a substrate. The results may be of pivotal importance for the explanation of the immune deficiency in rheumatoid arthritis patients: a defective natural killer cell mechanism prevents the removal of pathologically changed host cells. There are, however, patients with a less defective killer cell function. This group might be one kind of nonresponders in levamisole treatment and indicates, at the same moment, the heterogeneity of the rheumatoid arthritis population (148). In addition to chronic rheumatoid arthritis, levamisole has been used in the treatment of several other inflammatory diseases of the rheumatoid and nonrheumatoid type.

Behçet's disease responds to a normal levamisole regimen by clinical improvement (149-152). Mild and inactive lupus erythematosus can improve clinically under levamisole (130,153,154), and lymphocytes from treated patients show an enhanced PHA reaction (155). Active lupus tends to deteriorate under treatment (156). Normal therapeutic doses of levamisole are ineffective in active Crohn's disease (157,158), whereas extremely high, immunosuppressive doses may have some positive effect. This is, however, beyond the intention of an immunotherapeutic treatment (159). Nephrotic syndrome in children responded very well to a normal dosage given on 2 consecutive days every week: the ERF cell count reached normal levels and complete remission was induced after 1-6 months of treatment (160). Erythema-multiforme patients did not show any improvement in skin reactivity or immunological parameters in vitro, although in seven patients with a cyclic disease pattern out of a total number of 13, positive clinical results were obtained (161). The usefulness of levamisole in multiple sclerosis is uncertain. Although this inflammatory autoimmune disease should be a target for levamisole, neither particularly positive nor negative effects have been observed in the past (4). In an in vitro study with peripheral lymphocytes from multiple sclerosis patients, levamisole was unable to increase the suppressor cell activity (162).

C. Activity in Cancer

1. Experimental Cancer Models and Ex Vivo Investigations

The mechanism of action of levamisole in cancer is at least as complex as in other diseases, and numerous models have been developed in order to find an explanation for the therapeutic activity.

Normal as well as phagocytosing human leukocytes were not influenced in their glucose metabolism if the concentration of levamisole remained below 10^{-2} mg/ml. The metabolic activity of acute myeloblastic leukemia cells was inhibited by 5×10^{-3} mg/ml. This indicates a possible hypermetabolism of some malignant cells and a regulatory effect of levamisole (163). Lymphocytes of acute lymphoblastic or nonlymphoblastic leukemia patients under the influence of levamisole develop in vitro a natural cytotoxicity against leukemia blasts which seems to be based upon interferon production as well as specific T-cell mediated toxicity (164). The colony-stimulating activity of human bone marrow and peripheral blood granulocytes of leukemic or preleukemic patients is increased by in vitro addition as well as previous oral administration of levamisole. A stimulation of the hematopoietic progenitor cells is suspected which mimicks a remission (165). Neutrophils from patients with hematological malignancies and lymphoma are unable to kill *Candida guilliermondii* in vitro. Addition of levamisole corrects this failure in most of the cases (166).(166). In concentrations of 2×10^{-2} mg/ml, levamisole stimulates the adherence of leukocytes from patients with prostatic cancer (167).

The necessity to remove the tumor as much as possible before levamisole treatment has been concluded from experimental and clinical experiences, since levamisole is devoid of any direct antitumor effect. If mice with plasmocytoma were treated with aniline mustard for tumor eradication, a consecutive levamisole treatment increased the resistance against tumor rechallenge and improved tumor cell neutralization. This is a result of a faster recovery of the T-cell competence which is normalized but not stimulated to supranormal levels (168). Extirpation of murine spontaneous mammary tumors followed by levamisole treatment remained without any evidence of tumor inhibition, although a marked immune response upon the drug was recognized (169). Dimethylhydrazine-induced bowel carcinoma in rats responded favorably to a combination of levamisole and *Corynebacterium parvum* extract with at least signs of tumor rejection, if the therapy was installed at an early tumor stage (170). After implantation of the carcinogen dimethylbenzanthracene into the submandibular gland of rats, levamisole was unable to prevent carcinogenesis, but it delayed the process (171). When a combined therapy consisting of splenectomy, injection of unblocking serum and lymphocytes, *C. parvum* extract, and levamisole was used in the treatment of dimethylhydrazine-induced gastrointestinal tumors of rats, the progress of tumor growth was suppressed, and many animals showed signs of tumor destruction (172). Injection of methylcholanthrene-induced fibrosarcoma cells in mice resulted in an early tumor death of the animals. If five to nine doses of levamisole were given from the first day of inoculation on, a significant prolongation of the survival interval was observed after 10^3 cells, whereas 10^6 cells obviously exceeded the host defense (173). This is a good model for the necessity of tumor reduction. In rats with dimethylbenzanthracene-induced mammary tumors, it was shown that levamisole, as well as adriamycin alone, inhibited the growth of small tumors. Monotherapy against large tumors, however, appeared ineffective, whereas combined treatment inhibited tumor growth (174).

Levamisole was ineffective against implanted mammary adenocarcinomas in mice. A combination with cyclophosphamide improved slightly the antitumor effect but was without any influence upon the survival period (175). Levamisole alone slightly increased the metastasis formation after KHT sarcoma implantation in mice. If x-ray therapy was combined with levamisole, a significantly increased tumor control was obtained (176).

From a similar experimental setup, it was concluded that pure immunotherapy in cancer should be avoided, whereas a combination of cytostatic measures with not more than one immunostimulant looks very promising (177). Macrophages from mammary carcinoma-bearing mice showed a reduced colony formation. Low levamisole doses normalized this dysfunction, whereas high doses were suppressive. Colony formation parallels tumor inhibition if cyclophosphamide is given concomitantly; increased macrophage cytotoxicity alone is not related to any signs of tumor suppression (178). Experiments with fibrosarcoma cell-injected mice indicated the enhanced immune response after minimal doses of levamisole while excessive doses suppressed the defense (179). From a lymphoma experiment in chemotherapeutically treated mice, it is concluded that immunotherapy should be applied in the drug-free intervals after tumor surgery (180). A positive interaction with the cytocidal effect of 6-mercaptopurine riboside has been observed in L 1210 cell-bearing mice, although levamisole did not contribute to a life prolongation (181). Mice which received levamisole and fibrosarcoma cell vaccine, an immunoprophylactic antitumor agent, reached a higher tumor-specific resistance level than upon the vaccine alone (182).

This result is similar to that obtained by Renoux in the *Brucella* experiment. In a study with L 1210 tumor vaccine and levamisole in normal mice, it was shown that neither the vaccine nor levamisole alone was able to improve the outcome after a tumor challenge. If, however, the vaccine was bound to ConA, 0.38 mg/kg levamisole produced an optimal immunomodulation which resulted in some complete cures (183). In Wilms' tumor-implanted rats treated with high levamisole doses, the medication had an immunosuppressive effect; 4 mg/kg were neither tumoricidal nor preventively active while 1 mg/kg yielded a significant tumor reduction. This underlines the necessity of careful clinical dosage (184). The clinically used dosage delays the onset of transplanted transitional cell carcinoma growth as well as the growth velocity in mice. This results in a prolonged survival and can be interpreted by an increased tumor resistance (185). More survivors and a prolonged survival interval were also observed after lymphoma implantation in mice. The effect was comparable with that of a *Brucella* vaccine (186). In Ehrlich ascites carcinoma or S-180 sarcoma-bearing mice treated with bacterial preparations for immunostimulation alone or together with antitumor chemotherapy, further improvement was reached as indicated by a prolonged survival, if levamisole was given 1 to several days after the medication. The distance between administration of the bacterial extract and levamisole to reach a maximum survival was different in several therapeutic combinations. This indicates the importance of accurate timing of adjuvant levamisole treatment (187). Beyond a stimulation of normal murine lymphocytes in vitro, levamisole similarly stimulated the growth of some types of leukemia cells and reduced the survival of P1798-implanted mice. From this system a stimulation of the immune system as well as the tumor growth is derived (188).

Although results from experimental cancer models cannot be translated into clinical terms, some important aspects of the levamisole therapy can be derived. The outcome depends upon quality and quantity of the tumor. Slow proliferation and low cell numbers increase the efficacy of the immunotherapy. This underlines the importance of surgical, chemotherapeutic, or radiotherapeutic reduction of the tumor load. Moreover, the dosage has a key function, since high doses have an immunosuppressive effect and low doses are ineffective. Finally, the timing seems to be important as indicated by some experimental models, and an early start is always better than a later one.

2. Clinical Implications: Treatment of Cancer

As cancer has been recognized to be a syndrome of immune dysregulation and disturbed immunological monitoring, the use of the immunomodulator levamisole was a logical consequence. Many reports are available and the drug was one of the main subjects at the Second International Conference: "Immunotherapy of Cancer: Present Status of Trials in Man" in Bethesda, Maryland, April 1980.

In the past some reviews summarized the aspects of cancer treatment with levamisole (see Introduction), including the possible mechanisms of action and potential benefit (189). There is an absolute necessity of previous tumor reduction by chemotherapy, radiotherapy, or surgery (6). The clinical experience resulted in two standard schedules, that is, 150 mg or 2.5 mg/kg daily on 2 consecutive days a week or the same dose on 3 consecutive days every 2 weeks during the chemotherapy-free intervals (24). The latter tended to be superior and had a smaller risk of side effects. Such a fixed schedule reduces the danger of a sudden agranulocytosis and of immunosuppression instead of immunorestoration.

In the evaluation of the levamisole effect in cancer, two different approaches were followed: first the use of immunological parameters and their improvement as a more theoretical indicator and, second, the survival as a measure of the clinical efficacy as a more practical approach, particularly since the importance of certain immunological parameters in cancer remains an open question. In several cases, the survival rate is discussed in the light of improved immunological parameters (e.g., PPD and DNCB skin reaction) which were enhanced parallel with life prolongation (190). Since, however, the present contribution deals with the mechanism of action, trials which investigate survival will not be reviewed.

From a study including 50 patients with advanced cancer it has been questioned whether levamisole can outweigh the tumor-related depression of delayed cutaneous hypersensitivity (191), whereas a trial with chemotherapeutically or surgically treated patients indicated the best benefit in those where the circulating lymphocytes and, hence, cellular immunity were particularly damaged at start (192). Another parameter is the circulating α_2-globulin fraction which has immunosuppressive properties and increases with the progress of the disease. After surgery as well as levamisole therapy the α_2-globulin level drops (193). Levamisole produced in 10 patients with liver cell carcinoma after intake on 3 consecutive days a reactivation of the PPD skin test in three patients and a transient suppression of the α-fetoprotein level in six patients. Pure immunotherapy is said to be insufficient, since the transfer factor also yielded unsatisfactory results (194). Monocytes of levamisole treated bladder cancer patients showed a similar increase in motility and chemotaxis as monocytes from healthy donors in a levamisole solution, whereas drug intake was ineffective in healthy volunteers. The importance of this short-lived effect is not clear (195). Postsurgical colorectal cancer patients on chemotherapy showed during levamisole treatment an increased reactivity of lymphocytes in the PHA transformation test, whereas the PHA skin test remained unchanged (196). Postoperative immunosuppression after colorectal cancer surgery was partly neutralized by levamisole as indicated by a more rapid return to preoperative leukocyte migration inhibition in presence of tuberculin or tumor extract, whereas the lymphoblast transformation in the presence of PHA remained unchanged (197). In order to prevent the surgery-related drop in lymphocyte proliferation, gastric and colon cancer patients received from day -3 until 8 weeks after the operation 150 mg levamisole on 3 consecutive days every 2 weeks. They benefited from this treatment as indicated by the mitogen-induced blast formation, the stimulation index, the number of active T cells, and the enhanced PPD skin reaction after 2 weeks. This treatment aimed at reduction of postoperative metastasis liability (198). The same authors report a continuous increase in PHA blast formation after levamisole in postsurgical gastric cancer patients, whereas an untreated group needed 4 weeks to reach the preoperative level (199).

Although levamisole usually has a favorable effect on survival time, relapse-free interval, and seeding of metastases or, at least, no deteriorations are reported, one report mentions a higher incidence of nontumor death by cardiorespiratory failure in the levamisole group after surgery. This observation has been tentatively explained by the formation of antimyocardial antibodies (200). The formation of such antibodies seems rather improbable, and external factors might be responsible (201). Coincidence may be all the more likely in this study since its randomization was very heavily stratified. Excessive stratification may carry the risk of increasing the probability that randomization produces two different populations.

Finally, in Hodgkin patients who were in remission, levamisole increased in the beginning the number of positive skin tests and decreased the quantity of circulating immune complex. After a 3-month period of 150 mg three times weekly in 2 weeks, some decline was observed, particularly in some patients who received higher doses (202). In lymphocyte-deficient Hodgkin patients, levamisole was ineffective, whereas one patient with preserved T-cell function showed mitogen response (203).

D. Activity in Infectious Diseases

1. Experimental Infections and Ex Vivo Investigations

Immunorestoring effects have been studied in experimental models which cover the range from viral to helmintic infections.

The drug was ineffective against intranasal herpes simplex infections in newborn mice (204). Encephalomyocarditis-M virus in mice is known to be particularly suppressive against mitogen response of lymphocytes and produces at the same time glycosuria. Levamisole restored the blast formation as indicated by [^{3}H] thymidine incorporation, but exacerbated glycosuria, probably by stimulating T cells which attack the Langerhans' β cells (205).

An in vitro study with neutrophils from tuberculosis patients showed an impaired chemotaxis. The defect was corrected by addition of levamisole to the suspension (206). If *Escherichia coli* was preincubated with levamisole, an increased digestion of the bacteria was found in a meningitis model in rabbits (207).

It appeared impossible to yield a higher resistance against subsequent worm infections if *Schistosoma* preparations were combined with levamisole treatment in mice. This can be explained by the fact that levamisole has immunorestoring and not immunostimulating properties (208). Treatment of schistosomiasis in *Macaca fascicularis* tended to be more effective if killed schistosomula vaccine was combined with two doses of tetramisole on the first and third day after the vaccine injection. The suboptimal results might be a consequence of a suboptimal dosage of tetramisole, 1.25 mg/kg (209).

From all these results it can be concluded that the classic effect of levamisole which was observed for the first time by Renoux and Renoux (1) can be reproduced in some other vaccination models. Moreover, the drug has some positive influence upon the course of viral infections, while the immunotherapeutic concept in the treatment of worm infections or leishmaniasis was less favorable.

2. Clinical Implication: Treatment of Infectious Diseases

There is a close relation between many infections and a suppression of the host defense which, in turn, results in an increased liability to further infections. Moreover, nutritional deficiency increases the risk of infections and enhances the vicious circle. Therefore, levamisole might be useful to interrupt this sequence. Symoens et al. (4) give a good survey of trials and results of the past.

A short-term treatment of malnourished children during critical periods of stress (e.g., infections) might be useful because the impaired lymphocyte function is improved by this treatment (210). Infectious inflammatory skin diseases, for example, inflammatory acne (211), skin furunculosis (212), and recurrent chronic pyoderma (213), are a result of or occur at least concomitantly with impaired lymphocyte and neutrophil functions. Levamisole normalizes the blood cell functions in vitro and, at the same time, clinical improvement or cures were obtained. The treatment of some chronic bacterial infections, for example, brucellosis (214), meloidosis (215), tuberculosis (216-219), or leprosy (220, 221), appears promising insofar as levamisole improves the disease or treatment-dependent suppression of the cellular immunity. However, levamisole is not suitable for a monotherapy and must be used, as in cancer treatment, as an adjuvant to chemotherapy. It is compatible with the standard chemotherapeutics and has been shown to produce better clinical results in some studies than chemotherapeutics alone (215,218,221). In patients with chronic fungal infections, particularly in chronic mucocutaneous candidiasis (222,223) and aspergillosis (224), cellular immunity is frequently disturbed as indicated by in vitro tests with neutrophils and lymphocytes. Although cellular immunity was improved after some weeks in both trials, no clinical correlation was found.

Viral infections seem to be a more suitable target for levamisole since, in addition to the immunorestoration, some interferon-inducing properties were found. Although expectations frequently remained unverified in the past (225), some positive reports from controlled studies have become available. Recurrent infections, particularly of the upper respiratory tract, are in children a rather frequent condition associated with an impaired neutrophil function (i.e., chemotaxis, bacterial killing, and phagocytosis). Different treatment schedules were applied, but in all cases significantly fewer episodes of infection, with a shorter duration and less severity, were found, particularly if compared with a placebo (226-230). However, an increased recurrence rate in comparison with the placebo group was found in one herpes simplex trial, although levamisole clearly diminished duration and painfulness of the episodes (231). In herpetic keratitis, a combination of levamisole with a standard topical treatment was more effective than topical treatment alone. This was paralleled by a normalization of the ERF reaction (232). In a trial including various central and peripheral nervous diseases probably of viral origin, levamisole had a positive influence upon remission in herpes zoster (233). Although some normalization of immunological parameters is reported after levamisole treatment of patients with chronic HBsAg-positive hepatitis, this effect was never associated with any clinical improvement (234-238). Therefore, as earlier stated (225), levamisole is useless as a monotherapy in the treatment of chronic hepatitis.

IV. ADVERSE REACTIONS AND THERAPEUTIC BENEFIT

Because levamisole has already been used in a large number of patients, side effects have been reviewed in several reports (4,18,239-241). One of the greatest advantages of the drug is the absence of unwanted interactions with drugs which are an obligatory medication in some indications: antibiotics (215,218,221), antineoplastics (242) and acetylsalicylic acid (243,244). The most prominent side effect still is blood dyscrasia which occurs in the form of agranulocytosis, leukopenia, or thrombocytopenia. Several clinical reports in the recent literature describe the occurrence of agranulocytosis with uneventful recovery after cessation of the drug (245) and sometimes antibiotic protection of the patients (246-249).

The HLA genotype B 27 seems to be particularly predisposing to the development of agranulocytosis, especially in females with rheumatoid arthritis (250-252). Cases of agranulocytosis in diseases other than rheumatoid arthritis are rare, but this adverse reaction has been documented, for example, in a female scleroderma patient (253), a female cancer chemotherapy patient (254), and a male Behçet patient (255), all of the HLA-B-27 type. The risk of blood dyscrasia in cancer patients can be further reduced by a treatment schedule of 3-day treatment in a 2-week interval (190) or in rheumatoid arthritis patients by a single 150-mg dose weekly (136,139). Agranulocytosis is attributed to an antibody formation which results in granulocytotoxicity (256,257). The immune complexes are absorbed by granulocytes, and this process initiates complement activation and lysis (258,259). That reaction occurs although levamisole does not directly damage the granulopoiesis (242). It was suspected to be more frequent after discontinuing cancer chemotherapy (260), but this remained unconfirmed. The phenomenon depends upon a hapten mechanism which cannot be reproduced in vitro (256). Leukopenia is a less incisive side effect which occurs in rheumatoid arthritis patients at a similar percentage as in gold- or penicillamine-treated patients (261). Recovery is possible without withdrawal of the drug (262), and it must not be interpreted as a sign of an impending agranulocytosis.

A rather rare adverse reaction is thrombocytopenia (4,263). Some patients suffer from cutaneous side effects (e.g., lichenoid eruptions and rash). The supposed origin of these reactions is an increased T-cell activity (264) or an allergic reaction (265,266). Again, the phenomena disappear upon drug withdrawal. Active Crohn's disease may be particularly predisposing to side effects. Patients might react with exacerbation (267), arthralgia, and erythema (268). Case reports describe two cases of rheumatoid arthritis patients, one suffering from proteinuria and immunoglobulin deposits after a 10-month treatment (269) and the other showing ulceration of the rectal and oral mucosa after a 6-week treatment (270).

From these observations it can be concluded that the recent literature did not contribute to a more extended list of side effects but to the finding of criteria which allow to a certain degree their prevention, that is, selection of patients (4,18,239-241) and an appropriate dosage schedule (136,139,190). If all measures are taken to prevent serious consequences of agranulocytosis, levamisole is a safe drug whose therapeutic benefit outweighs in many indications the potential risks. Moreover, it is a scientifically stimulating drug, because it allows not only the treatment of some immunodeficiency diseases, but it initiated many studies and will continue to do so in the future to find out why and where it is therapeutically effective. And this is of great importance for the further development of immunopharmacology.

REFERENCES

1. G. Renoux and M. Renoux, *C.R. Acad. Sci. (D) (Paris)*, *272*:349 (1971).
2. P. A. J. Janssen, in *Progress in Drug Research* (E. Jucker, ed.), Vol. 20, Birkhäuser, Basel, 1976, p. 347.
3. D. A. Willoughby and C. Wood, *Forum of Immunotherapy*, Vol. 1(1), The Royal Society of Medicine, London, 1977.
4. J. Symoens, J. De Cree, W. F. M. Van Bever, and P. A. J. Janssen, in *Pharmacological and Biochemical Properties of Drug Substances* (M. E. Goldberg, ed.), Vol. 2, Am. Pharm. Assoc. Acad. Pharm. Sci., Washington, D. C., 1979, p. 407.
5. G. Renoux, *Drugs*, *19*:89 (1980).
6. W. K. Amery and D. A. Gough, *Oncology*, *38*:168 (1981).
7. A. G. Mowat and T. L. Vischer, *Eular Monograph Series*, Vol. 5, EULAR Publishers, Basel, 1979.
8. J. Symoens and M. Rosenthal, *J. Reticuloendothel. Soc.*, *21*:175 (1977).
9. J. Symoens and Y. Schuermans, *Clin. Rheum. Dis.*, *5*:603 (1979).
10. W. K. Amery, *J. Reticuloendothel. Soc.*, *24*:187 (1978).
11. W. K. P. C. Amery, *Ann. Clin. Res.* (Suppl. 27) *12*: (1980).
12. M. A. Chirigos, *Modulation of Host Immune Resistance in the Prevention or Treatment of Induced Neoplasia*, DHEW Publications, Washington, D.C., 1974.
13. M. A. Chirigos, *Progress in Cancer Research and Therapy*, Vol. 2, Raven Press, New York, 1977.

14. M. A. Chirigos, *Progress in Cancer Research and Therapy*, Vol. 7, Raven Press, New York, 1978.
15. D. A. Willoughby and C. Wood, *Forum on Immunotherapy*, Vol. 1(2), The Royal Society of Medicine, London, 1977.
16. D. A. Willoughby, A. J. Cochran, L. Israel, R. D. Thornes, E. M. Hersh, L. M. Jerry, and W. K. Amery, *Forum on Immunotherapy*, Vol. 2(1), The Royal Society of Medicine, London, 1978.
17. D. A. Willoughby and C. Wood, *Forum on Immunotherapy*, Vol. 2(2), The Royal Society of Medicine, London, 1979.
18. D. A. Willoughby and C. Wood, *Forum on Immunotherapy*, Vol. 3(1), The Royal Society of Medicine, London, 1979.
19. D. A. Willoughby and C. Wood, *Forum on Immunotherapy*, Vol. 3(2), The Royal Society of Medicine, London, 1979.
20. G. Renoux, *T.I.P.S.*, *2*:248 (1981).
21. G. Goldstein, *J. Rheumatol.* (Suppl. 4) *5*:143 (1978).
22. G. Graziani and G. L. De Martin, *Drugs Exp. Clin. Res.*, *2*:221 (1977).
23. G. Graziani and G. L. De Martin, *Drugs Exp. Clin. Res.*, *2*:235 (1977).
24. W. K. Amery and B. S. Butterworth, *Int. J. Immunopharmacol.*, *5*:1 (1983).
25. J. G. Adams, *J. Rheumatol.* (Suppl. 4) *5*:137 (1978).
26. W. H. Hsu, *J. Am. Vet. Med. Assoc.*, *176*:1166 (1980).
27. J. W. Hadden, A. Englard, J. R. Sadlik, and E. M. Hadden, *Int. J. Immunopharmacol.*, *1*:17 (1979).
28. Pham Huu Trung, *Biomedicine*, *30*.121 (1979).
29. F. Laghi Pasini, A. Auteri, L. Ceccatelli, and T. Di Perri, *Boll. Soc. Ital. Biol. Sper.*, *56*:317 (1980).
30. F. Laghi Pasini, A. Auteri, A. L. Pasqui, A. E. Speri, and T. Di Perri, *Int. J. Immunopharmacol.*, *2*:176 (1980).
31. A. Bertelli, M. I. Schinetti, and R. Greco, *Int. J. Tissue React.*, *1*:123 (1979).
32. D. A. Stringfellow, F. A. Fitzpatrick, F. F. Sun, and J. C. McGuire, *Prostaglandins*, *16*:901 (1978).
33. D. Del Principe, A. Menichelli, B. M. Tallarida, M. Gabriotti, F. Mastracchio, L. M. Colella, S. Del Vecchio, and C. D'Arcangelo, *Res. Commun. Chem. Pathol. Pharmacol.*, *25*:307 (1979).
34. Y. Hokama, A. H. Morita, M. A. Abad, B. S. Joyo, D. A. Uchida, and G. W. Fischer, *Res. Commun. Chem. Pathol. Pharmacol.*, *19*:141 (1978).
35. K. S. Kumar, C. R. Dobbs, J. F. Weiss, and M. A. Chirigos, *J. Immunopharmacol.*, *2*:73 (1980).
36. R. Anderson, R. Oosthuizen, and G. Grabow, *Int. J. Immunopharmacol.*, *3*:123 (1981).
37. R. Anderson, *Int. Arch. Allergy Appl. Immunol.*, *65*:257 (1981).
38. J. Van Wauwe and J. Goossens, *Ann. Immunol. (Paris)*, *130C*:756 (1979).
39. R. Anderson, A. Glover, and A. R. Rabson, *Immunology*, *35*:141 (1978).
40. T. Yoshikawa, *Int. J. Immunopharmacol.*, *2*:178 (1980).
41. H. Van Belle and P. A. J. Janssen, *Biochem. Pharmacol.*, *28*:1313 (1979).
42. K. S. Kumar, M. A. Chirigos, and J. F. Weiss, *Int. J. Immunopharmacol.*, *1*:85 (1979).
43. M. De Brabander, H. Van Belle, F. Aerts, R. Van de Veire, and G. Geuens, *Int. J. Immunopharmacol.*, *1*:93 (1979).
44. H. -G. Opitz, G. Hewlett, and H. -D. Schlumberger, in *Macrophage Regulation of Immunity* (E. R. Unanue and A. S. Rosenthal, eds.), Academic Press, New York, 1980, p. 415.
45. C. Eschenbach, W. Hahm, and D. Becker, *Blut*, *39*:383 (1979).
46. W. K. Amery, *J. Reticuloendothel. Soc.*, *24*:187 (1978).

47. L. Kalmár, P. Gergely, K. Nékám, I. Láng, and Gy. Petrányi, *Acta Med. Acad. Sci. Hung.*, *35*:21 (1978).
48. S. Hazama, K. Hirose, Y. Ishikawa, K. Saito, H. Enokihara, H. Komatsu, S. Furusawa, and H. Shishido, *Igaku no Ayumi*, *110*:220 (1979).
49. E. Jirillo, D. Colucci, A. De Santis, and I. Munno, *Ann. Sclavo*, *19*:1264 (1977).
50. P. Hersey, K. Ho, J. Werkmeister, and U. Abele, *Clin. Exp. Immunol.*, *46*:340 (1981).
51. T. Miyawaki, H. Seki, N. Moriya, T. Nagaoki, M. Kubo, N. Okuda, and N. Taniguchi, *Clin. Exp. Immunol.*, *40*:161 (1980).
52. N. Moriya, T. Miyawaki, H. Seki, M. Kubo, T. Nagaoki, N. Okuda, and N. Taniguchi, *Scand. J. Immunol.*, *10*:535 (1979).
53. A. O. Lyapon, K. A. Lebedev, and A. L. Mashkilleison, *Biull. Eksp. Biol. Med.*, *89*:630 (1980).
54. K. E. Schult and D. A. Powell, *Pediatrics*, *65*:501 (1980).
55. J. W. Kazura, W. Negendank, D. Guerry, and A. D. Schreiber, *Clin. Exp. Immunol.*, *35*:258 (1979).
56. G. Ippoliti, G. Marini, R. Invernizzi, M. Aloc-Spiriti, G. Cattaneo, and G. Di Noi, *Haematologica (Pavia)*, *63*: No. 5 (1978).
57. K. Meretey, G. Room, and R. N. Maini, *Agents Actions*, *11*:84 (1981).
58. G. S. Del Giacco, S. Tognella, A. L. Leone, F. Locci, P. Cornaglia, A. Sangiuolo, and V. Grifoni, *Blood*, *53*:1002 (1979).
59. L. C. Giraudo Conesa and G. Astaldi, *Sangre (Barc.)*, *24*:18 (1979).
60. R. Anderson, R. Oosthuizen, A. Theron, and J. N. Van Rensburg, *Clin. Exp. Immunol.*, *35*:478 (1979).
61. P. Palmblad and L. Engstedt, *Acta Pathol. Microbiol. Scand. (C)*, *87*:357 (1979).
62. A. Rhodes-Feuillette, M. Canivet, J. M. Andrieu, and J. Périès, *Biomedicine*, *31*:170 (1979).
63. H. Kato, N. Yokoe, S. Takemura, T. Yoshikawa, M. Matsumura, K. Nishida, T. Hotta, K. Watanabe, Y. Furukawa, Y. Wakamatsu, H. Tagami, and M. Kondo, *Rinsho Yakuri*, *11*:161 (1980).
64. J. Eskola, E. Soppi, O. Ruuskanen, and J. E. Fräki, *Arch. Dermatol. Res.*, *263*:335 (1978).
65. B. Serrou, J. Caraux, C. Thierry, and A. Goldstein, Abstract of *Meeting on Immunological Aspects of Experimental and Clinical Cancer*, Tel Aviv, October 28-November 1, 1979, p. 143.
66. E. M. S. Gatner, *S. Afr. Med. J.*, *59*:109 (1981).
67. M. Y. Gordon, J. A. King, and E. C. Gordon-Smith, *Clin. Exp. Immunol.*, *44*:117 (1981).
68. L. Ivanyi, *Clin. Exp. Immunol.*, *38*:370 (1979).
69. K. Nékám, H. H. Fudenberg, B. Mándi, I. Láng, P. Gergely, and Gy. Petrányi, *Immunopharmacology*, *3*:31 (1981).
70. A. R. Rabson, R. Anderson, and A. Glover, *Clin. Exp. Immunol.*, *33*:142 (1978).
71. J. L. Meakins and N. V. Christou, *Surg. Forum*, *29*:1 (1978).
72. N. V. Christou and J. L. Meakins, *Surgery*, *85*:543 (1979).
73. Kue-Hsiung Hsie, *Ann. Allergy*, *44*:91 (1980).
74. R. O'Connor, J. Ring, A. A. Jalowayski, and R. N. Hamburger, *Clin. Allergy*, *10*:705 (1980).
75. J. M. B. Kaneene, S. P. Kumar, D. W. Johnson, D. J. Klausner, E. D. Sloane, and C. C. Muscoplat, *Vet. Sci. Commun.*, *3*:237 (1979).
76. M. Mariano and B. E. Malucelli, *J. Pathol.*, *130*:33 (1980).
77. M. T. Kelly, *J. Reticuloendothel. Soc.*, *24*:139 (1978).
78. M. Pelletier, D. A. Willoughby, and J. P. Giroud, *J. Reticuloendothel. Soc.*, *24*:333 (1978).

79. K. Ogawa, T. Nakayama, and E. Tsubura, *Int. J. Immunopharmacol.*, *2*:165 (1980).
80. I. G. Otterness, M. L. Bliven, and H. E. Holden, Jr., *Immunopharmacology*, *1*:245 (1979).
81. I. G. Otterness, A. J. Torchia, and M. L. Bliven, *Cell. Immunol.*, *43*:62 (1979).
82. I. G. Otterness and M. L. Bliven, *Int. J. Immunopharmacol.*, *2*:23 (1980).
83. S. K. Tyring and S. S. Lefkowitz, *Experientia*, *36*:1323 (1980).
84. J. V. Fahey, B. M. Clancy, and F. S. Szmalc, Jr., *Immunol. Commun.*, *8*:241 (1979).
85. R. M. Bergoc, R. A. Caro, J. N. Feierstein, J. E. Ihlo, A. J. Olivari, and A. F. Rojas, *Int. J. Nucl. Med. Biol.*, *4*:209 (1977).
86. N. L. Astorri, R. M. Bergoc, R. A. Caro, H. N. Glait, J. E. Ihlo, and A. J. Olivari, *Int. J. Nucl. Med. Biol.*, *6*:124 (1979).
87. J. L. Turk and D. Parker, *Int. Arch. Allergy Appl. Immunol.*, *58*:237 (1979).
88. G. Renoux, M. Renoux, and J. -M. Guillaumin, *Int. J. Immunopharmacol.*, *1*:43 (1979).
89. D. E. Griswold and D. T. Walz, *Inflammation*, *3*:111 (1978).
90. E. Bramm, L. Binderup, and E. Arrigoni-Martelli, *Acta Pharmacol. Toxicol.* (*Copenh.*), *44*:75 (1979).
91. F. M. Cunningham, A. W. Ford-Hutchinson, A. M. Oliver, M. J. H. Smith, and J. R. Walker, *Br. J. Pharmacol.*, *63*:119 (1978).
92. S. Okubo, M. Morimoto, N. Nakamura, and M. Tanaka, *Cancer Chemother.* (*Japan*), *7*:1272 (1980).
93. D. Sampson, *J. Oral Pathol.*, *7*:383 (1978).
94. A. Cruchaud, M. Berney, and H. D. Welscher, *Int. J. Immunopharmacol.*, *1*:49 (1979).
95. D. N. Rush, A. R. Bridges, M. Skinner, A. S. Cohen, and R. M. Lindsay, *J. Immunopharmacol.*, *2*:553 (1980).
96. G. Griffiths and G. B. West, *Int. Arch. Allergy Appl. Immunol.*, *61*:107 (1980).
97. C. Morimoto, T. Abe, and M. Homma, *Clin. Immunol. Immunopathol.*, *12*:316 (1979).
98. R. L. Gross, N. Osdin, L. Fong, and P. M. Newberne, *Am. J. Clin. Nutr.*, *32*:1267 (1979).
99. S. O. Olusi, W. J. E. Jessop, and A. Shoroye, *Pediatr. Res.*, *13*:1237 (1979).
100. J. Niedworok, M. Offierska, and W. Lambrecht, *Z. Exp. Chir.*, *13*:151 (1980).
101. H. Sikorska, *Arch. Immunol. Ther. Exp.* (*Warsz.*), *28*:565 (1980).
102. S. Seo, J. Yasuhara, and K. Saeki, *Agents Actions*, *9*:344 (1979).
103. J. Gieldanowski, *Arch. Immunol. Ther. Exp.* (*Warsz.*), *29*:121 (1981).
104. A. Machoninová, Z. Rychter, M. Holub, L. Korčáková, and B. Mándi, *Folia Biol.* (*Praha*), *24*:424 (1978).
105. T. Ogita, T. Hayakawa, Y. Horiuchi, and Y. Mizushima, *Int. Arch. Allergy Appl. Immunol.*, *59*:222 (1979).
106. S. Matsubara, F. Suzuki, and N. Ishida, *Cell. Immunol.*, *43*:214 (1979).
107. S. Dolenská, M. Holub, and B. Mándi, *Folia Biol.* (*Praha*), *24*:421 (1978).
108. A. Alomar, J. M. Giménez-Camarasa, and J. M. de Moragas, *Arch. Dermatol.*, *114*: 1316 (1978).
109. C. R. White and J. M. Hanifin, *Arch. Dermatol.*, *114*:1314 (1978).
110. G. M. Halpern and C. Lévy, *Med. Hyg.*, *37*:110 (1979).
111. A. Rebora, E. Nunzi, M. Pezzuolo, F. Patrone, F. Dallegri, and C. Sacchetti, *Br. J. Dermatol.*, *99*:569 (1978).
112. G. Schlegel and M. Lüthgens, *Tumor Diagnostik*, *4*:219 (1980).
113. F. Mazzoleni, A. Chiarelli, A. Corsano, O. Dal Lago, and U. Fagiolo, *Riv. Ital. Chir. Plast.*, *11*:1 (1979).
114. G. Renoux, M. Renoux, and J. M. Greco, *Ann. Chir. Plast.*, *24*:57 (1979).

115. F. Puppo, G. Corsini, G. F. Adami, and J. Zattoni, *Br. J. Surg.*, *66*:599 (1979).
116. J. L. Meakins, N. V. Christou, H. M. Shizgal, and L. D. McLean, *Ann. Surg.*, *190*: 286 (1979).
117. N. Yokoe, H. Kato, S. Takemura, T. Yoshikawa, M. Kondo, K. Hosokawa, and M. Kodama, *Jpn. J. Clin. Oncol.*, *9*:209 (1979).
118. M. Kondo, H. Kato, and M. Masuda, *N. Engl. J. Med.*, *298*:1146 (1978).
119. P. J. Cole, K. M. Citron, P. N. Plowman, T. G. J. R. Evans, and R. M. Vick, *Br. J. Dis. Chest*, *73*:367 (1979).
120. Z. Katona, Zs. Bösze, I. Gajó, and Gy. Milassin, *4th European Immunology Meeting*, Budapest, April 12-14, 1978.
121. S. J. Proctor, M. M. Reid, and W. T. Low, *Postgrad. Med. J.*, *55*:39 (1979).
122. M. S. Koh and D. A. Willoughby, *Agents Actions*, *9*:284 (1979).
123. J. Bure and F. Degrand, *Agents Actions*, *9*:534 (1979).
124. J. P. Tarayre and H. Lauressergues, *J. Pharm. Pharmacol.*, *32*:584 (1980).
125. Z. Trnavská, D. Mikuliková, K, Trnavský, and J. Rovenský, *Z. Rheumatol.*, *37*:221, (1978).
126. N. D. Hall and A. H. Gillan, *J. Pharm. Pharmacol.*, *31*:676 (1979).
127. D. F. Horrobin, *Med. Hypotheses*, *6*:687 (1980).
128. B. H. Hahn and L. L. Knotts, *Arthritis Rheum.*, *22*:236 (1979).
129. J. A. Menchaca, S. S. Lefkowitz, S. Tyring, and B. Bartholomew, Abstract of *American Society of Nephrology Meeting*, November 1978.
130. A. Horiuchi, K. Irimajiri, Y. Kazuta, K. Hashimoto, and K. Tsubaki, *Kinki Daigaku Igaku Zasshi*, *4*:379 (1979).
131. A. Rabson, S. Blank, and R. Lomnitzer, *Immunopharmacology*, *2*:103 (1980).
132. A. O. Vladutiu, *Fed. Proc.*, *40*:1138 (1981).
133. T. Di Perri, A. Auteri, and F. Laghi Pasini, in *Advances in Inflammation Research* (G. Weissmann, ed.), Vol. 1, Raven Press. New York, 1979, p. 605.
134. P. Franchimont, G. Heynen, H. Berghs, J. Remans, and P. Vroninks, *Scand. J. Rheumatol.*, *8*:43 (1979).
135. P. J. Lewi and J. Symoens, *J. Rheumatol.*, *4*:17 (1978).
136. Multicenter Study Group, *Ann. Rheum. Dis.*, *41*:159 (1982).
137. Multicentre Study Group, *Lancet*, *ii*:1007 (1978).
138. E. M. Veys and H. Mielants, *J. Rheumatol.* (Suppl. 4) *5*:31 (1978).
139. E. M. Veys, H. Mielants, G. Verbruggen, E. Dhondt, L. Goethals, L. Cheroutre, and H. Buelens, *J. Rheumatol.*, *8*:45 (1981).
140. B. Miller, P. de Merieux, R. Srinivasan, P. Clements, Peng Fan, J. Levy, and H. E. Paulus, *Arthritis Rheum.*, *23*:172 (1980).
141. A. G. Mowat and A. M. Mowat, *J. Rheumatol.*, *8*:575 (1981).
142. Z. Husain and L. A. Runge, *J. Rheumatol.*, *7*:825 (1980).
143. K. M. Wynne, P. A. Dieppe, J. Scott, and E. C. Huskisson, *Ann. Rheum. Dis.*, *40*: 382 (1981).
144. K. L. Schmidt and V. R. Ott, *Verh. Dtsch. Ges. Rheumatol.*, *6*:143 (1980).
145. J. Levy, *J. Rheumatol.*, *4*:63 (1978).
146. J. Levy, *Cancer Treat. Rep.*, *62*:1715 (1978).
147. J. Tanaka, J. Yata, S. Irimajiri, Y. Matsuoka, M. Tomii, T. Sugano, and H. Tanaka, *Clin. Immunol. (Japan)*, *10*:828 (1978).
148. F. A. Barada, W. O'Brien, and D. A. Horwitz, *Arthritis Rheum.*, *25*:10 (1982).
149. P. de Merieux, L. E. Spitler, and H. E. Paulus, *Arthritis Rheum.*, *24*:64 (1981).
150. T. Lehner and J. M. A. Wilton, in *Behçet's Syndrome: Clinical and Immunological Features* (T. Lehner and C. T. Barnes, eds.), Academic Press, London, 1979, p. 291.
151. T. Lehner and J. M. A. Wilton, in *Drugs and Immune Responsiveness* (J. L. Turk and D. Parkers, eds.), Macmillan, London, 1979, p. 119.

152. B. Graisely, O. Margueritte-Renard, M. Cloarec, and J. Debray, *Nouv. Presse Med.*, *8*:867 (1978).
153. O. Scherak, J. Smolen, G. Kolarz, M. Kojer, and J. Menzel, *Wien. Klin. Wochenschr.*, *91*:758 (1979).
154. K. Ogawa, T. Sano, G. Hisano, and E. Tsubara, *Ann. Allergy*, *43*:187 (1979).
155. H. Hoshina, *J. Jpn. Soc. Intern. Med.*, *68*:16 (1979).
156. T. Hadidi, J. L. Decker, L. El-Nagdy, and M. Samy, *Arthritis Rheum.*, *24*:60 (1981).
157. E. T. Swarbrick and D. P. O'Donoghue, *Lancet*, *i*:392 (1979).
158. J. Villand and H. Carli, *Nouv. Presse Med.*, *8*:3271 (1979).
159. P. Tixier, J. B. Verger, M. Rabia, P. Bardeche, and L. Brodi, *Nouv. Presse Med.*, *7*:3942 (1978).
160. P. Tanphaichitr, D. Tanphaichitr, J. Sureeratanan, and S. Chatasingh, *J. Pediatr.*, *96*:490 (1980).
161. F. Lozada, L. Spitler, and S. Silverman, Jr., *Int. J. Immunopharmacol.*, *2*:63 (1980).
162. J. P. Antel, B. G. W. Arnason, and M. E. Medof, *Ann. Neurol.*, *5*:338 (1979).
163. G. W. Fischer, J. O'Brien, Y. Hokama, D. Maybee, and S. C. Chou, *Cancer Treat. Rep.*, *62*:1637 (1978).
164. B. Sharma, L. F. Odom, and J. Tilles, *Proceedings of the American Association of Cancer Research*, Vol. 21, 1980, p. 203.
165. J. S. Senn, C. C. Lai, and G. B. Price, *Br. J. Cancer*, *41*:40 (1980).
166. J. A. Child, S. Martin, J. C. Cawley, and A. T. M. Ghoneim, *Biomedicine*, *29*:159 (1978).
167. S. Zamora, R. A. Bhatti, R. J. Ablin, R. Rao, G. Baumgartner, and P. D. Guinan, *Cell. Mol. Biol.*, *25*:57 (1979).
168. M. L. Padarathsingh, J. H. Dean, J. L. McCoy, D. D. Lewis, and J. W. Northing, *Cancer Treat. Rep.*, *62*:1627 (1978).
169. D. Valdivia, R. H. Page, R. W. Talley, and R. A. Huseby, *Proceedings of 17th Annual Meeting of the American Association for Cancer Research*, May 16-19, 1979, p. 20.
170. H. O. Sjögren, *Cancer*, *45*:1229 (1980).
171. S. Pisanty, E. Eisenberg, and G. Shklar, *Arch. Oral Biol.*, *23*:131 (1978).
172. B. R. Bansal, J. Mobini, and S. C. Bansal, *Cancer*, *42*:2079 (1978).
173. T. Ashizawa, O. Shuji, M. Morimoto, N. Nakamura, K. Mineura, and M. Tanaka, *Cancer Chemother.* (*Japan*), *7*:707 (1980).
174. T. Tominaga, M. Kitamura, T. Saito, and I. Itoh, *Eur. J. Cancer*, *16*:1489 (1980).
175. D. M. Purnell, G. L. Bartlett, J. W. Kreider, T. G. Biro, and J. Kontra, *Cancer Res.*, *39*:4838 (1979).
176. D. Baker, Meng-lai Lim, D. Elkon, W. Constable, and H. Wanebo, *Proceedings of 17th Annual Meeting of the American Association for Cancer Research*, May 16-19, 1979, p. 269.
177. B. Fisher, J. Linta, J. Hanlon, and E. Saffer, *J. Natl. Cancer Inst.*, *60*:391 (1978).
178. B. Fisher and M. Gebhardt, *Cancer Treat. Rep.*, *62*:1919 (1978).
179. J. J. Gozzo and R. H. Hanson, *Transplant. Proc.*, *11*:1420 (1979).
180. M. C. Caprino, A. Barzi, L. De Vecchis, E. Menconi, and A. Bonmassar, *Abstract of 7th International Congress of Pharmacology*, Paris, July 16-21, 1978, p. 68.
181. T. Miura, E. Nogiwa, S. Kurashige, and T. Maekawa, *Cancer Res.*, *40*:4813 (1980).
182. M. Okabe, M. Morimoto, K. Mineura, N. Nakamura, and M. Tanaka, *Cancer Chemother.* (*Japan*), *7*:835 (1980).
183. T. Kataoka, S. Tsukagoshi, Y. Sakurai, and M. Okabe, *Gann*, *70*:515 (1979).
184. Z. Wajsman, P. D. Williams, and G. P. Murphy, *Oncology*, *35*:212 (1978).
185. D. L. Lamm, G. N. Yee, D. F. Reichert, and H. M. Radwin, *Invest. Urol.*, *16*:286 (1979).
186. M. A. Chirigos, R. M. Schultz, N. Pavlidis, D. S. Feingold, and J. S. Youngner, *Cancer Treat. Rep.*, *62*:1943 (1978).

187. S. Yamagata, T. Koh, M. Oride, and T. Hattori, *Cancer Immunol. Immunother.*, *7*:217 (1980).
188. W. C. Gordon and M. D. Prager, *J. Natl. Cancer Inst.*, *61*:415 (1978).
189. W. K. Amery, *Int. J. Immunopharmacol.*, *3*:339 (1981).
190. T. Okayasu, T. Takeoka, Y. Moriyama, N. Shinzato, M. Kawabata, M. Hashimoto, T. Tanabe, and S. Sugie, *Gan to Kagaku-Ryoho*, *7*:1479 (1980).
191. Y. Hirshaut, C. M. Pinsky, I. Frydecka, H. J. Wanebo, S. Passe, V. Miké, and H. F. Oettgen, *Cancer*, *45*:362 (1980).
192. E. M. Hersh, Y. Z. Patt, G. M. Mavligit, S. G. Murphy, J. U. Gutterman, K. Dicke, and G. Spitzer, in *Human Lymphocyte Differentiation: Its Application to Cancer* (B. Serrou and C. Rosenfeld, eds.), INSERM Symposium No. 8, Elsevier/North Holland, Amsterdam, 1978, p. 375.
193. T. Sakai, T. Ikeda, S. Kitamura, T. Mori, S. Kaseda, and I. Ito, *Int. J. Immunopharmacol.*, *2*:178 (1980).
194. M. Sano, M. Adachi, Y. Fukuda, T. Takeuchi, K. Ito, N. Waseda, T. Shimizu, and K. Nakajima, *Cancer Chemother.* (*Japan*) (Suppl. 3), *6*:95 (1979).
195. S. D. Nathanson, P. L. Zamfirescu, J. K. Portaro, J. B. deKernion, and J. L. Fahey, *J. Natl. Cancer Inst.*, *61*:301 (1978).
196. T. Akao, S. Fujimoto, B. Itoh, Y. Kitsukawa, M. Takahashi, H. Ishigami, T. Minami, and M. Miyazaki, *Cancer Chemother.* (*Japan*), *7*:1063 (1980).
197. R. Windle, R. F. M. Wood, and P. R. F. Bell, *Br. J. Surg.*, *66*:507 (1979).
198. H. Miwa, T. Kawai, H. Nakahara, and K. Orita, *Int. J. Immunopharmacol.*, *2*:31 (1980).
199. H. Miwa, T. Kawai, and K. Orita, *Okayama Igakkai Zasshi*, *90*:1151 (1978).
200. H. M. Anthony, A. J. Mearns, M. K. Mason, D. G. Scott, K. Moghissi, P. B. Deverall, Z. J. Rozycki, and D. A. Watson, *Thorax*, *34*:4 (1979).
201. W. K. Amery, *Thorax*, *34*:141 (1979).
202. E. Berényi, M. Kávai, M. Szabolcsi, and Gy. Szegedi, *Acta Med. Acad. Sci. Hung.*, *36*:177 (1979).
203. M. Björkholm, G. Holm, and H. Mellstedt, *Cancer Immunol. Immunother.*, *8*:205 (1980).
204. C. Strulovitch, M. I. Marks, A. Soneji, and S. Goldberg, *J. Antimicrob. Chemother.*, *5*:437 (1979).
205. G. A. Warchalowski and H. R. Strausser, *Immunol. Commun.*, *8*:443 (1979).
206. E. M. S. Gatner and R. Anderson, *Clin. Exp. Immunol.*, *40*:327 (1980).
207. T. R. Beam, Jr. and J.C. Allen, *J. Infect. Dis.*, *142*:72 (1980).
208. S. E. Maddison, S. B. Slemenda, F. W. Chandler, and I. G. Kagun, *J. Parasitol.*, *64*:986 (1978).
209. K. D. Murrell, S. S. Clark, D. A. Dean, and W. E. Vannier, *Exp. Parasitol.*, *48*:415 (1979).
210. R. K. Chandra, *Bull. WHO*, *57*:167 (1979).
211. J. De Cree, W. De Cock, and H. Verhaegen, *Biomedicine*, *31*:95 (1979).
212. J. I. Gallin, D. G. Wright, H. L. Malech, J. M. Davis, M. S. Klempner, and C. H. Kirkpatrick, *Ann. Intern. Med.*, *92*:520 (1980).
213. D. Djawari and O. P. Hornstein, *Dermatologica*, *161*:116 (1980).
214. M. Raptopoulou-Gigi, J. Kountouras, and G. Goulis, *J. Immunopharmacol.*, *2*:85 (1980).
215. D. Tanphaichitra, S. Vanwari, Y. Siristonpun, and K. Promjunyakul, *Chest*, *75*:646 (1979).
216. D. Tanphaichitra, *Bull. Int. Union Tuberc.*, *54*:175 (1979).
217. D. Tanphaichitra, Y. Siristonpun, and K. Promjunyakul, *International Congress of Inflammation*, Bologna, October 31, 1978.
218. M. M. Singh, P. Kumar, A. N. Malaviya, and R. Kumar, *Am. Rev. Respir. Dis.*, *123*:277 (1981).

219. G. Daddi, S. Ferrari, P. A. Mancini, and A. Contini, *Boll. Ist. Sieroter. Milan.*, *58*:104 (1979).
220. J. C. Souza Carvalho, W. M. Hildebrand, S. Migdal, and A. Wakamatsu, *Folho Med.*, *7*:193 (1979).
221. M. Galmarini, C. M. Riera, J. Ripoll, M. A. Orozco, and J. Katz, *Med. Cutan. Iber. Lat. Am.*, *6*:179 (1978).
222. A. C. Ferguson, H. E. Kershnar, W. K. Collin, and E. R. Stiehm, *Am. J. Clin. Pathol.*, *68*:499 (1977).
223. D. Djawari, *Z. Hautkr.*, *54*:403 (1979).
224. G. Daddi, G. De Ritis, P. A. Mancini, and A. Stefanini, *Boll. Ist. Sieroter. Milan*, *58*:273 (1979).
225. A. S. Russel, *Drugs*, *20*:117 (1980).
226. A. Rebora, F. Dallegri, and F. Patrone, *Br. J. Dermatol.*, *102*:49 (1980).
227. M. Van Eygen, F. Dils, J. Gillerot, and E. Verschueren, *Eur. J. Pediatr.*, *131*:147 (1979).
228. M. Hatala, *Cas. Lek. Cesk.*, *117*:467 (1978).
229. F. Dils, *J. Int. Med. Res.*, *7*:302 (1979).
230. F. De Loore, E. Heck, M. Van Eygen, and J. Casneuf, *Curr. Med. Res. Opin.*, *6*:142 (1979).
231. S. L. Spruance, G. G. Krueger, J. MacCalman, J. C. Overall, Jr., and M. R. Klauber, *Antimicrob. Agents Chemother.*, *15*:662 (1979).
232. M. C. Voci, P. Pivetti-Pezzi, I. Quinti, and F. Aiuti, *Int. J. Immunopharmacol.*, *2*:165 (1980).
233. A. Gentile, B. Pannone, A. M. Fasanaro, C. Mazza, and G. Scoleri, *Acta Neurol. (Napoli)*, *33*:365 (1978).
234. M. Masi, P. Paolucci, G. Timoncini, M. P. Fantini, F. Chiodo, and C. Franceschi, *Boll. Ist. Sieroter. Milan.*, *57*:471 (1978).
235. F. Milazzo, E. Ghezzi. M. Resta, M. A. Brugo, D. Vitali, G. M. Vigevani, and G. C. Tassi, *Boll. Ist. Sieroter. Milan*, *57*:477 (1978).
236. G. Giuliani Piccari, F. Sarti, N. D'Imperio, G. Formica, M. Milandri, and M. Soffritti, *Acta Gastroenterol. Belg.*, *41*:356 (1978).
237. R. G. Chadwick, S. Jain, B. J. Cohen, G. M. Scott, H. C. Thomas, and S. Sherlock, *Scand. J. Gastroenterol.*, *15*:973 (1980).
238. A. Pár, K. Barna, G. Bajtai, I. Hollós, M. Ambrus, M. Kovács, and T. Jávor, *Acta. Med. Acad. Sci. Hung.*, *37*:269 (1980).
239. J. Symoens, E. Veys, M. Mielants, and R. Pinals, *Cancer Treat. Rep.*, *62*:1721 (1978).
240. R. S. Pinals, *J. Rheumatol.* (Suppl. 4), *5*:71 (1978).
241. H. Mielants and E. M. Veys, *Acta Rhumatol. Belg.*, *3*:104 (1979).
242. W. Schreml and H. -P. Lohrmann, *Blut*, *38*:331 (1979).
243. H. R. Rumble, P. M. Brooks, and M. S. Roberts, *Br. J. Clin. Pharmacol.*, *7*:631 (1979).
244. P. M. Brooks, M. S. Roberts, R. Rumble, and N. Johnson, *Clin. Exp. Pharmacol. Physiol.*, *6*:176 (1979).
245. A. Du P. Heyns, F. P. Retief, and B. J. Vorster, *S. Afr. Med. J.*, *55*:177 (1979).
246. B. Kaplan, C. Cardarelli, and S. R. Pinnell, *Cutis*, *24*:429 (1979).
247. A. Rossard, J. Barrier, M. Audran, P. Dubigeon, J. -Y. Grolleau, and D. Hervouët, *Nouv. Presse Med.*, *8*:593 (1979).
248. A. Laurens, P. Schmit, R. Monteil, J. Meadeb, and R. Martoia, *Med. Armees*, *6*:319 (1978).
249. M. Krogh Jensen, J. Eriksen, H. Andersen, and P. A. Østergaard, *Dan. Med. Bull.*, *26*:14 (1979).

250. K. L. Schmidt, C. Mueller-Eckhardt, and H. Breithaupt, *Klin. Wochenschr.*, *56*: 1189 (1978).
251. K. L. Schmidt, C. Mueller-Eckhardt, H. Breithaupt, H. Löffler, and V. R. Ott, *Verh. Dtsch. Ges. Rheumatol.*, *6*:131 (1980).
252. L. Hodinka, P. Géher, K. Merétey, E. K. Gyódi, G. Gy. Petrányi, and S. Bozsóki, *Int. Arch. Allergy Appl. Immunol.*, *65*:460 (1981).
253. P. Choutet, G. Lorette, and M. Renoux, *Nouv. Presse Med.*, *8*:1262 (1979).
254. S. Gundersen and S. D. Fossa, *Cancer Immunol. Immunother.*, *7*:271 (1980).
255. M. Hamza and H. Ben Ayed, *Nouv. Presse Med.*, *8*:3167 (1979).
256. J. S. Thompson, J. M. Herbick, L. W. Klassen, C. D. Severson, V. L. Overlin, J. W. Blaschke, M. A. Silverman, and C. L. Vogel, *Blood*, *56*:388 (1980).
257. S. I. Drew, B. M. Carter, D. S. Nathanson, and P. I. Terasaki, *Ann. Rheum. Dis.*, *39*:59 (1980).
258. J. G. Pegels, A. E. G. Kr. von dem Borne, L. L. M. Thomas, G. N. Tytgat, and C. P. Engelfriet, *Clin. Lab. Haematol.*, *2*:339 (1980).
259. C. L. Vogel, M. A. Silverman, P. W. Mansell, A. M. Miller, J. S. Thompson, J. M. Herbick, D. E. Brunskill, D. C. Padgett, E. C. McKinney, and E. V. Sugarbaker, *Am. J. Hematol.*, *9*:171 (1980).
260. M. Silverman, J. Thompson, A. Miller, P. Mansell, E. Sugarbaker, C. McKinney, and C. Vogel, *Proceedings of 15th Annual Meeting of the American Society of Clinical Oncology*, May 14-15, 1979, p. 381.
261. W. Ebner, P. Petera, A. Dunky, G. Tausch, and R. Eberl, *Verh. Dtsch. Ges. Rheumatol.*, *6*:421 (1980).
262. G. T. Williams. S. A. N. Johnson, P. A. Dieppe, and E. C. Huskisson, *Ann. Rheum. Dis.*, *37*:366 (1978).
263. J. Lanng Nielsen, *Ugeskr. Laeger*, *142*:171 (1980).
264. J. D. Kirby, M. Black, and D. McGibbon, *J. R. Soc. Med.*, *73*:208 (1980).
265. L. Secher, H. Permin, P. Stahl Skov, S. Ullman, and P. Halberg, *Acta. Derm. Venereol. (Stockh.)*, *58*:372 (1978).
266. D. G. Macfarlane and P. A. Bacon, *Br. Med. J.*, *I*:407 (1978).
267. J. Villand and H. Carli, *Nouv. Presse Med.*, *8*:3753 (1979).
268. J. L. Dupas, J. P. Capron, J. Delamarre, and A. Lorriaux, *Nouv. Presse Med.*, *8*:1350 (1979).
269. T. M. Hansen, J. Petersen, P. Halberg, H. Permin, S. Ullman, C. Brun and S. Larsen, *Lancet*, *ii*:737 (1978).
270. G. V. H. Bradby, M. F. Shadforth, and A. M. Hoare, *Ann. Rheum. Dis.*, *38*:399 (1979).

19

Lentinan, a T-Cell-Oriented Immunopotentiator

Its Experimental and Clinical Applications and Possible Mechanism of Immune Modulation

Junji Hamuro Central Research Laboratories, Ajinomoto Co., Inc., Yokohama, Japan

Goro Chihara National Cancer Center Research Institute, Tokyo, Japan

I. INTRODUCTION

In spite of the enormous efforts made by numerous researchers in the world, a decisive pharmaceutical agent against cancer has not appeared except for a few that have been effective for some leukemias and for certain types of cancer having a special characteristic. Antitumor agents that attack cancer cells directly accompany detrimental toxic side effects to the host, and reduce the host resistance against cancer or infections, especially by destroying lymphoid cells and bone marrow cells, which have been recently considered to play an important role in host defense-surviellance mechanisms against cancer.

On the other hand, there are some reliable clinical evidences suggesting the existence of an intrinsic resistance against cancer in the human body, and the experimental evidence has also claimed that the host possesses a capability to attack even autochthonous tumors through a cell-mediated immune reaction.

From such a viewpoint, we have reexamined a great number of folk remedies said to be effective against cancer for a long time in Japan and Asian countries, and have found that lentinan, a polysaccharide isolated from the hot-water extract of fruit-body of *Lentinus edodes* (Berk.) Sing., the most popular edible mushroom in Japan, completely regresses sarcoma 180 (solid form) transplanted subcutaneously in Swiss or CD-1/ICR mice (1,2).

At present, lentinan not only stimulates the rejection of a foreign graft such as an allogeneic tumor, but also inhibits the growth of various kinds of syngeneic and autochthonous tumors, and prevents chemical and viral carcinogenesis. Lentinan is also effective in bacterial, viral, and parasitic infections. The results of phases I, II, and III trials of lentinan for patients with advanced or recurrent gastric, colorectal, breast, lung cancer, and malignant lymphoma are very hopeful. Among numerous immunomodulating agents, lentinan has drawn much attention from experimental and clinical oncologists as a potent immunotherapeutic agent against neoplastic diseases as well as against clonic obstinate infections.

Recently, the mode of action mechanism of lentinan has been extensively clarified in immunological and biological terms, and distinct characteristics of the action mode of lentinan to reject a wide scope of not-self have been claimed compared with other known immunomodulators. Main immunopharmacological characteristics of lentinan reside in the T-cell-dependent immunopotentiation and in the action of lentinan functioning as maturation factors of lymphoid cells.

This review concerns experimental and clinical application of lentinan and its possible mechanisms of immune modulation.

II. CHEMISTRY

In contrast to Bacillus Calmette-Guérin (BCG), *Corynebacterium parvum*, and many other immunopotentiators of polyanionic nature, lentinan is distinct in that it is chemically a strictly defined polysaccharide sufficiently purified after extraction and in that its physical and chemical characteristics are completely clarified (2). Therefore, biological activities of lentinan are reproducible, and no differences are observed from lot to lot; and this defined chemical nature of lentinan greatly promotes the further analysis of biological, physiological, and immunological characteristics of lentinan to know the real action mode against neoplastic diseases.

Lentinan is a β-1,3-glucan with average molecular weight of 500,000 daltons, and its repeating unit is composed of five β-1,3-glucopyranoside linkages with two β-1,6-glucopyranoside-linked branches (2,3). Thus, lentinan is composed of only glucose with no other sugar component. Elementary analysis verified the molecular formula as $(C_6H_{10}O_5)_n$ consistent with structural elucidation, and no nitrogen, phosphorous, and sulfur were detected. According to x-ray analysis, lentinan is shown to have a triple-helix structure (4). The higher-order structure or micelle formation in the solution seems to have an important role in their physiological activities. Pachyman and laminaran, which possess the same skeletal structure as lentinan, are devoid of the antitumor activity. However, pachymaran, a β-1,3-linear glucan obtained by chemical scission of β-1,6-branchings in pachyman, has a strong antitumor activity (5). In addition, pachyman with no antitumor activity has been derived to U-pachyman with strong antitumor activity by merely heating pachyman in 4 M aqueous urea at 45°C for 4 hr to modify the quarternary structure (6).

It is also interesting that a class of polysaccharide with antitumor activity only increases the content of α-helix structure in serum albumin or β-structure in serum globulin when incubated in vitro, while antitumor inactive polysaccharides or other polyanions are completely devoid of this effect, and exert the adverse effect (7).

The importance of higher-order structure of polysaccharides for the appearance of the activity suggests the presence of biological systems in the host recognizing conformational adaptability of polysaccharides. This finding led us to analyze the nature of host factors interacting with lentinan to cause the antitumor effect of lentinan, from immunological and physiological viewpoints, to know more decisively the host defense mechanisms playing a role against neoplastic diseases or in the rejection of non-self.

We also found that linear β-1,3-lentinan, obtained by chemical scission of β-1,6-branches (Smith degradation) (8), and small lentinan (mol wt, 6000-10,000), obtained by degradation of parent lentinan in formic acid, are also effective to inhibit tumor growth (9).

All of these experimental results favor the concept that the activity entity of lentinan is really a pure polysaccharide.

III. BIOLOGICAL ACTIVITIES

A. Antitumor Effects

Lentinan exerts prominent antitumor effects on various syngeneic tumors as well as on allogeneic tumors in animal models and is devoid of direct cytocidal effects on these tumors when tested in cell culture systems (10). Namely, lentinan does not possess any direct effects on tumor cells in terms of their growth rate and DNA and RNA synthesis. In this context, lentinan is said to be a potentiator of host defense mechanisms. Lentinan also exerts no direct cytocidal action on normal cells, while most of chemotherapeutic agents often show detrimental effects.

As already described, lentinan causes the prominent growth inhibition or sarcoma 180 at optimal dose range, while higher dosages show considerably decreased activity. Thus, one of the characteristic features of antitumor activity of lentinan resides in the presence of optimal dosage (6). The other relevant feature is that, depending on the responding character of host to lentinan action, optimal doses, frequency and timing of administration showing optimal activity differ greatly. Lentinan exerts its growth-inhibitory activity against sarcoma 180 to the same extent even injected 5 weeks before tumor transplantation as postinjection.

In order to know the antitumor action of lentinan on syngeneic tumors in detail, the effects of lentinan were investigated using the similar administration protocols now undertaken in clinical application, namely, lentinan was injected intravenously several days or weeks after tumor transplantation. Also, lentinan exerted prominent growth-inhibitory activity when administered 10-14 days after sarcoma 180 transplantation to the same extent as was observed when lentinan was injected just 1 day after sarcoma 180 transplantation. This fact suggests that injection of lentinan at the time when transplanted tumors are recognized by host also causes considerable effects.

The growth-inhibitory effects of lentinan on syngeneic P815, L5178Y, MM46, and MM102 tumors are illustrated in Fig. 1 and Table 1. As can be seen from the results shown in Table 1, the time of injection of lentinan seems to be critical for lentinan to exert significant antitumor activity in MM102-C3H/HeN system. The results suggest that lentinan demonstrates its action depending on the state of relative host-tumor immunological relationship. In contrast, the activity of lentinan on P815 is remarkable, regardless of the timing of administration. Interestingly, the later the injection of lentinan at the same dose and frequency, the stronger becomes the growth inhibition. Optimal timing of administration appears to be 2 to 3 weeks after P815 transplantation. The results showing the same tendency were obtained also in L5178Y-DBA/2 and MM46-C3H/He syngeneic systems (Fig. 1). The host immune responses triggered and modulated by tumor growth might probably have the same roles in these phenomena.

It can be safely said that lentinan shows antitumor effects also on syngeneic murine tumors, even when administered without any other chemotherapeutic agents, such as cyclophosphamide and 5-fluorouracil (5-FU), when we know the optimal timing of injection. Depending on the host-tumor relationship, however, the antitumor effects of lentinan become far less (EL4-C57BL/6 system). The results demonstrate that combined administration of lentinan and indomethacin resulted in synergistic growth inhibition of EL4, even when the sole injection of lentinan did not cause any effect (Fig. 2). The augmented growth inhibition observed may be attributed to the diminished suppression of

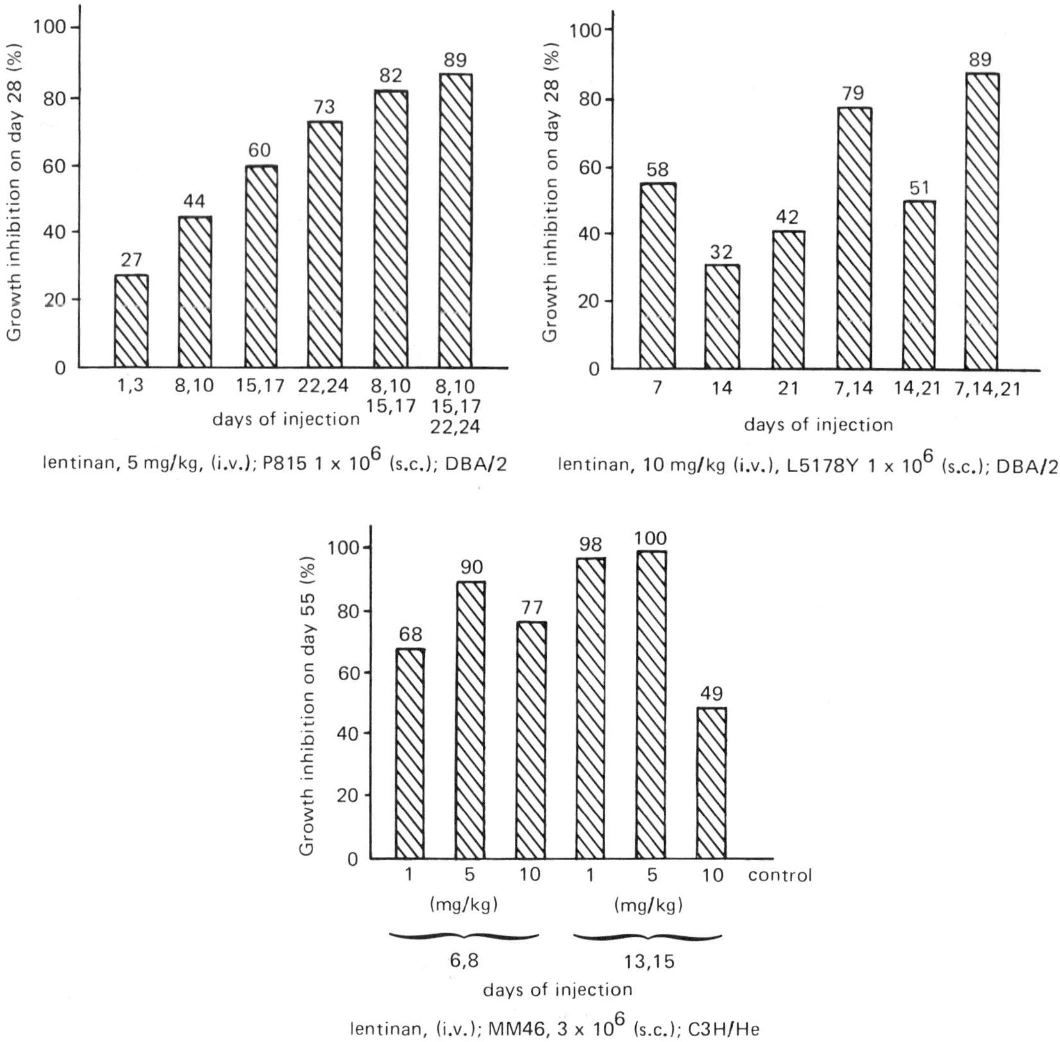

Figure 1 Effect of intravenous injection of lentinan on the growth of syngeneic tumors P815, L5178Y, and MM46. Numbers above shadowed columns show growth inhibition (%) compared with nontreated tumors. (From Ref. 46.)

immune responses dictated by prostaglandins, which may be released by tumor cells or by suppressor macrophages (11,12).

Lentinan also showed growth inhibitory action against other tumors such as Lewis lung carcinoma, B-16 melanoma (13), SR-C3H/He sarcoma, and colon 26 in syngeneic murine systems. Zákány et al. have reported that lentinan can completely regress methylchoranthrene-induced A/Ph. MC. S1 fibrosarcoma in an A/Ph syngeneic host in a dose of 1 mg/kg administered intraperitoneally for 10 consecutive days (Fig. 3). A/Ph mice in which these tumors have regressed can also reject a secondary challenge with the same tumor (14,15).

Table 1 Growth Inhibitory and Survival Effect of Lentinan on Mammary Carcinoma, MM-102 in C3H/HeN Mice

Treatment	Date of lentinan injection	Tumor size[c] (mm^2)	Survival[d]
Lentinan[a]	Day 0	458 ± 215	1/7
Lentinan	Day 7	529 ± 180	4/6
Lentinan	Day 14	198 ± 125	7/7
Lentinan	Day 21	637 ± 256	2/6
Lentinan	Day 28	477 ± 241	5/7
Control		425 ± 253	3/6

[a]Doses of lentinan (10 mg/kg) were injected IV.
[b]The date of lentinan injection after the transplantation of 3×10^6 MM-102 mammary carcinoma cells SC into C3H/HeN mice.
[c]Means ± SD on day 35.
[d]Proportion alive on day 70.

These results have prompted us to claim that lentinan is a true antitumor substance capable to potentiate host defense mechanisms against syngeneic tumors and, it is not merely a substance promoting the rejection of a foreign graft. Thus, immunogenetic analysis of the host would become an important issue in the future, as well as analysis of the common basis of host's response to transplantation antigens and tumor antigens.

It was also demonstrated that lentinan could prolong more than two times the survival of C3H/He mice bearing primary autologous tumors induced by methylcholanthrene when administered together with cyclophosphamide (13). In this context, it might be worthwhile to mention that lentinan prevents methylchoranthrene-induced carcinogenesis considerably when administered before or within 3 weeks after

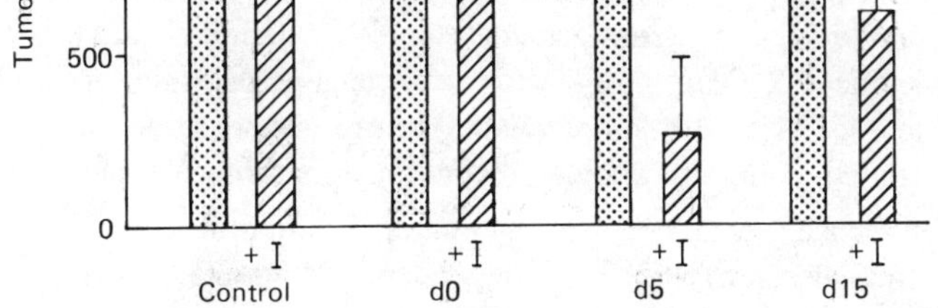

Figure 2 Synergistic growth inhibition of El4-C57B1/6 by lentinan (10 mg/kg IV) and indomethacin (I: 1 mg/kg IP). Shadowed and dotted columns show tumor size by treatment with and without indomethacin, respectively.

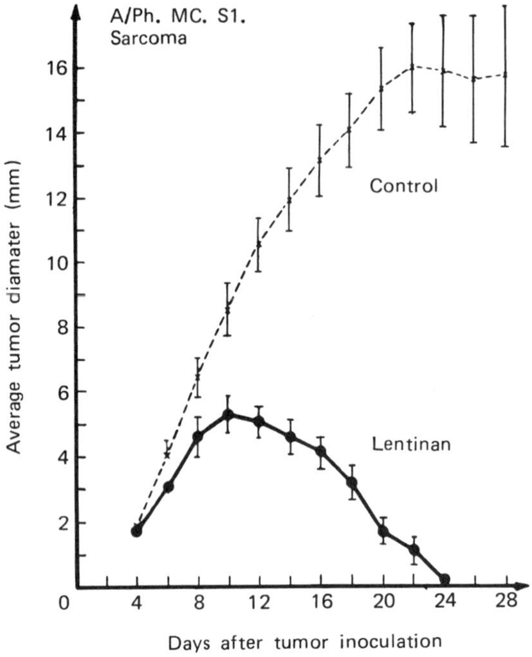

Figure 3 Growth of A/Ph. MC. S1 sarcoma in control and lentinan-treated A/Ph mice. Both groups of mice (15 and 18, respectively) received 2.5 X 10^4 tumor cells ID and treatment with lentinan (· —— ·) or solvent (x - - x).

methylcholanthrene inoculation (83-30%) (Fig. 4). Lentinan also prevents viral tumorigenesis induced by adenovirus type 12 in C3H/He mice (79-40%).

Antitumor effects and preventive effects of carcinogenesis by lentinan are summarized in Table 2.

B. Antibacterial, Viral, and Parasitic Effects

It has been recently demonstrated that lentinan possesses strong inhibitory action against various bacteria, viruses, and parasites (Table 3).

When lentinan was administered to thymus-intact mice by intraperitoneal injection, conspicuously enlarged lung granulomas were formed in response to either *Schistosoma mansoni* or *Schistosoma japonicum* eggs or to antigen-coated polyacrylamide beads (16). Liver granulomas in serratia-induced *S. mansoni* infections were augmented up to eightfold in volume. By contrast, nude mice showed a complete absence of hypersensitivity granulomas. Lentinan-potentiated granuloma shows a distinct histopathological picture characterized by frequent, extensive central necrosis, uncommon in unpotentiated *schistosome* foci. These findings also verify the T-cell dependency of lentinan against parasitic infection.

Recent studies also indicated that lentinan is effective in immunopotentiating effect, so as to reduce the frequency of postchemotherapy relapse in experimental tuberculosis (17). After termination of 5 months of intensive chemotherapy, one group

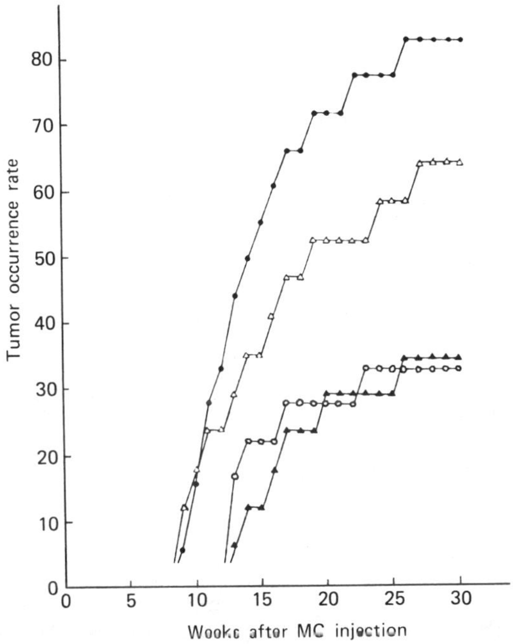

Figure 4 Preventive effect of lentinan on chemical carcinogenesis by 3-methylcholanthrene: ● - - - control (no injection); ○ - - -, pretreated with lentinan from 10 days before MC inoculation; ▼- - -, lentinan was injected from third week after MC inoculation; ▽- - -, from sixth week after MC inoculation. Dose of lentinan, 1 mg/kg X 10 days IP.

Table 2 Antitumor Effect of Lentinan in the Syngeneic Hosts and its Prevention of Chemical and Viral Carcinogenesis

Tumors[a]	Host	Dose[b]	Timing[c]	Inhibition[d] Ratio (%)	References
Syngeneic tumors					
A/PH, MC, S1 sarcoma	A/Ph(A/J)	1 X 10 (IP)	1-11	100	14
P-815 mastocytoma	DBA/2	5 X 4 (IV)	8,10,15,17	82	46
L-5178Y lymphoma	DBA/2	10 X 3 (IV)	7,14,21	89	46
MM-46 carcinoma	C3H/He	5 X 2 (IV)	13,15	100	46
MM-102 carcinoma	C3H/He	10 X 6 (IP)	7	60	46
Lewis lung carcinoma	C57BL/6	1 X 6 (IP)	1-7	59	13
Prevention of carcinogenesis				Tumor incidence	
MC induced	SWM/Ms	1 X 10 (IP)	21-31	83 → 33%[e]	13
Adenovirus induced	C3H/He	10 X 3 (IP)	14,16,18	79 → 40%[f]	19

[a]All tumors are solid form implanted subcutaneously.
[b]mg/kg x days.
[c]Days of lentinan administration after tumor (or MC, ad) inoculation.
[d]Tumor inhibition ratio = (C – T)/T x 100; (C = average tumor weight of control mice; T= that of lentinan-treated mice).
[e]Determination at 30 weeks after MC inoculation.
[f]Determination at 90 days after adenovirus type 12 inoculation.

Table 3 Increase of Host Resistance to Infections by Lentinan

	Reference
Bacteria	
Mycobacterium tuberculosis	17
Mycobacterium leprae	20
Listeria monocytogeneses	21
Streptococcus pneumoniae	47
Klebsiella pneumoniae	47
Virus	
VSV-encephalitis virus	18
Abelson virus	18
Adenovirus type 12	19
Parasites	
Schistosoma mansoni	16
Schistosoma japonicum	16
Mescocestoides corti	Thompson

of mice in a treated group (streptomycin, isoniazid, rifampcin) received lentinan for 4 weeks and again for 4 weeks after a 1-month interval. The results indicated that the later multiplication of the latent bacilli was strongly reduced by lentinan treatment during the advance of postchemotherapy period. These results clearly suggest the effectiveness of lentinan against chronic infectious diseases and various infections frequently observed among patients with neoplastic diseases.

Prophylactic effects of lentinan against mouse encephalitis caused by VSV, Abelson virus infection have been reported also in terms of its strong effect to prolong the survival of infected animals (18). The preventive effect on viral carcinogenesis by adenovirus type 12 was also reported (19). These kinds of prophylactic effects of lentinan suggest that lentinan is hopeful not only in curative but also in preventive utilization against oncogenesis, although application of lentinan in clinics in this context has not yet occurred.

IV. IMMUNOLOGICAL PROPERTIES

Several immunopotentiators such as the BCG strain of *Mycobacterium bovis* and *C. parvum* have been studied for their potency as antitumor immunotherapeutic agents. Among the well-known immunopotentiators, lentinan appears to represent a unique class of immunological adjuvants. Lentinan has little toxic side effects upon in vivo application. The antitumor effect of lentinan appeared to be mediated by the host, for it does not exert any cytocidal or cytostatic direct effects on the cultured tumor cell lines in vitro, while its growth-inhibitory effects on transplantable syngeneic tumors are distinct. One of the distinct characteristics of its immunological reactivity is its capacity to act as a T-cell-immune adjuvant.

Here we describe the major immunological properties of lentinan relevant for the biological activities of it as an immunotherapeutic agent against neoplasia, infections, and immunodeficiency, and the mechanism of its action.

A. Nonspecific Immunopotentiation

Lentinan exerts various effects on complicated macrophage functions. Among functions of macrophages in host defense mechanisms against cancer, the following are typical: phagocytic function, antigen-presenting function, various secretive functions, and cytotoxic (cytostatic) functions. Lentinan-induced peritoneal macrophages elicited almost no elevation of phagocytic activity than resident macrophages as assessed by carbon clearance tests. Macrophages harvested 7 days after injection of 0.1 mg/kg of lentinan IV only showed a slight increase of phagocytic index expressed by K value. On the contrary, injection of zymosan or lipopolysacharide (LPS) caused a strong elevation of phagocytosis by macrophages already 2 days after injection. Schizophyllan, which has similar structure to lentinan, also caused elevation as early as 2 days after injection (Fig. 5).

Therefore, lentinan seems to be distinct from zymosan, lipopolysaccharides, schizophyllan, and most of other immunopotentiators possessing a nature as reticuloendothelial system (RES) stimulants. Intravenous injection of lentinan at a dose of 10 mg/kg, where lentinan exerted the prominent growth-inhibitory action against syngeneic murine tumors, did not show any elevation of carbon clearance index of macrophages harvested from 2 to 7 days after injection, especially in inbred mice such as C3H/HeN, BALB/c, DBA/2, and C57Bl/6. These results clearly verify the absence of direct participation of phagocytic function of macrophages in the appearance of antitumor activity of lentinan.

It is well known that lipopolysaccharides, zymosan, poly I:C, pyran copolymer, *C. parvum*, BCG, and most of the immunopotentiators known so far cause elevated release

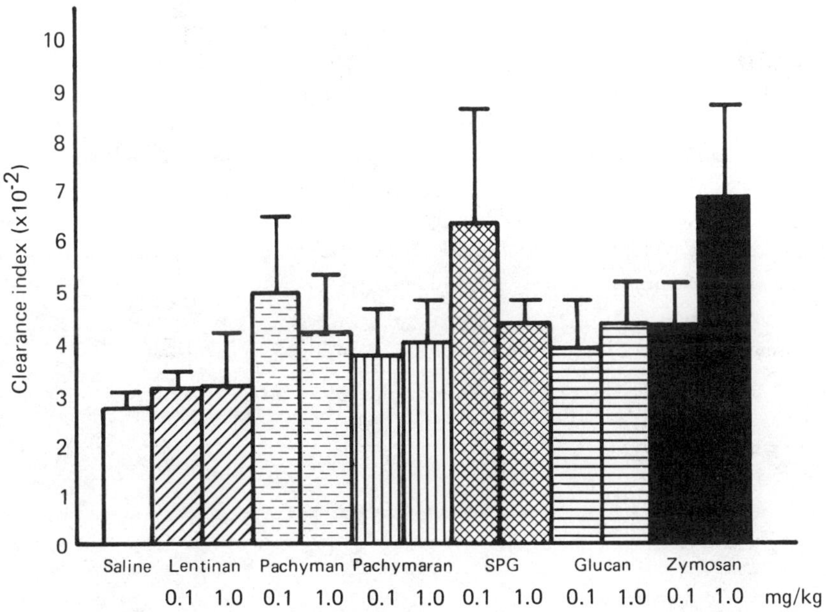

Figure 5 Effect of various polysaccharides on carbon clearance test. Each polysaccharide was injected intravenously into ICR female mice on day −2 and day 0. Assay was carried out on day 2.

of lysosomal enzymes from macrophages when cocultured in vitro (22). Again lentinan completely is devoid of this impact on cultured macrophages; however, in vivo application of lentinan results in the induction of macrophages possible to secrete more lysosomal enzymes than resident.

When peritoneal macrophages were harvested from mice which received IP lentinan 4 days before, the spontaneous release of prostaglandins E and F (PGE, PGF) was strikingly reduced from resident macrophages (23). The diminished spontaneous release of both PGE and PGF was still apparent when macrophages from mice were examined which had received lentinan 8 days before, in contrast to the restored normal release from macrophages induced by the antitumor-inactive polysaccharide, pachyman. Although immunopotentiators such as *C. parvum* and BCG have been shown to induce a high spontaneous release of prostaglandins from spleen cells and peritoneal macrophages (24), the results described here show that lentinan is distinct from them in the sense that it may lead to a depressed prostaglandin synthesis. This finding indicates a possible correlation between the observed depression of prostaglandin release by lentinan-induced macrophages and the augmenting effect of lentinan on T-cell functions. Thus, it is possible that the absence of an immune response inhibitory-acting compound such as prostaglandin E may facilitate the cytotoxic action of T cells and/or macrophages in cell-mediated immune responses.

On the other hand, lentinan was found to be a potent activator of alternative pathway of complement system (APC), and potency to activate APC was demonstrated not to be correlated with the potency of growth-inhibitory action on tumors, because antitumor-inactive pachyman activates APC to the same extent as lentinan (25).

Thus, lentinan could activate certain classes of serum components in vivo in the tumor antigen nonspecific manner, and it may be possible that thus activated serum components play a role in the antitumor action of lentinan by inducing nonspecific cytotoxic macrophages as effectors against tumor cells. A recent report described the participation of activated complement components in macrophage activation, leading to the release of lysosomal enzymes (26). This concept is consistent with the finding that in vivo application of lentinan can induce macrophages capable of secreting more amounts of lysosomal enzymes compared with resident (Table 4). At present, it is unclear whether lysosomal hydrolytic enzymes released from macrophages by exocytosis could participate in tumor-regressing activity of lentinan, but the possible participation of APC activation locally on tumor cell membranes cannot be excluded.

Table 4 Release of β-Glucuronidase from Macrophages Induced by Lentinan

Macrophage origin[a]	In Vitro	β-Glucuronidase total (mU/ml)	β-Glucuronidase release (%)
Normal	–	4.08	11.5
	Lentinan[c]	3.92	14.3
	Zymosan[c]	4.45	47.9
Lentinan induced[b]	–	11.6	30.6
	Lentinan[c]	11.5	29.6
	Zymosan[c]	10.0	54.8

[a]NMRI mice.
[b]Lentinan 2 mg/kg IP, PEC harvest day 3.
[c]Concentration 50 μg/ml.
Source: Ref. 46.

Lentinan is able to induce cytotoxic macrophages only when administered in vivo and is not able to mount cytotoxic macrophages upon in vitro coculture with macrophages, distinct from other immunopotentiators such as *C. parvum*, BCG, and lipopolysaccharides. These characteristics of lentinan are in accordance with our interpretation that induction of cytotoxic macrophages observed upon in vivo application of lentinan is due to the induction of activated serum components. In the meantime, most immunopotentiators have been demonstrated to induce in vitro cytotoxic macrophages by the induction of macrophage-activating fragment of the third component of complement, C3b, the production of which is amplified by the elevated release of lysosomal enzymes from macrophages during coculture in vitro, the activity absent for lentinan (27).

B. Specific Immunopotentiation

Since antitumor activity of lentinan against sarcoma 180 was markedly decreased by the administration of antilymphocyte serum (28), it seems likely that recirculating T lymphocytes have some role in the antitumor activity. Furthermore, antitumor activity of lentinan against sarcoma 180 completely disappeared in neonatally thymectomized mice (10, 29), and growth inhibition against syngeneic KKN-1 tumor was observed only in nu/+BALB/c but not in nu/nu (30). These experimental results support the concept that antitumor activity of lentinan requires intact immunocompetent T-cell compartments, and the activity is mediated through thymus dependent immune mechanism.

In vivo application of lentinan caused an increase in the level of certain types of serum proteins acutely or semiacutely (31). One of the increased serum proteins was functionally assigned as colony-stimulating factor (CSF). Upon in vitro incubation of nylon-column purified splenic T cells with lentinan, CSF is released into supernatant in five times a larger amount than control. Thus produced CSF then acts on immune regulatory Ia^+ macrophages, resulting in augmented production of Interleukin 1 (lymphocyte-activating factor = LAF) by a positive feedback mechanism. On the other hand, lentinan-induced peritoneal macrophages produced an increased amount of Interleukin 1 (Il-1). The augmented production of Il-1 was also observed when peritoneal macrophages were incubated in vitro with lentinan. Production of Il-1 from macrophages was also confirmed by cocultivation of macrophage cell line $P388D_1$ with lentinan (Fig. 6).

Recent studies clearly indicated that lentinan augments the generation of antigen-specific cytotoxic T lymphocytes (CTLs) against alloantigen and haptenated syngeneic cells in vivo (32) and in vitro (33). Namely, lentinan is an effective immune adjuvant of both alloreactive CTL responses and H-2 restricted CTL response specific to foreign antigens. In analyzing the mechanism of this adjuvant effect, it was noted that on in vitro incubation of splenic adherent cells or peritoneal exudate cells with a critical concentration of lentinan, a soluble product is generated, which in turn is able to augment the differentiation of antigenically triggered clonally distinct CTL precursors into highly reactive CTL (34). The complete failure to generate anti-$H\text{-}2^d$ allokiller cells was confirmed in the absence of adherent splenic accessory cells even in the presence of lentinan, and the successful transfer of augmenting effect on anti-$H\text{-}2^d$ allokiller cell generation by soluble factors from 24-hr culture supernatant of spleen cells or splenic adherent cells in the presence of lentinan was observed.

Recently, we have found that lentinan also exerted the augmentation of Il-1 production by macrophages even in syngeneic tumor-bearing murine systems, although controls showed considerable depression of Il-1 production from peritoneal macrophages (Table 5).

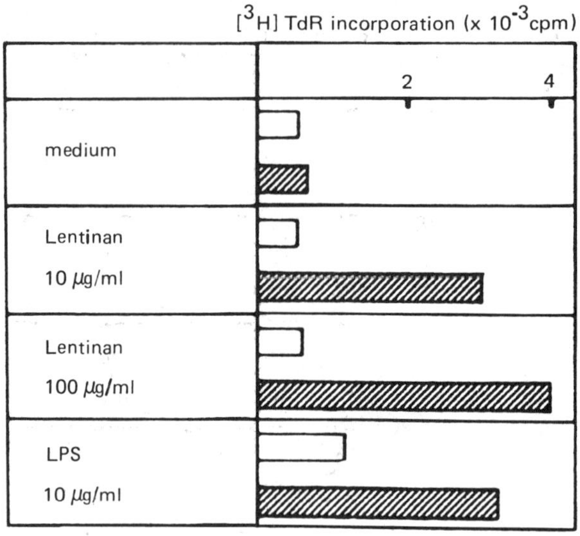

Figure 6 Direct effect of lentinan to macrophage cell line $P388D_1$ to produce Interleukin 1 (Il-1). Lentinan and LPS were incubated for 24 hr with $P388D_1$ cells, and the culture supernatants were assayed. Shadowed and open columns show [^{3}H] TdR incorporation into mouse thymocytes with and without $P388D_1$ cells, respectively.

It has been found also that lentinan is able to generate augmented CTL against LSTRA tumor cells in mixed syngeneic tumor-lymphocyte culture, and the effect was concluded by limiting dilution method to be due to the increase of CTL precursor cells in the presence of lentinan (38). All findings presented here are in favor of the interpretation that lentinan promotes differentiation of thymic-premature T cells into immunocompetent mature T cells recirculating in the periphery. This interpretation clearly

Table 5 Effect of Lentinan on the Production of Il-1 in L5178Y Tumor-Bearing Mice

	[^{3}H] TdR incorporation
Normal	1108
Tumor	856
Tumor + lentinan	2481
Tumor (d19)	543
Tumor + lentinan	3038

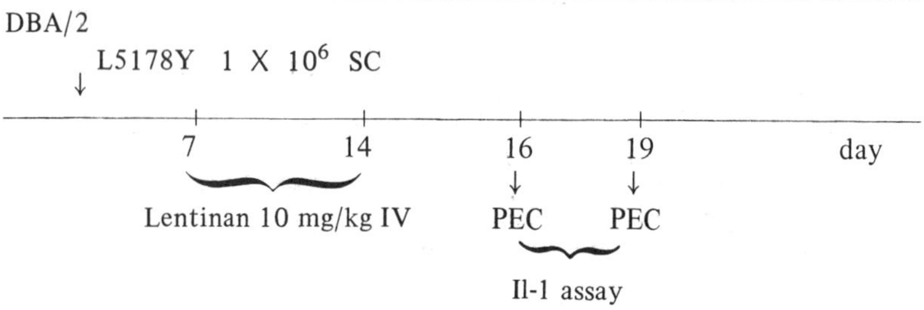

explains the requirement of an intact T-cell compartment for the appearance of antitumor activity of lentinan.

To evaluate the validity of the reaction scheme presented, generation of allokiller cells from thymocytes was tested. Thymocytes harvested from responder BALB/c mice treated with lentinan induce augmented generation of allokiller cells in the presence of Interleukin 2 (Il-2). This fact demonstrates that thymocytes of lentinan-injected mice are more reactive to Il-2. In a syngeneic tumor-bearing system such as P815-DBA/2, allokiller cell generation from thymocytes is considerably suppressed, even in the presence of Il-2. The generation, however, was restored to the level of tumor-nonbearing mice by the injection of lentinan. The generation of allokiller cells from splenocytes was also restored from null to around 40% in the absence of Il-2 (Table 6). These results are possible to explain by the augmented induction of mature T cells reactive to Il-2 as a second signal. Furthermore, most interestingly, spleen cells harvested from syngeneic tumor-bearing mice (P815-DBA/2) which received triple IP injection of lentinan 2 weeks after P815 transplantation were able to generate a significant level of antisyngeneic P815 tumor killer cells in the presence of Il-2.

Concerning the other important nonspecific effector, natural killer cells (NK), it was found that lentinan could augment NK activity in spleen cells and peritoneal exudate cells when administered into NK high-responder C3H/He mice, but could not when

Table 6 Augmented Allokiller T-Cell Generation by Lentinan in Syngeneic Tumor-Bearing Murine System

I. Allokiller generation from splenocytes: lysis of El-4 (%)

P-815	Lentinan dose (mg/kg x 3) 0	0.01	0.1	10
Bearing	0	46	43	20

II. Allokiller generation from thymocytes: lysis of El-4 (%)

P815	Il-2[a]	Lentinan dose (mg/kg x 3) 0	0.01	0.1	10
Bearing	–	1	2	0	3
	+	4	37	37	24
Nonbearing	–	1	4	2	9
	+	23	38	51	48

[a]Il-2: Interleukin-2.
E/T = 50 (culture base).
Killer assay: 3 hr, ^{51}Cr release.

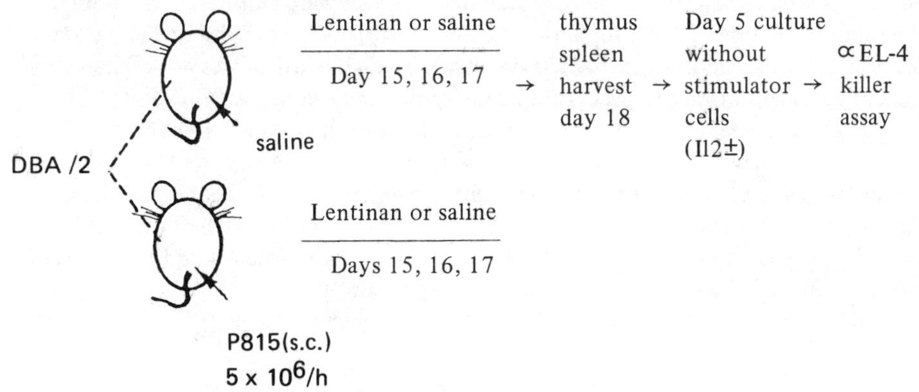

administered into BALB/c mice. However, lentinan did not activate NK cells when incubated in vitro as poly I:C and zymosan do. Augmented natural killer cell generation was also observed when lentinan-treated spleen cells were cultured with an interferon inducer, poly I:C, or with Il-2 generation from cloned murine or human T-cell leukemias, but not with α, β-interferon (IFN) (Fig. 7). Recent data showed that Il-2 activates NK cells as reported for α, β-IFN. At present, it is not clear whether the augmented NK activtion by lentinan would be due to the augmented reactivity of NK-cells to interferon or Il-2. Because we know lentinan does not induce interferon as other polyanionic immune adjuvants and does not activate NK cells in vitro, it seems likely that in vivo application of lentinan results in the augmentation of NK cell reactivity to Il-2. In relation to the above-described hypothesis, the fact that serum obtained from lentinan-treated mice lacking Il-2 activity is able to augment NK activation drew our attention to the future detailed analysis of NK cell activation by lentinan.

The doses required to activate NK cells were found to be relatively higher than the doses required for antitumor activity and for the other immunological reactivities of lentinan. Thus, it is difficult to ascertain the roles of NK cells in the antitumor activity of lentinan at present.

Lentinan not only augments antigen-specific cellular immune responses, but also is capable of triggering antigen-nonspecific immune responses against neoplastic cells. It was observed that lentinan and its related substances with antitumor activity could induce cytotoxic peritoneal macrophages after intraperitoneal injection, whereas antitumor-inactive polysaccharides showed only slight inducing activity (34). In spite of many experiments to date, all attempts to render normal or thioglycolate-induced peritoneal exudate cells cytotoxic by the in vitro addition of lentinan have failed. Thus, lentinan is capable of rendering peritoneal exudate cells cytotoxic only under in vivo conditions while most immunopotentiators could render peritoneal exudate cells cytotoxic upon in vitro incubation.

More interestingly, lentinan augmented the reactivity of macrophages to macrophage-activating factor(s) (MAFs) generated from activated T cells, resulting in the augmented generation of cytostatic and cytotoxic macrophages against tumor cells. Cell-free supernatants containing MAF were harvested from cultures of normal ICR mice spleen cells incubated in vitro for 72 hr with concanavalin A (5 μg/ml). As shown in Fig. 8, macrophages elicited by lentinan administered IV showed the augmented response to MAF.

In order to know whether this augmentation of responsiveness would occur after direct action of lentinan on macrophages, peritoneal adherent cells were cocultured with lentinan in vitro for 24 hr, and thus treated macrophages were cultured in the presence of a suboptimal dose of MAF for another 24 hr. Lentinan exerted the augmentation of responsiveness of macrophages to MAF in vitro, although lentinan was not capable of rendering resident macrophages cytotoxic under this condition.

In this context, in vitro lentinan-stimulated macrophages are neither cytotoxic nor cytostatic, but they possessed elevated reactivity to MAF. Recently, we have also found that in the syngeneic tumor-bearing mice, lentinan exerted the augmentation of responsiveness of peritoneal macrophages to MAF. The response of macrophages to MAF in L5187Y syngeneic tumor-bearing mice was significantly suppressed as compared with that in normal mice on day 25, but lentinan treatment of these L5178Y-bearing mice resulted in augmented response over that of the control level (Table 7).

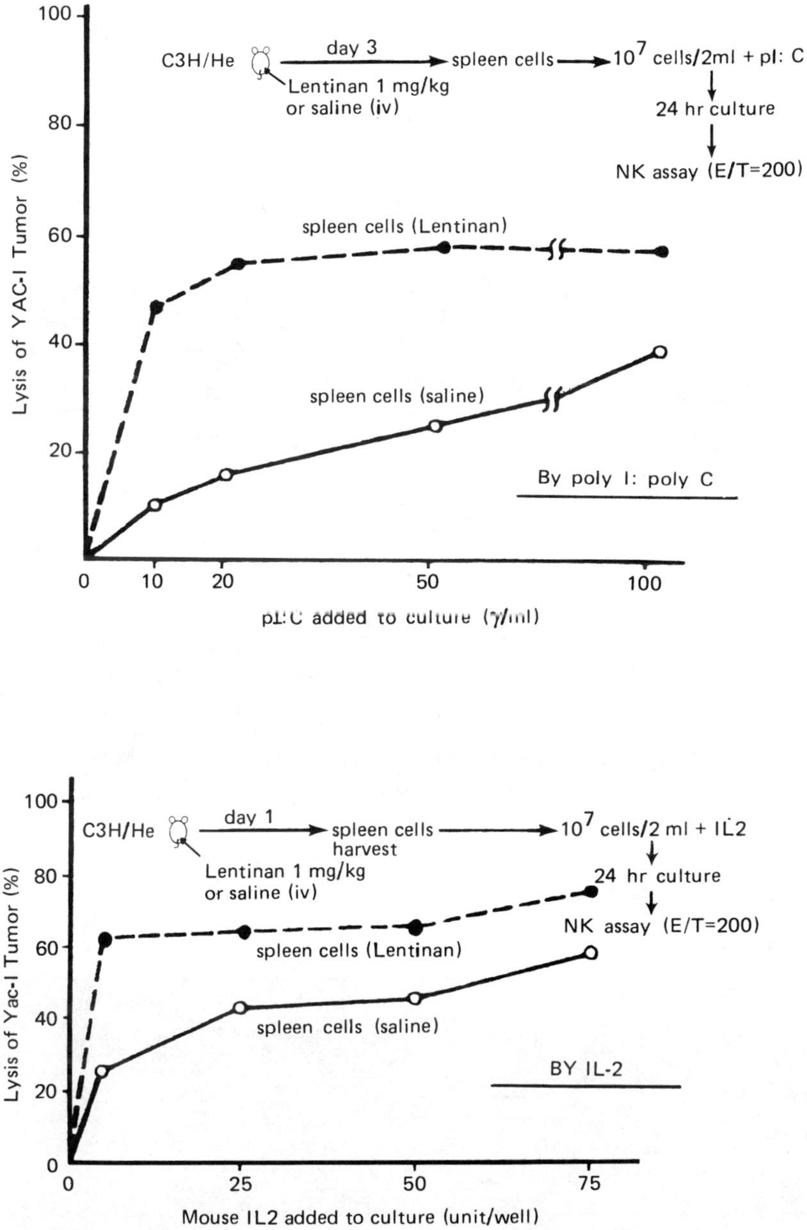

Figure 7 Synergistic augmentation of natural killer cells by lentinan with poly I:C and with Il-2. Experiments were carried out according to the protocols indicated. Natural killer cell activity was assayed using ^{51}Cr-labeled YAC-1 cells as a target cells in 4 hr ^{51}Cr-release assay at a ratio of effector/target = 200:1 (initial cell density basis). (From Ref. 46.)

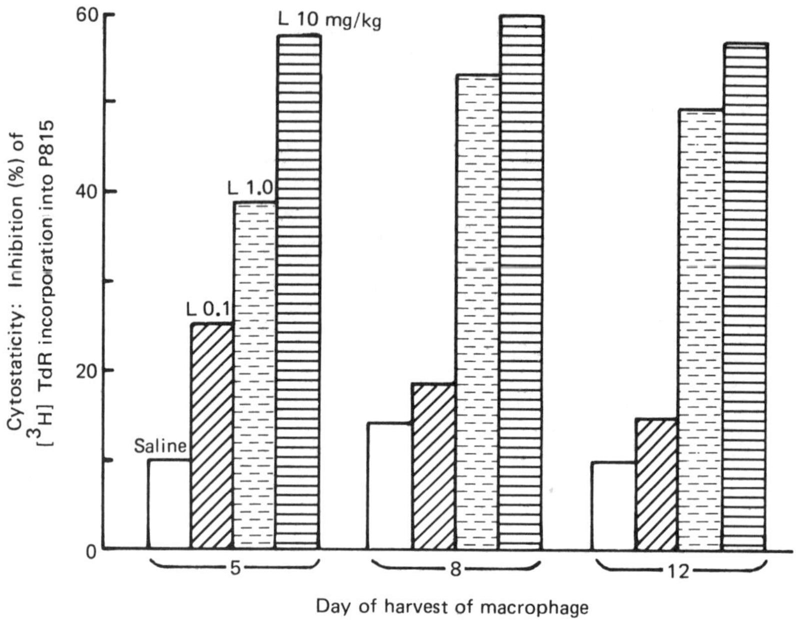

Figure 8 Augmentation by lentinan of macrophage-activating factor(s) induced cytostatic macrophage generation in vivo. Indicated doses of lentinan was intravenously injected into BALB/c mice on day 0. Peritoneal exudate cells were harvested on days 5, 8, and 12, respectively; 8 X 10^5 peritoneal exudate cell-derived adherent cells were incubated with macrophage-activating factor(s). (From Ref. 46.)

Table 7 Effect of Lentinan on the Response of Macrophages to Macrophage-Activating Factor(s) (MAF) in Tumor-Bearing Mice

	Inhibition (%) of tumor growth in the presence of MAF
Normal	30.1
Tumor (d20)	34.3
Tumor + lentinan	72.4
Tumor (d25)	8.1
Tumor + lentinan	74.6

DBA/2; L5178Y 1 X 10^6 SC (↓ day 0); lentinan 5 mg/kg IV (↓ days 7, 14); PC (↑ day 20)

0 — 7 — 14 — 20 — 21 — 25

lentinan 5 mg/kg IV (↑ days 7, 14, 21); PC (day 25)

PC $\xrightarrow{\text{3 hr}}$ adherent cells ± MAF $\xrightarrow{\text{24 hr}}$ [^{3}H] TdR incorporation inhibition into P815

As already mentioned, lentinan is not capable of rendering resident, or stimulated macrophages, cytotoxic under in vitro conditions, so it is suggested that the capacity of lentinan to render in vivo macrophage cytotoxic is related to the potency of lentinan to activate alternative pathway of complement system (APC) in so far as C3b may be the essential component required to render macrophages cytotoxic, or to the potency of lentinan to augment the reactivity of macrophages to activated T-cell-derived MAF.

Masuko and Mizuno (36) found that in MM46 syngeneic tumor-bearing mice lentinan augmented the antitumor delayed hypersensitivity reaction (DHR) measured by the footpad test and concluded that antibody-dependent macrophage-mediated cellular cytotoxicity (ADMC) was the effector mechanism in this case.

In order to elucidate the action mechanism of lentinan to augment antitumor DHR, we examined whether antitumor DHR was adoptively transferred into normal syngeneic C3H/He mice by extradermal injection of tumor antigen with sensitized lymphoid cells from donor mice. As shown in Fig. 9, lentinan-treated recipient mice alone showed a significant positive DHR, and the results are consistent with the previously described interpretation that lentinan stimulates effector macrophages so as to show augmented reactivity to activated T-cell-derived lymphokine MAF.

Lentinan not only augments antitumor effector cell generation, but also lentinan is well known as an immune adjuvant in humoral and cellular immune responses. Lentinan augments plaque-forming cell (PFC) induction against sheep red blood cells (SRBCs). Antigen SRBCs were injected on day 0 at several inoculum sizes, and lentinan was injected IP three times on days 0, 1, and 2 in a wide dose range from 0.02 to 100 mg/kg. Depending on the size of inoculated SRBCs, the augmenting and inhibiting effect of lentinan on PFC induction varied. In principle, the smaller the size of SRBCs, the larger the dose of lentinan showing optimal augmentation.

Yohikai et al. (37) reported that macrophage activators such as *C. parvum* usually depressed anti-SRBC PFC induction and delayed hypersensitivity reaction. In this context, the impact of lentinan on macrophages may be distinct from that of *C. parvum* and other macrophage activators, which usually enhance phagocytic activity of macrophages. It should be kept in mind that lentinan does not enhance phagocytic activity of macrophages as measured by carbon clearance. Augmentation of antibody production against SRBCs was also observed in an in vitro culture system in the presence of 0.1-1 μg/ml lentinan, and the augmenting effect was also explained by the augmented production of Interleukin 1, which in turn acts on helper T cells or B cells to augment antibody responses against T-cell-dependent antigens. Recently, we have observed lentinan also augments the reactivity of B cells to T-cell replacing factor (TRF), resulting in augmented anti-SRBC PFC induction (unpublished data).

Lentinan also augmented DHR to SRBCs measured by footpad swelling 1 day after SRBC rechallenge. Lentinan was injected IV according to protocols corresponding to those of standard antitumor assay on syngeneic tumors. In all strains of mouse tested, 5 mg/kg of lentinan clearly showed significant augmentation of DHR to SRBCs, consistent with the above-mentioned effect on PFC induction to SRBCs (Fig. 10). This augmenting effect exhibited by lentinan can be explained also by the augmenting effect of lentinan on reactivity of macrophages to MAF as demonstrated in tumor antigen-directed DHR.

There are several preliminary papers describing the specific impact of lentinan on T-cell compartments. One describes the augmentation of antibody-dependent cellular cytotoxicity (ADCC) in spleen cells as assessed by cytotoxicity against chicken red blood cells (CRBSs) as target cells (38). However, augmenting effect was observed only at a critical inoculum size of CRBSs as an immunogen (10^7 cells).

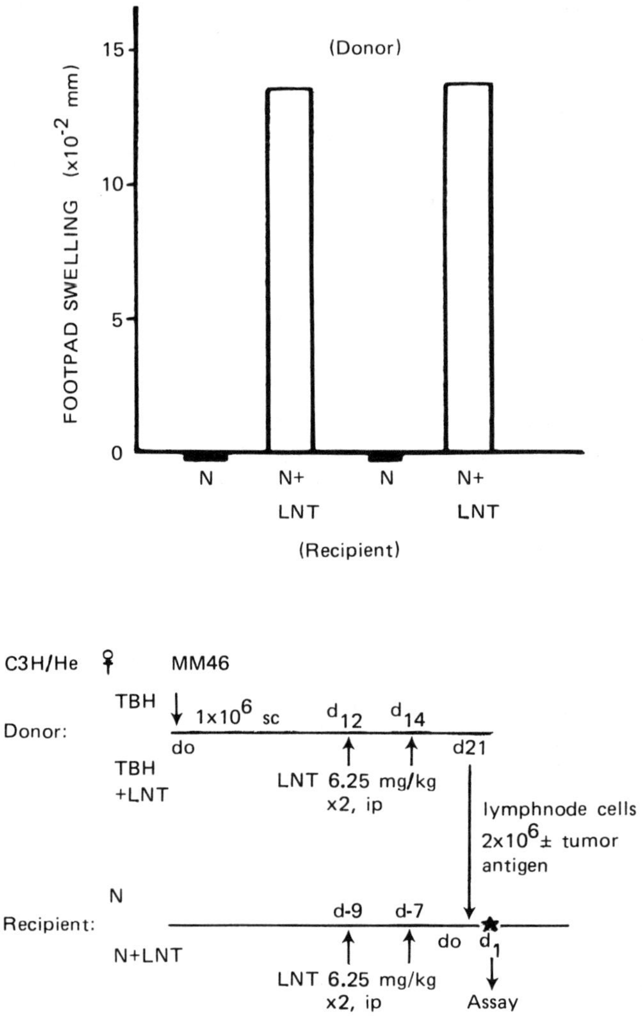

Figure 9 Effect of lentinan on adoptive transfer of delayed hypersensitivity reaction. Experiment was carried out according to the protocols indicated.

In the course of the analysis of augmenting effects of antibody generation by lentinan in hapten-carried conjugate systems, Dennert and Tucker (38) reported that lentinan seems to be a stimulator of helper T cells in normal murine systems. The same conclusion that lentinan stimulates helper T cells was demonstrated by Dresser and Phillips (39) by analyzing the details of lentinan effect on antibody production of distinct classes against SRBCs.

C. Lentinan-Induced Effector Cells against Tumors

After establishment of P815 or L5178Y tumors in DBA/2 mice, Lentinan was injected IV, and peritoneal cells and spleen cells were harvested when the tumor growth-inhibition ratios reached 51 and 70%, respectively. These cells were transplanted to recipient DBA/2 mice together with 1 X 10^6 tumor cells subcutaneously to test the neutralizing

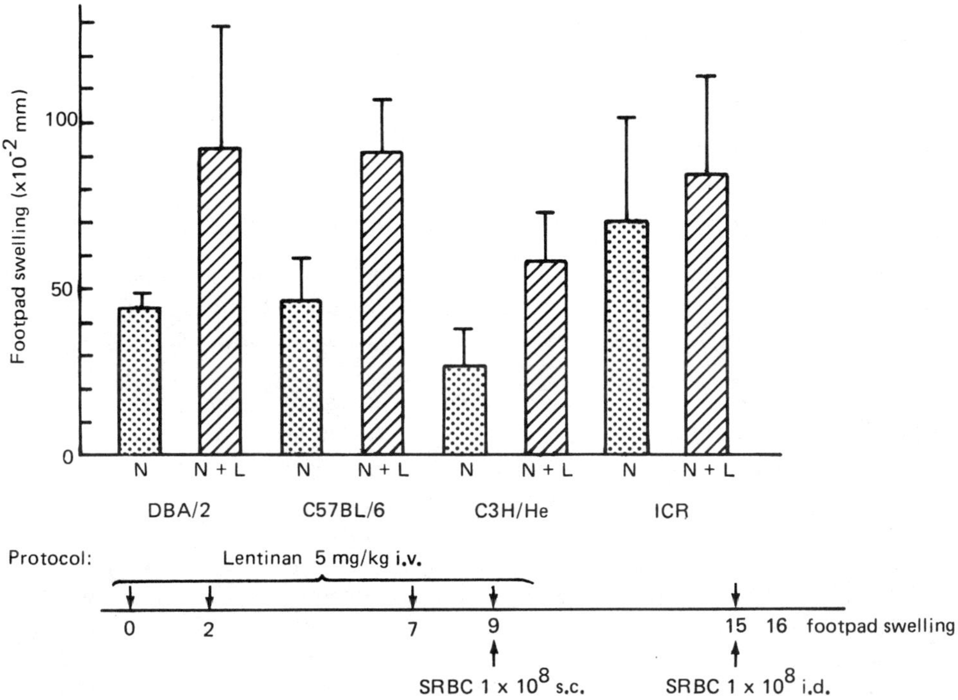

Figure 10 Augmentation by lentinan of delayed hypersensitivity reaction against SRBCs. Lentinan (5 mg/kg IV) was injected into various strains of mice on days 0, 2, 7, and 9. Mice were sensitized with SRBCs (1 X 10^8 SC) on day 9 and challenged by the same number of SRBCs on day 15. Footpad swelling was measured on day 16. (From Ref. 46.)

effects (cell ratio 1:8 for peritoneal cells, and 1:50 for spleen cells). In both P815 and L5178Y, spleen cells and peritoneal exudated cells obtained from tumor-regressing mice treated with lentinan exhibited more than 70% neutralizing effects, whereas both cells from control tumor-bearing mice elicited only marginal effects. The results clearly demonstrated the activation of host defense mechanisms by lentinan and the presence of lentinan-activated effector cells against syngeneic tumors in spleen cells and peritoneal exudated cells.

In an MM102-C3H/HeN system, the similar neutralizing effect was observed only when lentinan-treated spleen cells were transferred with serum from MM102-bearing mice and in an MM46-C3H/HeN system only when lentinan-treated peritoneal exudated cells were transferred with serum from MM46-bearing mice. Therefore, in these systems antitumor effector mechanisms exist as antibody-dependent cellular cytotoxicity reaction (ADCC) and lentinan clearly augments the ADCC effector mechanism.

Next was to examine the localization of cytotoxic effector cells in situ in the tumor-regressing site. Aiming to solve this problem we tried to isolate cytotoxic effector cells from tumor mass. In L5178Y and P815-DBA/2 systems, regressing solid tumors were extirpated at the same date with that of the Winn test and a single-cell suspension was prepared by collagenase-trypsin-DNase treatment. After cell fractionation by 1 X g velocity sedimentation on a gradient of Ficoll in culture medium, each cell fraction was tested for its cytotoxicity against corresponding target tumor cells. Again, cell fractions obtained from tumors under regression by lentinan treatment showed considerable cytotoxicity. Thus, isolated cells are negative in neutral red staining, and they are characterized as lymphoid cells on the basis of morphology. The presence of effector cells in the tumor-regressing local site was also confirmed by the observation that lentinan-treated mice showed augmented infiltration of lymphoid cells into tumor in a syngeneic P815-DBA/2 system.

V. NONIMMUNOLOGICAL POTENTIATION OF HOST DEFENSE

In the preceding section, we described the relevance of immunological action of lentinan. Here we would like to describe the roles of components newly generated or increased after in vivo application of lentinan as triggers or modulators of activation of succeeding immune responses.

It is of interest that various serum proteins are increased transiently after lentinan application. We have found that three major serum proteins in α- and β-globulin region markedly increased in serum 4-7 days after lentinan injection, and these three major components were tentatively named LA, LB, and LC (31).

There is a clear parallel between the antitumor activity of polysaccharides and the unique increase in these three serum protein components. Although there is a marked increase in serum proteins LA, LB, and LC after administration of antitumor-active polysaccharides such as lentinan, such a phenomenon is not detected entirely after administration of the polysaccharides lacking in antitumor activity. Lentinan appears to have an optimal dose for its antitumor activity, and the activity does not appear at all when a large dose of 80 mg/kg is applied in a sarcoma 180-ICR system. At the dose of 80 mg/kg, no increase in the serum protein components LA, LB, and LC were observed. As mentioned previously, growth-inhibitory action of lentinan differs from one mouse strain to the other mouse strain at the 1 mg/kg dose, namely, among different mouse strains, there exist high-responder mouse strains and low-responder mouse strains. As imagined, marked increases in these serum proteins were observed clearly in high-responder mice such as ICR, SWM/Ms, A/J, C57B1/6, and DBA/2, but not in low-responder mice such as BALB/c.

With reference to the results of polyacrylamide gel electrophoresis of other serum proteins reported so far, these components LA, LB and LC have been reported to include haptoglobin (50), ceruloplasmin, and hemopexin (40-42). The full assignments of these components wait for further detailed studies, but there exists the possibility of participation of the third component of complement C3, because it has been reported that C3 was also increased markedly after lentinan application. Based on the analysis of enzymatic activity, it has been concluded that antitrypsin is not included in these components. In addition, a marked increase of the amount of acute-phase proteins such as serum amyloid-P factor and α_2 HS-glycoprotein were also observed.

It should be kept in mind that these factors increased upon lentinan application may probably be synthesized in the liver and may have relevant roles to maintain biochemical hemeostasis of the host. Ceruloplasmin possesses a protective effect against the lowering of liver catalase activity triggered by toxohormone (40), and it can be used as a therapeutic agent for human aplastic anemia, cachexia, and others. In Table 8, various serum factors which increased after lentinan application are listed.

As has been stated above, lentinan has several characteristics which are considerably different from numerous known immunopotentiators, and it seems necessary to study its

Table 8 Various Serum Proteins or Factors Increased after Lentinan Application

		References
Compliment system		
Classic	Activation	58
Alternative	Activation	28,59
Total complement value	Increase	58
Absolute C3 value	Increase	A. J. S. Davies
Acute-phase proteins		
LA, LB, and LC	Increase	31
Haptoglobin	Increase	50
Hemopexin	Increase	55
Ceruloplasmin	Increase	56
Serum amyroid P	Increase	A. J. S. Davies
Enzymes		
Trypsin inhibitor	Not increase	57
Cyclooxygenase inhibitor	Increase	J. Hamuro
Lysozyme	Increase	57
Colony-stimulating factor	Increase	46
Cytokines as modulation factor	Increase	J. Hamuro
Tumor necrosis factor (TNF)	Not increase	G. Chihara

action from entirely different standpoints. In this sense, lentinan has some physiological and endocrinological effects.

Lentinan increases the histamine or serotonin sensitivity in mice in the same way as pertussis vaccine (43), but, by contrast, lentinan can also suppress the histamine shock of pertussis-treated mice. It seems to be relevant that lentinan prevents an indistinct toxic death due to the administration of cyclocytidine or vincristine (44). Toxic death by the administration of 500 mg/kg for 20 days of cyclocytidine alone occurred in 7 of 17 mice, but this toxic action is apparently suppressed when lentinan is used in combination with cyclocytidine. The effects of physiological active amines, such as vascular permeability, might play a part in the mechanism of lentinan in some form (6).

The difference between 25 and 70% in the tumor-inhibitory effect of lentinan against the LOU immunocytoma in rat, according to chronobiological best timing or worst timing, may be relevant to the action of serotonin, melatonin, or catecholamines (45).

What is most interesting is that the antitumor activity of lentinan is strongly inhibited by thyroxine, the activity lowering from 98 to 22% by the administration of thyroxine. Since thyroxine tends to enhance the growth of a tumor, there remains a possibility that this inhibition may be the result of antagonism between the action of lentinan and thyroxine (51). In any case, it is of interest that the thyroid gland takes part in tumor growth, because there is a report that cancer incidence is high in myxedema and low in hyperthyroidemia. Therefore, the role of the thyroid gland in tumor invasion is an inportant problem to be considered in future studies on the host defense against cancer.

The antitumor effect of lentinan is also inhibited by hydrocortisone (51). As the action of cortisol is synergistic with the action of antilymphocyte serum and this hormone is known to specifically attack the thymus-derived lymphocyte, it is natural that the antitumor effect of lentinan is inhibited by hydrocortisone acetate. Thus, the endocrinological homeostasis is affected by the action of lentinan.

VI. ACTION MODE OF LENTINAN

Lentinan augments the reactivity of precursor effector cells responding to major lymphokines, Interleukin 2, macrophage-activating factor, and T-cell replacing factor (TRF), produced by activated subsets of T lymphocytes. The augmentation of the reactivity of precursor effector cells in turn results in the augmented generation of cytotoxic T lymphocytes, natural killer cells, activated macrophages, and antibody.

Thus, lentinan exerts augmentation of T-cell-dependent immune responses by augmenting the generation of tumor-specific and nonspecific but selective effector cells triggered by T-cell activation.

We postulate that Interleukin 1 and Interleukin 2 act as two signals for the activation of cytotoxic T lymphocytes. For the activation of NK cells, a certain signal may act synergistically with Interleukin 2 as a second signal. Similarly, to activate macrophages, the second signal may play a role to activate macrophages synergistically with MAF. For the activation of B cells to produce antibody, Interleukin 1 and T-cell replacing factor may act synergistically. At present, it is unclear what kind of factors may act as second signals for NK cells and macrophage activation although we postulate the role of colony-stimulating factors as second signals. Our preliminary experimental results suggest the presence of these kinds of factors playing roles as second signals functioning as maturation factor for NK cells and macrophage activation in serum harvested from lentinan-administered mice. Although the validity of this postulation would be evidence in detailed future analysis, lentinan may act indirectly as a second signal with lymphokines such as Interleukin 2, MAF, and TRF to activate major antitumor effectors, namely, cytotoxic, T lymphocytes, NK cells, activated macrophages, and antibody.

Lentinan triggers increased production of Interleukin 1 by direct impact on immune regulatory macrophages or indirectly via augmented colony-stimulating factor (CSF) production from lentinan-stimulated alveolar macrophages. Thus, increased production of Interleukin 1 results in the augmented maturation of premature lymphoid cells into mature cells capable of responding to lymphokines; then in turn, mature cells are differentiated into effector cytotoxic T lymphocytes, NK cells, activated macrophages, and plasma cells in the presence of Interleukin 2, MAF, and TRF. In addition, lentinan-induced mature T cells can generate CSF upon lentinan stimulation to form an amplification loop to produce Il-1 (Fig. 11). Thus produced Il-1 may play a central role in increasing

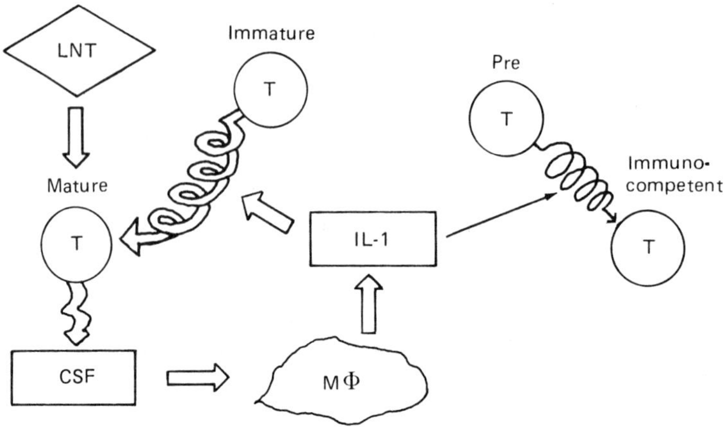

Figure 11 Action mode of lentinan mediated by T-cell-derived CSF.

acute-phase proteins or to increase a unique class of serum proteins, described in the preceding section. Then some of these increased serum proteins may trigger or modulate the specific or nonspecific immune response.

Many of the immunopotentiators of a polyanionic nature are said to activate macrophages and NK cells by inducing the production of interferon from stimulated macrophages. As mentioned, lentinan could not activate macrophages or NK cells upon in vitro exposure, therefore it might not be probable that interferon plays a central role in lentinan-augmented generation of effector cell induction. However, this concept does not necessarily exclude the possible participation of interferon in the activation of NK cells and macrophages in vivo by lentinan.

Lentinan is a neutral, well-characterized, purified, and nontoxic immunotherapeutic agent capable of positively influencing the immunological-specific limb of T-cell-mediated cytotoxic immune responses as well as the nonspecific limb of macrophage and natural killer cell-mediated responses.

The summarized possible mode of action described well explains several observed characteristics of the antitumor action of lentinan, such as the absence of antitumor activity in neonatally thymectomized mice, the lack of activity in nu/nu mice, the decrease of activity by carageenan treatment, loss of activity by 400-R irradiation at an early phase after transplantation, and loss of activity by administration of immunosuppressive agents.

The term *immune adjuvants* characterizes substances that either convert apparently nonimmunogeneic antigens into effective immunogens or lead to augmented humoral or cell-mediated immune responses, leading to more protective immunity. Adjuvants such as Freund complete adjuvant, BCG, *C. parvum*, or other adjuvants of bacterial origin are of remarkable complex and diverse chemical nature, which may be one of the explanations as to why their modes of action are so poorly understood. Because of a well-defined chemical nature, the modes of action of lentinan are relatively well understood. Among several immunological characteristics, lentinan is known to have relevant distinctive features as an immune adjuvant compared with other immune adjuvants, thus far known, with complex or polyanionic chemical natures. From time to time in the preceding sections, the distinctive characteristics of lentinan were described in detail, thus it is sufficient to generalize these as follows in order to gain a fuller understanding.

1. Chemically fully defined nature to produce reliable, reproducible activity.
2. Effectiveness by systematic administration comparable with actual protocol in clinical studies.
3. No activation of macrophages or NK cells during in vitro cocultivation, but efficient activation of these cells upon in vivo application.
4. No increase of interferon and lysosomal enzymes released from macrophages upon in vitro cultivation.
5. Depression of protaglandin release from macrophages induced by lentinan
6. Characteristic dependency on T cells as an immune adjuvant such as to augment reactivity of precursor effector cells to T-cell-derived lymphokines.
7. No activation of macrophages in vitro in terms of cytotoxicity, but stimulation of macrophages to increase reactivity to MAF.
8. No mitogenicity and absence of the character as a polyclonal activator.
9. Generation of serum factor (s) functioning as maturation factor for lymphoid cells by generation of Il-1.
10. Production of CSF from T cells.

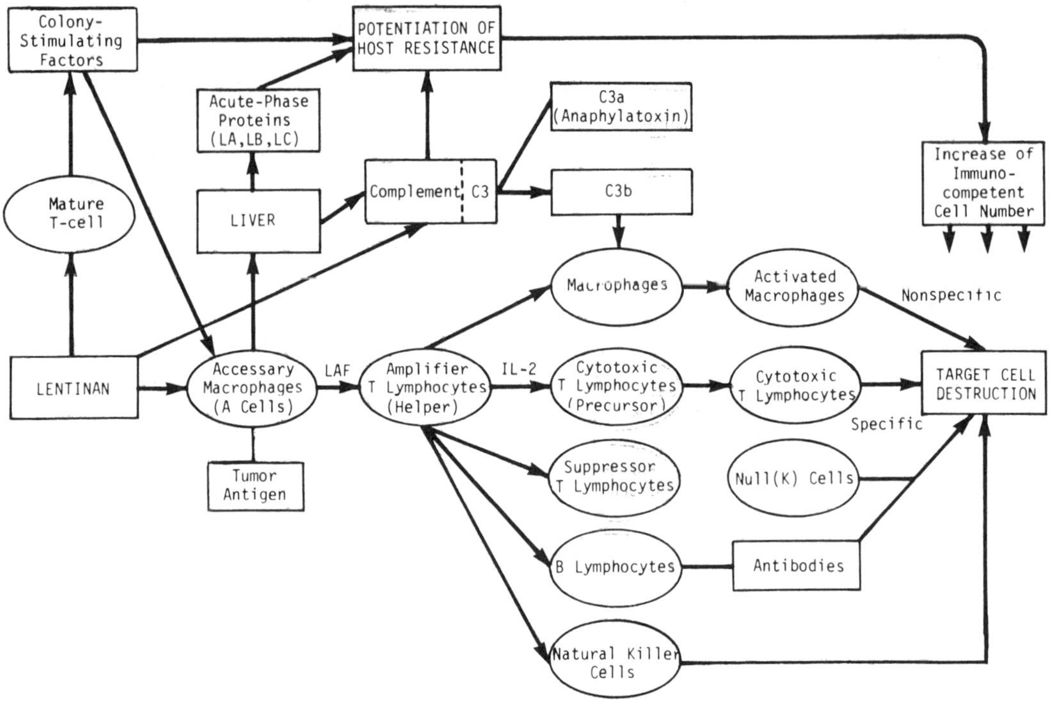

Figure 12 Possible mode of action of lentinan.

11. Synergistic potentiation of immune response with T-cell-derived lymphokines.
12. No increase of phagocytic activity of macrophages both in vivo and in vitro.

Possible mode of action of lentinan is summarized in Fig. 12.

VII. CLINICAL APPLICATION

As already mentioned, lentinan shows the distinct antitumor effects in allogeneic, syngeneic, and autologous hosts, and its unique mode of action has been precisely clarified. Toxicological studies have been completed in animal models, and LD_{50} is over 1500 mg/kg intraperitoneally in mice.

Therefore, lentinan has been expected to be effective in human cancer patients, and Taguchi and cooperative clinical study groups have performed phases I, II, III clinical trials of lentinan (48,49).

A phase I study has been conducted on 50 eligible patients with various types of advanced cancer, and side effects of lentinan have been observed in 3 of 50 cases; that is, slight liver dysfunction, feeling of mild oppression on the chest, and petechiae on the legs. These side effects are transitional and disappeared by the cessation or reduction of dosage of lentinan administration. A phase II clinical study has been performed to determine the optimal conditions of administration of lentinan. The recommended administration of lentinan would be at doses of 0.5-1 mg/day per person intravenously once or twice a week, in combination with chemotherapeutic agents such as tegaful (FT-207) or mitomycin C + 5-FU, according to its antitumor effect and improvement of host immune responses such as PPD skin test and lymphoproliferative response of peripheral blood lymphocytes (PBL) in the eligible 127 cases, in which advanced gastrointestinal cancer patients have been more than half.

According to these results, a phase III study has been conducted to evaluate clinical efficacy in patients with advanced or recurrent gastric cancer (52) and colorectal cancer (53). A randomized controlled trial has been performed under the following two kinds of treatments: one was the single administration of tegafur (FT-207) as control treatment (FT group), and the other was the combination administration of lentinan and tegafur (LTN group). Lentinan has been administered at the doses of 1 mg/day per person twice a week or 2 mg/day per person once a week by intravenous injection, Kaplan-Meier's method and generalized Wilcoxon's test have been employed for the assessment of life-span prolongation effect of lentinan. Eligible cases of gastric cancer patients were 72 in the FT-control group and 77 in the lentinan group. A remarkable life-span prolongation effect of lentinan has been observed with statistical significance ($p < 0.01$) (Fig. 13). In addition, the life-span prolongation effect of lentinan have been observed in the following stratifications: Zubrod's performance status of the patients at the commencement of the trial; with or without prior chemotherapy, with or without primary lesions. Thus, lentinan should be effective for patients with advanced and recurrent gastric cancer in combination with tegafur (52). Eligible cases of colorectal cancer patients were 17 in the

	No. of cases	Survival days at 50% survival
C: Tegafur (Control) :	72	105
L: Tegafur + LNT :	77	163

	No. of cases	Survival days at 50% survival
C: Tegafur (Control) :	17	94
L: Tegafur + LNT :	23	200

Tegafur (FT-207) : 400~1200 mg/person/day
LNT 1 or 2 mg/person/day, 2 mg/week

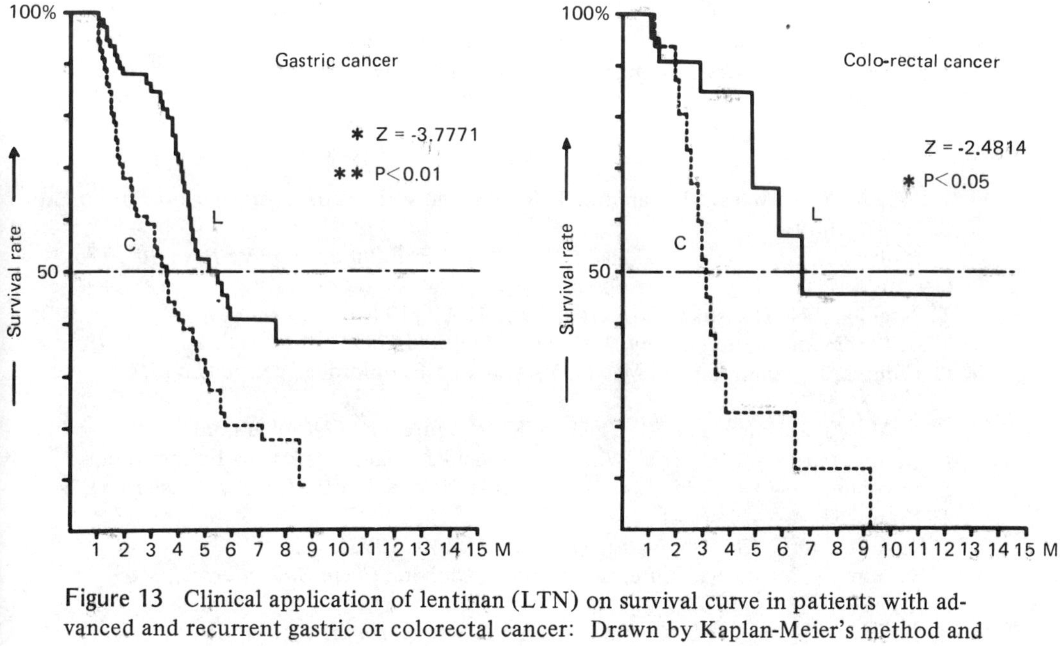

Figure 13 Clinical application of lentinan (LTN) on survival curve in patients with advanced and recurrent gastric or colorectal cancer: Drawn by Kaplan-Meier's method and examined by generalized Wilcoxon's test.

FT-control group and 23 in the lentinan group. A distinct life-span prolongation effect of lentinan has been observed with statistical significance ($p < 0.05$). In addition, patient survival over 9 months was 0% in the FT-control group and 45% in the lentinan group through the course of the trial. These results suggest that lentinan should be effective also for patients with advanced and recurrent colorectal cancer (53). Phase III studies are underway in patients with breast cancer (54), lung cancer, and malignant lymphomas. Clinical efficacy of lentinan on these types of cancer are to be assessed by prolongation of life span, antitumor effect, and side effects.

Next, as our future target, combination treatment of lentinan with curative operation is now planned for evaluating its effect on metastasis and/or recurrence after surgery. Besides cancer, lentinan is expected to be effective in bacterial, viral, and parasitic infectious diseases on the basis of the results of animal experiments. Therefore, clinical trials of lentinan on these diseases will be designed and conducted in the near future.

VIII. CONCLUSION

Lentinan, exhibiting prominent antitumor, antibacterial, antiviral, and antiparasitic effects, is a chemically well-defined neutral polysaccharide. It is characterized by its distinct immunological and biological activities from those of other immunostimulants, such as BCG, *C. parvum*, LPS, levamisole, pyran copolymer, poly I:C, interferons, and so on. Low toxicity showing $LD_{50} > 1500$ mg/kg (mice) is also an important characteristic of lentinan when compared with other chemotherapeutic agents possessing detrimental toxic side effects. Thus, lentinan with these characteristic features might be one of the potent candidates to apply in clinical studies for cancer patients.

We consider lentinan to be the most interesting and fascinating immunopotentiator among substances known thus far. To abstract as much as possible the characteristics of lentinan, it might be a more important and urgent task for clinical immunologists to find parameters of the host-tumor relationship beneficial for the indication of protocols to apply lentinan as an immunomodulating agent for therapeutic and prophylactic treatment against bacteria, viruses, parasites, neoplasias, and immunodeficiencies.

REFERENCES

1. G. Chihara, Y. Y. Maeda, J. Hamuro, T. Sasaki, and F. Fukuoka, *Nature (Lond.)*, *222*:687 (1969).
2. G. Chihara, J. Hamuro, Y. Y. Maeda, Y. Arai and F. Fukuoka, *Cancer Res.*, *30*:2776 (1970).
3. T. Sasaki and N. Takasuka, *Carbohyd. Res.*, *47*:99 (1976).
4. T. H. Bluhm and A. Sarko, *Can. J. Chem.*, *55*:293 (1977).
5. G. Chihara, J. Hamuro, Y. Y. Maeda, Y. Arai, and F. Fukuoka, *Nature (Lond.)*, *225*:943 (1970).
6. Y. Y. Maeda, J. Hamuro, Y. O. Yamada, K. Ishimura, and G. Chihara, in *Immunopotentiation* (G. E. W. Wolstenholm and J. Kight, eds.), Ciba Foundation Symposium, New Series 18, Elsevier, Excerpta Medica, North-Holland, Amsterdam, 1973, p. 259.
7. J. Hamuro and G. Chihara, *Nature (Lond.)*, *245*:40 (1973).
8. J. Hamuro, Y. Y. Maeda, F. Fukuoka, and G. Chihara, *Chem-Biol Interact.*, *3*:69 (1971).
9. T. Sasaki, N. Takasuka, G. Chihara, and Y. Y. Maeda, *Gann*, *67*:191 (1971).
10. Y. Y. Maeda and G. Chihara, *Int. J. Cancer*, *11*:153 (1973).

11. O. J. Plescia, A. H. Smith, and K. Grinwich, *Proc. Natl. Acad. Sci. USA*, *72*:1848 (1975).
12. J. I. Kurland and R. Bockman, *J. Exp. Med.*, *147*:952 (1978).
13. T. Shiio and Y. Yugari, *Int. J. Immunopharmacol.*, *2*:172 (1980).
14. J. Zâkâny, G. Chihara, and J. Fachet, *Int. J. Cancer*, *25*:371 (1980).
15. J. Zâkâny, G. Chihara, and J. Fachet, *Int. J. Cancer*, *26*:783 (1980).
16. J. E. Byrum, A. Sher, J. DiPietro, and F. von Lichtenberg, *Am. J. Pathol.*, *94*:201 (1979).
17. K. Kanai, E. Kondo, P. L. Jacques, and G. Chihara, *Jap. J. Med. Sci. Biol.*, *33*:283 (1980).
18. K. S. S. Chang, in *Manipulation of Host Defense Mechanisms* (T. Aoki, ed.), *Excerpta* Medica, Amsterdam, 1981, p. 76.
19. T. Hamada, in *Manipulation of Host Defense Mechanisms* (T. Aoki, ed.), Excerpta Medica, Amsterdam, 1981, p. 78.
20. J. Delville and P. L. Jacques, *Int. J. Immunopharmacol.*, *2*:183 (1980).
21. T. Kawamura and Y. Numasaki, *Proc. Jap. Cancer Assoc.*, *39*:134 (1980).
22. H. U. Schorlemmer, D. Bitter-Suermann, and A. C. Allison, *Immunology*, *32*:929 (1977).
23. J. Hamuro, M. Rollinghoff, H. Wagner, M. Seitz, W. Grimm, and D. Gemsa, *Z. Immun-Forsch.*, *155*:28 (1979).
24. M. Grimm, M. Seitz, H. Kierchner and D. Gemsa, *Cell Immunol.*, *40*:419 (1978).
25. J. Hamuro, U. Hadding, and D. Bitter-Seuermann, *Immunology*, *14*:695 (1978)
26. H. U. Schorlemmer, D. Bitter-Suermann, and A. C. Allison, *Immunology*, *32*:929 (1977).
27. H. U. Schorlemmer, P. Davies, and A. C. Allison, *Nature*, *261*:48 (1976).
28. Y. Y. Maeda, J. Hamuro, and G. Chihara, *Int. J. Cancer*, *8*:41 (1971).
29. Y. Y. Maeda, and G. Chihara, *Nature* (*Lond.*), *229*:634 (1971).
30. Y. Yamada, S. Matsumoto, K. Kumai, K. Hibiki, and O. Abe, in *Manipulation of Host Defense Mechanisms,* (T. Aoki, ed.), Excerpta Medica, Amsterdam, 1981, p. 219.
31. Y. Y. Maeda, G. Chihara, and K. Ishimura, *Nature* (*Lond.*), *252*:250 (1974).
32. J. Hamuro, M. Röllinghoff, and H.Wagner, *Cancer Res.*, *38*:3080 (1978).
33. J. Hamuro, H. Wagner, and M. Röllinghoff, *Cell Immunol.*, *38*:328 (1978).
34. J. Hamuro, M. Röllinghoff, and H. Wagner, *Immunology*, *39*:551 (1980).
35. J. P. Levy, E. Gomard, and J. Wibier-Franqui, in *Manipulation of Host Defense Mechanism* (T. Aoki, ed.), Excerpta Medica, Amsterdam, 1981, p. 268.
36. Y. Masuko, S. Abe, and D. Mizuno, *Proc. Jap. Cancer Assoc.*, *38*:92 (1979).
37. Y. Yohikai, S. Miake, T. Matsumoto, K. Nomoto, and K. Takeya, *Proc. Jap. Soc. Immunol.*, *9*:171 (1979).
38. G. Dennert and D. Tucker, *J. Natl. Cancer Inst.*, *51*:1729 (1973).
39. D. W. Dresser, and J. M. Phillips, *Immunoloby*, *27*:895 (1974).
40. O. Itoh, T. Torikai, M. Satoh, and T. Osawa, *Gann, 71*:644 (1980).
41. G. Chihara, in *The Mechanisms of Host Defense* (D. Mizuno, K. Takeya, and N. Ishida, eds.), Univ. of Tokyo Press, Tokoy, 1980, pp. 301.
42. T. Torikai, O. Itoh, M. Satoh, and T. Osawa, *Proc. Jap. Cancer Assoc.*, *39*:105 (1980).
43. R. Homma and K. Kuratsuka, *Experientia*, *29*:290 (1973).
44. R. Tokuzen, M. Okabe, and W. Nakahara, *Gann*, *67*:327 (1976).
45. G. Chihara, F. Carandente, and Halberg, *Proc. Am. Assoc. Cancer Res.*, *20*:111 (1979).
46. Y. Akiyama, S. Kashima, T. Hayami, M. Izawa, K. Mitsugi, and J. Hamuro, in *Manipulation of Host Defense Mechanisms* (T. Aoki, ed.), Excerpta Medica, Amsterdam, 1981, p.227.

47. T. Kawamura, Y. Taguchi, and Y. Numasaki, *Proc. Jap. Assoc. Cancer Res.*, *41*:163 (1982).
48. H. Furue, I. Ito, T. Kimura, T. Kondo, T. Hattori, N. Ogawa, and T. Taguchi, *Gan to Kagakuryoho* (*Cancer and Chemotherapy*), *8*:944 (1981).
49. G. Chihara and T. Taguchi, *Rev. Immunol. Immunopharmacol.*, *2*:93 (1982).
50. Y. Y. Maeda, S. Watanabe, M. Rokutanda, and G. Chihara, *Int. J. Immunopharmacol.*, *4*:263 (1982).
51. Y. Y. Maeda, K. Ishimura, N. Takasuka, T. Sasaki, and G. Chihara, in *Host Defense Against Cancer and Its Potentiation* (D. Mizuno, G. Chihara, F. Fukuoka, T. Yamamoto, and Y. Yamamura, eds.), University of Tokyo Press, Tokyo, 1975, pp. 181.
52. T. Taguchi, H. Furue, T. Kimura, T. Kondoh, T. Hattori, I. Itoh, and N. Ogawa, *Int. J. Immunopharmacol.*, *4*:272 (1982).
53. T. Taguchi, H. Furue, T. Kimura, T. Kondoh, T. Hattori, I. Itoh, and N. Ogawa, *Int. J. Immunopharmacol.*, *4*:271 (1982).
54. T. Taguchi, O. Abe, K. Enomoto, S. Kusama, J. Tomiyama, K. Tominaga and N. Ogawa, *Int. J. Immunopharmacol.*, *4*:271 (1982).
55. T. Torikai, O. Itoh, M. Satoh, O. Okamura, and T. Osawa, *Gann* (*Jap. J. Cancer Res.*), *72*:92 (1981).
56. O. Itoh, T. Torikai, M. Satoh, and T. Osawa, *Gann* (*Jap. J. Cancer Res.*), *71*:644 (1980).
57. G. Chihara, in *The Mechanisms of Host Defense* (D. Mizuno, K. Takeya, and N. Ishida, eds.), University of Tokyo Press, Tokyo, pp. 301 (1980).
58. M. Sakamoto and K. Nishioka, *Proc. Compl. Symp.*, *18*:46 (1981).
59. T. Okuda, Y. Yoshioka, T. Ikekawa, G. Chihara, and K. Nishioka, *Nature* (*New Biol.*), *238*:59 (1972).

20

Influence of Host-Tumor Relationships on Response to the Biological Response Modifiers, Glucan, and Methyl Palmitate

N. R. Di Luzio, Rose B. McNamee, Ernest L. Jones, and David L. Williams
Tulane University School of Medicine, New Orleans, Louisiana

I. INTRODUCTION

It is now generally conceded that clinical experience with such classic biological response modifiers (BRMs) as Bacillus Calmette-Guérin (BCG), methanol extraction residue of BCG (MER), and *Corneybacterium parvum* has been most disappointing. In part this is due to the fact that these agents have had relatively significant effects on the modification of tumor growth and development in a variety of experimental animals (1-4). Reasons for the possible diversity of effectiveness between experimental animals and humans may include (a) clinical employment of doses of these agents to the point of toxicity rather than to the point of immunobiological effectiveness; (b) inappropriateness of animal models which lack clinical relevance, such as the employment of allogeneic and xenogeneic tumor models; (c) the extensive employment of transplantable or chemically induced tumors rather than autochthonous tumors; (d) the nutritional, metabolic, and immune status of the employed experimental animals which are not generally impaired or altered as would be the case in the clinical setting; (e) the failure to effectively utilize experimental models of metastases; and (f) limited utilization of animal models employing multiple therapeutic procedures which could restrict effectiveness of BRMs.

Advances in the field of immunotherapy have taken immunomodulating agents from the Middle Ages to the Renaissance period (5). With the development of highly purified nontoxic water-soluble glucans, as well as synthetic agents such as muramyl dipeptides, immunotherapy is entering the era of modern biotechnology. It is now essential in the evaluation of these and other forthcoming BRMs that animal tumor models closely mimic the clinical situation where the immunoactivating agents may ultimately be employed. Only with appropriate animal tumor models can one begin to ascertain the clinical potential of newly developed biologic response modifiers. In support of this concept, several investigators have outlined various criteria for the selection of what might be more appropriate tumor models.

The review by Bartlett et al. (6) considers, in depth, the problems of transferring experimental findings to the clinical situation. Hewitt and colleagues (7,8), in an extensive study employing 27 different experimental tumors, stressed that isotransplants of spontaneously arising tumors are the most appropriate models of human malignancy. Alexander (9), in stressing the need for more realistic animal models in evaluating immunotherapeutic procedures, suggested that animal tumors which are not immunogeneic by standard transplantation tests are potentially the most valuable models with regard to transfer of information from experimental animals to humans. Weiss (10) has also reviewed the status of animal models and stressed that host-tumor relationships must be seriously considered in studies involving immunological intervention. Greager and Baldwin (11) have studied the influence of immunotherapeutic agents on the progression of spontaneously arising metastatic rat mammary adenocarcinomas of varying immunogenicity and concluded that the immunogenic nature of the tumor played an important role in the effectiveness of such biological response modifiers as *C. parvum* or BCG. Martin et al. (12) stressed the importance of employing autochthonous tumors, so that data derived in studies of immunotherapeutic modification may be transferable to the autochthonous tumors of man. These comments have initiated considerable controversy, as reflected by the response of Rapp to several of these articles (13,14) and the ensuing reply of the investigators (15,16).

In view of the significant controversy associated with employment of various animal models, studies were undertaken in our laboratory to establish the influence of glucan and methyl palmitate on tumor growth in murine models where genetically diverse host-tumor relationships existed. In these studies tumor progression was evaluated in allogeneic, syngeneic, and autochthonous tumor models, in the presence and absence of both positive and negative immunomodulation. The tumors that were selected in this comparative study had either a 100, 50, or 0% incidence of acceptances, depending upon host-tumor antigenic relationships.

These studies clearly indicate that the influence of biological response modifiers, such as glucan (17-19) and methyl palmitate (20-22), which diversely influence host defense mechanisms, had a quantitatively differential effect on tumor progression that was dependent upon the tumor-host model employed.

II. MATERIALS AND METHODS

Two transplantable murine tumor models were employed. Mammary adenocarcinoma (H2712), which is syngeneic for the C3H/HeJ mouse, was studied in allogeneic and syngeneic mice. It normally is completely rejected in the allogeneic C57BL/6J mice which were employed. The second mammary carcinoma employed (15091A) is syngeneic for A/J mice and was studied in allogeneic and syngeneic tumor systems. Both tumors were initially obtained from The Jackson Laboratory, Bar Harbor, Maine. In the C3H/HeJ mouse an approximate 50% acceptance of the 15091A tumor is normally observed. In the initial studies, the influence of glucan or methyl palmitate on tumor incidence and growth as well as phagocytic function was determined on days 5, 10, and 15 following the subcutaneous administration of 3×10^6 cells.

Additional studies were conducted to evaluate the influence of macrophage stimulation with glucan and macrophage suppression with methyl palmitate on the development of spontaneous leukemia in aging AKR/J mice. In these studies initial treatment with glucan or methyl palmitate began when the AKR/J mice were approximately 6 months of age. At this time extensive histopathological studies and peripheral leukocyte counts indicated no evidence of leukemia. Methyl palmitate (35 mg) or glucan (0.45 mg) were administered IV at biweekly intervals for the duration of the study. Isovolumetric dextrose (5% w/v) and water served as the control for the glucan-treated mice, while a Tween-20 solution served as a control for the methyl palmitate-treated group.

Analysis of the particulate glucan preparation, prepared from *Saccharomyces cerevisiae* (Red Star Yeast, Universal Floods, Milwaukee, Wisconsin) by previously outlined procedures (23), denoted a high degree of purity, with a mean 99.6% carbohydrate, and less than 0.01% phosphorus, 0.06% sulfate, and a 0.38% nitrogen (Galbraith Laboratories, Knoxville, Tennessee). Glucan was suspended in dextrose (5% w/v) and water and sterilized. The glucan suspension was endotoxin free as determined by Limulus lysate gelation.

An emulsion of methyl palmitate was prepared in dextrose (5% w/v) and water with 0.1% (v/v) Tween-20. The suspension was sonicated for 15 min. Tween-20 (0.1% v/v) in 5% dextrose and water served as the control for methyl palmitate experiments.

Phagocytic function, as measured by intravascular clearance, was evaluated in vivo employing colloidal carbon C11/1431A (Gunther-Wagner, Hanover, Federal Republic of West Germany), in the dose of 16 mg/100 g (17). Tail blood was sampled at 1, 3, 5, 7, and 9 min after IV injection of carbon. Blood samples, were diluted in 4 ml of (0.1%) sodium carbonate to lyse the cellular components of blood. The optical density of the resultant colloidal suspension was read at 650 μm and the intravascular half-time determined by semilogarithmic plots.

Statistical comparisons between groups were performed employing Student's t-test. A value of $p < 0.05$ was considered significant. Analysis of survival data was based on chi-square with one degree of freedom. A value representing a 95% confidence level was considered significant.

III. RESULTS

Studies concerning the growth of the adenocarcinoma (H2712) cells in allogeneic C57BL/6J mice indicated complete rejection in control animals (Table 1). In contrast, the methyl palmitate-treated animals showed a 100% incidence of tumor acceptance. Throughout the 15-day period of study the measurement of phagocytic function indicated an approximate 100% decrease in the intravascular half-life of colloidal carbon in the methyl palmitate-treated animals.

Similarly, the employment of the adenocarcinoma 15091A, which is partially accepted (33-71% incidence) in allogeneic C3H/HeJ control mice, showed 100% incidence in the methyl palmitate-treated group (Table 2). In addition to an enhanced incidence of tumor occurrence, a significant difference in the growth of the tumor occurred between the control and the methyl palmitate-treated group. The enhancement of tumor growth in methyl palmitate-treated mice was 1373, 344, and 675% at days 5, 10, and 15, respectively.

Similar findings were observed when methyl palmitate was administered to syngeneic A/J mice in which the adenocarcinoma 15091A was transplanted (Table 3). Here, again, at days 5 and 10, a significant enhancement in tumor growth occurred. However, the enhanced growth of the syngeneic tumor was not comparable with that observed in the allogeneic models.

Table 1 Influence of Methyl Palmitate-Induced Macrophage Suppression on Growth of Mammary Carcinoma (H2712) in Allogeneic C57BL/6J Mice[a]

Treatment	Days	Phagocytic function (t/2, min)	Tumor Weight (mg)	Tumor Incidence (%)
Control	0	8.1 ± 0.57	–	–
Methly palmitate	0	17.6 ± 0.67[d]	–	–
Control	5	10.9 ± 0.79	0	0
Methyl palmitate	5	17.6 ± 2.35[b]	330 ± 36.7	100
Control	10	10.8 ± 1.53	0	0
Methly palmitate	10	13.9 ± 1.78	466 ± 88.2	100
Control	15	9.6 ± 2.22	0	0
Methyl palmitate	15	18.5 ± 3.26[b]	466 ± 36.1	100

[a]The adenocarcinoma H2712 is a mammary tumor which spontaneously arose in a C3H/HeJ mouse. It normally is completely rejected in allogeneic C57BL/6J mice. Values are expressed as mean ± standard error and are derived from 48 mice (i.e., six mice per group). Methyl palmitate (35 mg per mouse) was administered −2 days before the subcutaneous transplantation of 3.0×10^6 cells and at days 5 and 10 posttumor cell administration. Control mice received isovolumetric injections of 0.2% Tween in 5% dextrose and water.

[b]$p < 0.05$.

[c]$p < 0.01$.

[d]$p < 0.001$.

Table 2 Influence of Methyl Palmitate Administration on Phagocytic Function and Growth of a Mammary Carcinoma (15091A) in Allogenic C3H/HeJ Mice[a]

Treatment	Days	Phagocytic function (t/2, min)	Tumor Weight (mg)	Tumor Incidence (%)
Control	0	8.0 ± 0.67	–	–
Methyl palmitate	0	31.1 ± 5.35[c]	–	–
Control	5	9.3 ± 0.75	49 ± 39	33
Methyl palmitate	5	22.9 ± 2.38[d]	673 ± 153[c]	100
Control	10	11.4 ± 0.94	94 ± 60	42
Methyl palmitate	10	33.6 ± 3.29[d]	327 ± 60[b]	100
Control	15	24.4 ± 3.41	136 ± 70	71
Methyl palmitate	15	40.3 ± 6.28[c]	919 ± 88[d]	100

[a]The mammary carcinoma is syngeneic in the A/J mouse. In allogeneic C3H/HeJ mice an approximate 50% tumor acceptance occurs. Values are expressed as mean ± standard error and are derived from six mice per group.

[b]$p < 0.05$.

[c]$p < 0.01$.

[d]$p < 0.001$.

Table 3 Influence of Methyl Palmitate Administration on Phagocytic Function and on Mammary Carcinoma (15091A) Growth in Syngeneic A/J Mice[a]

Treatment	Days	Phagocytic function (t/2, min)	Tumor weight (mg)
Control	0	11.8 ± 0.57	–
Methyl palmitate	0	32.8 ± 2.34[d]	–
Control	5	13.0 ± 2.33	294 ± 40
Methyl palmitate	5	23.4 ± 2.75[b]	454 ± 50[b]
Control	10	13.5 ± 1.23	641 ± 60
Methyl palmitate	10	28.2 ± 3.78[c]	864 ± 50[b]
Control	15	10.7 ± 0.90	1.602 ± 160
Methyl palmitate	15	20.6 ± 2.12[c]	1.724 ± 90

[a]Values are expressed as means ± standard error and are derived from 56 mice (i.e., 7 mice per group).
[b]$p < 0.05$.
[c]$p < 0.01$.
[d]$p < 0.001$.

In contrast to the detrimental effects of macrophage suppression on tumor acceptance and progression in the various syngeneic and allogeneic models employed, the administration of glucan to allogeneic C3H/HeJ mice bearing the adenocarcinoma 15091A revealed that the incidence of malignancy was materially reduced to where approximately one-third of the animals had detectable tumors (Table 4). The reduction in mean tumor weight in the glucan-treated animals was 95, 94, and 96% on days 5, 10, and 15, respectively. Inhibition of tumor growth, as well as the incidence of malignancy, appeared to be correlated with the enhancement of macrophage phagocytic function throughout the 15-day period of study.

In contrast to the very profound reduction in tumor growth induced by glucan in allogeneic models, glucan was not as effective in syngeneic models, even though a comparable degree of macrophage hyperfunction was achieved. The decrease in tumor growth induced by glucan in the syngeneic model approximated 64, 51, and 32% at days 5, 10, and 15, respectively (Table 5). Thus, the effectiveness of glucan on tumor progression can be materially altered depending upon host-tumor relationships.

In evaluation of the influence of glucan and methyl palmitate on the development of spontaneous leukemia in aging AKR mice, it was observed that the biweekly administration of glucan over a 6-month period of time resulted in a significant ($p < 0.01$) prolongation in survival (Table 6). Survival time was extended to 240 days in the glucan-treated mice in contrast to 210 days in the control group. Conversely, the biweekly administration of methyl palmitate resulted in a significant ($p < 0.01$) decrease in survival time to 150 days. Thus, an approximate 90-day difference in survival time occurred between the macrophage-stimulated and macrophage-depressed groups. These findings further accent the concept that survival appears to be generally directly related to macrophage functional status. That is, an increase in macrophage function is associated with enhanced survival while, conversely, depressed macrophage function is associated with decreased survival. Tumor growth and development appear therefore to be inversely related to macrophage functional status.

Table 4 Influence of Glucan Administration on Phagocytic Function and Mammary Tumor (15091A) Growth in Allogeneic C3H/HeJ Mice[a]

Treatment	Days	Phagocytic function (t/2, min)	Tumor Weight (mg)	Tumor Incidence (%)
Control	0	8.6 ± 0.57	–	–
Glucan	0	4.0 ± 0.49[b]	–	–
Control	5	10.1 ± 0.81	529 ± 43	100
Glucan	5	4.6 ± 0.22[b]	24 ± 16[b]	33
Control	10	8.3 ± 0.57	623 ± 54	100
Glucan	10	5.0 ± 0.23[b]	39 ± 19[b]	50
Control	15	8.1 ± 0.46	819 ± 149	100
Glucan	15	5.0 ± 0.24[b]	31 ± 26[b]	33

[a]The mammary carcinoma is syngeneic in the A/J mouse. Values are expressed as means ± standard error and are derived from seven mice per group.
[b]$p < 0.001$.

Table 5 Influence of Glucan-Induced Macrophage Activation on Mammary Tumor (15091A) Growth in Syngeneic A/J Mice[a]

Treatment	Days	Phagocytic function (t/2, min)	Tumor weight (mg)
Control	0	21.4 ± 8.14	–
Glucan	0	2.4 ± 0.34[c]	–
Control	5	8.5 ± 0.78	300 ± 15
Glucan	5	4.1 ± 0.45[b]	108 ± 20[c]
Control	10	3.7 ± 0.37	242 ± 70
Glucan	10	4.4 ± 1.10	119 ± 46
Control	15	7.6 ± 1.33	913 ± 91
Glucan	15	3.3 ± 0.29[d]	617 ± 83[e]

[a]Values are expressed as means ± standard error and are derived from six mice per group.
[b]$p < 0.001$.
[c]$p < 0.01$.
[d]$p < 0.02$.
[e]$p < 0.05$.

Table 6 The Influence of Glucan or Methyl Palmitate on Survival of Aging AKR/J Mice[a]

	Survival %		
Day	Control	Glucan	Methyl Palmitate
90	44 (22/50)	48 (24/50)	31 (14/44)
150	28 (14/50)	40 (20/50)	0 (0/44)[b]
210	0 (0/50)	28 (14/50)[b]	0 (0/44)

[a]Glucan (0.45 mg per mouse) or methyl palmitate (35 mg per mouse) was administered IV at 14-day intervals, beginning when the mice were approximately 6 months old. The numbers in parentheses represent the number surviving over the total N for each group.
[b]$p < 0.001$.

IV. DISCUSSION

These studies clearly denote that variant data can be generated employing biological response modifiers depending upon the nature of host-tumor systems which are utilized in the experimental study. These studies are in fundamental accord with the observations of Hewitt (16,24), Alexander (9), Weiss (10), Baldwin et al. (25), and Martin et al. (12) which stressed that, if data generated in experimental models are to be transferred to clinical situations, the model employed must be syngeneic in nature and preferably autochthonous. It is clear that employment of allogeneic tumors will lead to an overoptimistic evaluation of therapeutic agents and are therefore an inadequate index for immunotherapeutic agents.

The present findings are similar in nature to the observations obtained when radiation chimeras were established in mice by means of transplanting either syngeneic, allogeneic, or xenogeneic bone marrow and the animals subsequently injected with glucan to activate host macrophage populations (26). The greater the antigenicity of the transplanted bone marrow cells, the greater was the rejection process (26). In these studies (26) it was observed that mice that were lethally irradiated and subsequently transplanted with syngeneic bone marrow would not show any modification in survival when glucan was administered to activate their host defense mechanisms. In contrast to the unaltered survival pattern in syngeneic mice, the allogeneic bone marrow transplanted mice which received glucan showed a significant increase in mortality. The most rapid occurrence of death, reflecting complete rejection of the transplant, occurred when xenogeneic bone marrow was utilized.

It may be suggested that the differential effects which were observed with glucan and methyl palmitate on tumor growth and development are due to the modification of natural killer cell (NK) function (27) instead of macrophage activity. However, recent studies in our laboratory by Edwards and Di Luzio (unpublished data) have indicated that in contrast to glucan's ability to enhance macrophage function, glucan exerts a significant suppressant effect on NK cell activity. Additionally, methyl palmitate, which enhances tumor growth and development, appreciably enhanced NK cell function. These studies indicate that results obtained with the two biological response modifiers employed do not show a correlation between NK cell activity and tumor progression or regression. Indeed, with these agents, an inverse relationship of tumor growth to NK function is strongly suggested.

The increased survival of aging AKR mice, which develop spontaneous leukemia, by the administration of glucan is in basic accord with the observations of Mathé and Olsson (5) and Check et al. (28) employing *C. parvum*, and Ungaro et al., utilizing BCG (29). Likewise, the observation that methyl palmitate decreases longevity in AKR mice and generally promoted tumor growth in other models is in basic accord with the observations of Jones and Castor (1) and Keller (30) when silica was employed as the macrophage toxin. Additional evidence for the important role of macrophages in tumor development was our preliminary observation, that in methyl palmitate-treated mice where the growth of allogeneic tumors were significantly enhanced, the cessation of methyl palmitate administration was associated with restoration of macrophage function to normal and subsequent rejection of the tumor. Similarly, Jones and Castro (1) also concluded that metastatic spread of the Lewis lung carcinoma was inversely related to phagocytic activity. Keller, et al. (31) have recently implied a relationship between the tumor-promoting activity of diterpene esters and suppression of macrophage cytolytic function.

The present findings of the importance of macrophage function to growth and development was supported by our previous observations employing a murine mammary adenocarcinoma (BW10232) (32). Administration of glucan resulted in a decrease in tumor growth and enhanced the population of tumor macrophages. In contrast, methyl palmitate macrophage suppression was associated with enhanced tumor growth and a decrease in the number of tumor macrophages. These composite findings add further support to the concept that macrophages are essential effector cells in host resistance to neoplasia.

It can be anticipated that continued employment of biological response modifiers, glucan and methyl palmitate, which diversely affect macrophage function activity will contribute to delineating the cellular basis of tumor surveillance and rejection.

V. SUMMARY

The appropriateness of animal models in the evaluation of potentially clinically useful immunotherapeutic agents has been a matter of significant concern. The present study was undertaken to evaluate the effects of glucan, a macrophage stimulant, and methyl palmitate, a macrophage depressant, on tumor growth in conditions of genetically diverse host-tumor relationships. In allogeneic C3H/HeJ mice, glucan pretreatment resulted in a profound inhibition (95%) in the growth of adenocarcinoma (15091A). Tumor incidence, which was 100% in control groups, ranged from 33-50%, in the glucan-treated groups. In syngeneic A/J mice, however, the inhibition of tumor growth ranged from 34 to 64%. In contrast to complete rejection of the adenocarcinoma in allogeneic mice, the administration of methyl palmitate resulted in 100% incidence of tumor growth. In allogeneic C3H/HeJ mice where approximately a 50% incidence of growth of an anaplastic carcinoma (15091A) was manifested, a 100% incidence of tumor acceptance and enhanced growth (50-380%) occurred in macrophage-suppressed mice. However, in syngeneic A/J mice, only a 35-54% increase in tumor growth was manifested. In an autochthonous tumor model employing aging AKR/J mice which develop spontaneous leukemia, the biweekly intravenous administration of glucan for a 6-month period resulted in significant prolongation in survival. The biweekly administration of methyl palmitate resulted in decreased survival. While these studies denote that variant data can be generated employing biological response modifiers dependent on host-tumor relationships, tumor growth and development appear to be generally inversely related to macrophage functional status.

ACKNOWLEDGMENTS

This study was supported, in part, by the American Cancer Society, The National Cancer Institute, and the MECO Cancer Research Fund.

REFERENCES

1. P. D. E. Jones and J. E. Castro, *Br. J. Cancer, 35*:519 (1977).
2. G. Mathé, O. Halle-Pannenko, and C. Bourut, *Rev. Eur. Etudes Clin. Biol., 17*:997 (1972).
3. M. F. A. Woodruff, V. L. Whitehead, and G. Speedy, *Br. J. Cancer, 37*:345 (1978).
4. J. Zákány, G. Chihara, and J. Fachet, *Intl. J. Cancer, 25*:371 (1980).
5. G. Mathé and L. Olsson, *Cancer Immunol. Immunother., 6*:197 (1980).
6. G. L. Bartlett, J. W. Kreider, and D. M. Purnell, *J. Natl. Cancer Inst., 56*:297 (1976).
7. H. B. Hewitt, E. R. Blake, and A. S. Walder, *Br. J. Cancer, 33*:241 (1976).
8. H. B. Hewitt, *Cancer Res., 27*:149 (1978).
9. P. Alexander, *Cancer, 40*:467 (1977).
10. D. W. Weiss, *Cancer Immunol. Immunother., 2*:11 (1977).
11. J. A. Greager and R. W. Baldwin, *Cancer Res., 38*:69 (1978).
12. D. S. Martin, R. L. Stolfi, and R. A. Fugmann, *Cancer Immunol. Immunother., 2*:77 (1977).
13. H. J. Rapp, *Cancer, 3*:1208 (1978).
14. H. J. Rapp, *Cancer Res., 39*:4285 (1979).
15. P. Alexander, *Cancer, 3*:1214 (1978).
16. H. B. Hewitt, *Cancer Res., 39*:4286 (1979).
17. S. J. Riggi and N. R. Di Luzio, *Am. J. Physiol., 200*:297 (1961).
18. W. R. Wooles and N. R. Di Luzio, *J. Reticuloendothel. Soc., 1*:160 (1964).
19. N. R. Di Luzio, R. B. McNamee, W. Browder, and D. L. Williams, *Cancer Treat. Rep., 62*:1857 (1978).
20. W. R. Wooles and N. R. Di Luzio, *Science, 142*:1078 (1963).
21. W. R. Wooles and N. R. Di Luzio, *Am. J. Physiol., 206*:939 (1964).
22. D. A. Blickens and N. R. Di Luzio, *J. Reticuloendothel. Soc., 2*:60 (1965).
23. N. R. Di Luzio, D. L. Williams, R. B. McNamee, B. F. Edwards, and A. Kitahama, *Int. J. Cancer, 24*:773 (1979).
24. H. B. Hewitt, *Clin. Radiol., 30*:361 (1979).
25. R. W. Baldwin, F. R. C. Path, and M. R. Price, *Ann. Rev. Med., 27*:151 (1976).
26. W. R. Wooles and N. R. Di Luzio, *Proc. Soc. Exp. Biol. Med., 115*:756 (1964).
27. R. B. Herberman and J. R. Ortaldo, *Science, 214*:24 (1981).
28. J. H. Check, G. A. Silverman, R. L. Dryden, and L. W. Brady, *Cancer, 44*:488 (1979).
29. P. C. Ungaro, W. P. Drake, and N. R. Mardiney, *J. Natl. Cancer Inst., 50*:125 (1973).
30. R. Keller, *J. Natl. Cancer Inst., 57*:1355 (1976).
31. R. Keller, R. Keist, W. Adolf, H. J. Opferkuch, R. Schmidt, and E. Hecker, *Expl. Cell Biol., 50*:121 (1982).
32. N. R. Di Luzio, K. M. Gilbert, and M. A. Spanjers, *Cancer Immuno. Immunother., 9*:37 (1980).

21

Immunopharmacological Properties of 2-Cyanaziridine Derivatives

Uwe F. Bicker Boehringer Mannheim GmbH, Mannheim, Federal Republic of Germany

I. INTRODUCTION

In 1975 we described the antitumor efficacy of a 2-cyanaziridine derivative, N-2-cyanethylene urea (1). These substances were initially synthesized as aziridine derivatives with a view to their being potential cytostatics. The aziridine structure is a well-known component in a number of alkylating cytostatic substances. Surprisingly, however, it did not show, in contrast to cytostatic aziridine derivatives, any potent alkylating action, either in vitro or in vivo. Furthermore, instead of the expected leukocyte depression, there was a dose-dependent increase in the number of leukocytes. These striking pharmacological effects led early on to the working hypothesis that this class of substances exert their antitumor activity not via a direct cytostatic action, like that developed by the known aziridine derivatives, but rather by an effect on immunological mechanisms. In the course of the pharmacological characterization of this class of substances, this working hypothesis was confirmed, and it was found that these compounds represent very selectively acting immunopharmacological agents.

II. CHEMISTRY

In the course of our investigations of the 2-cyanaziridine class of substances, several 100 different derivatives have been synthesized and tested pharmacologically. The dose-dependent leukocytosis observed in rats first was used as a screening criterion although later on we learned that this leukocytosis might be caused by the hemolytic anemia induced by the 2-cyanaziridine derivatives (see below). It was found that 2-cyanaziridine structure is essential for the induction of the leukocytosis. Substitutions on the carbon atom of the three-membered ring led to loss of this special pharmacodynamic action, while substitutions on the nitrogen could be carried out in many different ways.

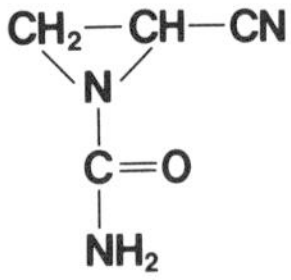

BA 1

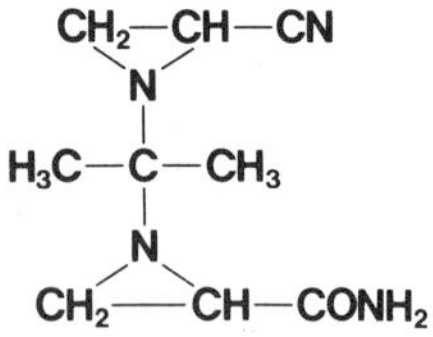

BM 12.531

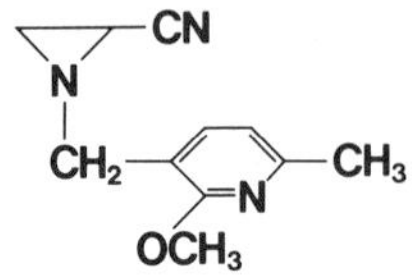

BM 41.332

In addition to the N-2-cyanethylene urea (BA 1), the derivatives BM 12.531 (azimexone, 2-[2-cyanaziridinyl-(1)]-2-[2-carbamoylaziridinyl-(1)]-propane) and BM 41.332 (2-cyan-1-[(2-methoxy-6-methyl-pyridin-3-yl)-methyl]-aziridine) were investigated.

From the chemical point of view, these substances have the aziridine structure in common. The stability of BM 41-332 in aqueous media at various pHs is greater than that of azimexone. Azimexone decomposes very quickly in aqueous solution to acetone, 2-cyanaziridine, and aziridine-2-carboxamid.

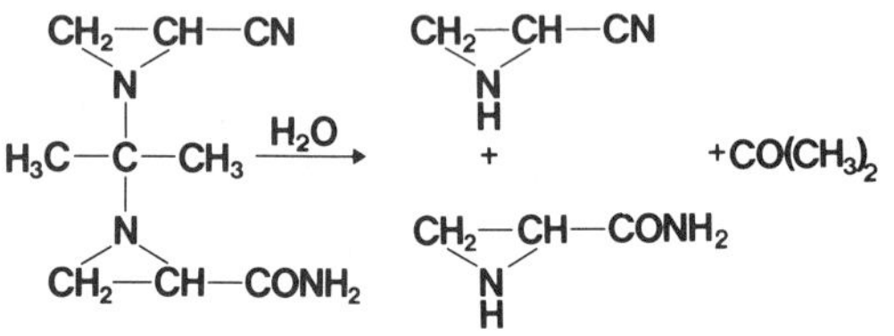

This low-molecular compound 2-cyanaziridine itself also induces leukocytosis in rats. However, BM 12.531 and BM 41.332 have, in comparison with 2-cyanaziridine itself, the advantage of crystalline structure and thus of greater chemical stability. 2-Cyanaziridine, which has been known for many years (2), is also unstable in the pure form and polymerizes in vitro to various products, some of which are undefinable.

The 2-cyanaziridine that arises is initially relatively stable at the pH of the stomach. In contrast to ethylenamine, 2-cyanaziridine reacts very slowly with many of the physiologically occurring amino acids. In contrast, the very rapid reaction with cystein is striking, and the chemical conversion take place preferentially by reaction with the nitrile group with maintenance of the three-membered ring.

The reaction products with cystein do not show the pharmacological action of 2-cyanaziridines. The selective reactivity of the 2-cyanaziridines and derivatives with cystein appears to us to be of special importance in relationship to the action of these compounds on the erythrocytes or on hemoglobin, as both human and rat hemoglobin bear a vulnerable cystein structure (3).

Furthermore, cyanaziridine itself decomposes slowly by incorporation of water into serine, isoserine, 2-cyanocarboxamide, and various, as yet, unidentified products.

After administration of BM 12.531 to beagles, the aziridine-2-carboxamid could be identified as the main metabolite. The 2-cyanaziridine itself is metabolized in bealges to cyanoacetic acid and oxalic acid amid.

III. ANTITUMOR ACTIVITY

The 2-cyanaziridine derivatives BM 12.531 (azimexone) and BM 41-332 showed antitumor effects against various experimental models in studies by different investigators. No direct tumor activity in vitro could be found for any of the substances investigated.

Azimexone was tested, for example, against the MethA sarcoma of the mouse in comparison with various other immunomodulators with respects to its antitumor activity. Tumor cells (10^4 MethA) (obtained from Prof. Munder, Max-Planck-Institut, Freiburg, Federal Republic of West Germany) were injected subcutaneously into the napes of female C57B1/6 X BALB/c (F1) mice. The different immunomodulators were administered either from day 3 or from day 7 after the transplantation on 3 consecutively days at the doses given in Table 1. As the values in Table 1 show, azimexone exerted an action, on triple doses of 25 mg/kg orally, especially if the tumor mass was not very large (start of the treatment 3 days after transplantation). BM 12.531 proved to be considerably better than levamisole, Bacillus Calmette-Guérin and cyclophosphamide and equivalent to *Corynebacterium parvum*. At higher tumor cell counts (i.e., if the treatment was started 7 days after the transplantation), an attenuated effect was shown. An increase of the dose above 25 mg/kg did not lead in this tumor model to any improvement of the therapeutic effect (4).

A good antitumor efficacy was also found after administration of azimexone to mice with an AKR leukemia (5). These spontaneously occurring AKR leukemia cells were inoculated into young AKR mice (the inoculation was intravenous and the number of cells inoculated was 10^3 per mouse). The tumor cells were characterized before inoculation into four antigenically different types (clones A, B, C, and D); clone D proved to be antigenically inert in AKR mice (6). Azimexone was injected at doses of 1-50 mg/kg IV in physiological saline solution. The optimum dose was found to be 25 mg/kg six times at 4-day intervals. Interestingly, both the immunogenic tumor cells and the cells of the nonimmunogenic clone D showed a good response to azimexone. The latter observation appears to us to be of particular importance as many spontaneous occurring tumors in humans have so far not been adequately antigenically characterized. In the investigation of azimexone in this tumor model, the bell-shaped dose-response curve is again apparent, that is, increasing the dose above 25 mg/kg led to an attenuation of the therapeutic effect. As investigations that will be discussed later show, this attenuation of the therapeutic effect can be attributed to a stimulation of the suppressor T cells.

Azimexone and BM 41.332 also show effects on the Lewis lung (LL) carcinoma in mice. In these experiments 5 X 10^5 cells of the Lewis lung tumor (National Cancer Institute, Bethesda, Maryland) were injected intramuscularly into the hindpaw. Azimexone was administered immediately after tumor inoculation twice a week at doses of 10, 20, 50, and 100 mg/kg orally by gavage. Twenty days after the tumor inoculation, the tumor-bearing right hindpaw was amputated under anesthesia. Eleven to thirteen days later the

Table 1 Growth of MethA Sarcoma Cells after Treatment with Various Immunomodulators

Immunomodulator	Treatment starting on day: +3 after transplantation (no. of tumor-free survivors on day 28/total)[a]	Treatment starting on day: +7 after transplantation (no. of tumor-free survivors on day 28/total)[a]
Control	0/20	0/20
Levamisole (3 X 5 mg/kg) orally	2/10[b]	1/16[b]
C. parvum (35 μg/kg) IP	12/20	0/20
BCG (10^7 cells/mouse) IP	5/20	3/20
BM 12.531 (3 X 25 mg/kg) orally	10/20	4/20
Cyclophosphamide (150 mg/kg) orally	0/20	0/20

[a] 10^5 cells/mouse SC in the neck.
[b] Ten and four mice, respectively, died immediately after treatment.

Table 2 Antitumor Effect of Azimexone in Spontaneous AKR Leukemia

Tumor type	No. of grafted tumor cells and route of administration	No. takes/no. grafted[a] Control	Azimexone[b]
Spontaneous AKR leukemia cells	10^3 IV	15/15	8/15
Clone A leukemia cells	10^3 IV	15/15	4/15
Clone B leukemia cells	10^3 IV	15/15	8/15
Clone C leukemia cells	10^3 IV	15/15	8/15
Clone D leukemia cells	10^3 IV	15/15	7/15

[a]Azimexone was administered in a dose of 25 mg/kg IV, given six times with 4-day interval; injections were started on day +1 after tumor challenge.
[b]Determined 80 days after tumor challenge.

animals were killed, and the number of metastases in the lungs determined by the injection of ink into the trachea by the method of Wexler (7). No clear effect of azimexone on the primary tumor was found at any of the doses investigated. A clear reduction in the number of metastases was, on the other hand, observed after azimexone administration (5). Table 3 shows the action of azimexone on the metastasing of LL tumors at the optimum dosage. If the animals were inoculated with tumor cells that were obtained from the lung metastases, then a greater therapeutic effect was obtained than after inoculation of cells that arose from the primary tumor. As we know that 2-cyanaziridine derivatives do not have any direct antitumor effect, this finding seems to us to be especially important as an immunological effect on the tumor growth could be clinically important, especially where there is threatened metastasis. Furthermore, these investigations show that the immunological effect on primary tumor cells and metastasizing cells can differ considerably. On closer investigation of the dose-response relationship of azimexone in this Lewis lung tumor model, a similar dose-response relationship was observed, that is, an increase of the dose above an optimum dose again led to an attenuation of the therapeutic effect.

Table 3 Antitumor Effect on Azimexone in Lewis Lung Tumor Cells

Tumor type	No. of grafted tumor cells and route of administration	No. takes/No. grafted[a] Control	Azimexone[b]	No. lung metastases in controls[c] / No. lung metastases in azimexone treated
Lewis lung tumor cells from primary tumor site	10^4 SC	15/15	15/15	$\frac{29 \pm 11}{11 \pm 3}$
Lewis lung tumor cells from lung metastatic foci	10^4 SC	15/15	15/15	$\frac{46 \pm 14}{9 \pm 8}$

[a]Determined 80 days after tumor challenge.
[b]Azimexone was administered in a dose of 25 mg/kg IV, given six times with 4-day interval; injections were started on day +1 after tumor challenge.
[c]Determined at day 28 after tumor challenge by counting metastatic foci on both lungs that were fixated in Bouvin's fixative; the countings were performed under stereomicroscope.

An almost identical dose-response relationship with respect to antitumor efficacy was also found in BALB/c fibrosarcoma of the mouse (5). As the values in Table 4 show, the six-fold injection of 25 mg/kg to mice that had been inoculated subcutaneously with 10^4 cells of the K-B-23 fibrosarcoma produced a cure in almost 100% of the animals.

Stylos, et al. (8) were able to show a clear antitumor effect of azimexone against Madison lung carcinoma (M109) in BALB/c mice. Azimexone was injected at doses of 100 mg/kg intraperitoneally on the ninth and sixteenth days after tumor inoculation, and this led to a significant prolongation of the mean survival time.

A dose of 300 mg/kg cyclophosphamide given 6 days after the inoculation of L1210 leukemia into CD2F1 mice showed a not quite significant prolongation of the mean survival time or the number of cured animals on day 45. If, however, azimexone was given additionally intraperitoneally from the eighth day after tumor inoculation at doses of 50 mg/kg at 4-day intervals, then 70% of the inoculated animals survived on the forty-fifth day (8). The mean survival time was prolonged to a highly significant degree. It is known that cyclophosphamide produces, in addition to the antitumor effect, a preferential action on the suppression of some suppressor T cells (9).

As, on the other hand, it is known that BM 12.531 at a dose schedule of 50 mg repeatedly at 4-day intervals produces a marked stimulation of suppressor T cells (see below), the good therapeutic effect observed in spite of this by the combined treatment with cyclophosphamide and azimexone may be explained by the fact that the undesired stimulation of suppressor T cells is abolished in this case by the cyclophosphamide.

Table 4 Effect of Azimexone on the BALB/c-Fibrosarcoma SC[a]

(mg/kg)	No. of injections at a 4-day interval	Take failure
Control		0/0
1	4	1/30
	6	2/30
	8	1/30
10	4	1/30
	6	1/30
	8	2/30
20	4	9/30
	6	17/30
	8	14/30
25	4	28/30
	6	27/30
	8	24/30
35	4	2/30
	6	12/30
	8	21/30
50	4	1/30
	6	1/30
	8	0/30

[a] 10^4 cells of K-B-23, 30 animals per group.

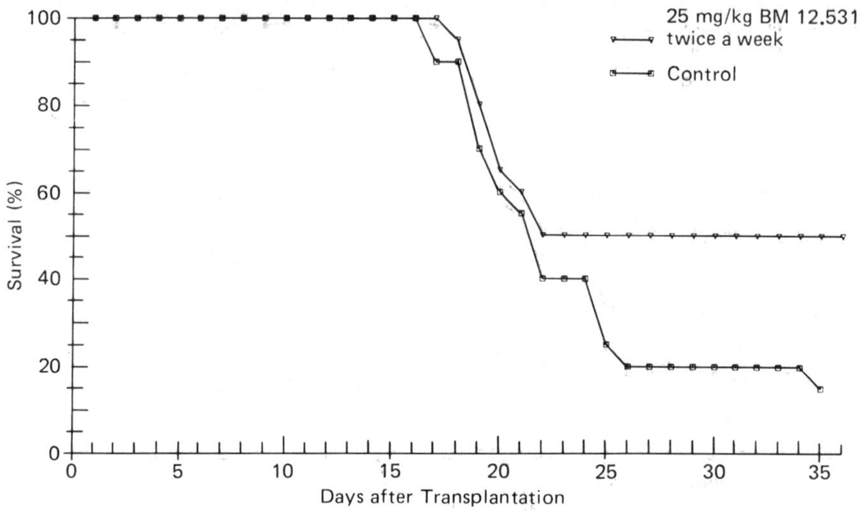

Figure 1 Antitumor effect on BM 12.531 against L1210 leukemia in DBA_2 mice.

Azimexone also showed a marked potentiating effect on using an L1210 vaccination (8). In this case, a single dose of 100 or 25 mg/kg intraperitoneally produced a prolongation of the survival time by 45 and 54%, respectively. A clear antitumor effect was also shown on oral administration of 25 mg/kg BM 12.531 administered twice weekly, following inoculation of 1×10^3 L1210 leukemia cells to female DBA mice (Fig. 1). Further antitumor actions of azimexone were observed against Friend virus leukemia in mice, DS carcinosarcoma in rats, and the Ehrlich ascites carcinoma of mice (unpublished data).

IV. INFLUENCE OF 2-CYANAZIRIDINE DERIVATIVES ON NATURAL KILLER (NK) CELLS AND LYMPHOCYTE SUBPOPULATIONS

The 2-cyanaziridine derivatives have, as already mentioned, no direct cytostatic action on tumor cells or other proliferating or nonproliferating normal cells in concentrations which can be expected in vivo. On the other hand, clear antitumor effects have been described by numerous authors. To find an explanation of these in vivo effects against experimental tumors, the action of azimexone or other 2-cyanaziridine derivatives on NK cells was investigated. These natural killer (NK) cells are thought to play an important role in the defense against tumors. Not only the growth of experimental transplantation tumors of animals, but also the growth of spontaneously occurring human tumors are thought to be regulated by NK cells (10). NK cells are considered to be lymphoid cells (10) that do not possess T-cell markers. The antitumor activity of NK cells is not dependent on antibodies.

According to preliminary investigations by Chirigos et al. (11), a single intraperitoneal administration of 25 mg/kg azimexone produces a significant stimulation of NK cell activity of mice lymphocytes against YAC cells. It is striking that a significant potentiation of the NK cell activity is observed only 6 days after the treatment with BM 12.531 (11).

Other nonspecifically acting immunostimulants, in contrast, produce, in most cases, a very rapid activation of NK cells (e.g., already 1 or 2 days after administration) (11).

More precise investigations have shown that azimexone, like other 2-cyanaziridine derivatives, stimulates dose depently the activity of cytotoxic autoreactive cells. The antineoplastic potential of these cytotoxic autoreactive cells, which are identical to the NK cells (12), is independent of the comparison of the tumor cell population with respect to antigenicity and is thus independent of the occurrence of surface noeantigens. The antitumor activity of azimexone against the nonimmunogenic clone D of AKR leukemia (Table 2) shows that in vivo such cytotoxic autoreactive cells are probably activated by azimexone.

The NK cell activity was determined by means of the ^{51}Cr-release assay. In this, 10^7 tumor cells were incubated for 1 hr with 200 μCi. The NK cells were obtained from the spleen cell population which had been freed of erythrocytes, dead cells, and mononuclear phagocytes by means of iron phagocytosis and subsequent magnetic removal. The NK cells were mixed with the target cells in microtiter plates in 0.1 ml medium with the desired ratio of target and attacker cells. The spontaneous release did not exceed 15% in any of the experiments. In some experiments, theta-antigen-bearing cells were removed in addition from these spleen cells suspensions by the addition of antitheta-antibody and complement.

As the values given in Fig. 2 show, the optimum dose of 25 mg/kg azimexone in mice produced a marked increase in NK cell activity. As Fig. 2 also shows, the dose-response profile of the activation of NK cells agrees completely with the dose-response relationship of the antitumor activity of azimexone (Table 4). A maximum activation of NK cells is seen in both AKR mice and in C57B1/6 mice after sixfold injection of 25 mg/kg each at 4-day intervals. An increase of the dose led to a reduction of the therapeutic effect (5).

If the lymphocytes of the mice treated with azimexone were treated in the NK cell assay additionally with antitheta-antigen-antibodies and complement, then there was, on

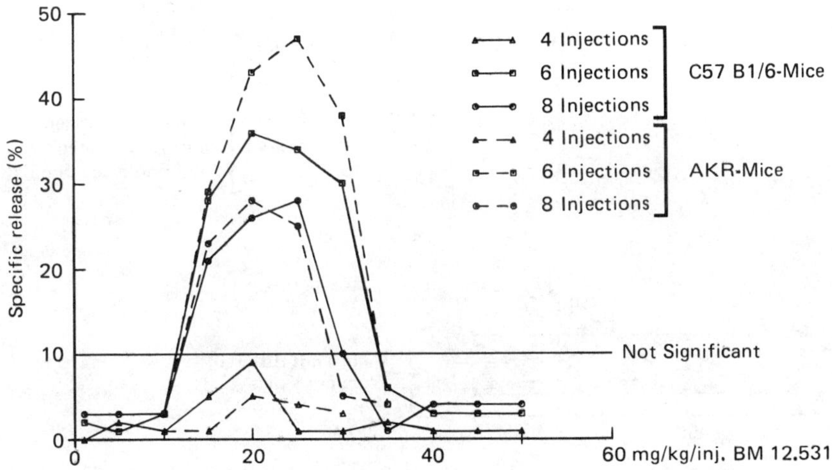

Figure 2 Activity of cytotoxic autoreactive cells (CAuC) in young healthy AKR mice and in young healthy C57B1/6 mice in relation to dose of azimexone per injection and the number of injections. CAuC activity was tested against AKR leukemia cells. All tests were performed 4 days after last azimexone injection. Each point represents the mean of four to six mice, and vertical bars indicate standard deviations.

raising the dose above 25 mg/kg, no attenuation of the NK cell activity, but in contrast a clear increase (5). These investigations suggest that higher doses of azimexone activate lymphocytes that bear antitheta-antigens and that these T lymphocytes paralyze the NK cell activity. By definition, therefore, one can speak of suppressor T lymphocytes (Fig. 3).

The observation by Stylos et al. (8) that azimexone also shows synergistic effects with cyclophosphamide at high doses can be readily harmonized with this finding, as cyclophosphamide at the doses selected preferentially suppresses suppressor T lymphocytes (9) and thus increases the therapeutic range of azimexone against tumor cells.

The influence of the 2-cyanaziridine derivatives azimexone and BM 41.332 on the percentage of total T lymphocytes, helper T cells, and the cytotoxic and suppressor cells was determined with the aid of monoclonal antibodies and a cell sorter. (All three antibodies were supplied by Beckton Dickinson, Mountain View, California, conjugated with fluorescein.) The cell suspensions were obtained from spleen single-cell suspensions from treated and control animals (13). To determine the functioning of the cells, Ly 1^-, 2^+ cells were isolated with a cell sorter and tested for their suppressive effect on lymphocyte blastogenesis induced with phythemagglutinin (13). As can be seen from the values in Table 5, neither BM 41.332 nor azimexone showed any change in the percentage of Thy 1, 2 cells from C57B1/6 mice. As the values in Table 5, however, also show in contrast, azimexone induced, with an unchanged percentage of total T lymphocytes, a fall in the percentage of Ly 1^+, 2^- lymphocytes and a mirrow-image rise of the suppressor/cytotoxic cells (Ly 1^-, 2^+ cells). BM 41.332 behaved completely analogously.

With respect to the induction of Ly 1^-, 2^+ cells (suppressor and cytotoxic cells), no differences were found in AKR, C57B1/6, or BALB/c mice. Analogously, in the investigations with respect to the fall in NK cell activity, significant rises in suppressor T cells were observed, especially at doses greater than 25 mg/kg given six times at 4-day intervals.

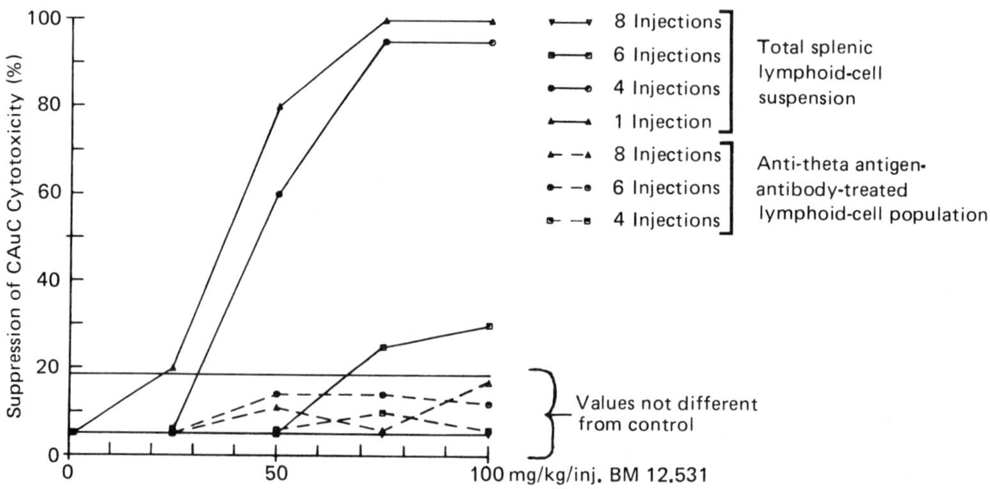

Figure 3 Suppression of CAuC activity by spleen lymphoid cells from mice treated with azimexone in various doses and with various numbers of injections. All tests were performed 4 days after last azimexone injection, and each point represents the mean of suppression (%) of four to five spleen cell populations tested. Vertical bars indicate standard deviations.

Table 5 Effect of the 2-Cyanaziridine Derivatives BM 12.531 and BM 41.332 on the Percentage of Lymphocyte Subsets in Mice

Strain of mice	Lymphocite subset (%)[a]	Doses of 2-cyanaziridine derivatives (IV mg/kg) (given six times at a 4-day interval)								
		0	5	15	25	35	45			Bm 12.531
	Thy 1,2	34	33	34	33	34	32			
C57B1/6	Lyt $1^-, 2^+, 3^+$	10	9	13	17	19	20			
	Lyt $1^-, 2^+, 3^+$	31	22	19	15	12	12			
		0	1	3	6	12	25	50	75	BM 41.332
C57B1/6	Thy 1,2	36	34	32	34	36	30	36	33	
	Lyt $1^-, 2^+, 3^+$	12	15	12	11	19	26	31	29	
AKR	Lyt $1^-, 2^+, 2^+$	12	11	12	13	16	19	23	24	
BALB/c	Lyt $1^-, 2^+, 3^+$	15	16	19	21	29	36	33	33	

[a]Percentage of Thy $1, 2^-$, Lyt $1^-, 2^+, 3^+$ –, and Lyt $1^+, 2^-, 3^-$ - cells in the spleen. Standard variation is max. 3%. Twenty-four hours after the last injection spleen single-cell suspensions were prepared from individual mice. The viable cells were incubated with fluorescein-conjugated rat antibody against Thy 1,2, Lyt $1^-, 2^+, 3^+$ and Lyt $1^+, 2^-, 3^-$ (Becton Dickinson) and analyzed using a cell-sorter (FACS III, Becton Dickinson). These experiments were carried out in cooperation with Dr. L. Olsson, Copenhagen. Details will be published elsewhere (13).

After isolation of the Ly 1^-, 2^+ cells in the cell sorter it was found that the rise in the percentage of these T cells is accompanied by a potentiation of the suppressive function. As the values in Table 6 show, the sixfold injection of 25 mg/kg BM 41.332 produced both a direct inhibition of the PHA stimulation of lymphocytes of C57B1/6 mice, which had been previously treated, and also an inhibition of the thymidine incorporation of PHA-stimulated nonpretreated spleen lymphocytes. The direct inhibition of the [^{3}H] thymidine incorporation of mice lymphocytes after PHA stimulation can be explained by the fact that PHA stimulates preferentially the Ly 1^+, 2^- (helper) cells (14). This clear and dose-dependent stimulation of suppressor T cells by 2-cyanaziridine derivatives could be of therapeutic importance, especially in the treatment of those illnesses that are characterized by reduced functioning of suppressor T cells (see below).

The Ly 1^-, 2^+ cells include, in addition to the suppressor T lymphocytes, the cytotoxic T lymphocytes. In the delayed-type hypersensitivity reaction, such as is found after immunization with sheep red blood cells (SRBCs) or oxazolone, these cytotoxic T lymphocytes are said to play a major role, along with the macrophages (16,17). There is, in fact, after administration of azimexone and other 2-cyanaziridine derivatives a marked potentiation of this delayed-type hypersensitivity reaction. Stylos et al. (8) found, for example, a significant increase of the delayed-type hypersensitivity reaction after injection of 10^8 SRBCs and subsequent intraperitoneal administration of azimexone 4 days later. This effect was shown even more clearly if 7 days elapsed between immunization and challenge. Here, too, there was a highly significant potentiation of the DTH at doses of 2.5 and 25 mg/kg, but an attenuation of the therapeutic effect on increasing the dose to 250 mg/kg (4) (Fig. 4).

Most immunostimulants show clear effects on macrophages, and the antitumor activity of such compounds as BCG or *C. parvum* is attributed partially to an activation of macrophages (18-20). Macrophages are also said to play a decisive role in the delayed-type hypersensitivity (17).

The action of the 2-cyanaziridine derivative azimexone on macrophages is not quite clear. While some authors report weak to marginal potentiation of macrophage activities (4,21,23), these could not be confirmed in investigations by others (8), so that an action of azimexone on macrophages almost certainly does not occupy a prime place in the pharmacological action of 2-cyanaziridine derivatives. We found, in contrast, a reduction of the clearing function of the reticuloendothelial system, measured according to the method of Biozzi et al. (24) (Table 7). If BM 12.531 or BM 41.332 was admin-

Table 6 Effect of Mononuclear Spleen Cells from Mice Treated with BM 41.332 (25 mg/kg/inj.) on PHA Stimulation of Mononuclear Spleen Cells from Conventional Mice

PHA stimulation of 10^6 cells from conventional mice (cpm)	PHA stimulation of 10^6 cells from BM 41.332-treated mice (cpm)	PHA stimulation of 5 x 10^5 normal spleen cells plus 5 x 10^5 spleen cells from BM 41.332-treated mice (cpm)	Suppression (%)
28.4 X 10^3	1 inj.: 21.4 X 10^3	1 inj.: 12.8 X 10^3	49[a]
	6 inj.: 14.3 X 10^3	6 inj.: 9.3 X 10^3	59

[a]Control cpm was calculated as: 0.5 x 28.4 x 10^3 + 0.5 x 21.4 x 10^3, and 28.4 x 10^3 x 0.5 + 0.5 x 14.3 x 10^3, respectively

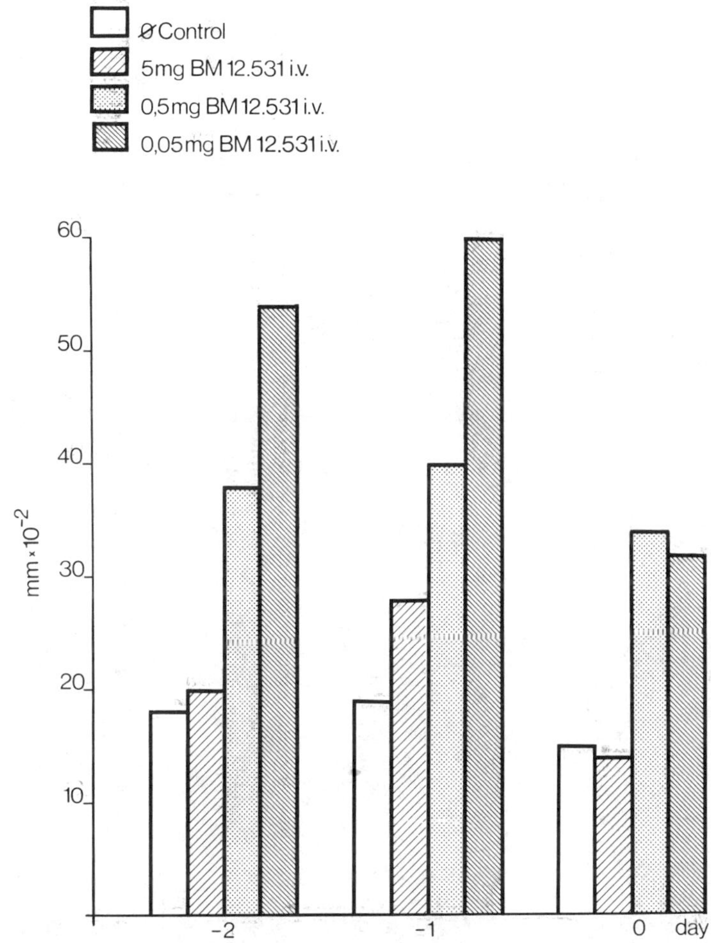

Figure 4 Delayed-type hypersensitivity reaction (footpad swelling). Seven mice per group were injected on day −7 with 10^7 SRBCs, on day −1 and day −2 and day 0 injected IV with BM 12.531 as indicated. The animals were challenged with 10^8 SRBCs in the right footpad on day +1.

istered at various doses orally for 2 or 3 weeks and then the RES function as measured by clearance of intravenously administered charcoal subsequently determined, then a dose-dependent reduction of RES function (Tables 7 and 10) with a parallel reduction in the [^{3}H] thymidine incorporation in PHA-stimulated lymphocytes was found. The reduction of the PHA-induced [^{3}H] thymidine incorporation can again be explained by a reduction of the percentage or activity of helper T cells. Moreover, it seems that there is a close interaction between RES and helper T-cell activity (25). This interaction be-appears to be of particular importance, especially in autoaggressive diseases such as rheumatoid arthritis in which both an increased helper T cell activity and a potentiated RES or macrophage activity has been described (26). The reduced antibody-dependent cellular cytotoxicity (ADCC) can also be explained by an inhibition of the helper T-cell

Table 7 Effect of BM 12.531, BM 41.332, and Methylprednisolone on the Number of Lymphocytes, Erythrocytes, Hb, Heinz Bodies, PHA-Induced Spleen Cell Proliferation, and the RES Clearance in Mice (C57B1/6, N = 10, ♀)

		BM 12,531[b], PO		BM 41.332[b], PO		Methylprednisolone[b], PO
	Control	5 mg/kg	25 mg/kg	5 mg/kg	25 mg/kg	5 mg/kg
Lymphocytes						
Peripheral blood ($x10^3$ μl)	8.5 ±0.3	8.1 ±0.5	9.0 ±0.4	8.5 ±0.3	8.8 ±0.2	6.8 ±0.4[a]
Spleen ($x10^7$ spleen)	17.76	13.68	27.04	19.50	22.40	12.32[a]
Erythrocyte ($x10^6$)	3.93 ±0.06	4.13± 0.10	3.98± 0.15	3.88± 0.9	3.86± 0.07	3.91± 0.06
Hb (g/L)	14.00 ±0.19	14.54± 0.18	14.54± 0.15	13.94± 0.36	14.11± 0.26	14.73± 0.16
Heinz bodies (%)	0	0	25	0	0.5	0
Relative response of agent-treated spleen cells						
Without mitogen	1[c]	0.75	0.61	1.16	0.54[a]	1.23
With PHA	1	1.47[a]	0.27	0.79	0.16[a]	1.36[a]
Slope of the regression curves in the carbon clearance test	-0.0422[d]	-0.0288[a]	-0.0272[a]	-0.0366[a]	-0.0333[a]	-0.0354[a]

[a] $p \leqslant 0.05$.
[b] The compounds were given orally daily for 21 days. On day 23 blood from the retroorbital venous plexus was taken and the number of peripheral lymphocytes was counted, mice were killed, spleens were removed and pooled (N = 5), single cell suspensions were made, lymphocyte number was counted, lymphocytes were separated by means of a Percoll gradient (d = 1.09), erythrocytes were lysed with 11m NH_4Cl-solution, and lymphocyte transformation test was carried out in the usual way.
[c] $\frac{\text{Mean cpm in cultures of } 0.5 \times 10^6 \text{ agent-treated spleen cells/well}}{\text{Mean cpm in cultures of } 0.5 \times 10^6 \text{ normal spleen cells (control)/well}}$
[d] After 21 days of treatment five mice per group were injected 0.2 ml Pelikan-C11-1431a ink, and the clearance of the carbon particles was measured according to the method of Biozzi et al. (24). Details will be published elsewhere.

activity (23). Azimexone treatment produces a clear reduction of ADCC when administered 1, 3, and 14 days before testing (23).

The 2-cyanaziridine derivatives show in vitro, with respect to an effect on mitogen-induced lymphocyte transformation, an action only at concentrations above 100 μg/ml in the form of a reduction of [^{3}H] thymidine incorporation. These effects are probably nonspecific and generally of a cytotoxic type. An increase in [^{3}H] thymidine incorporation of the mitogen-stimulated lymphocytes after in vitro incubation with azimexone was reported by some authors (22,41), but could not be reproduced generally, so that this direct action on the lymphocyte proliferation is scarcely central to the pharmacological action of 2-cyanaziridine derivatives. Similar, macrophages are scarcely affected in vitro, and there is no significant effect on cyclic AMP (cAMP) or cyclip GMP (cGMP) levels (22).

V. EFFECT OF 2-CYANAZIRIDINES ON BONE MARROW AND ERYTHROCYTES

As already described in 1975, various 2-cyanaziridine derivatives induce leukocytosis in rats (27). As the figures in Table 8 show, BM 41.332, for example, produce a marked rise in the number of leukocytes after oral administration of 200 mg/kg. These investigations indicate that the 2-cyanaziridine derivatives produce a direct stimulation of bone marrow cells, so that an increase in the number of leukocytes results. On the other hand, it was found that the doses that led to an increase in the number of leukocytes in the peripheral blood led to a fall in the number of erythrocytes and hemoglobin (Table 8) especially after azimexone administration. Very similar phenomena were observed in mice and in dogs after treatment with 2-cyanaziridines. These changes in the RBCs could be explained as a direct toxic action of 2-cyanaziridines. If reticulocyte staining is carried out, we found a dose-dependent rise in the number of erythrocytes with Heinz inclusions (Table 8) which finally results in hemolytic anemia. In parallel, there is a massive enlargement of the spleen after azimexone treatment, but not after BM 41.332 administration.

Histologically, quite clear hemosiderosis is detectable in the spleen and liver. On the other hand, it is known that in the presence of hemolytic anemias there is a reactive leukocytosis (28). In splenectomized rats, a hemolytic anemia also could be found (Table 8). These findings indicate that the leukocytosis should be seen in association with the hemolytic anemia.

The formation of Heinz bodies could be explained by a direct reaction of the 2-cyanaziridines with hemoglobin, but also by enzyme inhibition of those enzymes that are responsible for the integrity of the hemoglobin molecule. The shift of the p_{50} value, that is, of the partial oxygen pressure producing 50% oxygen saturation of the hemoglobin (Table 9), after in vitro incubation with high concentrations of azimexone with human blood indicates that a direct reaction with hemoglobin might take place.

The increase in CFUs or CFUc reported by various authors (29-31) could consequently be the result of a reaction to the hemolytic anemia or to the peripheral hypoxia-arising from the reaction with the hemoglobin. BM 41.332 in rats also shows a leukocytosis and a hemolytic anemia, but in mice this occurs only after doses of more than 100 mg/kg orally daily for 2 weeks (Table 10). In agreement with this, we were unable to observe, in contrast to azimexone, a rise in the number of CFUs with BM 41.332 at lower doses.

Table 8 Influence of the 2-Cyanaziridine Derivative BM 41.332 on the Leukocytes, Erythrocytes, Hb, and Heinz Bodies in Rats (200 mg/kg PO, N = 10)

	Normal							
	Leukocytes ($x10^3/\mu l$)		Erythrocytes ($x10^6/\mu l$)		Hb (g%)		Heinz Bodies (%)	
Time	Control	BM 41.332	Control	BM 41.332	Control	BM 41.332	Control	BM 41.332
0	9.25 ±0.50	8.21 ±0.44	7.60 ±0.12	8.20 ±0.12	15.39 ±0.26	15.23 ±0.19	0	0
4 hr	10.48 ±0.60	7.30 ±0.40	7.09 ±0.18	7.16 ±0.14	14.80 ±0.52	13.61 ±0.21	0	10
24 hr	8.97 ±0.22	9.21 ±0.30	7.03 ±0.13	6.94 ±0.12	14.48 ±0.41	13.58 ±0.28	0	15
Day +2	9.50 ±0.41	11.30 ±0.75	6.80 ±0.14	6.18 ±0.09	13.98 ±0.43	13.28 ±0.21	0	40
Day +6	10.93 ±0.65	18.36 ±1.02[a]	7.11 ±0.10	6.14 ±0.14[a]	14.59 ±0.32	12.77 ±0.30[a]	0	40
Day +10	10.42 ±0.42	10.1 ±0.88	7.71 ±0.23	7.57 ±0.33	15.76 ±0.37	15.86 ±0.52	0	25
Day +16	13.54 ±0.74	11.45 ±0.44	8.34 ±0.22	8.22 ±0.22	14.90 ±0.31	15.60 ±0.31	0	10
	Splenectomized							
	Leukocytes ($x10^3/\mu l$)		Erythrocytes ($x10^6/\mu l$)		Hb (g%)		Heinz Bodies (%)	
Time	Control	BM 41.332	Control	BM 41.332	Control	BM 41.332	Control	BM 41.332
0	7.38 ±0.36	7.66 ±0.41	8.09 ±0.11	8.34 ±0.06	14.94 ±0.25	15.37 ±0.10	5	0
4 hr	11.32 ±0.73	6.41 ±0.41	7.45 ±0.13	7.36 ±0.05	13.93 ±0.28	13.79 ±0.15	5	0
24 hr	8.60 ±0.30	6.74 ±0.22	7.32 ±0.11	6.91 ±0.05	13.82 ±0.25	13.30 ±0.10	0	16
Day +2	9.26 ±0.25	12.68 ±0.69[a]	7.02 ±0.09	5.90 ±0.10	14.03 ±0.24	13.08 ±0.15	0	52
Day +6	11.08 ±0.56	17.75 ±0.97[a]	7.54 ±0.18	5.95 ±0.08[a]	14.26 ±0.41	12.86 ±0.20[a]	0	50
Day +10	7.9 ±0.36	8.37 ±0.56	8.14 ±0.15	6.59 ±0.21	15.58 ±0.16	14.3 ±0.35	0	40
Day +16	9.87 ±0.74	9.77 ±0.55	8.70 ±0.21	7.93 ±0.08	15.38 ±0.31	15.32 ±0.15	0	10

[a] $p \leq 0.05$.

Table 9 In Vitro Influence of the O_2 Saturation of Human Hemoglobin after Incubation with Azimexone

Incubation time		P_{50} (Torr)	Methemoglobin (%)
30 min	Control	24.7	0.5
	0,1 mg/ml	24.9	0.65
	1 mg/ml	25.3	0.65
	10 mg/ml	24.9	0.85
24 hrs	Control	15.3	1.6
	0,1 mg/ml	15.5	1.3
	1 mg/ml	15.5	1.4
	10 mg/ml	13.2[a]	15.2[a]

[a] $p \leqslant 0.05$ compared with control.

Detailed investigations by Jeng et al. (31) have shown that the single intraperitoneal administration of 25 mg/kg azimexone leads to a clear rise in the stem cells in the spleen and in the bone marrow of mice that are determined in the direction of granulocytes and macrophages. The stem cells of the bone marrow which mature into macrophages (MM-CFC) rise only 7 days after treatment. This behavior of 2 cyanaziridine stands in contrast to other immunostimulants such as *C. parvum*, BCG, glucan, or pyran (32-35), all of which induce hematopoietic stem cells directly 24 hr after treatment, while there is a lag phase of 7 days with the 2-cyanaziridine derivative azimexone. This rise in GM-CFC and MM-CFC after azimexone treatment is used by some authors (30,31) to explain the therapeutic action of azimexone in irradiation damage or the reduction of the toxicity of cytostatics such as cyclophosphamide (36).

This increase was found by Jeng et al. (31) after a single dose of 25 mg/kg azimexone which does not induce Heinz bodies or anemia. However, Schlick et al. (30) only found a significant increase in CFUs after 12 doses of 25 and 50 mg/kg, respectively, which also induce Heinz bodies and anemia (Table 11). Maybe azimexone at low, nontoxic doses increases selectively the GM-CFU and MM-CFU; however, the increase of pluripotent stem cell CFU is only the result of the anemia.

Azimexone and BM 41.332 at very high doses lead, as a result of the above-mentioned reaction with hemoglobin, to deposition of hemosiderin both in the spleen and in the liver (i.e., in the reticuloendothelial system). This should lead to a blockage of the RES, which can be readily tested with the aid of the carbon clearance method. On the other hand, Yoshikai et al. (37) have reported that the blockade of the RES leads to inductions of suppressor T cells. We investigated the action of the 2-cyanaziridine derivatives azimexone and BM 41.332 at doses of 5 and 25 mg/kg orally, administered over 3 weeks on the number of lymphocytes in the peripheral blood and on the spleen and on the mitogenic response and the induction of nonantigen-specific suppressor cells, and the action of this dosage of BM 41.332 on the clearing function of the RES. As the values in Tables 7 and 10 show, there was a blockade of the RES and, in parallel, a decrease in $[^3H]$thymidine incorporation in PHA-stimulated spleen, and lymphocytes (Table 7), especially after treatment with azimexone which leads to Heinz bodies and slight splenomegaly. From these investigations it might be concluded in association with the findings of Yoshikai et al. (37) that this suppressive effect (Table 5 and 7) of 2-cyanaziridine de-

Table 10 Influence of BM 12.531 and BM 41.332 on the Number of Erythrocytes, Leukocytes, and the Percentage of Heinz Bodies and RES Functioniin Mice after 14-Day Treatment (C57B1/6 Mice, N = 15, ♀)

	Leukocytes ($x10^3/\mu l$)	Erythrocytes ($x10^6/\mu l$)	Heinz Bodies (%)	Hb (g%)	Spleen weight (mg)	Slope of the regression curves in the carbon clearance test[a]
Control	8.62 ± 0.91	4.81 ± 0.22	0	14.8 ± 0.34	600	-0.04935
BM 12.531						
50 mg/kg	13.96 ± 0.74[b]	4.02 ± 0.20[b]	60	15.8 ± 0.35	814	-0.02260[b]
100 mg/kg	14.82 ± 0.61[b]	3.59 ± 0.06[b]	90	14.18 ± 0.16	1.200	-0.03260[b]
BM 41.332						
50 mg/kg	10.49 ± 0.65	4.54 ± 0.65	1.5	14.36 ± 0.14	690	-0.04005[b]
100 mg/kg	11.28 ± 0.61[b]	4.36 ± 0.09[b]	2.5	15.06 ± 0.25	780	-0.02645[b]

[a]According to the method of Biozzi et al. (24).
[b]$p < 0.05$ compared with control.

Table 11 Effect of BM 12.531 on the Pluripotent Bone Marrow Stem Cells in Mice

Group	No. of CFUs/femur (mean ± SEM) After 3 days[a] 3 doses of azimexone ($x10^3$)	After 16 days[a] 12 doses of azimexone ($x10^3$)
Controls (solvent)	20.22 ± 1.11	24.71 ± 2.04
Azimexone 25 mg/kg PO	24.10 ± 1.47	30.45 ± 2.28[b]
Azimexone 50 mg/kg PO	21.34 ± 2.11	35.85 ± 1.26[c]

[a]Day of sacrifice.
[b]$p < 0.05$ in comparison with control.
[c]$p < 0.05$ in comparison with control and with 25-mg/kg azimexone group.

rivatives might be the result of RES blockade by hemosiderin deposits. However, the 5- and 25-mg/kg doses of BM 41.332 only have a marginal effect in induction of Heinz bodies, anemia (Table 7), or splenomegaly, so that the reduction of RES activity cannot be explained only by the RES blockade by hemosiderin. Unfortunately, the doses of azimexone which induce suppressor cell activity are only slightly below those that produce toxic changes in the erythrocytes, so that both actions cannot be precisely separated from each other.

VI. OTHER PHARMACOLOGICAL ACTIONS OF 2-CYANAZIRIDINES

Both azimexone and BM 41.332 produce a marked reduction of the toxicity of x-irradiation. The investigations by Stylos et al. (8) show that the single administration of 50 mg/kg azimexone in mice that have received an x-irradiation dose of 500 R produced a 100% survival after 20 days, while a high percentage of the untreated control animals died as the result of the irradiation. These investigations have been reproduced by various authors (30,36). The toxicity of cyclophosphamide in rats could also be markedly reduced by the administration of azimexone (36). The LD_{50} of cyclophosphamide in rats without azimexone treatment is about 190 mg/kg, but after administration of 3 × 10 mg/kg azimexone it is 220 mg/kg and after 3 × 25 mg/kg azimexone it is 250 mg/kg. To what extent this effect is caused by a stimulation of the stem cells damaged by the x-rays and cyclophosphamide or a restoration of the T-cell functions has so far not yet been clearly determined, especially as there is a suspicion that the bone marrow stimulation might be at least partially the result of a toxic action of the substances on the erythrocytes.

Azimexone and BM 41.332 (38) also show a good action on adjuvant arthritis in the rat. This model is usually used for the pharmacological testing of antirheumatics and immunosuppressants (39). This adjuvant arthritis in the rat is characterized by a T-cell defect and can be transferred, for example, by the injection of lymphocytes from sick animals to healthy animals. Rheumatoid arthritis in humans is also associated with a T-cell defect (40) in which there is subfunctioning of the suppressor T lymphocytes and a hyperfunctioning of the helper T lymphocytes with a resultant continuous, but insufficient, monocyte activation (26). A substance such as BM 41.332, which selectively inhibits the helper T-cell activity and stimulates suppressor cells with simultaneous inhibition of the macrophages, could consequently show a direct action on the clinical

Table 12 Effect of BM 41.332 and Methylprednisolone on Adjuvant Arthritis in Rat[a] (N = 15)

	Paw volume on left and right hindpaw (cm^3) and score ($\bar{x} \pm s_{\bar{x}}$) Day 0		Day +6		Day +14		Day +20		Lymphocytes on day 20 x $10^3/\mu l$	Weight on Day +22 (mg)		Popliteal lymph nodes	
	Left	Right	Left	Right	Left	Right	Left	Right		Spleen	Thymus	Left	Right
BM 41.332													
5 mg/kg oral	1.74	1.74	1.71	2.21	1.97[b]	2.91[b]	2.30[a]	3.31[a]	9.5	1000.27	505.13[b]	26.20[b]	48.40
daily	0.04	0.03	0.03	0.04	0.09	0.16	0.12	0.20	0.58	91.38	31.00	4.10	5.19
Score	0		0		35[b]		95[b]						
Methylprednisolone													
1 mg/kg oral	1.75	1.76	1.72	2.13	1.88[a]	2.42[a]	1.97[a]	2.65[a]	6.5[a]	600.07[b]	302.14[b]	11.36[b]	54.07
daily	0.03	0.02	0.03	0.04	0.05	0.11	0.07	0.15	0.28	33.66	24.24	1.47	8.05
Score	0		0		12[b]		46[b]						
Arthritis													
control	1.72	1.72	1.75	2.24	2.20	3.14	3.17	4.36	11.0	989.36	413.50	32.79	41.46
Tylose, oral	0.02	0.01	0.03	0.04	0.09	0.17	0.16	0.19	0.47	69.67	27.52	5.20	9.61
daily													
Score	0		0		72		150						
Healthy	1.80	1.78	1.90	1.87	1.81	1.89	1.85	1.87	7.7	482.3	654.4	6.2	6.5
Control	0.03	0.04	0.03	0.03	0.03	0.03	0.04	0.03	0.28	20.3	43.8	0.8	0.6

[a]The adjuvant arthritis is induced by injection of *M. tuberculosis* in the right hindpaw of male SIV rats according to the method described in Ref. 36. The paw volume was measured with the aid of a balance by volume displacement. The clinical findings were described by alloting scores to the swelling of the forepaws, the tails, the ears, eyes, and nose. The animals were killed on day 22, and the organ weights of popliteal lymph nodes, spleen, and thymus were determined.
b$\leqslant$0.05 compared with the arthritis control.

development of rheumatoid arthritis. We were, in fact, able to show that azimexone and BM 41.332 had a clear action on adjuvant arthritis in the rat in a dose (5 mg/kg daily) which does not induce an anemia in rats. Both the paw weight and the weight of the lymph nodes could be significantly reduced by treatment with BM 41.332 (Table 12), and the clinical symptoms, such as swelling and infiltration of the ears, eyes, nose, and tails, were considerably attenuated by the treatment.

VII. PHARMACOKINETIC INVESTIGATIONS

The pharmacokinetics of the 2-cyanaziridines were determined in male Sprague-Dawley rats by means of determination of ^{14}C-activity (42). There is no direct chemical method of detection for azimexone because of the known chemical instability of this substance. Rapid and complete absorption could be demonstrated after oral administration. The elimination of the radioactivity from the plasma after intravenous use can best be described with the aid of an open four-compartment model with a terminal half-life of 74.5 hr. This long half-life indicates the existence of a deep compartment for azimexone or its metabolites; 50-60% of the radioactivity administered was recovered in the urine in 24 hr, both after parenteral and oral administration, and less than 1% in the feces. Distribution investigations show that even 12 days after injection there is enrichment of the radioactivity in the organs of the reticuloendothelial system. However, as we suspect a direct reaction of azimexone with hemoglobin, it cannot be ruled out that this enrichment of the radio activity in the RES is solely a deposition of the hemoglobin or hemosiderin that has reacted with radioactively labeled 2-cyanaziridines.

On the other hand, the enrichment of the radioactivity takes place precisely in those organs that are responsible for the immune response, so that it is conceivable that the ^{14}C-labeled azimexone has reacted with the receptors in the RES-forming cells and thus produced the corresponding pharmacodynamic changes.

VIII. TOXICOLOGICAL STUDIES

The two aziridine derivatives BM 12.531 (azimexone) and BM 41.332 have been investigated toxicologically in rats and mice. Azimexone showed a very low acute toxicity (LD_{50} in mice after oral administration about 1 g/kg and after IP administration about 1.5 g/kg; in rats after oral administration about 3 g/kg and after IP administration about 2.5 g/kg).

BM 41.332 showed a similarly low acute toxicity in mice (e.g. more than 1 g/kg after oral administration, about 1.2 g/kg after intraperitoneal administration) but in rats it showed an LD_{50} of about 600 mg/kg on intraperitoneal administration and about 1.2 g/kg after oral administration.

The following toxic effects were found during the chronic toxicity test (i.e., on daily administration of the two substances for 3 months to rats). The high dose of 25 mg/kg daily was found to be at the limit of tolerance. After the second week of the experiment, there was a fall in the hematocrit and erythrocyte count. As already found with the single administration, the fall in erythrocytes is accompanied by leukocytosis from the second week of the experiment onward. Histologically, there is marked hyperplasia of the lymph follicles in the spleen and rich deposits of hemosiderin and occasional hemopoietic foci. The relative weight of the spleen was increased. In addition, there was an increase in the relative weight of the liver in some animals. In the animals that were treated with a middle dose of 5 mg/kg for 3 months there was a reduction of the hemoglobin values from the fourth week of the experiment onwards. The relative weight of the spleen was again increased and there was also a deposition of hemosiderin. In the animals in the lowest dose group (1 mg/kg) no changes whatsoever could be found. In the animals in all dose groups, a cell-rich active bone marrow was present. None of the other parameters of blood chemistry showed any changes.

Very similar changes were found in the 3-month oral toxicity test of azimexone in dogs. For this, both male and female beagles were used. In the high-dose group (25 mg/kg orally, daily) there was a fall in hemoglobin and erythrocytes from the very start. The animals of the middle-dose group (3.5 mg/kg) also showed a fall in erythrocytes and in hemoglobin, but this was not so marked. The lowest-dose group (0.5 mg/kg) did not show any differences from untreated control groups. Here, too, hemosiderin deposits were found histologically in both the liver and the spleen in both of the higher-dose groups.

Very similar changes were also found in the chronic toxicity tests of the 2-cyanaziridine derivative BM 41.332. In the highest-dose group (25 mg/kg), there was both a fall in the hematocrit and erythrocyte count and hemoglobin and a parellel rise in the leukocyte count. In the differential blood count, a dose-dependent increase in hypersegmented neutrophilic leukocytes was found. A dose-dependent hemosiderosis of the spleen is also detectable histologically after administration of BM 41.332.

The changes found after BM 41.332 administration are not quite as marked as those of azimexone at the highest dose (25 mg/kg).

Similar changes in the red and white blood pictures were found after 3-month daily oral administration of BM 41.332 to male and female beagles at doses of 1.5, 6, and 25 mg/kg. Here, too, hemosiderosis of the spleen, liver, and lungs was detected histologically. No other toxic effects could be found for either of the two substances.

In summary it can be said that both 2-cyanaziridine derivatives are well tolerated and that only a reversible toxic anemia is to be observed. To what extent changes in erythrocytes are related to the immunomodulating action of these substances cannot so far be definitely clarified.

Azimexone (BM 12.531) proved, however, to be mutagenic. At a dose of 1000 mg/kg, azimexone proved to be mtuagenic in the dominant lethal test, in the AMES test with and without liver homogenate in test strains TA 100 and TA 1535, and also in the micronucleus test in Chinese hamsters at a dosage of 2 × 1000 mg/kg. It should, however, be borne in mind that the doses selected for the mutagenicity are extremely high. In a subsequently carried out carcinogenicity study, no indication of a possible carcinogenic action of azimexone could be found. No effect of azimexone could be found in the transformation test, which provides good predictions about the carcinogenicity of a substance, so that altogether it can be said that only extremely high doses, which are at the extreme limit of acute tolerance, produce a mutagenic effect.

The second 2-cyanaziridine derivative tested, BM 41.332, proved, in contrast, to be nonmutagenic in all the mutagenicity investigations, even at extremely high doses.

IX. CLINICAL TRIALS OF AZIMEXONE AND BM 41.332

After finishing tolerance studies, azimexone was tested in cancer patients in a double-blind study in 30 patients with various types of tumor (43). In this study, azimexone was administered at a dose of 300 mg orally for 7 days, while 15 other patients received a placebo. The effects found in animal studies on erythrocytes and hemoglobin were also clearly detected in this study. On increasing the dose to 900 mg, the effects were even more marked.

A significant rise in the percentage of activated T lymphocytes, measured by means of the rosette test (44), was found after intravenous administration of 200 mg on 5 consecutive days or after oral administration of 300 mg on 7 consecutive days. In contrast, no definite effect on lymphocyte transformation induced by various PHA concentrations could be found in these patients after Ficoll separation. In the double-blind study mentioned above, too, no clear effect of the substance on the transformation test could be found. It must, however, be remembered that these lymphocyte transformation tests after Ficoll separation provide very poorly reproducible values. Even in healthy subjects without treatment with drugs, the intra- and interindividual scatters of the [^{3}H] thymidine incorporation in the concanavalin A (ConA)- or phytohemagglutinin (PHA)-stimulated Ficoll-separated lymphocytes are so large that a nonoptimized test can scarcely supply any reasonable information on the effect of immunomodulator on the lymphocyte reactivity (45,46). Even the values obtained with the aid of the active rosette test should be treated with caution as here, too, Ficoll separation is necessary, and this is known to damage the lymphocytes and also leads under certain circumstances, to very artificial conditions.

Kreienberg et al. (47) were able to detect significant immunorestorative effects with azimexone in female patients having mammary carcinoma being treated with cytostatics. In this investigation, 10 women with metastasizing mammary carcinoma who were undergoing polychemotherapy with cyclophosphamide, methotrexate, 5-fluoruracil, and vincristin were given an additional 100 mg/kg azimexone IV once a week for 8 weeks and subsequently 400 mg/kg azimexone IV weekly for a period of 4 weeks. A significant restorative effect could be detected both with respect to the leukocyte count and the mitogen-induced lymphocyte transformation (47).

Goutner et al. (48,49) were able to show that the intravenous administration of 200 mg three times weekly for 2 weeks clearly restored the delayed-type hypersensitivity reaction in anergic cancer patients. Skin tests with tuberculin, candidin extracts, tetanus tetanus toxoid, and diphtheria toxoid, which are contained in a Merieux multipuncture apparatus, were used to characterize the delayed-type hypersensitivity. This immunorestoration was accompanied by a potentiated lymphocyte reactivity to tetradecanoylphorbol acetate (TPA). This TPA is said to stimulate preferentially those lymphocytes that form active rosettes (50), so that this finding is in agreement with the observation that azimexone increases the percentage of active T lymphocytes.

Azimexone administered twice weekly at a dose of 200 mg IV for 5 weeks also produced a clear increase in cellular immunoreaction in patients with chronic lymphatic leukemia who exhibit a constantly lowered T-cell function in vitro. Furthermore, a significant increase in immunoglobulin secretion, especially in IgG and IgM, could be detected (51).

No final statement is possible at present on the actual therapeutic efficacy of azimexone in various tumor diseases. Only after completion of the studies running in various hospitals will an assessment of the use of azimexone as an immunostimulant in tumor diseases be possible.

As BM 41.332 has no mutagenic activity, we were able to carry out a phase I investigation with this substance in healthy subjects. BM 41.332 has furthermore the major advantage that it is chemically very stable, and an HPLC method of detection in serum and urine could be developed. According to preliminary investigations with rats, BM 41.332 only was absorbed to about 50%. In humans increasing doses of up to 400 mg per subject have been administered. No side effects of either subjective or objective types (e.g., changes in the blood chemistry) were found.

As BM 41.332 in mice produces a clear effect on the percentage of suppressor T lymphocytes, lowers the percentage of helper T lymphocytes, and inhibits the PHA-induced lymphocyte proliferation in the spleen lymphocytes, it was tested in initial studies in healthy subjects with respect to the changes in these parameters.

Unfortunately the different methods used for determination of the immune status in man are not very reproducible so we could not find a clear effect of BM 41.332 on the lymphocyte subpopulation or PHA-induced lymphocyte transformation in healthy volunteers. On the other hand, BM 41.322 was found to have a larger therapeutic ratio so there is the hope to find clinical efficacy at non-toxic doses.

X. SUGGESTED MODE OF ACTION OF 2-CYANAZIRIDINES

The 2-cyanaziridines that we have synthesized and tested are characterized by three pharmacological actions in mice and rats.

1. Stimulation of NK cells at doses of up to 25 mg/kg
2. Stimulation of suppressor T-cell activities at doses greater than 25 mg/kg
3. Changes in erythrocytes in the form of Heinz inclusion body formation and subsequent hemolytic anemia and splenomegaly at doses greater than about 25 mg/kg

In vitro, the 2-cyanaziridines show virtually no effects at concentrations that can be achieved in vivo. Macrophages are only marginally activated by the 2-cyanaziridines, the RES tends to be inhibited rather than stimulated, and the antibody production is inhibited at higher doses. On the basis of these immunopharmacological characteristics, the following mode of action for 2-cyanaziridines is conceivable.

The 2-cyanaziridines affect the differentiation and maturation of lymphocytes in the form that initially the NK cell activity is potentiated, assuming that the NK cells are of a lymphoid nature (10). At higher doses, these NK cell activities are counteracted by the increasing activation of suppressor T-cell mechanisms, which also lead to a mirror-image fall of the helper T-cell count and activity. It is still not clear whether this stimulation of the suppressor T cells is caused by a direct action of the 2-cyanaziridines on the T lymphocytes, or whether the stimulation of these suppressor lymphocytes is the result of the RES blockade by hemosiderin. Our investigations in mice showed very clearly (Table 7) that at doses at which we found a clear stimulation of the suppressor mechanisms, as measured by means of the inhibition of [^{3}H] thymidine incorporation after PHA stimulation, there was also an inhibition of the RES function, as measured by means of the carbon clearance method. At these doses also there was a certain percentage of Heinz inclusion bodies and slight splenomegaly. The leukocytosis observed at higher doses is undoubtedly related to the hemolytic anemia, so that the feedback to the bone marrow can easily be explained rather as a toxic than as an immunopharmacological action of the 2-cyanaziridines. The actions of 2-cyanaziridine derivatives [e.g., in adjuvant arthritis of the rat in which a suppressor cell defect is suspected (52)], contradict the hypothesis that the therapeutic effect in this model is solely a result of the RES blockade by deposited hemosiderin.

Here, doses already have a clear therapeutic effect that do not show any toxic actions on the erythrocytes with a subsequent hemosiderin deposition in the RES. As a single parenteral administration of 25 mg/kg, according to investigations of Chirigos et al., already has a significant stimulant action on GM-CFC and MM-CFC and this single dose does not show any damage to the erythrocytes with subsequent hemosiderin deposition, the action of the 2-cyanaziridines on the bone marrow proliferation could also be independent of the action on the erythrocytes. As, however, a clear delineation of the dose between bone marrow-stimulating and hemoglobin-altering actions for the 2-cyanaziridine derivatives is not possible, the question to what extent the undoubtedly existing feedback between bone marrow stem cells and peripheral T lymphocytes is altered directly or only via involvement of the hemosiderin-storing cells of the RES cannot be explained. The clearly found inhibibition of the helper T-cell activity in animal experiments should be seen in association with the stimulation of the suppressor T cells and here, too, the question must remain open as to whether a direct action of 2-cyanaziridine on the T lymphocytes or the interaction with hemosiderin-storing RES cells plays the main role. The interaction with other cells that are not present in lymphocyte cultures in vitro could, incidentally, be a reason for the fact that 2-cyanaziridines scarcely show any effects in vitro.

The decrease in [^{3}H] thymidine corporation in PHA-stimulated lymphocytes after 2-cyanaziridine treatment might be the result of the decreased helper T-cell activity, but also might be caused by remains of an unspecific cytotoxic alkylating activity of these aziridine compounds at high doses.

In summary, the action of the 2-cyanaziridines can be conceived as follows. After stimulation of NK cells, there is a shift in the T-cell compartment in such a manner that the percentage and activity of helper T cells is reduced and the suppressor T cells increase in a mirrorlike manner. The changes in these T-cell compartments lead to a number of other immunological phenomena, for example, inhibition of antibody production by B lymphocytes and the retarded increase in GM-CFC and MM-CFC. At doses which are only a little over the doses which induce these immunological events, the Heinz bodies and hemolytic anemia occur.

The investigations presented here show clearly that 2-cyanaziridine derivatives are very selectively acting immunomodulators. On the basis of our working hypothesis, which has been supported by a number of investigations mentioned above, a possible clinical use for 2-cyanaziridines can be clearly delineated. The 2-cyanaziridines are not nonspecifically acting adjuvants such as, for example, BCG, *C. parvum* or levamisol, which affect both B-cell and T-cell functions and macrophages. The 2-cyanaziridines are characterized, in contrast, by an inhibition of helper T-cell activity, so that these compounds cannot be used as nonspecific adjuvants. The clearly demonstrable stimulation of NK cells predestines these substances to be additional therapy for tumor diseases in which an NK cell defect is postulated by most authors (10). As it has been suggested for very many autoaggressive diseases [e.g. rheumatoid arthritis (26)] that a continuous, but insufficient, stimulation of macrophages and helper T cells, which leads to underfunctioning of the suppressor T cells, is responsible for the maintenance of the illness, it is conceivable that the selective inhibition of the helper T-cell activity and of macrophages or RES activity with simultaneous stimulation of suppressor T cells could represent a completely new point of attack for the treatment of these diseases. The 2-cyanaziridines could be such selectively acting immunomodulators, especially as a therapeutic effect is detectable in adjuvant arthritis of the rats, which has a large degree of similarity with rheumatoid arthritis.

It is assumed by most authors that the potentiation of tumor growth observed with many immunomodulators at certain dosages is attributable to stimulation of suppressor T cells (53). There are, however, some papers that show fairly clearly that the production of blocking antibodies is responsible for such tumor enhancement, for example, following BCG or *C. parvum* administration (54). The nonspecific activation by macrophage activators such as BCG or *C. parvum* can lead, via stimulation of helper cells and B cells, to synthesis of blocking antibodies, so that one must ask the question to what extent a nonspecific immunostimulation is more damaging than helpful. Furthermore, it is known that such a nonspecific immunostimulation with BCG, for example, produces autoaggressive diseases both in animals (55) and in humans (56). In addition, progressively growing malignant tumors are very frequently associated with autoaggressive syndromes, and it is repeatedly observed under clinical conditions that an initially successful cytostatic therapy can favorably influence such autoaggressive paraneoplastic syndromes. From this point of view there are many immunological similarities between autoaggressive diseases and malignant tumors. One could postulate a disorder of the immunological homeostasis for both diseases of the form in which a vicious circle exists between continuously, but insufficiently, stimulated macrophages and helper T lymphocytes and leads to the formation of blocking antibodies that paralyze other immune mechanisms that are necessary for the removal of harmful structures (i.e., of tumor cells also). If one accepts this working hypothesis, the aim of an immunological therapy should be to stimulate those mechanisms that can suppress excessive reactions.

However, it must be admitted that the stimulation of suppressor T lymphocytes in those tumors that are removed via antibody-dependent cytotoxicity raise the possibility of enhancement. However, antigen-specific monitoring of immunity has been questioned for most spontaneous tumors, as specific tumor-associated antigens that cause a specific immune reaction have not been found with these tumors. One must therefore assume that if an antineoplastic activity can be ascribed to the immune system it must be sought in those components that react independently of antigens and possibly also of antibodies.

Acute illnesses are characterized by the fact that constituents of bacterial cell walls or membranes activate macrophages. Simultaneously, it should be borne in mind that the glucocorticoid levels are also increased in such acute stress reactions, so that a nonspecific damage of the T lymphocytes is to be expected. However, Bradley and Mishell (25) have reported that the T-helper cells are protected by products of activated macrophages, while the suppressor cells are damaged by the increased glucocorticoids induced by stress. These activated macrophages, helper T lymphocytes, and B lymphocytes, in the presence of simultaneously impaired suppressor T activity, lead to an optimum acute specific immunosuppression which is necessary in such life-threatening situations. The additional pharmacological stimulation with nonspecific immunoadjuvants could be extremely worthwhile in these diseases.

At the end of the acute phase of the disease, the steroid level and the nonselective macrophage stimulation normally decrease and the immunological homeostasis can be restored maybe by T-suppressor cells. In this "reconvalescence phase" T-suppressor cells not only restrain the helper cells, but also might put an end to the mutual stimulation between helper T cells and macrophages. However, when T-suppressor cells are insufficient and macrophages are consistently stimulated, chronic autoaggressive diseases (and maybe cancer?) can develop. A low-dose glucocorticoid treatment would not be optimum in this phase of disease because the suppressor cells, which are already insufficient, are additionally damaged, whereas the helper T lymphocytes are protected by the consistently stimulated macrophages, so that a vicious circle can develop. Moreover, these diseases should not be treated with nonspecific immunoadjuvants, which are mostly potent macrophage activators. The harmful role of directly activated macrophages in the induction of autoaggressive diseases is supported by the fact that immunoadjuvants promote induction of adjuvant arthritis (55) in rats or induce arthritis in cancer patients (56). This, however, would mean that the present policy of immunosuppression with cytostatic compounds might immunologically be more rational than a nonspecific immunostimulation, because the persistent mutual stimulation of macrophages and helper T cells mentioned above is suppressed by cytostatic compounds. The immunosuppressive activity of cytostatic compounds would therefore form an important part of its antitumor activity. The clinical efficacy of cytostatic therapy has already been demonstrated, both against certain types of cancer and autoaggressive diseases, whereas the current vogue for nonspecific immunostimulation has not been clearly shown to be effective. Unfortunately, most cytostatic compounds are not very selective and can also damage other proliferating cells, so that the therapy is very often limited. A selective influence on the balance between T-helper and T-suppressor lymphocytes in favor of T-suppressor cells, which ends the mutual stimulation between macrophages and T-helper cells, might therefore be an interesting new approach to the treatment of some chronic diseases.

REFERENCES

1. U. Bicker, *Exp. Pathol.*, *10*:106 (1975).
2. K. Burzin and K. Enderer, *Angew. Chem.*, *84*:3, 108 (1972).
3. H. S. Jacob, M. C. Brain, J. V. Dacie, R. W. Carrell, and H. Lehmann, *Nature*, *218*: 1214 (1968).
4. G. A. Luckenbach, D. Cortez-Campeao, M. L. Modolell, P. G. Munder, and U. Bicker, *Exp. Pathol.*, *19*:1, 37 (1981).
5. U. Bicker, in *Augmenting Agents in Cancer Therapy* (E. M. Hersh, eds.), Raven Press, New York, 1981, p. 523.
6. L. Olsson and P. Ebbesen, *J. Immunol.*, *122*:3, 781 (1979).
7. H. Wexler, *J. Natl. Cancer Inst.*, *36*:4, 641 (1966).
8. W. A. Stylos, M. A. Chirigos, V. Papademetriou, and L. Lauer, *J. Immunopharmacol.*, *2*:1, 113 (1980).
9. F. L. Shand, *Int. J. Immunopharmacol.*, *1*:165 (1979).
10. R. B. Herberman and H. T. Holden, *J. Natl. Cancer Inst.*, *62*:3, 441 (1979).
11. M. A. Chirigos, V. Papademetriou, A. Bartocci, and E. Read, in *Advances in Immunopharmacology* (J. Hadden, eds.), Pergamon Press, New York, 1981, p. 217.
12. L. Olsson, N. Kiger, and G. Mathé, *Science*, in press (1982).
13. L. Olsson and U. Bicker, *J. Immunopharmacol.*, in press (1982).
14. C. D. Platsoucas and R. A . Good, *Proc. Natl. Acad. Sci. USA*, *78*:7, 4500 (1981).
15. P. H. Lagrange, G. B. Mackaness, and T. E. Miller, *J. Exp. Med.*, *139*:1529 (1974).
16. G. B. Mackaness, P. H. Lagrange, and T. Ishibashi, *J. Exp. Med.*, *139*:1540 (1974).
17. P. H. Lagrange, G. B. Mackaness, and T. E. Miller, *J. Exp. Med.*, *139*:528 (1974).
18. R. N. Germain, R. M. Williams, and B. Benacerraf, *J. Natl. Cancer Inst.*, *54*:3, 709 (1975).
19. J. B. Weinberg and J. B. Hibbs, *Clin. Res.*, *25*:2, 163A (1977).
20. S. Riisgaard, J. Bennedsen, and J. W. Rhodes, *Acta Path. Microbiol. Scand. Sect. C*, *85*:233 (1977).

21. B. Bonfert, U. Bicker, G. Hebold, and W. Maus, *IRCS Med. Sci.*, *5*:523 (1977).
22. J. W. Hadden and R. G. Coffey, in *Recent Results in Cancer Research*, *Cancer Chemo- and Immunopharmacology*, Vol. 75, (G. Mathé, eds.), Springer Verlag, Heidelberg, 1980, p. 162.
23. I. Florentin, J. Schulz, M. Bruley-Rosset, N. Kiger, J. Martinez, and G. Mathé, in *Recent Results in Cancer Research*, *Cancer Chemo- and Immunopharmacology*, Vol. 75 (G. Mathé, eds.), Springer Verlag, Heidelberg, 1980, p. 153.
24. G. Biozzi, B. Benacerraf, and B. N. Halpern, *Br. J. Exp. Pathol.*, *34*:441 (1953).
25. L. M. Bradley and R. I. Mishell, *Proc. Natl. Acad. Sci. USA*, *78*:5, 3155 (1981).
26. G. Janossy, O. Duke, L. W. Poulter, G. Panayi, M. Bofill, and G. Goldstein, *The Lancet*, :839 (1981).
27. M. V. Ardenne and P. G. Reitnauer, *Arzneim.-Forsch.* (*Drug Res.*), *25*:9, 1369 (1975).
28. A. Ganzoni, in *Das Knochenmark* (W. Queisser, ed)), Georg Thieme Verlag, Stuttgart, 1978, p. 438.
29. W. D. Gassel, H. Laukel, R. Braun, T. Werner, and U. Bicker, *Exp. Pathol.*, *20*:105 (1981).
30. E. Schlick, K. Mengel, U. Bicker, and K. D. Friedberg, *IRCS Med. Sci.*, *10*:147 (1982).
31. J. C. Jeng, K. F. McCarthy, M. A. Chirigos, and J. F. Weiss, *Experientia*, *38*:132 (1982).
32. R. S. Foster, Jr., B. R. MacPherson, and D. A. Browdie, *Cancer Res.*, *37*:1349 (1977).
33. T. J. MacVittie, in *Experimental Hematology Today* (S. J. Baum and G. D. Ledney, eds.), Springer Verlag, New York, 1979, p. 3.
34. B. Fisher, S. Taylor, M. Levine, E. Saffer, and E. R. Fisher, *Cancer Res.*, *34*:1668 (1974).
35. A. R. Zander, K. A. Dicke, D. Verma, S. Ginzbarg, and G. Spitzer, *Exp. Hematol.* (Suppl. 5), *7*:116 (1979).
36. U. Bicker, K. D. Friedberg, G. Hebold, and K. Mengel, *Experientia*, *35*:1361 (1979).
37. Y. Yoshikai, S. Miake, T. Matsumoto, K. Nomoto, and K. Takeya, *Immunology*, *43*:241 (1981).
38. U. Bicker, *Arzneim.-Forsch.* (*Drug Res.*), *7*:746 (1982).
39. K. F. Swingle, in *Medicinal Chemistry*, Vol. 13-II (R. A. Scherrer et al., eds.), Academic Press, New York, 1974, p. 33.
40. H. Deicher, *Münch. Med. Wschr.*, *123*:15, 603 (1981).
41. M. Colot, M. Micksche, and U. Bicker, *Cancer Immunol. Immunother.*, *6*:175 (1979).
42. B. Wölfel, K. Hartung, A. Haak, B. Kaufmann, K. Koch, and U. Abshagen, *Intern. J. Immunopharmacol.*, *3*:2, 133 (1981).
43. M. E. Heim, B. Massner, L. Knebel, U. Stosiek, D. Boerner, and U. Bicker, *Cancer Immunol. Immunother.*, *12*:87 (1981).
44. D. Boerner, U. Bicker, A. E. Siegler, U. Stosiek, and H. J. Peters, *Cancer Immunol. Immunother.*, *6*:237 (1979).
45. U. Bicker, W. Schaumann, and V. Haas, *J. Immunopharmacol.*, *5,162*:1-12 (1983).
46. W. Schaumann, U. Bicker, and V. Haas, *J. Immunopharmacol.*, *5,162*:13-30 (1983).
47. R. Kreienberg, D. Boerner, F. Melchert, and E.-M. Lemmel, in *Wiss. Infos* (Wiss. Abteilung Milupa AG), Milupa AG, Friedrichsdorf, 1981, p. 199.
48. A. Goutner, F. Nasrat, D. Bornadelle, and G. Ramenau, in *Recent Results in Cancer Research*, *Cancer Chemo- and Immunopharmacology*, Vol. 75 (G. Mathé, eds.) Springer Verlag, Heidelberg, 1980, p. 47.
49. A. Goutner, Y. Thomas, R. Huchet, and G. Mathé, *C. R. Soc. Biol.* *174*:750 (1980).
50. J. L. Touraine, J. W. Hadden, F. Touraine, E. M. Hadden, R. Estensen, and R. A. Good, *J. Exp. Med.*, *145*:468 (1977).
51. N. Niederle, N. Butin, H. J. Illiger, L. Labedzki, R. E. Schmidt, J. Stroehmann, and

D. Boerner, *Verhandlungen der Deutschen Gesellschaft für innere Medizin*, *85*: (1979).
52. L. Binderup, E. Bramm, and E. Arrigoni-Martelle, *Agents Actions* (Suppl.), *7*:199 (1980).
53. S. Broder and T. A. Waldmann, *N. Engl. J. Med.*, *299*:23, 1281 (1978).
54. T. Ishibashi, H. Yamada, S. Harada, Y. Harada. M. Takamoto, and K. Sugiyama, *Int. J. Cancer*, *21*:67 (1978).
55. T. Koga, S. Sakamoto, K. Onoue, S. Kotani, and A. Sumiyoshi, *Arthritis Rheum.*, *23*:9, 993 (1980).
56. M. Torisu, T. Miyahara, N. Shinohara, K. Ohsato, and H. Sonozaki, *Cancer Immunol. Immunother.*, *5*:77 (1978).

22

NPT 15392
A New Chemically Defined Biological Response Modifier

Lionel N. Simon, Fred K. Hoehler, and Theodore Ginsberg Newport Pharmaceuticals International, Inc., Newport Beach, California

John W. Hadden University of South Florida Medical Center, Tampa, Florida

I. INTRODUCTION

The synthesis of NPT 15392, erythro-9-(2-hydroxy, 3-nonyl)-hypoxanthine, was performed under the aegis of a joint development program carried out by Memoral Sloan-Kettering Cancer Center and Newport Pharmaceuticals International, Inc. The existence of this compound was first announced in 1980 at the International Congress of Immunology in Paris (1) and at the International Conference on Immunopharmacology in Brighton (2). NPT 15392 was evaluated as an immunomodulator because of its structural similarity to Isoprinosine (both substances contain a 9-substituted hypoxanthine moiety) and because of the nature of the 9-substituent, (the 2-hydroxy-3-nonyl radical) which has also been found in the adenosine deaminase (ADA) inhibitor erythro-9 (2-hydroxy-3-nonyl)-adenine (EHNA). The information obtained to date supports the conclusion that NPT 15392 is a relatively nontoxic immunomodulator and, therefore, deserves consideration for further preclinical and clinical evaluation. This chapter will review the biological effects of NPT 15392.

II. TOXICOLOGY

A. Acute Toxicity

The acute toxicity of NPT 15392 was evaluated in rats and mice (1,2). All animals were observed for 14 days following subcutaneous intraperitoneal or oral administration of NPT 15392. The LD_{50} values obtained in these studies are shown in Table 1.

Table 1 LD_{50} Values for NPT 15392

Species	Route	LD_{50} value	Signs
Rats	IP	1275 mg/kg	Ptosis, piloerection, bradypnea, lethargy, decreased muscle tone, decreased activity
	SC	> 5000 mg/kg	Decreased activity, ptosis
	PO	> 5000 mg/kg	Decreased activity, ptosis
Mice	IP	1510 mg/kg	Ptosis, bradypnea, piloerection, lethargy, decreased muscle tone, decreased activity
	SC	> 5000 mg/kg	Decreased activity, ptosis
	PO	> 5000 mg/kg	Decreased activity, ptosis

B. Subchronic Toxicity

NPT 15392 was tested for subchronic toxicity in rats and dogs during 13 weeks of repeated oral administration. These trials (employing dosage levels as high as 250 times the anticipated human dose of 0.01 mg/kg), failed to reveal any significant toxicity (1,2).

1. Rats

A group of 120 albino rats was divided into eight subgroups of 15 animals each (four gropps of males and four groups of females). The animals were treated daily with either 0 (control), 0.25, 1, or 2.5 mg/kg NPT 15392 by oral gavage. NPT 15392 had no significant effect on body weight gain, food consumption, hematological parameters, or clinical chemistry values at any of the intervals of measurement. After 12 weeks of drug administration, female rats receiving 2.5 mg/kg had significantly higher blood glucose levels than the controls. No significant alterations were noted in gross or microscopic histopathological examinations conducted after 3 months of drug administration.

2. Dogs

A group of 32 pure-bred beagles (16 males and 16 females) was divided into eight subgroups of four dogs per groups. Animals received daily oral doses of 0 (control), 0.25, 1, or 2.5 mg/kg of NPT 15392. Clinical laboratory tests were performed at 1, 4, 8, and 13 weeks. No dogs died during the study, nor were there any effects of NPT 15392 on appearance, behavior, body weight changes, food consumption, or hematological data. There were no ocular changes at any of the examination intervals, and no consistent alterations were noted in gross examination of tissue at necropsy. Significantly higher levels of fasting glucose at week 4 and bilirubin and total globulin at week 13 were observed in the high-dose females. There was a significantly greater relative spleen weight in the mid- and high-dose males sacrificed at termination of the study. No treatment-related histomorphological alterations were observed in any of the tissues examined microscopically.

III. PHARMACOLOGY

NPT 15392 was evaluated using a total of 48 different in vitro and in vivo screening procedures to assess its pharmacological profile of activity (1,2). Potential activity as a central nervous system (CNS) agent was assessed using reflex or behavioural depression, muscle relaxant activity, cataleptic activity, amphetamine antagonism, acute convulsive activity, motor stimulant activity, anorexic properties, analgesic properties, and antiparkinsonism properties. No CNS effects were noted at any of the doses studied (25-300 mg/kg).

Cardiovascular properties of NPT 15392 were assessed by in vivo measurement of acute hypertensive, pressor, antiarrhythmic, and cardiotropic activity. No antihypertensive or pressor activity was noted at any of the doses studied (up to 100 mg/kg). β-Adrenergic inhibition or stimulation and anticoagulant activity or platelet aggregation were assessed in vitro. No effects were noted in these systems.

A number of tests were designed to evaluate the effects of NPT 15392 in selected organ systems. Administration of 200 mg/kg of NPT 15392 had no significant effect on hypocholestoremic activity; 100 mg/kg had no effect on hypoglycemic activity and 20 mg/kg had no effect on diurectic activity.

NPT 15392 was not found to inhibit the growth of a number of different microorganisms (*Staphylococcus aureus*, *Escherichia coli*, *Mycobacterium ranae*, *Pseudomonas aeruginosa*, *Proteus vulgaris*, *Klebsiella pneumoniae*, *Candida albicans*, *Trichophyton mentagrophytes*, *Tritrichomonas foetus*).

IV. IMMUNOPHARMACOLOGY

This section presents data indicating that NPT 15392 enhances the immune response in vitro and in vivo and that the target cells include T lymphocytes, macrophages, natural killer (NK) cells, and polymorphonuclear (PMN) cells.

A. T-Cell Mitogen Response

1. In Vitro Administration of NPT 15392

NPT 15392 induces a small but consistent augmentation of the concanavalin A (ConA) and phytohemagglutinin (PHA)-induced lymphoproliferative response when added directly to normal C57B1/6 mouse spleen cell cultures (1,3). Ikehara et al. (3) found that the response was maximal at 0.1-1.0 μg/ml with considerably less augmentation observed at lower (0.1 μg/ml) or higher (10 μg/ml) concentrations. They also found that, as a proportion of the control level, the response to NPT 15392 was greater in cells from aged (18 month old) mice with a depressed mitogen response than in cells from younger (3 month old) mice.

Tsang et al. (4) reported that the addition of NPT 15392 to mononuclear cells from normal hamsters had no effect on the PHA response although augmentation did occur in cells from hamsters immunosuppressed by methotrexate. Hadden et al. (5) have shown that PHA-induced proliferation in human peripheral blood lymphocytes (PBLs) is variably influenced by the presence of NPT 15392. Of 24 individuals tested, only 9 responded with more than a 10% increase in thymidine incorporation as compared with control. Likewise, only 3 cultures out of 14 receiving NPT 15392 showed a similar augmentation of the response to ConA. In responding individuals the ability of NPT 15392 to enhance the PBL mitogen response was optimal at 0.01 μg/ml. Drug concentrations of 10 μg/ml or above inhibited the mitogenic response. Hadden et al. (5) noted that, in contrast to previous studies that employed spleen cells from C57B1/6 mice (1,3) the effects of NPT 15392 on human PBLs are "subtle, small in magnitude and variable in direction." Jones et al. (6) have also investigated the effects of NPT 15392 on in vitro human PBL response to PHA. In individual subjects, the effects ranged from a 6% inhibition to a 36% stimulation relative to baseline. Lymphocytes from 7 of 13 subjects exhibited a 10% or greater increase in mitogen-induced responses as a result of treatment with NPT 15392 in vitro. The average increase in the stimulation index was 12%. Touraine et al. (7,8) and Vecchi et al. (9) have essentially confirmed these observations. NPT 15392 has also been reported to enhance the mitogenic response of lymphocytes from cancer patients (1,9).

2. In Vivo Administration of NPT 15392

In mice treated with a single dose of NPT 15392 (0.01 mg/kg) a significant augmentation of the ConA-induced lymphoproliferative response was observed in spleen cells from normal animals or animals immunosuppressed with Friend leukemia virus (FLV) (1). Jones et al. (6) examined mitogen responses in normal and thymectomized adult BALB/c mice which had received multiple administration of NPT 15392 (0.1-0.3 mg/kg, IP or PO). In experiments characterized by low levels of thymidine incorporation in spleen cells from control animals, NPT 15392 enhanced the mitogenic response. Conversely, high control-group responses were always accompanied by slightly depressed responses in cells from treated animals. ConA responses were enhanced by NPT 15392 in BALB/c mice thymectomized at 9 weeks of age and assessed for in vitro immunocompetence at 12 and 14 weeks. Adult thymectomy resulted in a diminished ConA response that was normalized by NPT 15392. Florentin et al. (10,11) reported inconsistent effects on the ConA response in BALB/c mice 1-14 days after a single IP injection (0.1 mg/kg) of NPT 15392. PHA responses in these animals were consistently depressed. Over the 14-day period following injection, PHA-induced mitogenic responses were diminished by as much as 45%. Tsang et al. (4) observed that treatment with NPT 15392 augmented the PHA response in young, mature, and aged hamsters and found that the responses of young and aged animals (in which PHA responses were initially depressed) showed a relatively greater augmentation with NPT 15392.

B. Suppressor Cells

Hadden et al. (5) obtained consistent evidence that in vitro treatment with NPT 15392 (0.01-10 μg/ml) induces suppressor cells in cultures of PBLs. This suppressor activity was manifested in the response of autologous lymphocytes to ConA or to allogeneic stimulation in a one-way mixed-lymphocyte culture (MLC). Maximal inhibition (approximately 30%) occurred with 1 μg/ml of NPT 15392. This inhibitory effect of NPT 15392 was less in magnitude than the 49% suppression of the MLC response and the 61% suppression of the ConA response induced by prior treatment with ConA alone. In combination with ConA, NPT 15392 (0.01-1.0 μg/ml) enhanced the ConA-induced suppression of the MLC by 16-27% and the ConA lymphoproliferative response by 8-15%. The maximal suppressive effect of ConA and NPT 15392 was observed at 0.1 μg/ml of NPT 15392. The effects of NPT 15392, ConA, or NPT 15392 plus ConA were not prevented by indomethacin or cimetidine, indicating these effects are not mediated by the induction of prostaglandin. Neither did NPT 15392, with or without ConA, induce detectable levels of interferon which might have accounted for the observed suppression. Touraine et al. (7,8) have confirmed these observations and shown further that, with the cells of some individuals, NPT 15392 and Isoprinosine show a synergistic potentiation of ConA-induced suppressor cell function. However, following in vivo administration of NPT 15392 in mice, Florentin et al. (10) were unable to demonstrate suppressor cell activation.

C. Delayed-Type Hypersensitivity

Pretreatment of BALB/c mice with a single IP dose of NPT 15392 (0.1 mg/kg) significantly augmented their delayed-type hypersensitivity (DTH) reaction to a secondary ear lobe challenge with oxazolone (10). The maximal response (a 1.9-fold augmentation) was observed when NPT 15392 was given 7 days prior to sensitization. NPT 15392 has also been shown to augment DTH in mice bearing sarcoma 180, L-1210, Ehrlich lung metastases, or Ehrlich ascites carcinoma (12).

D. B-Cell Mitogen Response

1. In Vitro Administration of NPT 15392

Ikehara et al. (3) reported that spleen cells from 18-month-old C57B1/6 mice, cultured in the presence of lipopolysaccharide (LPS) and NPT 15392 (0.1 μg/ml), incorporate up to 50% more thymidine than control cultures. In 3-month-old mice, the improvement in the response was only 20%. As with the ConA and PHA responses, the LPS response was initially depressed in the older mice. In agreement with these observations, Vecchi et al. (9) reported enhancement of the LPS response by 0.01-1.0 μg/ml NPT 15392.

2. In Vivo Administration of NPT 15392

Florentin et al. (10) have found that NPT 15392 augments the mitogenic response of spleen cells from BALB/c mice to the B-cell mitogen, dextran sulfate. A single intraperitoneal injection of NPT 15392 on day 0 was followed by a 14-day period during which the response increased as much as 100%. The dextran sulfate response, and its augmentation by NPT 15392, were reduced if adherent cells were eliminated from the cultures.

The effect of NPT 15392 on the response of lymphocytes to the B-cell mitogen LPS is not clearly delineated. In contrast to the in vitro results of Ikehara et al. (3), which showed augmentation of the LPS response of murine spleen cells, Florentin et al. (10) have been unable to demonstrate augmentation of the BALB/c LPS response by in vivo treatment with NPT 15392.

E. Plaque-Forming Cells

Plaque formation of spleen cells (PFCs) in either the Mishell-Dutton or the Jerne plaque assay is augmented by NPT 15392. Merluzzi et al. (13) found that the T-cell-dependent PFC response to sheep red blood cells (SRBCs) was elevated two- to threefold in C57B1 mice which had received six daily injections of 0.3-3 mg/kg NPT 15392 prior to in vitro antigen exposure. The response to the T-cell-independent trinitrophenylated-lipopolysaccharide (TNP-LPS) antigen was not affected in animals on the same drug regimen, suggesting that the effects of NPT 15392 on B-cell function are mediated by T helper cells. Jones et al. (6) found that BALB/c mice treated with NPT 15392 (0.05-0.5 mg/kg IP) mounted a 2.5-fold higher PFC response than animals treated with saline prior to SRBC immunization.

Florentin et al. (10) have measured PFCs in BALB/c mice given a single intraperitoneal injection of NPT 15392 up to 14 days prior to SRBC immunization. They observed an enhanced PFC response in spleen cells from NPT 15392-treated animals. On the average, the maximum drug-induced enhancement occurred when 0.1 mg/kg NPT 15392 was administered 1 day prior to antigen. Higher (1.0 mg/kg) or lower (0.01 mg/kg) doses tended to suppress the PFC response. In order to determine the mechanism of PFC enhancement, mice were given a T-dependent antigen, trinitrophenylated-hemocyanin (TNP-KLH), or a T-independent antigen, TNP-LPS, 0-14 days after treatment with

NPT 15392. The PFC response to TNP-KLH was increased threefold when NPT 15392 was administered 1 day prior to antigen. In contrast, PFC responses in animals receiving NPT 15392 1 day prior to TNP-LPS were inhibited 26% relative to the control culture. However, increasing the time between NPT 15392 and TNP-LPS administration not only reversed the inhibition but resulted in an augmented response. The maximal augmentation (2.4-fold) was recorded when 10 days elapsed between NPT 15392 administration and TNP-LPS immunization. However, Florentin et al. (11) observed that a similar single treatment with NPT 15392 inhibited PFC responses of C57B1/6 mice to TNP-LPS over a 14-day period. Anti-SRBC responses in tumor-bearing mice also appear to be enhanced by prior treatment with NPT 15392 (12,14).

F. Cytocidal and Cytostatic Activity

NPT 15392 modulates a variety of cytocidal functions. Florentin et al. (10,11) measured NK cell activity in spleen or peritoneal cells harvested from BALB/c mice following a single IP or IV injection of NPT 15392 (0.1 mg/kg) 1-14 days prior to cytotoxicity testing. In both cell populations the ability to lyse the YAC-1 tumor target cells was increased at least threefold by NPT 15392. The response was maximal 3-7 days after treatment with NPT 15392. As might be expected, the degree of augmentation was related to the route of administration. Higher levels of NK cell activity were exhibited by peritoneal cells following an IP injection of NPT 15392, while spleen cells expressed a higher level of NK cell activity when NPT 15392 was administered IV. Faanes et al. (15) have also reported enhancement of NK cell activity following in vivo administration of NPT 15392 in mice while Tsang et al. have reported similar effects in hamsters (4). The magnitude of the effect of NPT 15392 is comparable with that produced by interferon; however, Hadden et al. (16) have been unable to demonstrate induction of serum interferon by NPT 15392. Moreover, Hadden et al. (5) were unable to affect NK cell function by in vitro administration of NPT 15392 either alone or in combination with interferon. Antibody-mediated cellular cytotoxicity (ADCC) of human mononuclear cells was also unaffected by NPT 15392. In contrast Goutner (17) reported that NPT 15392 potentiated the effects of suboptimal doses of exogenous interferon on spontaneous cytotoxicity of human mononuclear cells. Furthermore, Tsang and Fudenberg (18) have shown that NPT 15392 appears to induce interferon in an assay in which culture fluid from stimulated lymphocytes is incubated in human foreskin fibroblasts and infected with vesicular stomatitis virus. Florentin et al. (11) have shown that combinations of interferon and NPT 15392 in vivo appear to produce at least an additive effect on NK cell activity. The level of T-lymphocyte-mediated cytotoxicity expressed by spleen cells imminized in vitro with allogeneic tumor cells is also increased by NPT 15392 (10,13). As compared with matched controls, spleen cells taken from mice which received single or multiple doses of NPT 15392 possess higher lytic activity against tumor cell lines. At an effector/target ratio of 100:1, spleen cells from animals which received multiple doses of NPT 15392 (0.1 mg/kg) exhibited 2.6-fold higher cytotoxic activity against the P815 mastocytoma (13). Against another tumor line, the EL-4 lymphoma, increases in the maximum lytic activity (2.7-fold) were noted in mice which received a single IP injection of 0.1 mg/kg NPT 15392 (10).

G. Induction of Cell Surface Markers

Prothymocytes from 8-week-old athymic (nu/nu) mice treated in vitro with concentrations of 0.1-10.0 μg/ml of NPT 15392 acquired a high degree of the T-cell marker Thy 1 (3). A maximum induction of 27-34% was observed at 0.1 μg/ml NPT 15392. Similar results with human prothymocytes have been obtained by Touraine et al. (8). This activity was similar to that observed in the augmentation of active rosettes of human T lymphocytes by Hadden et al. (5) and Wybran (19). Wybran (19) has further shown that NPT 15392, like thymic hormones, increased the percentage of active rosettes in vivo following administration of the drug to cancer patients.

H. Miscellaneous Measures of Immune Function

In addition to its effects on lymphocytes, NPT 15392, at low concentrations, augmented zymosan-induced chemiluminescence of human buffy coat cells (1). Wybran reported that NPT 15392 (0.001-10 μg/ml) augmented leukocyte adherence inhibition and phagocytosis of zymosan by granulocytes (19). Hadden et al. (20) found that 0.001 μg/ml of NPT 15392 augmented lymphokine-induced guinea pig macrophage proliferation in vitro, but Faanes et al. (15) reported no effect on macrophage phagocytosis and Vecchi et al. (9) reported no modification in nonspecific macrophage cytotoxicity. Pompidou et al. (21) have demonstrated that NPT 15392 in vitro promotes the induction of plasma cells and plasmablasts. NPT 15392 also enhanced pokeweed mitogen induced B-cell differentiation. Pompidou (22) has also shown that NPT 15392 (0.2 μg/ml) alone or in combination with ConA decreased nuclear refringence of lymphocytes after 20 min of incubation. This suggested a mechanism of action involving RNA synthesis. Hadden and Coffey (23) have presented preliminary evidence that NPT 15392 selectively inhibits cyclic GMP phosphodiesterase, an action consistent with the nuclear mechanism involving RNA synthesis.

V. MODELS OF HUMAN DISEASE

A. Animal Models of Autoimmune Disease

New Zealand Black (NZB) mice develop a disease resembling human autoimmune hemolytic anemia. This disorder is characterized by splenomegaly, anemia, and the development of antierythrocyte antibody. Jones et al. (24) have shown that daily injections of 0.1 mg/kg NPT 15392 significantly retarded the development of antierythrocyte antibody in young (11 week old) mice and 0.4 mg/kg NPT 15392 reduced the levels of antierythrocyte antibody in older (38 week old) mice. Anemia and splenomegaly were also slightly reduced in the older mice. This indicates that NPT 15392 may be useful in the treatment of autoimmune diseases.

B. Tumor Models

Table 2 shows the tumor models in which the antineoplastic and immunorestorative properties of NPT 15392 have been evaluated. The results obtained in each model are discussed below.

Experiments performed by Jones (25) demonstrated that IP injections of Friend leukemia virus (FLV) caused splenomegaly and subsequent death in BALB/c mice. Accompanying the splenomegaly was leukemia, with the infected mice showing greatly elevated white blood counts. The presence of this leukemia severely depresses the immunoresponsiveness of the host and in this aspect parallels leukemia in humans. NPT 15392 administered IP at 0.01 mg/kg/day produced a reduction in splenomegaly as demonstrated by the lower spleen weights in FLV-infected BALB/c mice. Comparable results were obtained with doses as low as 0.001 mg/kg/day. Animals receiving NPT 15392 were also

Table 2 Tumor Models Used to Investigate NPT 15392 Action

Tumor	Parameter measured
FLV-induced leukemia	Reduction in spleen weight
Lewis lung carcinoma	Number of lung metastases
T241 fibrosarcoma	Number of lung metastases
Sarcoma 180 (solid)	Tumor weight
NF sarcoma	Tumor weight
Sarcoma 180 (ascitic)	Survival
P-388 leukemia	Survival
BC-47 carcinoma	Survival
AH series hepatoma	Survival
L1210 lymphoma	Survival
	Immune function
Ehrlich ascitic carcinoma	Plaque assay (PFC)
Ehrlich ascitic carcinoma	ConA mitogen response
Ehrlich ascitic carcinoma	DTH
Ehrlich lung metastatic	Plaque assay (PFC)
Ehrlich lung matastatic	DTH
Sarcoma 180	DTH
NF sarcoma	DTH
L1210 lymphoma	DTH
BC-47 carcinoma	Cytotoxic activity

able to partially overcome the immunosuppression produced by the FLV infection. Spleen cells taken from NPT 15392-treated mice exhibited enhanced mitogenic responses to controls (Table 3).

The effects of NPT 15392 on tumor development and metastatic potential have been investigated in a Lewis lung carcinoma (LLC) model (11). Groups of mice were each given 10 IP injections of NPT 15392 (0.1 mg/kg) over a 25-day period beginning 1 day after tumor implantation. The mean diameter of the implanted tumor was determined on each day of drug treatment. At the end of 25-days, animals were sacrificied and the mean number of lung metastases were measured in animals treated with NPT 15392 and controls. In these experiments, NPT 15392 had no demonstrable effect on the rate of tumor growth. However, significant reductions (30%) in the mean number of metastases were observed in mice receiving NPT 15392.

Jones (25) conducted a series of experiments with a fibrosarcoma (T-241) implanted into the dorsal aspect of the foot of C57B1/6 mice. NPT 15392 was given by IP injection at a dose level of 0.3 mg/kg beginning on the day of implantation and continuing until day 28, the day of sacrifice. The number and size of lung metastases were determined on day 28 using the method described by Deodhar (26). A control group received saline injections daily. The results are presented in Table 4A. Independent verification of this result was achieved by Deodhar (26) using two different dosage levels of NPT 15392. Drug was administered 5 days out of 7 (weekends excluded) for 4 weeks. The animals were sacrified 28 days after tumor implantation and metastases were counted. Results are presented in Table 4B.

Measurement of tumor weight has been utilized in the evaluation of NPT 15392 action against two model sarcomas, sarcoma 180 (solid form) and NF sarcoma (27).

Table 3 Enhancement of the In Vitro Mitogen Response of Spleen Cells from FLV-Infected, Immunosuppressed Mice

Mitogen	NPT 15392 dose (mg/kg)				
	0.0[b]	0.001	0.01	0.10	1.0
ConA 1 μg/ml	100 (±7)	108[a] (±10)	212 (±20)	327 (±20)	195 (±14)
PHA 40 μg/ml	100	92.7 (± 6.3)	241 (±22)	314 (±31)	173 (±11)
LPS 50 μg/ml	100	45.4 (± 6.0)	290 (±9	210 (±17)	141 (±14)

[a]Activity is expressed as percent of the response from the infected control animals.
[b]The response of infected control animals as percent of the uninfected controls are: ConA, 2.7%; PHA, 13.7%; LPS, 11.1%.

Using a number of different treatment protocols including (a) treatment prior to tumor inoculation, (b) treatment after inoculation, and (c) treatment before and after inoculation, using a variety of drug concentrations, NPT 15392 was shown to exhibit no clear influence on tumor weight.

Variable extension of survival in tumor-bearing animals has resulted from treatment with NPT 15392 as a single therapy. In the ascites form of sarcoma 180, animals receiving 0.01 mg/kg NPT 15392 prior to and following tumor implantation exhibited a significant increase in their mean survival time in some experiments but not in others. Similarly, NPT 15392 treatment of DBA/2 but not CDF_1 mice bearing P388 tumors yielded increased survival in some experiments (27).

Sato (27) has also utilized the AH series of hepatomas as a model system for evaluating NPT action in vivo. Groups of six female Sprague-Dawley rats were inoculated (IV) with 107 cells from 1 of 10 hepatoma types, followed by a series of IP (0.5 mg/kg) or PO (5 mg/kg) administrations of NPT 15392. Survival was followed in control and drug-treated animals for a period of 60 days. The drug was judged of positive efficacy if the increased life span (ILS) was greater than 200% relative to the untreated control and

Table 4 Effect of NPT 15392 on Metastases in T-241-Implanted C57B1/6 Mice

Treatment (dosage)	Metastases No. ± SE	Inhibition (%)	(p)
A. Control (N = 10)	43.0 ± 8.8		
NPT 15392 (0.3 mg/kg/day) Day 0 to +28 (N = 10)	27.8 ± 3.9	36	(<0.05)
B. Control (N = 10)	57.6 ± 6.6		
NPT 15392 (0.1 mg/kg) N = 10	21.0 ± 7.0	64	(<0.01)
NPT 15392 (1.0 mg/kg) N = 10	37.6 ± 5.8	35	(<0.05)

mixed if the improvement was between 50 and 100%. All untreated animals, regardless of AH tumor type received, died within 20 days.

NPT 15392 administered PO was found to be a positive treatment against AH-44. More than 50% of these animals survived to the 60-day test limit. The response in animals with the AH-66 and AH-130 hepatoma types was mixed. Two animals with AH-66 and one animal with AH-130 remained alive at the end of the study.

In animals which received IP injections of NPT 15392, the effect on survival was not as dramatic. Animals bearing the AH-44 or AH-66 tumor type were the only ones whose survival curves were improved by NPT 15392. The magnitude of the improvements was only sufficient to qualify drug efficacy as mixed.

Sato and Tsurufuji (12) have measured NPT 15392-mediated restoration of immune function in tumor-bearing mice. In all experiments, mice were administered NPT 15392 IP, either prior to tumor inoculation or before and after exposure to the tumor. As a result of the drug treatment, the suppressed DTH response in the Ehrlich ascitic tumor, Ehrlich lung tumor, sarcoma 180, and L1210 leukemia models was partially reversed. The ordinarily depressed mitogenic response in Ehrlich ascitic tumor or L1210 leukemia models was normalized by treatment with NPT 15392. In mice with Ehrlich lung metastic tumor, the number of PFCs was increased from 27 to 97% (relative to untreated controls) by NPT 15392. PFC levels, in NPT 15392-treated Ehrlich ascitic carcinoma-bearing animals, were elevated two- to threefold over untreated tumor-bearing controls. The degree of improvement in the PFC response depended on the drug dose and administration regimen. In general, the most effective dose of NPT 15392 was 0.1 mg/kg. No immune functions in NF sarcoma-bearing animals were modified by NPT 15392.

In rats, chemically induced bladder carcinoma was treated with NPT 15392 (27). A significant increase in survival was reproducibly obtained in drug-treated animals compared with saline-treated controls. In addition, 10-20% of the animals in the drug-treated group appeared to exhibit cures (survival ⩾ 51 days). Enhancement by NPT 15392, of a depressed cytotoxic T-cell response of spleen cells isolated from tumor-bearing animals was also noted.

In these tumor studies, NPT 15392 was employed as a monotherapy. Given the negative effects of levamisole in such tests, the results are encouraging. As with levamisole, it will be important in the future to study NPT 15392 as an adjunctive therapy following cytoreductive therapy with surgery, chemotherapy, or radiation.

VI. CLINICAL STUDIES

A. Tolerance: Human Safety Studies

Single- and multiple-dose tolerance studies have been carried out in human volunteers. The results of the single-dose tolerance studies have been discussed elsewhere (28). In a recent study, three groups of normal male volunteers received 0.7, 3.5, or 0 mg of NPT 15392 on days 0, 3, 6, and 9 and were compared with a group receiving placebo. Clinical chemistry, complete blood count, urinalysis, and physical evaluation were performed initially and throughout the study. The doses chosen represented 1, 5, and 10 times the anticipated effective dose in humans. No changes in mean values outside normal limits were observed in any of the drug treatment groups. In addition, by use of a recently developed radioimmune assay (29), we were able to detect serum and urinary levels of NPT 15392 that were present in a dose-responsive fashion and were detectable at all dosage levels administered.

B. Immunopharmacological Effects in Cancer Patients

A multicenter study has been performed by the tumor immunology group of the European Organization for the Research and Treatment of Cancer (EORTC) (30,31). In this study, patients with various cancers, who were not currently receiving other therapy, were treated with 0.4 or 0.7 mg/kg oral NPT 15392 on days 0, 4, 7, and 10 of the study. Various immune tests were performed at the discretion of the participating investigator before, during, and after therapy. A statistical analysis of the data capable of being compared has been presented (30,31). NPT 15392 appeared to augment T-lymphocyte counts, percentage of E rosettes, NK cell activity, and autologous rosettes. No effect on DTH was observed. These effects were usually observed in patients with initially depressed immune function. Patients with normal or high values were essentially unaffected. These data allow the tentative conclusion that NPT 15392 is a modifier of human biological (immunological) responses and indicate that further clinical testing is warranted.

VII. CONCLUSION

NPT 15392 is a novel heterocyclic compound with complex immunopharmacological activity. It is active at low doses and shows a remarkable lack of toxicity. Cellular targets of its actions, either direct or indirect, include T and B lymphocytes, prothymocytes, NK cells, macrophages, and granulocytes. For prothymocytes and NK cells it induces differentiation or function in a manner similar to thymic hormones or interferon, respectively. For mature cells, it potentiates the effects of other primary stimulants (e.g., mitogen, antigen, or lymphokine) for functions of proliferation, secretion, and cytotoxicity. Its in vitro effects translate well in vivo with augmentation of T-cell function and NK cell activation in both animals and humans. Its immunopharmacological effects are clearly restorative in mice immunologically depressed by chemotherapy, aging, or cancer, and in humans with cancer. Effects in normal animals are variable and, in selected cases, immunosuppressive. Immunosuppression by NPT 15392 was also apparent in animals with autoimmune disease. Experimental clinical indications in the future are expected to be in humans immunosuppressed spontaneously, iatrogenically, or as a result of cancer.

REFERENCES

1. L. Simon, A. Giner-Sorolla, and J. Hadden, *4th International Congress of Immunology*, Paris, France, July, 1980.
2. L. Simon, R. Settineri, E. Pfadenhauer, C. Jones, K. Maxwell, and A. Glasky, *Int. J. Immunopharm.*, *2*:200 (1980).
3. S. Ikehara, J. Hadden, R. Good, D. Lunzer, and R. Pahwa, *Thymus*, *3*:87 (1981).
4. K. Y. Tsang, C. B. Phillips, M. J. Gnagy, and H. H. Fudenberg, *Fed. Proc.*, *41*:812 (1982).
5. J. Hadden, E. Hadden, T. Spira, R. Settineri, L. Simon, and A. Giner-Sorolla, *Int. J. Immunopharm.*, *4*:235 (1982).
6. C. Jones, B. Binko, R. Settineri, and K. Maxwell, unpublished data.
7. J. L. Touraine, F. Touraine, K. Sanadji, O. Othmane, G. Ferret, and G. Fournie, *Int. J. Immunopharm.*, *4*:235 (1982).
8. J. Touraine, G. Gay-Ferret, K. Sanadji, O. Othmane, G. Fournie, and F. Touraine, in *Current Concepts in Human Immunology and Cancer Immunomodulation* (B. Serrou, C. Rosenfeld, and J. Daniels, eds.), Elsevier Biomedical, Amsterdam, 1982.

9. A. Vecchi, M. Sironi, N. Serraglia, A. Mantovani, and F. Spreafico, *Int. J. Immunopharm.*, *2*:204 (1980).
10. I. Florentin, E. Taylor, M. Davigny, G. Mathé, and J. Hadden, *Int. J. Immunopharm.*, *4*:225 (1982).
11. I. Florentin, L. Kraus, G. Mathé, and J. Hadden, in *Current Concepts in Human Immunology and Cancer Immunomodulation* (B. Serrou, C. Rosenfeld, and J. Daniels, eds.), Elsevier Biomedical, Amsterdam, 1982.
12. S. Sato and M. Tsurufuji, *Int. J. Immunopharm.*, *2*:200 (1980).
13. V. Merluzzi, M. Walker, N. Williams, B. Susskind, J. Hadden, and R. Faanes, *Int. J. Immunopharm.*, *4*:219 (1982).
14. R. B. Faanes, unpublished data.
15. R. B. Faanes, V. J. Merluzzi, M. Walker, N. Williams, P. Ralph, and J. Hadden, *Int. J. Immunopharm.*, *2*:197 (1980).
16. J. Hadden, M. Ito, and A. Stewart, unpublished data.
17. A. Goutner, *Int. J. Immunopharm.*, *2*:197 (1980).
18. K. Y. Tsang and E. H. Fudenberg, *Clin. Res.*, *30*:564A (1982).
19. J. Wybran, *Int. J. Immunopharm.*, *2*:201 (1980).
20. J. Hadden, E. M. Hadden, T. Spira, and A. Giner-Sorolla, *Int. J. Immunopharm.*, *2*: 198 (1980).
21. A. Pompidou, in *Advances in Immunopharmacology* (J. Hadden, L. Chedid, P. Mullen, and F. Sreafico, eds.), Pergamon Press, Oxford, 1981.
22. A. Pompidou, B. Mace, N. Duchet, J. Leymeyer, and M. Cooper, *Int. J. Immunopharm.*, *4*:286 (1982).
23. J. W. Hadden and A. R. G. Coffey, unpublished data.
24. C. Jones, C. Lee, F. Hoehler, P. Koyama, W. Skinner, and J. Lamott, *Int. J. Immunopharm.*, *5*:85 (1983).
25. C. Jones, unpublished data.
26. D. Deodhar, unpublished data.
27. S. Sato, unpublished data.
28. J. Hadden and A. Giner-Sorolla, in *Augmenting Agents in Cancer Therapy* (E. M. Hersh, ed.), Raven Press, New York, 1981.
29. E. Pfadenhauer, C. Jones, and K. Maxwell, *J. Pharm. Sci.*, *72*:914 (1983).
30. J. Wybran, in *Current Concepts in Human Immunology and Cancer Immunomodulation* (B. Serrou, C. Rosenfeld, and J. Daniels, eds.), Elsevier Biomedical, Amsterdam, 1982.
31. M. Micksche, E. M. Kokoschka, H. Rainer, and A. Uchida, *Int. J. Immunopharm.*, *4*:283 (1982).

Section C

Induction of Cytotoxicity

Interferon, Natural Killer Cells, and Macrophages

23

Interaction of Interferon and Chemotherapeutic Agents in Modulation of Natural Killer Cell Activity

Julie Y. Djeu and Keith M. Ramsey Center for Drugs and Biologics, Food and Drug Administration, Bethesda, Maryland

I. INTRODUCTION

A variety of chemotherapeutic agents are in common use for two purposes: (a) to alter the direction of the immune response in preparation for acceptance of bone marrow or organ grafts in transplant recipients and (b) to reduce tumor load in cancer patients. On a clinical level, the goal is to achieve minimal graft rejection and maximal elimination of tumor without profound impairment of the immune system. Some retention of the host defense mechanism is necessary to prevent new infections or reactivation of latent ones which are often the leading causes of death in the immunocompromised individual. Thus, for effective chemotherapy, an understanding of the mechanism of action of the drugs at the cellular level is vital. In addition to gaining knowledge of its antitumor efficacy, each drug should be monitored for its selective adverse effect on a particular lymphocyte subset. It is also important to gain information on the stage of the lymphocyte maturation or activation process which is most vulnerable to drug inhibition.

Of the immune responses that have been studied, natural killer (NK) cells are believed to play a major role in immunosurveillance of neoplasia and control of metastatic spread (1). The evidence for this comes from studies of mice. In nude mice, transplanted tumors rarely have been shown to spread, most likely due to the existence of high NK activity in these T-cell-deficient mice (2-4). The reverse is also true in that NK-deficient beige mice readily show metastates of transplanted tumors and also have a high incidence of spontaneous lymphomas (5-7). Moreover, there is a good correlation between the levels of NK activity in different mouse strains and their ability to clear radiolabeled tumor cells in vivo (8). In humans, patients with Chediak-Higashi syndrome that have a selective defect in spontaneous NK activity have been shown to be prone to development of lymphoproliferative diseases (9). In addition, an X-linked genetic abnormality that is associated with lymphoproliferative disease also appears to correlate with low NK function (10).

Besides a role in antitumor immunity, NK cells may be important in mediating microbial immunity. Viruses such as influenza (11,12), cytomegalovirus (13), herpes simplex (14), and measles virus (15) cause a rise in NK levels against virus-infected targets in humans and mice while bacteria such as Bacillus Calmette-Guérin and *Corynebacterium parvum* are known to enhance NK cell function in mice (16). Moreover, mouse strains with high spontaneous NK activity are better able to resist lethal cytomegalovirus infection than those with low NK activity (17). A genetic link may therefore exist between NK activity and resistance to viral infection, at least in the case of cytomegalovirus. Clinical data have recently become available which suggest that survival from cytomegalovirus infection correlates with the presence of circulating NK cells in bone marrow transplant recipients (18).

This chapter summarizes our efforts to study the adverse effects of various chemotherapeutic agents on NK activity and the ability of interferon (IFN) to overcome the inhibitory process. In mice, both in vivo and in vitro data are presented to show the effects of these drugs on spontaneous NK cells and their augmentation by poly I:C. Data concerning the interaction of IFN and drugs in modulation of human NK activity are from in vitro experimentation of normal-donor lymphocytes.

II. MATERIALS AND METHODS

A. Drugs

For effective inhibition in vivo (19), hydrocortisone (HC) an anti-inflammatory and lympholytic agent, was administered intraperitoneally (IP) at 250 mg/kg in mice. Cyclophosphamide (CYP), an alkylating agent often used in cancer therapy, was administered IP at 200 mg/kg. Silica and carrageenan, which are primarily used in research to curb macrophage function, were administered at 15 mg per mouse IP and 1 mg per mouse intravenously (IV), respectively.

For effective inhibition in vitro (19), lymphocytes were incubated with HC at a final concentration of 100-250 μg/ml, CYP at 1000-2000 μg/ml, silica at 100-150 μg/ml, and carrageenan at 100 μg/ml. Cyclosporin A (CSA), used frequently in immunosuppression of transplant recipients, was dissolved in ethanol and diluted more than 1000-fold in medium for final use at 1-10 μg/ml (20). Diethylstilbestrol (DES), used to control prostate and breast cancer, was dissolved in dimethylsulfoxide and diluted in medium to 1-10 μg/ml (20).

Poly I:C, a double-stranded RNA used for the induction of IFN, was inoculated IP at 100 μg per mouse or used at 100 μg/ml in vitro. With human lymphocytes, cells were incubated with IFN-β at 250 U/ml.

B. Measurement of Mouse NK Activity

Mouse spleen cells were incubated with ^{51}Cr-labeled RLM1 tumor cells for 4 hr at 37°C at effector/target ratios of 200:1 to 50:1. The supernatants from these cultures were then collected and counted for the radioactive label released from lysed tumor target cells. The background release was determined from the incubation of labeled tumor cells with unlabeled cells used in the place of lymphocytes (19).

C. Measurement of Human NK Activity

Human peripheral blood lymphocytes (PBLs) were separated from buffy coats obtained from the National Institutes of Health Blood Bank by centrifugation on a Ficol-Hypaque gradient. For further purification of NK cells that are characteristically large granular lymphocytes (LGLs), adherent cells were first depleted from PBLs by successive plastic adherence and nylon-wool passage before the nonadherent cells were placed on a discontinuous Percoll gradient (21). The LGLs that were obtained from 42.5-45% Percoll contained virtually all of the NK activity and comprised about 5-10% of the starting PBLs.

The NK cell-enriched LGL fraction was incubated with ^{51}Cr-labeled K562 tumor cells at 30:1-3:1 effector/target ratios. Four hours after incubation at 37°C, the supernatants were collected and counted for released Cr (11).

$$\text{Percent cytotoxicity} = \frac{\text{Experimental release - background release}}{\text{Total cpm incorporated}} \times 100$$

III. MOUSE STUDIES

A. Hydrocortisone

Earlier studies from our laboratory (19) indicated that mice, inoculated IP with HC the day prior to testing their spleens for NK activity, displayed lower levels of cytotoxicity than those of untreated mice (Table 1). The dose-dependent inhibition was highest at 100-250 μg/kg. This effect was short-lived with full NK function recovered 7 days after a single dose of HC. Long-term depression of NK activity, however, could be maintained by repeated doses of HC on alternate days (19). Similar inhibitory action of HC has also been reported by Hochman and Cudkowicz (22), and they have further shown that the induction of adherent suppressor cells by in vivo administration of HC was responsible for the observed low NK activity. This mechanism may not be the only one in effect since splenic NK activity can be directly inhibited in vitro by short incubation with

Table 1 Inhibition of Mouse NK Activity by Hydrocortisone

Treatment		NK activity[a] (%)		
Type	Dose	Day 1	Day 3	Day 7
In vivo[b]		36	28	20
	250 mg/kg	10	14	20
	100 mg/kg	11	19	22
	10 mg/kg	18	36	27
In vitro[c]		28		
	500 μg/ml	3		
	250 μg/ml	1		
	125 μg/ml	14		

[a]Effector/target ratio of 200:1.
[b]Mice were treated with hydrocortisone on day 0 and then tested for NK activity, 1, 3, and 7 days later.
[c]Mouse spleen cells were incubated with hydrocortisone for 1 hr at 37°C before they were tested for NK activity.

250 μg/ml of HC (Table 1). This becomes even more apparent when human LGL-NK cells, exhaustively depleted of adherent cells by plastic adherence and nylon-wool passage, are shown to be inhibited by 2-4 hr incubation with HC, as discussed below.

B. X-Irradiation

Using an x-ray apparatus with Cu and Al filters, we consistently obtained decreased splenic NK levels of more than 50% in mice exposed the previous day to whole body irradiation at 900 R (Table 2). This is in agreement with the data of Stutman et al. (23) of the relative radiosensitivity of mouse spleen NK activity. Kiessling et al. (24), on the other hand, have conflicting data, perhaps due to their use of a gamma ^{137}Cs-machine for irradiation. It was noted by Stutman and his colleagues (23), however, that NK activity in bone marrow appeared initially to be radioresistant and declines only after 5-7 days of irradiation. The radiosensitivity of NK cells may differ in various parts of the lymphoid system, but as yet there is no clear explanation for the differences seen from laboratory to laboratory. In vitro irradiation of mouse NK spleen cells had no effect on their function (Table 2).

C. Cyclophosphamide

Administration of 220 mg/kg of CYP to mice caused depressed splenic NK activity within 1 day (Table 3). This effect is similar to that reported by Mantovani et al. (25) who also showed that the effect of a single dose of CYP was overcome within 7 days. As in the case of HC, repeated doses of CYP tended to maintain low NK levels in mice (25).

D. Silica and Carrageenan

Mice receiving 15 mg/mouse IP of silica or 1 mg/mouse IV of carrageenan exhibited low splenic NK activity after 1 day of administration (Table 3). The initial interpretation had been that these agents eliminated macrophages which were required for the maintenance of NK function in vivo because these same agents had no effect on mouse NK cells in vitro (Table 3). It appears, however, that silica has a direct effect on human NK cells in vitro (11), and a closer examination of the mouse NK susceptibility to silica may be in order. Cudkowicz and Hochman, on the other hand, have shown that adherent suppressor cells induced by carrageenan may be contributing to the observed low NK activity in mice (26).

Table 2 Inhibition of Mouse NK Activity by X-Irradiation

Type	Dose	NK activity[a] (%)
In vivo[b]	–	36
	900 R	16
	300 R	24
In vitro[c]	–	33
	900 R	38
	300 R	38

[a]Effector/target ratio of 200:1
[b]Mice were irradiated on day 0 and then tested for NK activity 1 day later.
[c]Mouse spleen cells were irradiated 1 hr before testing for NK activity.

Table 3 Inhibition of Mouse NK Activity by Cyclophosphamide, Silica, and Carrageenan

Treatment		NK activity day 1[a]
Type	Dose	(%)
In vivo[b]	–	31
	Cyclophosphamide, 220 mg/kg	13
	Silica, 15 mg	15
	Silica, 6 mg	14
	Silica, 3 mg	28
	Carrageenan, 2 mg	8
	Carrageenan, 1 mg	13
In vitro[c]	–	22
	Silica, 400 μg/ml	22
	Silica, 40 μg/ml	21
	Carrageenan, 1000 μg/ml	22
	Carrageenan, 100 μg/ml	23

[a]Effector/target ratio of 200:1.
[b]Mice were treated with each drug and tested for NK activity the following day.
[c]Mouse spleen cells were incubated with silica or carrageenan for 3 hr at 37°C before they were tested for NK activity.

E. Resistance of Poly I:C-Augmented NK Activity to Drug Inhibition

It has been of interest to us to determine whether the boosting of NK activity by IFN or an IFN inducer was also sensitive to inhibition by chemotherapeutic agents. Because of the scarcity of mouse IFN, poly I:C was used in conjunction with the immunosuppressive agents. It was found that irradiation or drug treatment did not interfere with subsequent NK boosting by poly I:C. Administration of 100 μg/ per mouse of poly I:C in mice 4 hr after 900 R, HC or CYP treatment produced similar enhancement of NK activity as that in mice receiving poly I:C alone (Table 4). The activation of NK activity was associated with the presence of serum IFN. This led us to postulate that there exists a drug and radioresistant precursor NK cell population that could be activated by poly I:C.

Table 4 Drug and Radioresistance of Poly I:C Boosting of Mouse NK Activity

Treatment		NK activity	Serum IFN titer
-4 hr	0 hr	(%)	(U/ml)
–	–	2	0
–	Poly I:C	19	356
900 R	Poly I:C	19	400
Hydrocortisone	Poly I:C	19	486
Cyclophosphamide	Poly I:C	18	391
Silica	Poly I:C	6	50
Carrageenan	Poly I:C	2	124

[a]Mice were treated with irradiation or drugs 3 hr before poly I:C administration and then tested for NK activity the following day.
[b]Effector/target ratio of 200:1.

In contrast, silica- and carrageenan-treated mice could not be subsequently boosted by poly I:C, suggesting the need for macrophage in the boosting process. Indeed, in vitro analysis showed that macrophages responded to poly I:C by production of IFN which was necessary for activating NK cells (27).

From the mouse model we thus learned of a drug- and radioresistant NK precursor cell that could be activated by IFN while the spontaneous NK cell is sensitive to irradiation, HC, and CYP. Similar experiments in the rat have also suggested the coexistence of drug- and radioresistant NK precursor cells which responded to poly I:C boosting and drug-sensitive spontaneously active NK cells (28).

IV. HUMAN STUDIES

More recently we have begun to study the effects of drugs on human NK activity and to determine whether similar patterns of drug resistance and sensitivity exist for human pre-NK and active NK cells (20). More importantly, we set out to determine whether IFN could reverse the immunosuppressive effect of these chemotherapeutic agents and thus provide for some reconstitution of the defense mechanism in the immunocompromised host. In addition to CYP and HC, other clinically useful drugs such as CSA and DES were also investigated. We have also chosen to study the response to drugs and IFN of purified LGL-NK cells rather than unseparated PBLs to avoid the complicating effects of cells that might positively or negatively regulate NK activity, such as macrophages or T-suppressor cells.

A. Hydrocortisone

Within 2-4 hr of exposure to HC, human LGL showed a dose-dependent loss of NK activity (Table 5). At 250 μg/ml, HC inhibited more than half of the NK activity present in untreated LGL. Cell viability was not affected by any of the doses used, and yet NK function of these cells was lost to a large degree. These observations confirm earlier reports by Parrillo and Fauci (29) using dexamethasone on human PBL in vitro. In vivo inhibition of NK activity was also shown to be possible by oral administration of dexamethasone (29).

B. Cyclosporin A

Extremely low doses of CSA were capable of suppressing NK activity in LGL (Table 5), similar to the findings of Introna et al. (30). However, the inhibition seen by us takes place more rapidly than that reported by these investigators who could not detect significant inhibition until after 8 hr of drug treatment. Incubation of LGL with 5-10 μg/ml of CSA for 2-4 hr was sufficient for NK function to be blocked.

C. Silica

Unlike mouse NK cells, human NK cells were susceptible to inhibition by silica (Table 5). In vitro incubation of LGL-NK cells for 4 hr at 37°C with 100-150 μg/ml of silica caused a dose-dependent reduction of their ability to lyse K562 target cells. The susceptibility to silica therefore appears to be another characteristic that human NK cells share with monocytes in addition to the OKM-1 surface antigen.

Table 5 In Vitro Inhibition of Human NK Activity by Hydrocortisone, Cyclosporin A, and Silica

		NK activity[a] (%)	
Drug	Dose	2 hr	4 hr
–	–	23	25
Hydrocortisone	500 μg/ml	14	7
	250 μg/ml	15	12
	100 μg/ml	19	19
Cyclosporin A	10 μg/ml	2	0
	5 μg/ml	2	2
	1 μg/ml	12	13
Silica	150 μg/ml	ND[b]	10
	100 μg/ml	ND	18

[a]LGL-NK cells were incubated with the various drugs at 37°C for 2 hr or 4 hr before they were tested against K562 tumor cells at effector/target ratios of 10:1.
[b]Not done.

D. Cyclophosphamide

Cyclophosphamide, added at 1000-5000 μg/ml to LGLs, caused a dose-dependent inhibition of NK activity, again without affecting cell viability (Table 6). The effect is seen within 2-4 hr of incubation with the drug. To our knowledge, this is the first demonstration of the ability of CYP to inhibit human NK activity in vitro.

E. Diethystilbestrol

The hormonal agent, DES, was found to inhibit NK activity in vitro at low doses of 1-10 μg/ml (Table 6). The time of incubation necessary for inhibition to occur was short,

Table 6 In Vitro Inhibition of Human NK Activity by Cyclophosphamide and Diethylstilbestrol

		NK activity[a] (%)	
Drug	Dose	2 hr	4 hr
–	–		30
Cyclophosphamide	5000 μg/ml		0
	2500 μg/ml		11
	1000 μg/ml		24
Diethylstilbestrol	10 μg/ml	0	0
	5 μg/ml	4	2
	1 μg/ml	11	12

[a]LGL-NK cells were incubated with the various drugs at 37°C for 2 hr or 4 hr before they were tested against K562 tumor cells at effector/target ratios of 10:1

within 24 hr. Kalland and Haukaas had earlier reported that prostate cancer patients on a DES regimen exhibited depressed NK activity significantly below the pretreatment level (31). Our results indicate that this inhibition can also be achieved in vitro.

F. Modulation of NK Activity by IFN and Chemotherapeutic Agents

Earlier mouse experiments had predicted that there were temporal factors related to the inhibition of NK activity (19). As discussed before, there appears to be a drug-resistant NK precursor, but the spontaneously active NK cell is drug sensitive. To determine whether such differences in drug sensitivity occur in human LGLs, we treated LGLs with IFN before exposure to immunosuppressive agents or in the reverse order (i.e., immunosuppressive treatment before IFN incubation). The usual procedure was to treat LGLs with IFN for 1 hr and immunosuppressive agents for 4 hr. Some significant differences were observed. LGLs pretreated with HC, CYP, CSA, or silica and then incubated with IFN showed higher reconstitution of activity than those that were first exposed to IFN and subsequent drug treatment (Table 7). The LGLs activated by IFN thus appeared more drug sensitive than the precursor NK cell.

V. CONCLUSIONS

Studies in the mouse have shown that the precursor NK cell that is subject to activation by IFN is resistant to inhibition by irradiation, HC, and CYP, whereas the spontaneous NK cell is drug- and radiosensitive. Similarly, in humans, the precursor NK cell which is resistant to HC, CYP, and CSA inhibition appears to acquire drug sensitivity after IFN activation. The IFN-activated cells are, therefore, much like the spontaneously active NK cells in being drug-sensitive, indicating perhaps that the circulating spontaneous NK cells are themselves the result of in vivo activation by IFN, which can be induced by foreign antigens of various types (e.g., viruses, bacteria, allogeneic cells).

Table 7 Reconstitution of Human NK Activity by Interferon

Drug	NK activity (%) Without IFN[a]	Drug before IFN[b]	IFN before drug[c]
None	19	39	38
Hydrocortisone	3	18	7
Cyclophosphamide	11	31	20
Cyclosporin A	5	25	11
Silica	14	35	18
Diethystilbestrol	7	28	25

[a]LGL-NK cells were incubated with each drug alone for 4 hr before testing for NK activity at effector/target ratios of 10:1.
[b]LGL-NK cells were incubated with each drug for 4 hr and then re-incubated with IFN for 1 hr before testing for NK activity.
[c]LGL-NK cells were incubated with IFN for 1 hr and then re-incubated with each drug for 4 hr before testing for NK activity.

From a clinical point of view, the data presented here signify that it is possible to reconstitute a large portion of the NK activity that is lost during treatment with immunosuppressive agents. Clinical trials are in progress using IFN as an antitumor agent, and the recent trend has been to combine IFN with other chemotherapeutic agents. It should be borne in mind that the sequence of drug/IFN administration may make some difference in the efficacy of the treatment regimen. Because of the liability of active NK cells and IFN-activated NK cells to chemotherapeutic agents, it would seem more beneficial to expose patients to immunosuppressive agents before IFN therapy rather than in the reverse order. A washout period after IFN administration might also be instituted before a second cycle of the bimodal therapy. In addition to cancer patients, bone marrow and renal transplant recipients who are on a chemotherapy regimen may benefit from IFN therapy which could aid in reconstituting some host responses to infections.

REFERENCES

1. R. B. Herberman, *Natural Cell-Mediated Immunity Against Tumors*, Academic Press, New York, 1980.
2. O. Haller, M. Hansson, R. Kiessling, and H. Wigzell, *Nature*, *270*:609 (1977).
3. M. Kasal, J. C. Le Clerc, L. McVay-Boudreau, F. W. Shen, and H. Cantor, *J. Exp. Med.*, *149*:1260 (1979).
4. N. Hanna and I. J. Fidler, *Cancer Res.*, *41*:438 (1981).
5. K. Karre, G. O. Klein, R. Kiessling, G. Klein, and J. C. Roder, *Nature*, *284*:624 (1980).
6. J. E. Talmadge, K. M. Meyers, D. J. Prieur, and J. R. Starkey, *Nature*, *284*:622 (1980).
7. J. F. Loutit, K. M. S. Townsend, and J. F. Knowles, *Nature*, *285*:66 (1980).
8. C. Riccardi, P. Puccetti, A. Santoni, and R. B. Herberman, *J. Natl. Cancer Inst.*, *63*:1041 (1979).
9. J. C. Roder, T. Haliotis, M. Klein, S. Korec, J. R. Jett, J. Ortaldo, R. B. Herberman, P. Katz, and A. S. Fauci, *Nature*, *284*:553 (1980).
10. J. L. Sullivan, K. S. Byron, F. E. Brewster, and D. T. Purtilo, *Science*, *210*:543 (1980).
11. J. Y. Djeu, N. Stocks, K. Zoon, G. J. Stanton, T. Timonen, and R. B. Herberman, *J. Exp. Med.*, in press.
12. F. A. Ennis, A. S. Baere, D. Riley, G. C. Schild, A. Maeger, Y. H. Qi, G. Schwarz, and A. H. Rook, *The Lancet*, *ii*:891 (1981).
13. G. V. Quinnan and J. Manischewitz, *J. Exp. Med.*, *150*:1549 (1979).
14. C. Lopez, in *Genetic Control of Natural Resistance to Infection and Malignancy* (E. Skamene, P. A. L. Kongshaw, and M. Landy, eds.), Academic Press, New York, 1980, p. 253.
15. N. Minato, L. Reid, H. Cantor, P. Lengyel, and B. R. Bloom, *J. Exp. Med.*, *152*:124 (1980).
16. R. B. Herberman, M. E. Nunn, H. T. Holden, S. Staal, and J. Y. Djeu, *Int. J. Cancer*, *19*:555 (1977).
17. G. J. Bancroft, G. R. Shellam, and J. E. Chalmer, *J. Immunol.*, *126*:988 (1981).
18. G. V. Quinnan, N. Kirmani, A. H. Rook, J. F. Manischewitz, L. Jackson, G. Moreschi, G. W. Santos, R. Saral, and W. H. Burns, *N. Engl. J. Immunol.*, *307*:7 (1982).
19. J. Y. Djeu, J. A. Heinbaugh, W. D. Vieira, H. T. Holden, and R. B. Herberman, *Immunopharmacology*, *1*:231 (1979).
20. K. M. Ramsey, N. Stocks, and J. Y. Djeu, submitted for publication.
21. T. Timonen, J. R. Ortaldo, and R. B. Herberman, *J. Exp. Med.*, *153*:569 (1981).

22. P. S. Hochman and G. Cudkowicz, *J. Immunol.*, *123*:968 (1979).
23. O. Stutman, E. F. Figarella, D. J. Paige, and E. C. Lattime, in *Natural Cell-Mediated Immunity Against Tumors* (R. B. Herberman, ed.), Academic Press, New York, 1980, p. 187.
24. R. Kiessling, P. S. Hochman, O. Haller, G. M. Shearer, H. Wigzell, and G. Cudkowicz, *Eur. J. Immunol.*, *7*:591 (1977).
25. A. Mantovani, W. Luini, G. Peri, A. Vecchi, and F. Spreafico, *J. Natl. Cancer Inst.*, *61*:1255 (1978).
26. G. Cudkowicz and P. S. Hochman, *Cell. Immunol.*, *53*:395 (1980).
27. J. Y. Djeu, J. A. Heinbaugh, H. T. Holden, and R. B. Herberman, *J. Immunol.*, *122*:182 (1979).
28. J. R. Oehler and R. B. Herberman, *Int. J. Cancer*, *21*:221 (1978).
29. J. E. Parrillo and A. S. Fauci, *Scand. J. Immunol.*, *8*:99 (1978).
30. M. Introna, P. Allavena, F. Spreafico, and A. Mantovani, *Transplantation*, *31*:113 (1981).
31. J. Kalland and S. Haukaas, *Invest. Urol.*, *18*:437 (1981).

24

Modulation of the Immune Response by Muramyl Dipeptide

William E. Fogler* and Isaiah J. Fidler* Cancer Metastasis and Treatment Laboratory, National Cancer Institute–Frederick Cancer Research Facility, Frederick, Maryland

I. INTRODUCTION

Forty years have elapsed since Freund and McDermott demonstrated the immunoadjuvant properties of *Mycobacteria* with water-in-oil emulsion (1). Since then many investigations have been carried out to determine the minimal structure inherent in the *Mycobacterium* that is responsible for these properties. Early studies clearly demonstrated that cell wall preparations (2) or a peptidoglycolipid fraction named Wax D (3,4) could replace whole microorganisms in Freund complete adjuvant (FCA). Soon, however, it became apparent that the lipid moiety was not essential and that a water-soluble preparation of glycopeptides could be substituted for mycobacteria to induce the stimulation of delayed hypersensitivity (5-7). Two groups of investigators have independently demonstrated that the minimum active unit which can replace *Mycobacteria* in FCA is N-acetylmuramyl-L-alanyl-D-isoglutamine, hereafter referred to as muramyl dipeptide (MDP) (8,9; Fig. 1).

Since MDP was first described in 1974, its immunopotentiating effects have been extensively studied, and its adjuvant capabilities, toxic reactions, and ability to stimulate host defense mechanisms against infections and neoplastic growth have been reported. The purpose of this brief review is to describe some of these studies and to introduce the reader to the biological effects associated with the administration of MDP.

*Current affiliation: University of Texas System Cancer Center, M.D. Anderson Hospital and Tumor Institute, Houston, Texas.

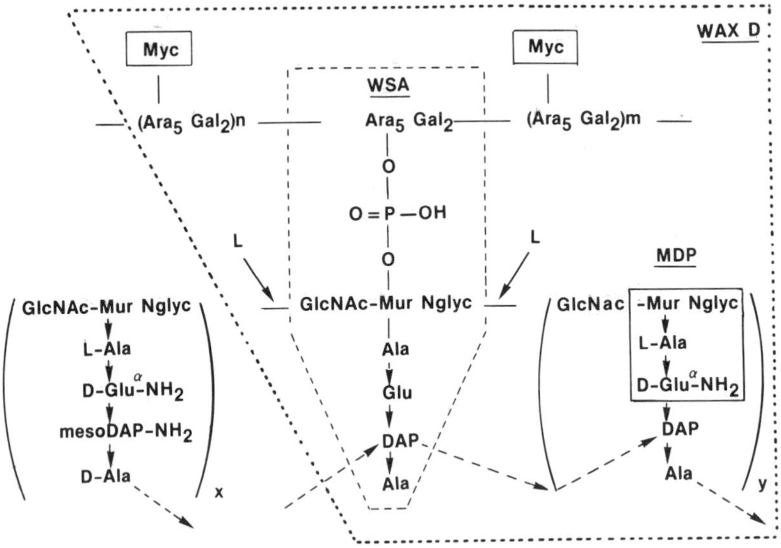

Figure 1 Simplified scheme of the *Mycobacterial* cell wall and its components that exhibit adjuvant activity, Wax D, water-soluble adjuvant (WSA), and MDP. L, lysozyme; MYC, mycolic acid; N + M, ~8-10; X + Y, ~8-10.

II. PROMOTION OF IMMUNE RESPONSIVENESS BY MURAMYL DIPEPTIDE

Ellouz and co-workers demonstrated that MDP admixed with a protein antigen and Freund incomplete adjuvant (FIA) can enhance immune responsiveness (8). In their study, a water-in-oil emulsion of either ovalbumin-MDP-FIA or ovalbumin-FCA was injected intradermally into both hind footpads of Hartley guinea pigs. A significant increase in the level of precipitating antibodies and of induced delayed hypersensitivity to ovalbumin was observed in the MDP-treated group; the antibody level was commensurate with that achieved with FCA (8). In another study, the antibody response to ovalbumin, which consisted of IgG_2 immunoglobulins (both the primary and secondary response), was found to be faster and higher in animals treated with MDP-FIA than in animals treated with FCA (10). MDP was also found to act as an adjuvant in the induction of delayed hypersensitivity to the haptenic group of azobenzene-arsonate N-acetyl-L-tyrosine (11); challenge with MDP alone evoke no response. Moreover, FCA was found to sensitize guinea pigs to tuberculin and to native mycobacterial water-soluble adjuvant but not to MDP (11). Rat (12) and mouse (13) models have also been used to study the immune adjuvant properties of synthetic MDP. These studies showed that water-soluble MDP can augment the humoral immune response, whereas mycobacterial adjuvant preparations function only when administered as water-in-oil emulsions. Finally, MDP need not be administered with the antigen by the same route to exact its adjuvant effect, and it is active even when given orally (13).

Experimental studies on the mechanism of action by which MDP promotes immune responsiveness have yielded contradictory results. MDP increased the primary response of CBA mice to a T-cell-dependent antigen, sheep red blood cells (14). Whether MDP affected the function of T lymphocytes by a direct manner was not clear. In mice given whole body irradiation and then reconstituted with appropriate bone marrow cells, cooperation between T and B lymphocytes was required for the expression of adjuvant activity (14). Treatment of sensitized donor spleen cells with antithymocyte serum abrogated the response, suggesting that the T lymphocyte is the immediate target cell of MDP (14). However, spleen cells from T-cell-deficient nude mice incubated with MDP responded to sheep red blood cells, as measured by an increase in plaque-forming cells (15). Moreover, MDP-induced activation of polyclonal antibodies to the T-cell-independent antigen trinitrophenyl polyacrylamide (15). In limiting dilution analyses with excess helper T cells or MDP, the frequency with which B-cell precursors responded to sheep red blood cells was similar (16). Collectively, these studies (15,16) suggest that MDP interacts directly with B cells, mimicking a helper T-cell signal. Other work using cell separation techniques and the plaque-forming cell response to sheep red blood cells showed that MDP directly interacts with T and/or B lymphocytes and that subsequent interaction between macrophages and lymphocytes is involved in the activation of helper T cells and/or B cells by adjuvants (17).

Although these reports are in apparent contradiction, they do not rule out the possibility that the adjuvant activity of MDP could be exerted by multiple mechanisms or that a single mechanism could be mediated by cells of the mononuclear phagocyte system. The studies of MDP administered in vivo have tested the production of humoral antibody (8-13). However, MDP administered parenterally can also stimulate macrophage function, as measured by colloidal carbon clearance (18-21), and investigators have studied whether the macrophage is primarily an accessory cell in the adjuvant response (14-17) or whether it represents the immediate target cell of MDP (22). Spleen cells incubated with MDP released a soluble factor capable of increasing the ability of fresh spleen cells to form plaques when cultured with sheep red blood cells (22). Although pretreatment of spleen cells with antitheta antigen serum entirely suppressed their reaction to sheep red blood cells despite the presence of MDP, supernatants from these cultures were as active as supernatants from cultures of MDP-stimulated normal spleen cells (22). Pretreatment of spleen cells with specific antimacrophage serum entirely suppressed both the response to sheep red blood cells and the supernatant activity (22). These results suggested that the target cell for MDP action is the macrophage, which, upon stimulation, releases factors (Interleukin 1?) that act on helper T cells regulating B-cell production of antibodies (22). Matter (23) compared the results obtained in in vitro and in vivo studies of the effects of MDP in cell-mediated immunity and concurred with this conclusion.

Indeed, there is now extensive experimental data demonstrating that MDP influences various macrophage activities in vitro (22-44) as summarized in Table 1. Many of the phenotypic alterations accompanying macrophage activation require a prolonged incubation of this glycopeptide with the cell (24-72 hr). In our laboratory we have concentrated on investigating the activation of tumoricidal properties in macrophages by MDP (39-44). Under optimal in vitro conditions, significant tumor cytotoxicity required an 8 hr macrophage-glycopeptide interaction (40) as measured by a radioactive release assay (45). Maximal activation was achieved only after a continuous 72-hr incubation with MDP (40). These data suggest that for MDP to be equally effective in modulating macrophage function in vivo, a similar period of interaction between MDP and the macrophages would be required. However, in vivo, more than 90% of parenterally administered MDP is cleared from the body within 2 hr and excreted, unmodified, in the urine (46). Hence, the administration of water-soluble MDP may not be a feasible way to activate macrophages in situ.

Table 1 In Vitro Effects of MDP on Biological Activities Associated with Macrophage Activation

	Macrophage source	MDP concentration	Reference
Enhancement of pseudopod formation	Guinea pig PEM[a]	1-10 μg/ml	24
	Murine PEM	1 μg/ml	25
Stimulation of [14-C] glucosamine incorporation	Guinea pig PEM	1-10 μg/ml	26
Increase in intracelluar cAMP and cGMP	Guinea pig PEM	1-10 μg/ml	24,27
Increase in O_2-generating capacity	Murine PEM	1 μg/ml	25
Increase in secretory products			
Collagenase	Guine pig PEM	1-10 μg/ml	24
Prostaglandin E_2	Guinea pig PEM	1-10 μg/ml	24
Fibroblast mitogenic factor	Guinea pig PEM	1-10 μg/ml	24
Lymphocyte-activating factor	Murine PEM	200 μg/ml	23,28
Enhancement of PFC	Murine splenocytes	5 μg/ml	22
Thymocyte mitogenic factor	Murine PEM	10 μg/ml	29
Increase in phagocytic capability	Guinea pig PEM	1.2-12 μg/ml	27,30
Inhibition of lymphokine-induced proliferation	Guinea pig PEM	0.1 μg/ml	27,30
Inhibition of migration	Guinea pig PEM	0.1-1 μg/ml	31-34
	Rat PEM	0.1-1 μg/ml	33
Increase in microbicidal properties			
Listeria monocytogenes	Guinea pig PEM	1.2-12 μg/ml	27,30
Candida parapsilosis	Murine PEM	100 μg/ml	35
Increase in tumor cytotoxic properties			
Cytostatic activity	Murine PEM	1.2 μg/ml	36
	Murine PEM	10 μg/ml	29
Cytolytic activity	Tumor associated murine macrophages	10 μg/ml	37
	Guinea pig KC[b]	Not reported	38
	Rat AM[c]	10-50 μg/ml	39-41
		0.25 μg encapsulated in liposomes	39-41
	Murine AM	50 μg/ml	42-44
		0.25 μg encapsulated in liposomes	42-44

[a]Peritoneal exudate macrophages.
[b]Kupffer cells.
[c]Alveolar macrophages.

III. USE OF LIPOSOMES AS CARRIERS FOR MURAMYL DIPEPTIDE

Several methods have been proposed to potentiate the activity of MDP in vivo (23,47,48). Recent attention has focused on the use of liposomes, multilamellar phospholipid vesicles separated by aqueous compartments, as a carrier for the transport of active materials into target cells in vitro and in vivo (42-52). Recent studies from our laboratory have shown that MDP encapsulated within liposomes can render macrophages tumoricidal much more efficiently than free, unencapsulated MDP (39-44). Liposome-encapsulated MDP, in contrast to free MDP, required less time (2 hr) to activate macrophages, and maximum cytolytic capacity was achieved after an 8-hr incubation (40,41). Furthermore, the total amount of liposome-encapsulated MDP delivered to macrophages was at least 4000 times lower than the total amount of free MDP that is needed to render macrophages tumoricidal (39-41). Moreover, after the initial activation period, the liposome-encapsulated MDP, in comparison with free MDP, prolonged the duration of tumoricidal properties in the macrophages (41).

These findings raised the possibility that MDP encapsulated within liposomes could be similarly efficient in activating macrophages in vivo. An attractive feature of liposomes as a carrier of MDP to macrophages in situ is that most of the liposomes injected intravenously are taken up by cells of the reticuloendothelial system. This passive targeting of liposomes to macrophages offers a means of enhancing uptake of therapeutic agents that stimulate macrophage activity. Moreover, liposomes prepared from natural phospholipids are nonimmunogenic, and thus they offer a means to avoid the elicitation of allergic reactions commonly associated with the systemic administration of immune adjuvants (53).

We have recently studied the organ distribution and retention of free and liposome-encapsulated MDP (^{3}H-labeled) following intravenous administration in the mouse. In agreement with the studies of Parent and co-workers (46), we found that by 2 hr after its administration, more than 90% of free MDP is cleared from the body and excreted in the urine; however, the excretion rate of liposome-encapsulated MDP is 3-6% per hr. Moreover, the percentage of the total dose of liposome-encapsulated MDP that localizes in the liver, spleen, and lung is increased 10- to 30-fold over that of free MDP. In this regard, the injection of MDP in saline did not render alveolar macrophages of mice tumoricidal, whereas injection of MDP encapsulated in liposomes did activate the macrophages to become tumoricidal against B16-BL6 melanoma cells (41-44). The systemic activation of macrophages by liposome-encapsulated MDP can be maintained by repeated injections (43) and can be accomplished in athymic nude mice and in adult thymectomized or x-irradiated mice (44). These results argue for the macrophage as a principal target cell for MDP and suggest the possibility that when appropriately administered, MDP may enhance the natural resistance of the host to infection and neoplasia.

IV. STIMULATION OF HOST DEFENSE AGAINST INFECTIOUS DISEASES BY MURAMYL DIPEPTIDE

Infectious diseases continue to be a major cause of death throughout the world, despite the fact that more is known about their cause and treatment than any other form of disease. The pathogenicity of a microbe depends on the ability to invade and destroy host cells and tissue. Invasiveness, in turn, is a complex of many variables which include a portal of entry, establishment of a microenvironment suitable for survival and replication, and capability of evading host defense mechanisms, both natural and acquired. The natural resistance of the host to infection can be stimulated by the prophylactic administration of various bacterial products. The ubiquitous nature of the MDP moiety in bacterial cell walls coupled with its immune-stimulating properties prompted studies of the potential of MDP to increase host resistance to both extracellular and intracellular pathogens (54-64; Table 2).

The effectiveness of MDP in the stimulation of host resistance to infection is not clearly established in the literature. MDP (and various analogs) administered in saline to adult mice enhanced their nonspecific immunity toward infection by *Klebsiella pneumoniae* (54). MDP was active when given by various routes and was also effective when administered after challenge with the organism (54). Of the 21 analogs of MDP tested, 11 were active adjuvants; however, only 4 afforded protection against *Klebsiella* (54). In a subsequent report, the same investigators found that MDP also definitively protected murine neonates against bacterial challenge with *K. pneumoniae*, whereas other immune stimulants (lipopolysaccharide) had no effect (55). However, other investigators reported that the intraperitoneal injection of MDP at a dosage identical to that in the previous studies resulted in only marginal protection against *K. pneumoniae* (56). However, those investigators found that MDP markedly increased resistance to infection by *Escherichia coli* and that it was active when administered by various routes (56). The optimal interval between MDP treatment and infection in that study was 24 hr when the treatment was carried out before infection (56). In addition, prophylactic treatment with MDP resulted in a moderate level of protection toward *Pseudomonas aeruginosa* (56). In contrast, another study (57) demonstrated no significant stimulation of host defense against

Table 2 Stimulation of Murine Resistance to Bacterial and Fungal Infections by the Administration of MDP

Infectious agent	MDP dose[a]	Route of administration	Protective effect[b]	Reference
Klebsiella pneumoniae	0.1 mg	IV, SC, IM, oral	++	54, 55
	0.1 mg	IP	+	56
Trypanosoma cruzi	0.1 mg	IP	+++	59
Pseudomomas aeruginosa	0.1 mg	IP	++	56
	80 mg/kg	IP	-	57
Streptococcus pneumoniae	0.5 mg	SC	+++	60
Listeria monocytogenes	0.5 mg	IP, SC, IV	-	60
	80 mg/kg	IP	-	57
Escherichia coli	0.1 mg	IP, SC, IV	+++	56
Toxoplasma gondii	80 mg/kg	IP	+	71
Schistosoma mansoni	0.2 mg	IV	-	64
Candida albicans	0.05 mg	SC	++	58
	80 mg/kg	IP	++	57
Mycobacterium leprae	80 mg/kg	SC	-	63

[a]Unless otherwise noted, values represent total dose per mouse.
[b](-), Not significantly different from control; (+) $\leq$ 33% increase in survival; (++), 34-66% increase in survival; (+++), > 67% increase in survival (all values taken at $p < 0.1$).

P. aeruginosa, even when MDP was administered for 4 consecutive days prior to infection; however, this report confirmed the initial observation by Cummings and co-workers (58) that treatment of mice with MDP significantly prolonged their survival to a lethal challenge with *Candida albicans*. MDP has been shown to enhance the resistance of mice to other pathogens, including *Trypanosoma cruzi* (59), *Streptococcus pneumoniae* (60), *Toxoplasma gondii* (61), and *Salmonella typhimurium* (62). Yet reports also demonstrate that MDP fails to protect mice to a challenge with *Mycobacterium leprae* (63) or the multicellular organism, *Schistosoma mansoni* (64). In several experiments conditions in which MDP gave either no or minimal protection against pathogens, structural analogs of this glycopeptide did enhance host resistance to infection (65,66).

Possible reasons for these disparate findings are differences in the dosage, treatment schedule, bacterial strain, and challenge level of pathogen, and in the genetic and environmental influences on the host. The mechanism(s) by which resistance is conferred must also be considered a factor in the effectiveness of MDP, as evidence by attempts to protect mice against infection with *Listeria monocytogenes* (57,60). Resistance to *Listeria* is effected solely by the enhanced microbicidal capacity of activated macrophages (67,68), but under optimal conditions, macrophages must interact with MDP for 24 hr in order to acquire microbicidal properties against *L. monocytogenes* (27,30). Given the rapidity with which MDP is cleared from the body (46, Sect. II), the inability of MDP to offer significant protection against *Listeria* infection is not surprising (57,60).

In addition to using MDP to augment natural host defense mechanisms, investigators have taken advantage of the adjuvant properties of MDP and its analogs to develop new vaccines aimed at the prevention and control of infectious diseases. Owl monkeys have been successfully immunized against the human malarial parasite, *Plasmodium falciparum*, following intramuscular vaccination with merozites admixed with a lipophilic derivative of MDP (69). Mice have exhibited significant protection against experimental *P. aeruginosa* infection following active immunization with exotoxin A toxoid and MDP (70). Moreover, results of a recent study demonstrated that the covalent attachment of MDP to a synthetic viral antigen converts the synthetic antigen into a conjugate that is capable of triggering an antiviral immune response when it is injected in aqueous form into rabbits (71). Only continued experimentation can reveal the full potential of MDP and its analogs for the stimulation of host natural defense to pathogens.

V. MANIPULATION OF THE HOST DEFENSE SYSTEM BY MURAMYL DIPEPTIDE FOR TREATMENT OF CANCER METASTASIS

Clearly, the most serious aspect of cancer therapy concerns the treatment of metastases. There are several reasons for the lethality of disseminated solid malignancies, the foremost being the heterogeneous nature of malignant neoplasms and the rapid emergence of metastases that are resistant to conventional forms of therapy (72-74). Although tumor cell populations are heterogeneous with regard to many characteristics, they appear to be susceptible to destruction by activated (tumoricidal) macrophages. The intravenous injection of activated mononuclear phagocytes into mice bearing metastases has been shown to inhibit tumor growth both in the primary site (75) and in metastases (76-78). Intravenous administration of activated macrophages thus might be useful in augmenting host resistance to disseminated neoplastic disease; however, for clinical use, this strategy presents the serious problem of requiring the transfusion of a large number of histocompatible or autologous macrophages. The development of methods to activate autologous macrophages in situ would circumvent the problem.

Mononuclear phagocytes can be activated to the tumoricidal state by various natural and synthetic materials, which include MDP (29,36-44) but, again, therapeutic use of water-soluble MDP is hindered by the rapid clearance of this glycopeptide from the body (46). As noted in Sec. III, we have recently shown that the phagocytic uptake by macrophages of liposome-encapsulated MDP results in highly efficient activation of rodent macrophages in vitro and in vivo (39-44). These findings raised the possibility that the in vivo activation of mononuclear phagocytes with liposome-encapsulated MDP might provide a therapeutic modality for the treatment of cancer metastases.

The results of our studies indicate that the multiple intravenous injections of liposome-encapsulated MDP, but not free MDP or control liposome preparations, eradicated spontaneous visceral metastases in C57BL/6 mice from which a syngeneic melanoma had been surgically removed (42). Each mouse was given an intrafootpad injection of viable B16-BL6 melanoma cells. When the primary tumor reached a size of 0.8-1 cm in diameter (4 weeks of growth), the tumor-bearing leg, including the draining popliteal lymph node, was amputated. Treatment of mice began 3 days after leg amputation and consisted of an intravenous injection of 2.5 μmol liposomes (phosphatidylcholine and phosphatidylserine admixed at a 7:3 mol ratio) containing 10 μg of water-soluble MDP. At the dose used here, these liposomes have been shown to be nontoxic when administered intravenously (70), and a significant proportion is retained in the lung (80). Mice were treated twice weekly for 4 weeks (total of eight injections). The B16-BL6 tumor routinely metastasizes to the lungs and lymph nodes in about 90% of untreated mice, and at the start of therapy, the metastatic tumor burden in the lungs and lymph nodes may have exceeded a total body burden of 10^7 cells. Nonetheless, 65% of mice treated with liposome-encapsulated MDP survived at least 200 days. The median life span of mice implanted with 10 viable B16 cells is 40-50 days (81); therefore, in these successfully treated mice, the tumor burden was probably reduced to fewer than 10 viable cells. Thus, the intravenous injection of liposome-encapsulated MDP brought about the complete regression of established pulmonary and lymph node metastases.

The mechanism(s) responsible for the regression of established metastases after the systemic administration of liposomes containing MDP probably involved the activation of macrophages to become tumoricidal. Several lines of evidence tend to support this conclusion. First, lung macrophages are not activated by macrophage-activating agents encapsulated within liposomes that are not retained in the lung (82). Second, the pretreatment of tumor-bearing animals with agents that are toxic for macrophages (silica, carrageenan, hyperchlorinated drinking water) before systemic therapy with liposome-encapsulated MDP abrogates the response to liposome therapy, and such animals rapidly die of metastatic disease (82). Third, the possible involvement of T lymphocytes as effector cells is excluded by the finding that systemic activation of macrophages by liposome-encapsulated MDP can be accomplished in athymic nude mice and in adult thymectomized or x-irradiated mice (44). Finally, direct evidence that macrophages activated by liposome-encapsulated MDP are effective in augmenting host resistance to metastases comes from adoptive transfer experiments. Intravenous injections of macrophages activated in vitro by incubation with liposome-encapsulated MDP produces a reduction in metastatic burden comparable with that achieved by systemic administration of liposome-encapsulated activators (82).

Antitumor activity of MDP has also been observed in other laboratories. Intralesional injection of an emulsion of MDP and trehalose-dimycolate in the present of 2% squalene into strain 2 guinea pigs bearing the line 10 hepatocarcinoma was shown to result in complete regression of the primary tumor and lymph node metastases and resulted in acquired immunity of the animals to a second challenge with the same tumor (83,84).

VI. UNDESIRABLE SIDE EFFECTS ASSOCIATED WITH MDP ADMINISTRATION

Any therapeutic application of an immunostimulant such as MDP must be weighed against potential deleterious effects on the host (85). The clinical utilization of FCA has been precluded both by the need for a nonmetabolizable mineral oil and by the toxic effects of the *Mycobacteria*. In 1947 Freund wrote, "it would be of great interest to identify the fraction or fractions which exert the adjuvant effect of *Mycobacteria* and to know whether the effect could be produced without sensitization to tuberculin" (cited in 48). The demonstration of MDP as the minimum unit that can replace *Mycobacteria* in FCA was followed shortly by the demonstration that MDP did not sensitize to tuberculin (11). This prompted further studies of whether the substitution of MDP for *Mycobacteria* in FCA could alleviate the problem of toxic reactions.

The histological finding associated with the injection of FCA containing *Mycobacterium* is the formation of epithelioid granulomas (86,87). Chronic granulomas are also formed following injection of the peptidoglycolipid component, Wax D, into guinea pigs (88); furthermore, the injection of MDP as a water-in-oil emulsion into rats or guinea pigs resulted in granulomas which often accompany abscesses at the site of injection and at the draining lymph nodes (89,90). MDP dissolved in saline and injected into animals evoked no granulomatous reaction (89-91). The inoculation of MDP (water-in-oil) into rats evoked massive granuloma formation in neonatally thymectomized animals treated with rat thymocyte antiserum to the same extent as in untreated controls (91). Thus, MDP seems to be essential for granuloma formation, but inoculation with a nonmetabolizable oil is also required for it to express granulomagenic activity. These studies suggest that allergic reaction plays no important role in the development of the MDP-induced granuloma (89-91), in marked contrast to the allergic granuloma induced by *Mycobacterium* (87).

The single intradermal injection into rats of FCA containing *Mycobacterium* (92) or peptidoglycolipid (93) results in the disease process termed adjuvant-induced arthritis, indicating that an adjuvant is considered necessary to produce the syndrome. The demonstration of MDP as the minimum moiety with adjuvant activity prompted investigations into its possible arthritogenic effects. In studies in which MDP was administered as a water-in-oil emulsion to Lewis rats (94), there was no indication that it was able to induce arthritis. Subsequently, MDP was found to produce an arthritic reaction when (a) injected with a copolymer of polyriboinosinic acid and polyribocytidylic acid as a water-in-oil emulsion (95); (b) injected as a water-in-oil emulsion prepared from Bayol F and Arlacel A (FIA), but not with emulsions prepared from Arlacel A plus Drackeol, liquid paraffin, or heavy mineral oil (96-98); or (c) administered repeatedly dissolved in saline (99). The polyarthritis induced following the administration of MDP in saline differed substantially from the disease process which occurred following the inoculation of MDP as a water-in-oil emulsion: clinical symptoms dissappeared 5 days after cessation of treatment, and histological lesions were reversed 23 days later. Also, the disease process occurred only in the Lewis strain of rats and not in the AVA strain.

When administered with an antigen, MDP has also been implicated in the induction of certain autoimmune diseases. Allergic encephalomyelitis occurred in guinea pigs following the injection of an encephalitogen peptide and MDP as a water-in-oil emulsion

(100,101); however, this too occurred only in the presence of Bayol F and Arlacel A. An orchiepididymitis was induced in guinea pigs by injection of a water-in-oil emulsion containing MDP and a sperm autoantigen (102). Specific antibodies and delayed hypersensitivity were produced aganst the sperm antigen but did not occur in the absence of the emulsion.

Finally, MDP has been shown to have a pyrogenic effect when administered as a large dose in saline and to elicit the production of endogenous pyrogen (103-106). The fever response in rabbits was completely abolished by indomethacin treatment, although endogeneous pyrogen production was not (107). One derivatized MDP that is devoid of pyrogenicity retians the immunostimulant activities of the parental molecule (108).

Many of the toxic reactions found with MDP appear to result from its administration in the form of a water-in-oil emulsion. Whether this is caused by the prolonged retention of MDP in the body when administred in an emulsion or by the emulsion itself is not known. However, toxicity studies in which liposome-encapsulated MDP was injected intravenously into beagles failed to reveal any adverse reactions in recipient animals, even after repeated injections (Ian Hart, personal communication). This result and the potential of synthetic derivatives devoid of pyrogenicity (108) offer promising approaches to circumvent deleterious reactions following treatment with MDP.

VII. FUTURE PROSPECTIVE

In the 8 years since the description of MDP as the minimum adjuvant unit in FCA, a large body of data has accumulated on its adjuvant capabilities, toxicological reactions, and potential for stimulating host defense mechanisms against infectious disease and neoplastic growth. Many laboratories are now devising novel methods for potentiating the immune adjuvant and/or immune stimulatory effects of MDP (23,47,48).

Our studies have shown clearly that MDP encapsulated within liposomes renders macrophages tumoricidal much more effectively than does unencapsulated MDP (39-44). Moreover, once macrophages have phagocytosed liposomes containing MDP, they remained cytotoxic for 2-3 days (41-43). Investigators are working to find ways to sustain this cytotoxicity beyond 3 days. Recent studies have suggested that lipophilic derivatives of MDP, in which acyl chains are attached to the molecule, enhance the effectiveness of MDP for priming peritoneal macrophages to release superoxide anion. Because low molecular weight solutes (109) such as hydrophilic MDP can leak out of liposomes, we examined the possibility of whether a lipophilic derivative of MDP, N-acetylmuramyl-L-alanyl-D-isoglutamyl-L-alanyl-2(1′,2′-dipalmitoyl-snglycero-3′phosphoryl)-ethylamide (MTP-PE) inserted in the phospholipid bilayers of liposomes could be retained more efficiently within macrophages, thereby promoting sustained periods of tumoricidal activity (110).

In our studies, the superiority of liposomes containing the lipophilic MTP-PE over liposomes containing water-soluble MDP for in vitro and/or in vivo activation of macrophages was demonstrated in several experiments (110). First, the intravenous injection of liposomes containing a dose of MTP-PE equal to MDP led to higher levels of alveolar macrophage-mediated cytotoxicity (110). Second, alveolar macrophages harvested from mice given intravenous injections of liposomes containing MTP-PE maintained their tumoricidal activity for a longer period (5 days) than macrophages harvested from mice inoculated with liposome-encapsulated MDP (3 days; 110). Similar results were obtained from experiments on macrophage activation in vitro (110).

It has been suggested that once macrophages phagocytose liposomes containing MDP, the liposomes function as a slow-release depot from which encapsulated material is released over a sustained period of time (39,41,42). The extent of release and the possible equilibration of MDP with the extracellular medium are determined by the integrity of liposome membranes. However, MTP, which is insoluble in water, would remain active for longer periods, until it is degraded. Since liposomes can be seen inside macrophages for several days after phagocytosis (111,112), the degradation of MTP-PE incorporated into the liposomal phospholipid bilayer is apparently relatively slow and inefficient.

The ability to activate alveolar macrophages in situ with liposomes containing MTP-PE is attractive for several reasons. First, the systemic injection of this agent leads to a consistent and reproducible activation of macrophages. Second, because MTP-PE is firmly associated with the phospholipid bilayer of liposomes, it is distributed to macrophages that phagocytose the liposomes. Once phagocytosed, liposomes containing MTP-PE maintain tumoricidal activity in macrophages for longer periods of time than do liposomes containing water-soluble MDP. In addition, on a molar basis, MTP-PE (mol wt, 1166) is approximately 2.5 times more efficient than MDP (mol wt, 492) in eliciting comparable levels of macrophage tumoricidal activity. The significance of these findings in the therapy of spontaneous metastases in murine tumor systems is now under investigation.

ACKNOWLEDGMENT

This research was sponsored by the National Cancer Institute, DHHS, under contract no. NO1-CO-2309 with Litton Bionetics, Inc. The contents of this publication do not necessarily reflect the views or policies of the Department of Health and Human Services, nor does mention of trade names, commercial products, or organizations imply endorsement by the U.S. Government.

REFERENCES

1. J. Freund and K. McDermitt, *Proc. Soc. Exp. Biol.*, *49*:584 (1942).
2. S. Raffel, L. E. Arnaud, D. C. Dukes, and J. S. Huang, *J. Exp. Med.*, *90*:53 (1949).
3. R. G. White, L. Bernstock, R. G. Johns, and E. Lederer, *Immunology*, *1*:54 (1958).
4. R. G. White, P. Jolles, D. Samour, and E. Lederer, *Immunology*, *7*:158 (1964).
5. A. Adam, R. Ciorbaru, J. F. Petit, and E. Lederer, *Proc. Natl. Acad. Sci. USA*, *39*: 851 (1972).
6. D. Migliore-Samour and P. Jolles, *FEBS Lett.*, *25*:301 (1972).
7. I. J. Hiu, *Nature (New Biol.)*, *238*:241 (1972).
8. F. Ellouz, A. Adam, R. Ciorbaru, and E. Lederer, *Biochem. Biophys. Res. Commun.*, *59*:1317 (1974).
9. S. Kotani, Y. Watanabe, T. Shimono, T. Narita, K. Kato, D. E. S. Stewart-Tull, K. Kinoshita, S. Yokogogawa, S. Katawa, T. Shiba, S. Kusumoto, and Y. Tarumi, *Z. Immunitaetsforsch. Immunobiol.*, *147*:302 (1975).
10. V. Souvannavong, A. Adam, and E. Lederer, *Infect. Immun.*, *19*:966 (1978).
11. F. Audibert, L. Chedid, P. Lefrancier, and J. Choay, *Cell. Immunol.*, *21*:243 (1976).
12. A. Tanaka, R. Saito, K. Sugiyama, I. Morisaki, S. Kotani, S. Kusumoto, and T. Shiba, *Infect. Immun.*, *15*:331 (1977).
13. L. Chedid, F. Audibert, P. Lefrancier, J. Choay, and E. Lederer, *Proc. Natl. Acad. Sci. USA*, *73*:2472 (1976).

14. I. Lowy, C. Bona, and L. Chedid, *Cell. Immunol.*, *29*:195 (1977).
15. C. Leclerc, E. Bourgeois, and L. Chedid, *Immunol. Commun.*, *8*:55 (1979).
16. J. Watson and C. Whitlock, *J. Immunol.*, *121*:383 (1978).
17. K. Sugimura, M. Uemiya, I. Saiki, I. Azuma, and Y. Yamamura, *Cell. Immunol.*, *43*:37 (1979).
18. A. Tanaka, S. Nagao, R. Saito, S. Kotani, S. Kusumoto, and T. Shiba, *Biochem. Biophys. Res. Commun.*, *77*:621 (1977).
19. A. Tanaka, S. Nagao, R. Nagao, S. Kotani, T. Shiba, and S. Kusumoto, *Infect. Immun.* *24*:302 (1979).
20. R. V. Waters and R. W. Ferraresi, *J. Reticuloendothel. Soc.*, *28*:457 (1980).
21. E. B. Fraser-Smith, R. V. Waters, and T. R. Matthews, *Infect. Immun.*, *35*:105 (1982).
22. M. Fevrier, J. L. Birrien, C. Leclerc, L. Chedid, and P. Liacopoulos, *Eur. J. Immunol.*, *8*:558 (1978).
23. A. Matter, *Cancer Immunol. Immunother.*, *6*:201 (1979).
24. S. M. Wahl, L. M. Wahl, J. B. McCarthy, L. Chedid, and S. E. Mergenhagen, *J. Immunol.*, *122*:2226 (1979).
25. M. J. Pabst and R. B. Johnston, Jr., *J. Exp. Med.*, *151*:101 (1980).
26. H. Takada, M. Tsujimoto, K. Kato, S. Kotani, S. Kusumoto, M. Inage, T. Shiba, I. Yano, S. Kawata, and K. Yokogawa, *Infect. Immun.*, *25*:48 (1979).
27. J. W. Hadden, *Cancer Treat. Rep.*, *62*:1981 (1978).
28. J. J. Oppenheim, A. Togawa, L. Chedid, and S. Mizel, *Cell. Immunol.*, *50*:71 (1980).
29. J. P. Tenu, E. Lederer, and J. F. Petit, *Eur. J. Immunol.*, *10*:647 (1980).
30. J. W. Hadden, A. Englard, J. R. Sadlik, and E. M. Hadden, *Int. J. Immunopharmacol.*, *1*:17 (1979).
31. Y. Yamamoto, S. Nagao, A. Tanaka, T. Koga, and K. Onoue, *Biochem. Biophys. Res. Commun.*, *80*:923 (1978).
32. A. Adam, V. Souvannavong, and E. Lederer, *Biochem. Biophys. Res. Commun.*, *85*:631 (1970).
33. S. Nagao, A. Tanaka, Y. Yamamoto, T. Koga, K. Onoue, T. Shiba, K. Kusumoto, and S. Kotan, *Infect, Immun.*, 24:*308* (1979).
34. Y. Homma, K. Onozaki, T. Hashimoto, K. Miura, S. Nagao, and A. Tanaka, *Int. Archs. Allergy Appl. Immunol.*, *65*:27 (1981).
35. R. Nozawa, R. Sekiguchi, and T. Yokota, *Cell. Immunol.*, *53*:116 (1980).
36. D. Juy and L. Chedid, *Proc. Natl. Acad. Sci. USA*, *72*:4105 (1975).
37. T. Taniyama and H. T. Holden, *Cell Immunol.*, *48:369* (1979).
38. J. M. Plummer, D. E. Thor, H. Cronenberger, and W. Magee (Abstr.), *Proc. Fed. Amer. Soc. Exp. Biol.*, *65*:1118 (1981).
39. S. Sone and I. J. Fidler, *J. Immunol.*, *145*:2454 (1980).
40. S. Sone and I. J. Fidler, *Cell Immunol.*, *57*:41 (1981).
41. A. J. Schroit and I. J. Fidler, *Cancer Res.*, *42*:161 (1982).
42. I. J. Fidler, S. Sone, W. E. Fogler, and Z. L. Barnes, *Proc. Natl. Acad. Sci. USA*, *78*: 1680 (1981).
43. W. E. Fogler and I. J. Fidler, *Fed. Proc.*, *40*:761 (1981).
44. I. J. Fidler, *J. Immunol.*, *127*:1719 (1981).
45. A. Raz, W. E. Fogler, and I. J. Fidler, *Cancer Immunol. Immunother.*, *7*:157 (1979).
46. M. Parant, F. Parant, L. Chedid, A. Yapo, J. F. Petit, and E. Lederer, *Int. J. Immunopharmacol.*, *1*:35 (1979).
47. E. Lederer, *J. Med. Chem.*, *23*:819 (1980).
48. L. Chedid, C. Carelli, and F. Audibert, *J. Reticuloendothel. Soc.*, *26*:631 (1979).
49. H. K. Kimelberg and E. Mayhew, *CRC Crit, Rev. Toxicol.*, *18*:25 (1978).
50. R. E. Pagano and J. N. Weinstein, *An. Rev. Biophys. Bioeng.*, *7*:435 (1978).
51. G. Poste, in *Liposomes in Biological Systems* (G. Gregoriadis and A. C. Allison, eds.), John Wiley and Sons, Inc., New York, 1980.

52. D. A. Tyrell, T. D. Heath, C. M. Holley, and B. E. Ryman, *Biochim. Biophys. Acta*, *457*:259 (1976).
53. A. C. Allison, *J. Reticuloendothel. Soc.*, *26*:619 (1979).
54. L. Chedid, M. Parant, F. Parant, P. Lefrancier, J. Choay, and E. Lederer, *Proc. Natl. Acad. Sci. USA*, *74*:2089 (1977).
55. M. Parant, F. Parant, and L. Chedid, *Proc. Natl. Acad. Sci. USA*, *75*:3395 (1977).
56. K. Matsumoto, H. Ogawa, O. Nagase, T. Kusama, and I. Azuma, *Microbiol. Immunol.*, *25*:1047 (1981).
57. E. B. Fraser-Smith and T. R. Matthews, *Infect. Immun.*, *34*:676 (1981).
58. N. P. Cummings, M. J. Pabst, and R. B. Johnston, Jr., J. Exp. Med., 152:*1659 (1980)*.
59. F. Kierzenbaum, and R. W. Ferraresi, *Infect. Immun.*, *25*:273 (1979).
60. R. C. Humphres, P. R. Henika, R. W. Ferraresi, and J. L. Krahenbuhl, *Infect. Immun.*, *30*:462 (1980).
61. J. L. Krahenbuhl, S. D. Sharma, R. W. Ferraresi, and J. S. Remington, *Infect. Immun.*, *31*:716 (1981).
62. F. M. Dietrich, W. Sackmann, O. Zak, and P. Dukor, *Curr. Dev. Chemother. Infect. Dis.*, *2*:1730 (1980).
63. J. L. Krahenbuhl, R. C. Humphres, and R. W. Ferraresi, *Int. J. Leprosy*, *48*:504 (1980).
64. G. R. Olds, L. Chedid, E. Lederer, and A. A. F. Mahmoud, *J. Infect. Dis.*, *141*:473 (1980).
65. K. Yamamoto, M. Kakinuma, K. Kato, H. Okuyama, and I. Azuma, *Immunology*, *40*:557 (1980).
66. K. Yamamoto, K. Kato, M. Kakinuma, H. Okuyama, and I. Azuma, *Immunology*, *46*:473 (1982).
67. G. B. Mackaness, *J. Exp. Med.*, *116*:381 (1962).
68. R. J. North, *J. Exp. Med.*, *130*:299 (1969).
69. W. A. Siddiqui, D. W. Taylor, S. C. Kan, K. Kramer, S. M. Richard-Crum, S. Kotani, T. Shiba, and S. Kusumoto, *Science*, *201*:1237 (1978).
70. O. R. Pavlovskis, D. C. Edman, S. H. Leppla, B. Wretlind, L. R. Lewis, and K. E. Martin, *Infect. Immun.*, *32*:681 (1981).
71. R. Arnon, M. Sela, M. Parant, and L. Chedid, *Proc. Natl. Acad. Sci. USA*, *77*:6769 (1980).
72. I. J. Fidler, *Cancer Res.*, *37*:2481 (1978).
73. G. Poste and I. J. Fidler, *Nature*, *283*:139 (1979).
74. I. J. Fidler and M. L. Kripke, *Antibiot. Chemother.*, *28*:123 (1980).
75. W. Den Otter, F. J. Dullens, H. Van Lovern, and E. Pels, in *The Macrophage and Cancer* (K. James, B. McBride and A. Stuart, eds.), Econoprint, Edinburgh, 1977.
76. I. J. Fidler, *Cancer Res.*, *34*:1074 (1974).
77. L. A. Liotta, C. Gattozzi, J. Kleinerman, and G. Saidel, *Br. J. Cancer*, *36*:639 (1977).
78. I. J. Fidler, W. E. Fogler, and J. Connor, in *Immunobiology and Immunotherapy of Cancer* (W. D. Terry and Y. Yamamura, eds.), Elsevier, New York, 1979.
79. I. R. Hart, W. E. Fogler, G. Poste, and I. J. Fidler, *Cancer Immunol. Immunother.*, *10*:157 (1981).
80. I. J. Fidler, A. Raz, W. E. Fogler, R. Kirsh, P. Bugelski, and G. Poste, *Cancer Res.*, *40*:4460 (1980).
81. D. P. Griswold, Jr., *Cancer Chemother. Rep.*, *3*:315 (1972).
82. I. J. Fidler, Z. Barnes, W. E. Fogler, R. Kirsh, P. Bugelski, and G. Poste, *Cancer Res.*, *42*:496 (1982).
83. C. A. McLaughlin, S. L. Schwartzman, B. L. Horner, G. H. Jones, J. G. Moffatt, J. J. Nestor, and D. Tegg, *Science*, *208*:415 (1980).
84. E. Yarkoni, E. Lederer, and H. J. Rapp, *Infect. Immun.*, *32*:273 (1981).
85. R. H. Gisler, F. M. Dietrich, G. Baschung, in *Drugs and Immune Responsiveness* (J. L. Turk and D. Parker, eds.), The Macmillan Press, Ltd., London, 1979.

86. W. L. Epstein, *Prog. Allergy*, *11*:36 (1967).
87. D. O. Adams, *Am. J. Pathol.*, *84*:164 (1976).
88. A. Delaunay, J. Asselineau, and E. Lederer, *C. R. Soc. Biol.*, *145*:650 (1951).
89. K. Emori and A. Tanaka, *Infect. Immun.*, *19*:613 (1978).
90. A. Tanaka and K. Emori, *Am. J. Pathol.*, *98*:733 (1980).
91. S. Nagao, F. Ota, K. Emori, K. Inoue, and A. Tanaka, *Infect. Immun.*, *34*:993 (1981).
92. C. M. Pearson, *Proc. Soc. Exp. Biol. Med.*, *91*:95 (1956).
93. O. Kohashi, C. M. Pearson, Y. Watanabe, S. Kotani, and T. Koga, *J. Immunol.*, *116*: 1635 (1976).
94. T. Koga, K. Maeda, K. Onoue, K. Kato, and S. Kotani, *Mol. Immunol.*, *116*:153 (1979).
95. O. Kohashi, S. Kotani, T. Shiba, and A. Ozawa, *Infect. Immun.*, *26*:690 (1979).
96. O, Kohashi, A. Tanaka, S. Kotani, T. Shiba, S. Kusumoto, K. Yukogawa, S. Kawata, and A. Ozawa, *Infect. Immun.*, *29*:674 (1980).
97. S. Nagao and A. Tanaka, *Infect. Immun.*, *28*:624 (1980).
98. Y. Chang, C. M. Pearson, and L. Chedid, *J. Exp. Med.*, *153*:1021 (1981).
99. Z. Zidek, K. Masek, and Z. Jiricka, *Infect. Immun.*, *35*:674 (1982).
100. Y. Nagai, K. Akiyama, K. Suzuki, S. Kotani, Y. Watanabe, T. Shimono, T. Shiba, S. Kusumota, F. Ikuta, and S. Takeda, *Cell. Immunol.*, *35*:158 (1978).
101. Y. Nagai, K. Akiyama, S. Kotani, Y. Watanabe, T. Shimono, T. Shiba, and S. Kusumoto, *Cell. Immunol.*, *35*:168 (1978).
102. F. Toullet, F. Audibert, G. A. Voisin, and L. Chedid, *Ann. Immunol.*, *128*:267 (1977).
103. S. Kotani, Y. Watanabe, T. Shimono, K. Harada, T. Shiba, S. Kusumoto, K. Yokogawa, and M. Taniguchi, *Biken J.*, *19*:9 (1976).
104. K. Masek, O. Kadlecova, and P. Petrovicky, in *Toxins: Animal, Plant and Microbial* (P. Rosenberg, ed.), Pergamon Press, New York, 1978.
105. C. A. Dinerello, R. J. Elin. L. Chedid, and S. M. Wolff, *J. Infect. Dis.*, *138*:760 (1978).
106. M. Parant, G. Riveau, and L. Chedid, *Agents Actions*, in press.
107. M. Parant, G. Riveau, F. Parant, C. A. Dinarello, S. M. Wolff, and L. Chedid, *J. Infect. Dis.*, *142*:708 (1980).
108. L. Chedid, M. A. Parent, F. M. Audibert, G. J. Riveau, F. J. Parant, E. Lederer, J. P. Choay, and P. L. Lefrancier, *Infect. Immun.*, *35*:417 (1982).
109. M. J. Pabst, N. P. Cummings, T. Shiba, S. Kusumoto, and S. Kotani, *Infect. Immun.*, *29*:617 (1980).
110. I. J. Fidler, S. Sone, W. E. Fogler, D. Smith, D. G. Braun, L. Tarcsay, R. H. Gisler, and A. J. Schroit, *J. Biol. Response Modifiers*, *1*:43 (1982).
111. A. Raz, C. Bucana, W. E. Fogler, G. Poste, I. J. Fidler, and G. Poste, *Cancer Res.*, *41*:495 (1981).
112. I. J. Fidler, A. Raz, W. E. Fogler, L. C. Hoyer, and G. Poste, *Cancer Res.*, *41*:495 (1981).

25

The In Vitro Induction of Colony-Stimulating Factor, Prostaglandin E, and Interferon in Macrophages and Tumor Cells by Biological Response Modifiers

Erich Schlick,* Klaus Hartung,† Mario Piccoli,‡ Anna Bartocci, and Michael A. Chirigos National Cancer Institute–Frederick Cancer Research Facility, Frederick, Maryland

I. INTRODUCTION

Infections associated with granulocytopenia and monocyte/macrophage dysfunctions are a major cause of morbidity and mortality in cancer patients (1). Antineoplastic treatment regimens with chemotherapeutic agents and/or irradiation reduces dose dependently the number of uncommitted stem cells (CFU-S), of granulocyte-macrophage precursors (GM-CFU-C), and their progenies (2-6). Several days after such a treatment, a spontaneous recovery of the hematopoietic stem cell function may occur, depending upon the extent of the prior hematopoietic dysfunction (7,8). Several humoral factors such as colony-stimulating factors (CSFs) seem to be involved in this recovery (9,10). CSFs are growth factors which stimulate the in vitro formation of colonies of granulocytes and/or macrophages by precursor cells in hemopoietic tissues (11-13). There is now considerable evidence to suggest that CSFs may act also in vivo to regulate granlopoiesis and/or macrophage formation (14-16). Elevated levels of CSFs as well as increases in the stem cell compartment in hematopoietic tissues are associated with different immunological situations, including host response to antigen administration, allograft and tumor rejection, bacterial and viral infections, as well as some lymphoproliferative diseases (17). The elaboration of CSFs by mononuclear phagocytes (18,19),

*Supported by Deutsche Krebshilfe e.V., Bonn, Federal Republic of Germany.
Current affiliations:
†Bundeswehrkrankenhaus, Klinische Medizin. Labor, Koblenz, Federal Republic of Germany
‡Institute of General Pathology, State University of Rome, Rome, Italy.

especially after their in vitro exposure to agents like lipopolysaccharides (20) that increase also serum CSF levels and stimulate granulocyte/macrophage formation in vivo (21), has implicated blood monocytes and tissue macrophages as the primary CSF-producing cell types. CSFs, however, are also found in culture media conditioned by certain tumor cell lines, such as Wehi-3, a myelomonocytic leukemia (22,23), and L1210, an undifferentiated lymphoma (23). Besides the secretion of CSFs, monocytes/macrophages are known to produce also prostaglandins, which exert a variety of effects on numerous cell types and tissues. They are known to elevate intracellular levels of cyclic AMP (24), to influence macrophage functions (25,26), to modulate cellular responses to antigens (27), mitogens (28), and proliferative factors including CSFs (29,30).

Considerable effort has been devoted to the development of preventive or therapeutically active drugs to minimize the duration and extent of hematopoietic dysfunction induced by antineoplastic treatment (31-33). Animal studies suggest that several biologicals, such as Bacillus-Calmette-Guérin (31), *Corynebacterium parvum* (32,34), and glucan (35), increase the concentration of hematopoietic precursors in bone marrow and spleen. The effects of other agents used in immunotherapy like maleic anhydride divinyl ether copolymer (MVE-2), poly ICLC, and interferon (FI) on hematopoiesis are not yet clear.

The present study describes the effects of six biological response modifiers (BRMs), interferon, poly ICLC, MVE-2, lipopolysaccharide, azimexone, and diethyldithiocarbamate on the secretion of CSFs, prostaglandin E, and interferon by resident peritoneal macrophages and two tumor cell lines, Wehi-3 and L1210, in an in vitro system.

II. MATERIALS AND METHODS

A. Macrophages

Peritoneal macrophages were aseptically harvested from male BALB/c mice, 6-8 weeks old, supplied by the Mammalian Genetics and Animal Production Section, Division of Cancer Treatment, NCI, NIH, Bethesda, Maryland. Peritoneal macrophages (8×10^5) were seeded onto 16-mm wells (Costar, Cambridge, Massachusetts) in 1 ml of RPMI-1640 medium (GIBCO, Grand Island, New York), supplemented with 10% heat-inactivated fetal calf serum (GIBCO, Grand Island, New York), 125 μg/ml gentamycin (Sigma Chemical Co., St. Louis, Missouri and 292 μg/ml L-glutamine (GIBCO, Grand Island, New York (RPMI-FCS). The cultures were incubated for 2 hr and the adherent macrophage monolayers were washed twice with medium before being used in experiments.

B. Murine Tumor Cell Lines

Weh-3 cells, originally obtained from BALB/c mice after induction of a myelomonocytic leukemia with mineral oil (36), are phagocytic, contain F_c receptors, and synthesize lysozyme and CSFs (22). L1210, a chemically induced lymphoma, contains no theta or kappa determinants (37) and synthesizes CSFs (23). Both cell lines grow in culture with doubling times of 12-24 hr.

C. Drugs

Polyriboinosinic-polycytidylic acid poly-L-lysine stabilized with carboxymethylcellulose (poly ICLC) was kindly supplied by Dr. H. B. Levy (NIAID, NIH, Bethesda, Maryland). Maleic anhydride divinyl ether copolymer (MVE-2) was kindly obtained from Dr. R.

Corrano (Adria Laboratories, Columbus, Ohio). Azimexone, a 2-cyanoaziridine, was a generous gift from Dr. U. Bicker (Boehringer, G.m.b.H., Mannheim, Federal Republic of West Germany). Mouse L-cell interferon (IF) with a specific activity of 3.5×10^7 U/mg protein and anti-L-cell interferon antibodies (IF-NA) were purchased from Dr. K. Paucker (Medical College of Pennsylvania, Philadelphia, Pennsylvania). Sodium diethyldithiocarbamate (DTC) was generously provided by Dr. G. Renoux (Laboratory of Immunology, Faculty of Medicine, Tours, France). Lipopolysaccharide (LPS) from *Salmonella typhimurium* was purchased from Difco (Detroit, Michigan).

D. Macrophage Activation Assay

The macrophage activation assay has been previously described (38). Briefly, monolayers of 8×10^5 Mϕ were pretreated in vitro with various concentrations of the BRMs tested for 24 hr. The Mϕ were then overlaid with 8×10^4 MBL-2 leukemia cells in RPMI-FCS. All cultures were incubated for a further 48 hr at 37°C, and 5% CO_2 in air and viable MBL-2 cells were then determined by trypan blue dye exclusion. The percent inhibition of MBL-2 cells by Mϕ was calculated by

$$\%\ \text{Inhibition} = 1 - \frac{\text{Mean of MBL-2 cells from drug-treated M}\phi}{\text{Mean of MBL-2 cells from control M}\phi} \times 100$$

E. In Vitro Inhibition of Tumor Cell Growth

In vitro inhibition of tumor cell growth in the presence of BRMs was measured as previously described (39). Briefly, 10^3 or 10^4 tumor cells were prepared in 1 ml of 0.3% agar, supplemented with 10% horse serum (GIBCO, Grand Island, New York), and 125 μg/ml gentamycin and plated over 1 ml of a 0.5% agar bottom layer (10% fetal calf serum and 125 μg/ml gentamycin) in 35-mm Petri dishes (Falcon, Oxnard, California). The drugs to be tested were added to the top layer. After a 10-day incubation period at 37°C and 5% CO_2, the number of tumor cells and/or colonies per plate were scored.

F. GM-CSF Assay

For the GM-CSF assay 2×10^5 tumor cells per milliliter of RPMI were incubated in 16-mm wells for up to 6 days under serum-free conditions at 37°C and 5% CO_2. The drugs to be tested were added to the cells on day 0. The final volume was 2 ml per well. Alternatively, 8×10^5 peritoneal Mϕ were incubated in 2 ml of RPMI-10% FCS for up to 4 days at 37°C and 5% CO_2. The drugs were added on day 0. Cell-free supernatants were harvested from both the tumor cells and Mϕ at different times and kept at -20°C until assayed. The supernatants to be tested (0.2 ml) for CSF were then added to each 35-mm petri dish containing 10^5 unfractionated bone marrow cells from normal mice in 2 ml of 0.3% agar, supplemented with 15% horse serum, 15% fetal calf serum, and 125 μg/ml gentamycin. At the end of the culture period (10 days at 37°C and 5% CO_2), the colonies (>40 cells) and clusters (3-40 cells) were counted, and then histologically classified according to a method previously described (40).

No colony formation was noted in the absence of either the standard CSF contained in the supernatant from the Wehi-3 cell line or a supernatant from the tumor cells or Mϕ. GM-CSF is expressed as units per milliliter (41), calculated from the number of myeloid colonies formed by 10^5 normal bone marrow cells in the presence of 1.0 ml of the CSF source (e.g. the formation of 20 colonies in the presence of 0.2 ml supernatant defines the CSF activity of that supernatant as 100 U/ml). These quantities of supernatants were chosen for testing because they gave results in the linear portion of the dose-response curve of myeloid colony formation as a function of both CSF concentration per petri dish and number of bone marrow cells cultured.

G. Prostaglandins of the E Series

PGEs were determined by radioimmunoassay (RIA) as previously described (42). Briefly, the assay consisted of incubating 100 μl of the experimental samples with 50 μl rabbit antiprostaglandin PGE_2, for 2 hr at room temperature, followed by the addition of 50 μl ^{3}[H]PGE_2 (8000 cpm), with further incubation at 4°C for 12-16 hr [final volume 200 μl; Trizma (0.012%), NaCl (0.083%), and gelatin (0.1%); pH 7.4]. The bound [^{3}H]PG was separated from the uncomplexed tracer after the addition of 0.25 ml iced Tris-NaCl-1.0% gelatin by adding 0.5 ml iced charcoal (0.5%)-dextran (0.5%) in Tris-NaCl buffer and incubating at 4°C for 20 min. After centrifugation (200 × g for 12 min), the supernatant was decanted into scintillation vials, 10 ml Ultrafluor were added, and radioactivity determined in an LS-350 (Beckman Corp., Fullerton, California).

The Student's t-test was used for statistical analysis.

III. RESULTS

A. Peritoneal Macrophages

Preincubation of peritoneal Mϕ for 24 hr in the presence of 10 μg/ml LPS, 500 U/ml IF, 50 μg/ml poly ICLC, or 50 μg/ml MVE-2 rendered the cells cytotoxic for MBL-2 cells (Table 1). Other drugs tested (azimexone and DTC) failed to stimulate in vitro Mϕ cytotoxicity (data not shown).

Table 1 Effect of Biological Response Modifiers on Different Macrophage Functions

Drug concentration		Control	LPS (10 μg/ml)	IF (500 U/ml)	Poly ICLC (50 μg/ml)	MVE-2 (50 μg/ml)
Macrophage tumoricidal activity[a]	%	0	42[e]	56[e]	72[e]	51[e]
IF titer (U/ml)[b]	D1	–	–	–	660[e]	–
	D2	–	–	–	190[e]	–
	D3	–	–	–	200[e]	–
PGE_2 (pg/ml)[c]	D1	610	6050[e]	890	3880[e]	420
	D2	1020	3700[e]	1840[e]	2430[e]	1390
	D3	260	3990[e]	760	2030[e]	180
CSF (U/ml)[d]	D1	31	80[e]	99[e]	101[e]	14
	D2	51	151[e]	125[e]	145[e]	37
	D3	42	119[e]	124[e]	124[e]	33

[a]Preincubate 8 × 10^5 Mϕ with BRMs for 24 hr. They were then overlaid with 8 × 10^4 MBL-2 tumor cells in RPMI-FCS and incubated for further 48 hr.
[b]Virus CPE-inhibition assay (VSV; L929).
[c]Specificity for PGE_2: PGE_2 (100%); PGE_1 (60%); PGA (< 12%); PGB (< 1.5%); $PGF_{2\alpha}$ (< 4%).
[d]Incubate 10^5 BMC + 0.2 ml supernatant of Mϕ treated with BRM in 2 ml of 0.3% agar (15% FCS + 15% HS) for 10 days.
[e]$p < 0.001$.

Incubation of Mϕ in RPMI-10% FCS resulted in a spontaneous secretion of about 30-50 U/ml GM-CSF, a level maintained over a 4-day incubation period. LPS in concentrations of 1-10 μg/ml resulted in a stimulation of up to a threefold increase in GM-CSF secretion (Fig. 1). The optimal concentration was found to be 10 μg/ml. The peak activity occurred on day 2 of the incubation period. LPS (1 μg/ml) also stimulated significantly the Mϕ, reaching a plateau activity on day 2. By incubating Mϕ with IF, a similar strong increase in GM-CSF secretion was obtained (Fig. 2). IF (500 U/ml) proved to be the optimal concentration, reaching a plateau of activity on days 2-4. The 100- and 1000-U/ml concentrations also significantly stimulated the GM-CSF secretion. Poly ICLC at the optimal concentration of 50 μg/ml stimulated a secretion of about 140 U/ml GM-CSF on day 2 (Fig. 3). With 10 or 100 μg/ml poly ICLC a plateau activity with about 100 U/ml GM-CSF was reached on days 2-4. Other drugs tested: Azimexone (1-50 μg/ml), DTC (1-50 μg/ml), or MVE-2 (1-50 μg/ml) failed to stimulated the secretion of GM-CSF by Mϕ (Fig. 4).

A histological classification of the colonies induced by control Mϕ-derived GM-CSF showed about 28% being pure granulocyte and 72% pure monocyte/Mϕ colonies (Table 2). By using the supernatants of Mϕ which were incubated for 2 days in the presence of poly ICLC (50 μg/ml), IF (500 U/ml), or LPS (10 μg/ml), the number of pure granulocyte colonies was reduced, whereas the number of pure monocyte/Mϕ colonies was simultaneously increased by about 10%. No mixed-colony formation was noted.

The incubation of control Mϕ with different amounts of neutralizing antibodies (IF-NA) directed against L-cell IF for 3 days at 37°C and 5% CO_2 did not alter their GM-CSF secretion (Fig. 5). The ability of IF to stimulate the GM-CSF secretion by Mϕ, however, was abrogated by IF-NA. When IF and IF-NA were added together at day 0,

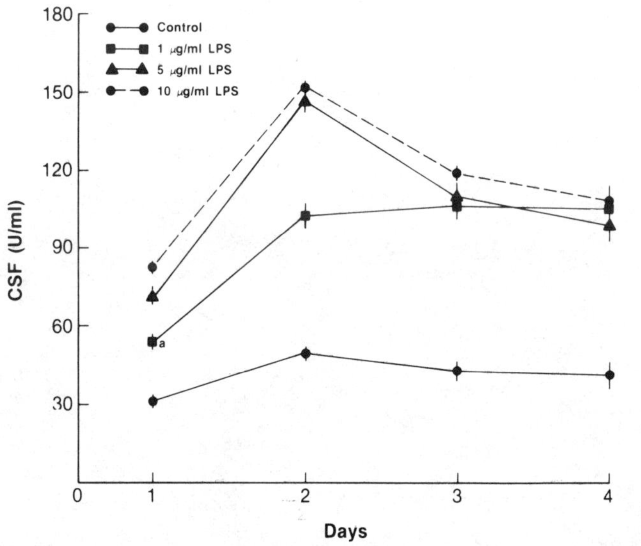

Figure 1 Resting peritoneal Mϕ (8×10^5) were incubated in the presence of LPS in RPMI–(10%) FCS in a total volume of 2 ml. At daily intervals, supernatants were tested for GM-CSF. Each value represents the mean ± SE of three separate experiments with four cultures each. All experimental values significant above controls ($p < 0.001$) except a = $p < 0.02$.

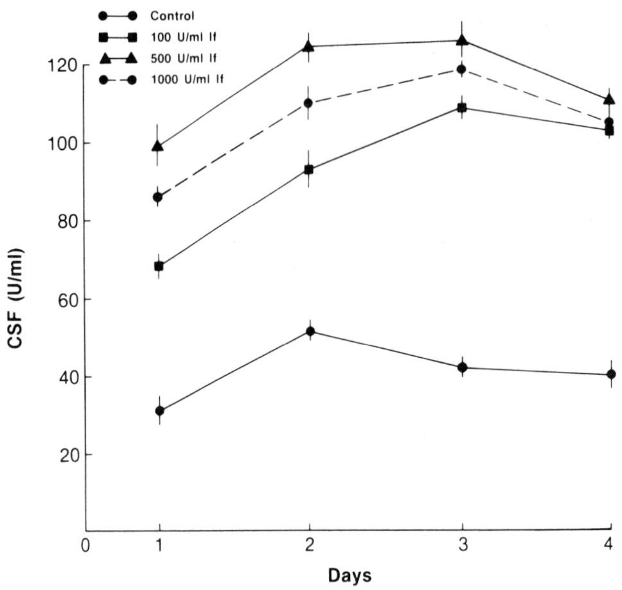

Figure 2 Resting peritoneal Mϕ (8 × 10^5) were incubated in the presence of IF in RPMI-(10%) FCS in a total volume of 2 ml. At daily intervals, supernatants were tested for GM-CSF. Each value represents the mean ± SE of three separate experiments with four cultures each. All experimental values significant above controls ($p < 0.001$).

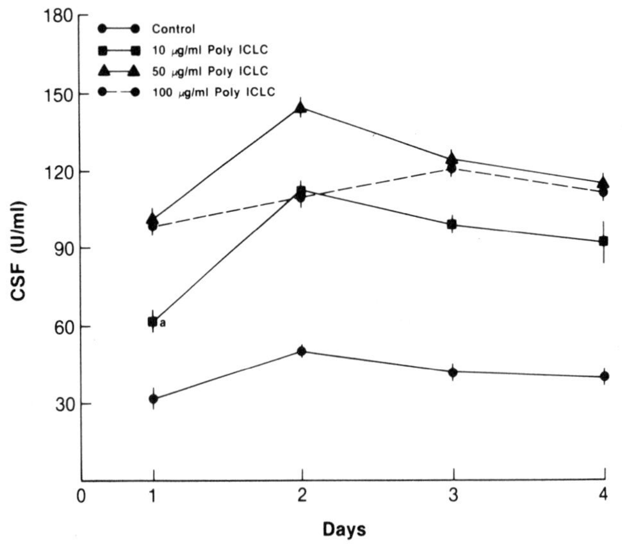

Figure 3 Resting peritoneal Mϕ (8 × 10^5) were incubated in the presence of poly ICLC in RPMI-(10%) FCS in a total volume of 2 ml. At daily intervals, supernatants were tested for GM-CSF. Each value represents the mean ± SE of three separate experiments with four cultures each. All experimental values significant above controls ($p < 0.001$) except a = $p < 0.01$.

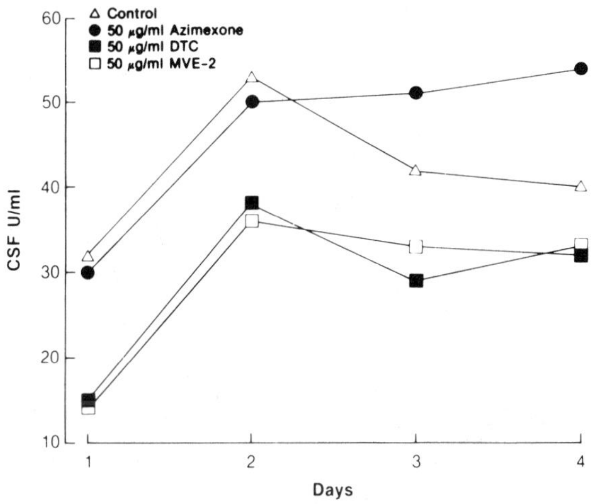

Figure 4 Resting peritoneal Mφ (8×10^5) were incubated in the presence of azimexone, DTC, or MVE-2 in RPMI-(10%) FCS in a total volume of 2 ml. At daily intervals, supernatants were tested for GM-CSF. Each value represents the mean ± SE of three separate experiments with four cultures each. No significant differences between control Mφ and drug-treated Mφ.

the amount of CSF secreted was reduced to control level by IF-NA neutralizing 70 U/ml IF. Higher concentrations of IF-NA even completely suppressed any GM-CSF secretion by the Mφ (Fig. 5). In contrast, IF-NA at concentrations able to neutralize up to 2000 U/ml IF did not interfere with the stimulatory effect of 10 µg/ml LPS or 50 µg/ml poly ICLC on GM-CSF secretion by Mφ, when cocultured for 3 days (Fig. 5).

Peritoneal Mφ spontaneously secretes PGE, when kept in RPMI-10% FCS at 37°C and 5% CO_2 (Table 1). The peak of secretion of 1000 pg/ml PGE occurred on day 2 of

Table 2 Histological Type of Colonies Induced by Macrophage and Tumor Cell-Derived CSF

	Macrophage supernatant[a]		Wehi-3 supernatant[a]			L1210 supernatant[a]		
Drug concentration	Gr (%)	Mono/Mφ (%)	Gr (%)	Mono/Mφ (%)	Mixed (%)	Gr (%)	Mono/Mφ (%)	Mixed (%)
Control	28	72	54	31	15	49	38	13
Poly ICLC (50 µg/ml)	19	81	50	38	12	45	46	9
LPS (10 µg/ml)	17	83	48	43	9	39	52	9
IF (500 U/ml)	15	84	45	46	9	35	57	8

[a]Incubate 10^5 BMC + 0.2 ml supernatant in 2 ml of 0.3% agar (15% FCS + 15% HS) for 10 days. Score the histological type of the BMC colonies, using the method of Salmon and Buick (40).

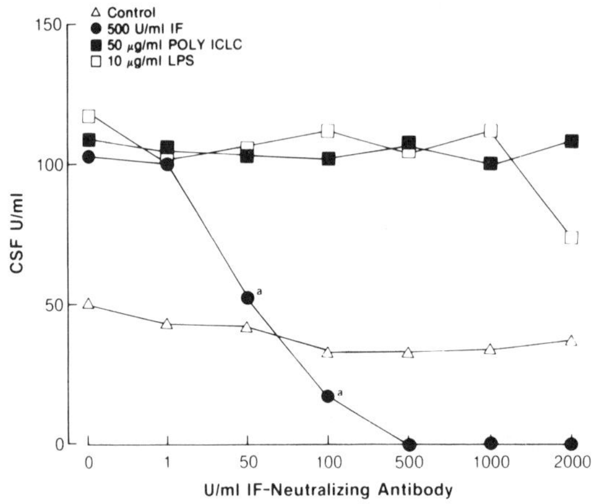

Figure 5 Resting peritoneal Mϕ (8×10^5) were incubated in the presence of different amounts of IF-neutralizing antibody (IF-NA) in RPMI-(10%) FCS in a total volume of 2 ml. IF, poly ICLC, or LPS was added to the cultures as well. Supernatants were tested for GM-CSF at day 3 of the incubation period. Each value represents the mean ± SE of three separate experiments with four cultures each. All values differ significantly from controls ($p < 0.001$) except a = not significant.

the incubation period. LPS at a concentration of 10 μg/ml stimulated a 10-fold increase in PGE secretion with a maximum of 6000 pg/ml on day 1; 50 μg/ml poly ICLC was also able to increase secretion of PGE by Mϕ. The peak activity with about 3900 pg/ml PGE occurred at day 1 of the incubation period. IF (500 U/ml) stimulated a small increase in PGE secretion and reached its peak activity with about 1800 pg/ml PGE at day 2. MVE-2 (50 μg/ml) failed to stimulate the PGE secretion of Mϕ. Among all the drugs tested in vitro, only poly ICLC induced considerable amounts of IF. The maximal secretory activity of the Mϕ with about 660 U/ml IF was found at day 1 of the incubation period (Table 1).

B. Wehi-3 and L1210 Tumor Cells

Incubation of the tumor cells with poly ICLC (50 μg/ml), IF (500 U/ml), LPS (10 μg/ml), and MVE-2 (50 μg/ml) resulted in a partial inhibition of tumor cell growth (Table 3).

The incubation of Wehi-3 cells resulted in a spontaneous production and secretion of GM-CSF which reached a plateau with a concentration of about 90 U/ml GM-CSF lasting from days 3 to 6 of the incubation period (Fig. 6). By adding different concentrations of IF (100-1000 U/ml) to the cells on day 0, the secretion of GM-CSF was significantly increased above control values (Fig. 6). An optimal effect was achieved with either 500 or 1000 U/ml IF between days 4 and 6 with a doubling of the amount of GM-CSF secreted, whereas 100 U/ml IF resulted in a lower stimulation of GM-CSF secretion.

By using poly ICLC, a similar strong increase in GM-CSF secretion by Wehi-3 cells was obtained (Fig. 7). Poly ICLC (50 μg/ml) was the optimal concentration to

Table 3 Inhibition of Tumor Cell Growth by Biological Response Modifiers

Drug concentration	Wehi-3[a]		L 1210[a]	
	b	c	b	c
Poly ICLC (50 μg/ml)	19[d]	22[d]	22[d]	25[d]
LPS (10 μg/ml)	18[d]	20[d]	25[d]	22[d]
IF (500 U/ml)	22[d]	15	20[d]	18
MVE-2 (50 μg/ml)	10	8	11	15

[a]Cell reduction compared with controls (%).
[b]Tumor cells 10^3 + BRM in a Salmon test for 10 days; count colonies.
[c]Tumor cells 10^4 + BRM in a Salmon test for 10 days; solubilize the agar with 5 ml PBS and count cells.
[d]$p < 0.05$

stimulate a twofold increase in GM-CSF. The maximal stimulatory effect lasted from day 3 to 6. Poly ICLC (10 or 100 μg/ml) resulted in a lower, still significant stimulation of the GM-CSF secretion. MVE-2 (50 μg/ml) failed to enhance the GM-CSF secretion by Wehi-3 cells (Fig. 8); other concentrations of MVE-2, ranging from 1 to 100 μg/ml, gave the same negative results (data not shown). LPS (10 μg/ml), a known inducer of CSF secretion by Wehi-3 (22), served as a positive internal control for the assay procedure (Fig. 8).

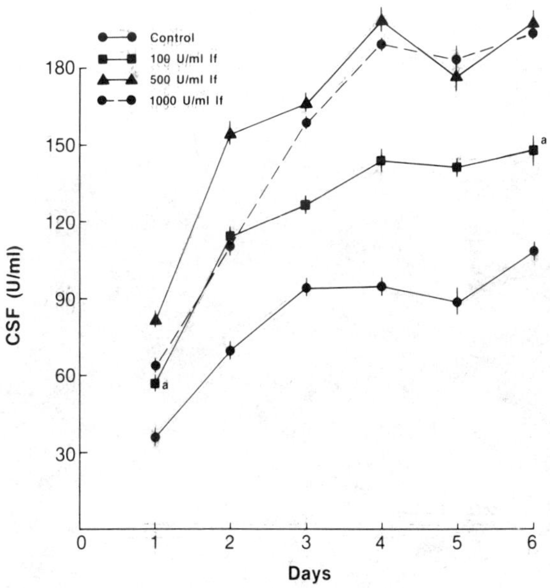

Figure 6 Wehi-3 tumor cells (2×10^5) were incubated in the presence of IF in RPMI in a total volume of 2 ml. At daily intervals, supernatants were tested for GM-CSF. Each value represents the mean ± SE of three separate experiments with four cultures each. All values significant above controls ($p < 0.002$) except a = $p < 0.02$.

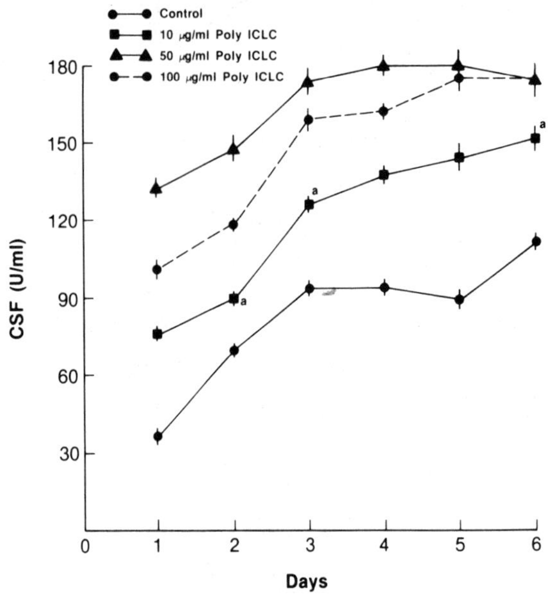

Figure 7 Wehi-3 tumor cells (2×10^5) were incubated in the presence of poly ICLC in RPMI in a total volume of 2 ml. At daily intervals, supernatants were tested for GM-CSF. Each value represents the mean ± SE of three separate experiments with four cultures each. All values significant above controls ($p < 0.002$) except a = $p < 0.01$.

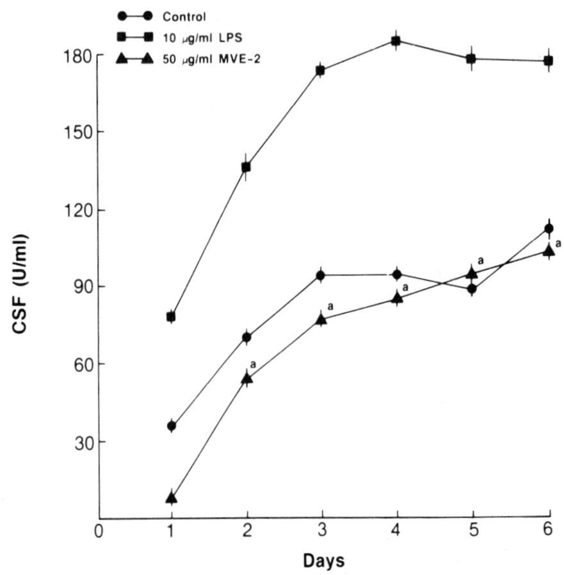

Figure 8 Wehi-3 tumor cells (2×10^5/ml) were incubated in the presence of LPS or MVE-2 in RPMI in a total volume of 2 ml. At daily intervals, supernatants were tested for GM-CSF. Each value represents the mean ± SE of three separate experiments with four cultures each. All values significant above controls ($p < 0.001$) except a = not significant.

L1210 cells spontaneously secreted GM-CSF at a relatively low concentration with a maximum of 20 U/ml GM-CSF at day 4 of the incubation period (Fig. 9). IF at a concentration of 500 U/ml stimulated up to a threefold increase in GM-CSF secretion with an optimal effect on day 3 (Fig. 9). Other concentrations of IF (100 or 1000 U/ml) tested also resulted in a significant stimulation of the GM-CSF secretion, which was, however, less marked.

Similarly to IF, poly ICLC at concentrations between 10 and 100 μg/ml induced a strong increase in GM-CSF secretion by L1210 IFig. 10). The optimal effect was achieved with 50 μg/ml poly ICLC on day 3. The other drug concentrations tested resulted in a lower, but significant stimulation of the GM-CSF secretion. But the total amount of GM-CSF secreted by L1210 cells never reached the level of the one secreted by Wehi-3 cells. None of the MVE-2 concentrations used (e.g., 50 μg/ml; Fig. 11) stimulated L1210 cells to increase their CSF secretion. LPS at a concentration of 10 μg/ml served as internal positive control (Fig. 11).

A histological classification of the colonies induced by supernatant containing GM-CSF from either one of the tumor lines incubated in medium alone (=control) showed about 50% being pure granulocyte, 31-38% being pure monocyte/Mϕ and about 14% being mixed colonies (Table 2). The supernatants of the tumor cells, incubated for 3 days with optimal concentrations of poly ICLC, LPS, and IF, however, gave rise to an increased percentage of pure granulocyte and mixed colonies compared with control values.

Wehi-3 and L1210 cells, when incubated for up to 6 days at 37°C and 5% CO_2, secreted between 50 and 100 pg/ml PGE, which is the detection limit for our RIA. No one of the drugs tested, IF (100-1000 U/ml), MVE-2 (1-50 μg/ml), poly ICLC (10-100 μg/ml), or LPS (1-10 μg/ml), was able to change significantly the secretory activity of both tumor cell lines for PGE (data not shown).

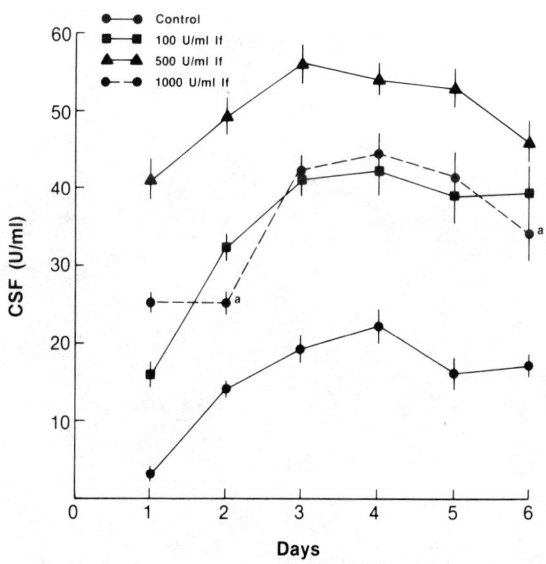

Figure 9 L1210 tumor cells (2×10^5/ml) were incubated in the presence of IF in RPMI in a total volume of 2 ml. At daily intervals, supernatants were tested for GM-CSF. Each value represents the mean ± SE of three separate experiments with four cultures each. All experimental values significant above controls ($p < 0.001$) except a = not significant.

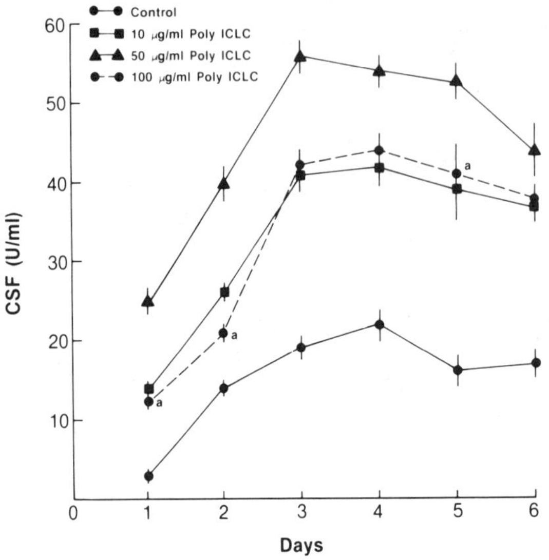

Figure 10 L1210 tumor cells (2×10^5/ml) were incubated in the presence of poly ICLC in RPMI in a total volume of 2 ml. At daily intervals, supernatants were tested for GM-CSF. Each value represents the mean ± SE of three separate experiments with four cultures each. All experimental values significant above control ($p < 0.01$) except a = $p < 0.05$.

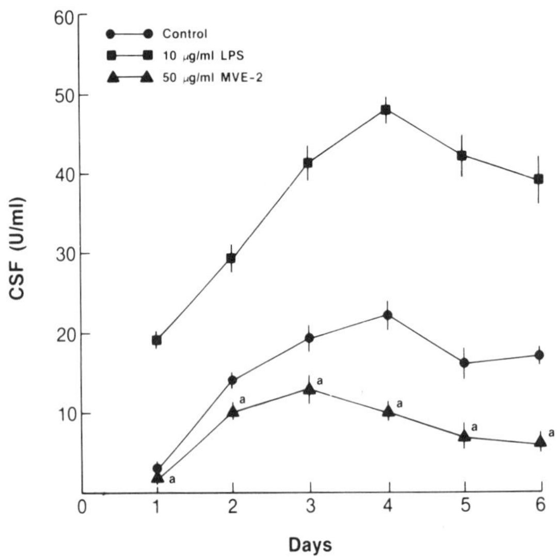

Figure 11 L1210 tumor cells (2×10^5/ml) were incubated in the presence of LPS or MVE-2 in RPMI in a total volume of 2 ml. At daily intervals supernatants were tested for GM-CSF. Each value represents the mean ± SE of three separate experiments with four cultures each. All experimental values significant above controls ($p < 0.002$) except a = not significant.

Both tumor cell lines did not spontaneously secrete any IF during a 4-day incubation period. Only poly ICLC at a concentration of 50 μg/ml consistently stimulated both tumor cell types to secrete marginally titers of about 10 U/ml IF. The other drugs tested, MVE-2 (1-50 μg/ml) and LPS (1-10 μg/ml), failed to stimulate the IF secretion by the tumor cells (data not shown).

IV. DISCUSSION

Macrophages can be activated in vitro and in vivo by a variety of agents to increase their metabolism, enzyme synthesis, membrane activity, and antitumor effects (43-45). Some of these agents are potent immunological adjuvants or immunopotentiators, such as BCG and *C. parvum* (46,47). LPS has also been found to exert a variety of direct effects on macrophages, including enhancement of killing capacity and secretion of proteolytic enzymes and of CSF (20,48-50). LPS, at concentrations ranging from 1 to 10 μg/ml, served as an internal positive control throughout all our experiments and increased the in vitro Mϕ tumoricidal activity, stimulated the PGE production, and increased significantly GM-CSF secretion by Mϕ, thus confirming the prior reports. In contrast to its potential to induce in vivo the secretion of IF by Mϕ and lymphocytes (51), it had no such activity on Mϕ in vitro.

The chemically well-defined biological response modifiers poly ICLC and MVE-2, as well as mouse IF, are potent in vivo stimulators of Mϕ and NK activity (43,45). All three drugs, at their optimal concentrations, also rendered Mϕ tumoricidal in vitro after a 24-hr preincubation period, exhibiting therefore a comparable in vivo/in vitro activity. Azimexone, an in vivo Mϕ activator (38), has no such in vitro capacity, due probably to its instability in solutions and to the lack of metabolic changes probably required for its in vivo activity. DTC, reported as being a macrophage activator (52,53), had at least in our hands no such capacity either in vivo or in vitro (54).

The obligatory requirement of CSF for the in vitro clonal proliferation of the GM-CFU-C is well established (55). The elaboration of this group of stimulatory macromolecules mainly by cells of the monocyte/Mϕ series has led to suggestions that granulopoiesis and Mϕ/monocyte function are controlled by a positive feedback mechanism involving CSF (12,13,18). On the other hand, PGE also produced by Mϕ has the ability to initiate a decreased responsive state of the progenitor cells to the actions of CSF, thus serving as a negative feedback regulator in the GM-CFU-C system (29,30,56). Peritoneal Mϕ are in vitro spontaneously secreting GM-CSF, as well as PGE. In our experiments they maintained a relatively stable level of about 35 U/ml GM-CSF over a 4-day incubation period, when kept under optimal culture conditions, including 10% FCS. Without FCS available in the culture medium, they are not secreting any CSF, nor do they respond to a CSF inducer, such as LPS (data not shown). During the first 2 days of the culture period they also secrete relevant levels of PGE. From the three drugs tested in our experiments, which stimulate in vitro Mϕ tumoricidal activity, only two, poly ICLC and IF, were potent GM-CSF inducers as well, whereas MVE-2 did not change significantly the spontaneous secretion of GM-CSF by Mϕ. The reason(s) for this dissociation in the in vitro activity of MVE-2 on Mϕ (tumoricidal status versus GM-CSF secretion) are not yet understood. Differences in the activation pathway of Mϕ to reach a tumoricidal status and/or to secrete GM-CSF could require different signals, not provided by MVE-2 in vitro, but by poly ICLC and IF. Metabolic changes of MVE-2, more likely to occur in vivo, may also play an important role for its lack of in vitro activity. These explanations are supported by preliminary results of in vivo experiments, which show that MVE-2 may well stimulate GM-CSF secretion by Mϕ (data not shown).

The results obtained so far with poly ICLC confirm and extend prior experiments, showing an increase in GM-CSF secretion by Mϕ, due to poly I:poly C stimulation (57,58). In our experiments, there seems to exist a bell-shaped dose-response relationship for both active drugs, by reaching a plateau at 50 μg/ml poly ICLC and 500 U/ml IF, and a somewhat lower response at higher drug concentrations. The colonies induced by the Mϕ supernatants were either pure granulocyte or pure Mϕ colonies. By treating control Mϕ with one of the active drugs, there was a tendency to reduce the number of granulocyte colonies and simultaneously to increase the number of pure Mϕ colonies. From the histological data presented one could speculate that the supernatants of the Mϕ contained two different subclasses of GM-CSF, namely CSF_M and CSF_G (12) or CSF_1 and CSF_3 (59). Depending upon the stage of Mϕ activity and/or the type of stimulus used, there seemed to be a change in the ratio of these two subclasses. Conclusive results, however, could only be obtained by means of a specific radioimmunoassay, capable of measuring both subclasses.

Since poly ICLC and LPS are reported to be IF inducers (51,60), one could speculate that the mechanism of GM-CSF induction consists of two steps: (a) the stimulation of Mϕ to secrete IF, which then (b) in turn may activate the Mϕ to also secrete GM-CSF. By using IF-NA, directed against IF used in our experiments, we could only completely abrogate the stimulatory effect of IF, but not of LPS or poly ICLC. This result and the findings of our experiments, in which we determined IF levels in the supernatants, make it rather unlikely that there is such a two-step activation of Mϕ. The reason(s) for the total suppression of any CSF secretion in the group treated with IF and higher concentrations of IF-NA are not yet clear.

Two sets of experiments were carried out to exclude a possible direct effect of the remaining drugs in the supernatants on the GM-CFU-C growth in the agar culture assay: (a) We did not obtain any significant changes in the number of colonies counted by using Mϕ-depleted bone marrow cells as indicator cells for the agar culture assay rather than using unfractionated bone marrow cells, thus indicating that the remaining drug concentrations had no further (stimulatory/inhibitory) effect on the Mϕ present in the agar culture. (b) We also incubated unfractionated or Mϕ-depleted bone marrow cells with supernatants from control Mϕ and added analog drug concentrations directly to the agar culture, which did not change the colony counts obtained, indicating that the drug concentrations used had no direct effect on GM-CFU-C present in the culture (data not shown).

Interestingly, there was a coincidental increase in both GM-CSF and PGE production by Mϕ. Only those drugs able to stimulate GM-CSF production by Mϕ were also inducers of elevated PGE levels (LPS, poly ICLC, and IF), whereas the drugs which did not change GM-CSF secretion by Mϕ had no effect on PGE synthesis (DTC, MVE-2 and azimexone). The peak activity of PGE secretion is reached at days 1 and 2, followed by slowly decreasing PGE levels thereafter, whereas the GM-CSF levels reach a relatively consistent plateau, lasting from day 2 to 4. This production and secretion of PGE and GM-CSF by Mϕ at the same time may be due to the stimulation of two different types of Mϕ, responsible for either the synthesis of PGE or CSF alone (61). There are also some indications that PGE may be an inducer of GM-CSF secretion by Mϕ in long-term bone marrow cultures (62). However, from the results presented here, it seems more likely to be a concomitant effect of the drugs on probably two subsets of Mϕ, rather than an induction of PGE secretion in a first step, which then in turn stimulates (a second subset of) Mϕ to secrete GM-CSF also.

A variety of agents (e.g., LPS, BCG, zymosan) known to stimulate Mϕ activity have cytostatic and/or cytotoxic effects on monocytic, macrophage, or histiocytic tumors in culture (63,64). By using the 10-day Salmon assay, which in the presence of the drugs measures mainly cytostatic effects (39), we could show that the in vitro Mϕ-activating drugs LPS, poly ICLC, and IF are significantly inhibiting the growth of the myelomonocytic Wehi-3 cell line and also the lymphoma L1210, whereas MVE-2 had no significant cytostatic or toxic effect on both tumor lines. These results confirm and extend a previous report on the effect of several immunopotentiators (e.g., LPS) on Wehi-3 cells (63); in contradiction, however, our findings show a sensitivity of L1210 cells, especially to LPS (63). Presently it is not clear whether the cytostatic effects on both tumor lines are reversible upon removal of the drug (63) or irreversible, and whether the inhibition of tumor growth is accompanied by an induction of tumor cell differentiation, as already reported for another murine myeloid leukemia (Ml) cell line (65,66).

Both tumor lines are constitutive producers of GM-CSF (our data and 23,63), which do not require the presence of any FCS in the culture (in contrast to Mϕ), an advantage for a possible further purification for GM-CSF. Differences within the tumor lines are found in the absolute amounts of GM-CSF secreted, with a higher spontaneous synthesis of GM-CSF by Wehi-3 cells than by L1210 cells (our data and 23).

According to a histological classification of the colonies obtained with GM-CSF from the tumor cells, both tumor types seem to secrete also CSF_{GM} (12), in addition to CSF_M and CSF_G, the only two subclasses found in the supernatants of Mϕ. There are no significant differences concerning the amount of GM-CSF subclasses secreted by both tumor lines. All inhibitors of tumor cell growth used in our experiments, poly ICLC, LPS, and IF, are potent stimulators of GM-CSF secretion by Wehi-3 or L1210 cells as well, thus confirming previous findings on the effect of LPS on GM-CSF secretion by both tumor lines (23). The dose-response relationship resembles much that one obtained with Mϕ, and the drug concentrations inducing optimal GM-CSF synthesis are virtually the same. The percent increase in GM-CSF secretion above control values after drug contact is very similar for each drug in both tumor lines, whereas the absolute amounts of GM-CSF secreted by L1210 cells are still significantly lower than those secreted by Wehi-3 cell.

Analogous to the situation with Mϕ, there was a tendency for an increase in the number of pure Mϕ/monocyte colonies and simultaneously to reduce the number of pure granulocyte and mixed colonies induced by supernatants of both tumor lines after treatment with one of the active drugs. MVE-2, similar to its lack of in vitro activity on GM-CSF synthesis by Mϕ, also failed to stimulate the GM-CSF synthesis by both tumor lines for unknown reasons.

In contrast to the situation with Mϕ and some Mϕ tumor lines, including Wehi-3 (67), both tumor lines tested by us produced only minimal amounts of PGE ($<$ 100 pg/ml), which were not further increased by any of the drugs used. This would support previous reports indicating that the GM-CSF production is not absolutely dependent upon PGE synthesis, because the former occurred also in the absence of PGE synthesis, as seen with murine or human mononuclear phagocytes treated with indomethacin (29,30). The synthesis of GM-CSF by both tumor lines seemed also to be independent from any constitutive or reactive IF secretion, which would support our findings obtained with Mϕ.

REFERENCES

1. G. P. Bodey, M. Buckley, Y. S. Sathe, and E. Freireich, *Ann. Intern. Med.*, *64*:328-340 (1966).

2. A. C. Eaves and W. R. Bruce, *Cancer Chem. Rep.*, *58*:813-820 (1974).
3. J. H. Hendry, N. G. Testa, and L. G. Lajtha, *Radiat. Res.*, *59*:645-652 (1974).
4. W. Chu-Tse and L. G. Lajtha, *Int. J. Radiat. Biol.*, *27*:41-50 (1975).
5. N. M. Blackett, J. C. Marsh, M. Y. Gordon, S. F. Okell, and M. Aguado, *Exp. Hemat.*, *6*:2-8 (1978).
6. G. E. Francis and G. A. Tuma, *Brit. J. Haematology*, *49*:259-267 (1981).
7. N. G. Testa, J. H. Hendry, and L. G. Lajtha, *Biomedicine, 21*:431-434 (1974).
8. K. F. Hübner, N. Gengozian, and T. A. Gilman, *Int. J. Radiat. Biol.*, *28*:301-312 (1975).
9. H. Croizat and E. Trindel, *Exp. Hemat.*, *8*:185-191 (1980).
10. M. Onoda, M. Shinoda, K. Tsuneoka, and M. Shikita, *J. Cell. Physiol.*, *104*:11-19
11. T. R. Bradley and D. Metcalf, *Aust. J. Exp. Biol. Med. Sci.*, *44*:287-299 (1966).
12. D. Metcalf, *Hemopoietic Colonies. In Vitro Cloning of Normal and Leukemic Cells*, Springer Verlag, Berlin, 1977.
13. A. W. Burgess, D. Metcalf, and S. M. Watt, *J. Supramol. Struct.*, *8*:489-500 (1978).
14. E. R. Stanley, G. Hansen, J. Woodcock, and D. Metcalf, *Fed. Proc.*, *34*:2272 (1975).
15. R. N. Apte and D. H. Pluznik, *J. Cell. Physiol.*, *89*:313-323 (1976).
16. R. K. Shadduck, A. L. Carsten, G. Chikkappa, E. P. Cronkite, and E. Gerard, *Soc. Exp.. Bio. Med., 158*:542-549 (1978).
17. J. W. Parker and D. Metcalf, *J. Immunol.*, *26*:1039-1049 (1974).
18. M. A. S. Moore and N. Williams, *J. Cell. Physiol.*, *80*:195-206 (1972).
19. P. A. Chervenick and A. F. LoBuglio, *Science*, *178*:164-166 (1972).
20. M. J. Cline, B. Rothman, and D. W. Golde, *J. Cell. Physiol.*, *84*:193-196 (1974).
21. H. E. Broxmeyer, *Blood*, *51*:889-901 (1978).
22. P. Ralph, M. A. S. Moore, and K. Nilsson, *J. Exp. Med.*, *143*:1528-1533 (1976).
23. P. Ralph, H. E. Broxmeyer, M. A. S. Moore, and J. Nakoinz, *Cancer Res.*, *38*:1414-1419 (1978).
24. D. R. Webb, *Prostaglandin Med.*, *1*:441-453 (1978).
25. E. Razin, S. Bauminger, and A. Golberson, *Res. J. Reticuloendothel. Soc.*, *23*:237-242 (1978).
26. R. M. Schultz, N. A. Pavlidis, W. A. Stylos, and M. A. Chirigos, *Science*, *202*:320-321 (1978).
27. D. R. Webb and I. Nowowiejski, *Cell Immunol.*, *33*:1-10 (1977).
28. R. Lomnitzer, A. R. Rabson, and H. J. Koornhof, *Clin. Exp. Immunol.*, *24*:42-48 (1976).
29. J. I. Kurland, H. E. Broxmeyer, L. M. Pelus, R. S. Bockman, and M. A. S. Moore, *Blood*, *52*:388-407 (1978).
30. R. N. Moore, R. Urbaschek, L. M. Wahl, and S. E. Mergenhagen, *Infect. Immun.*, *26*:408-414 (1979).
31. P. Pouillart, T. Palangié, L. Schwarzenberg, H. Brugerie, I. Lhéritier, and G. Mathé, *Cancer Immunol. Immunother.*, *1*:163-169 (1976).
32. R. S. Foster, B. MacPherson, and D. A. Browdie, *Cancer Res., 37*:1349-1355 (1977).
33. J. R. Maisin, G. B. Gerber, M. Lambiet-Collier, and G. Mattelin, *Radiat. Res.*, *82*: 487-497 (1980).
34. M. Y. Gordon, M. Aguado, and N. M. Blackett, *Eur. J. Cancer*, *13*:229-233 (1977).
35. C. Burgaleta and D. W. Golde, *Cancer Res.*, *37*:1739-1742 (1977).
36. H. E. Broxmeyer and P. Ralph, *Cancer Res.*, *37*:3578-3584 (1977).
37. E. M. Shevach, J. D. Stobo, and I. Green, *Immunology*, *108*:1146-1152 (1972).
38. W. A. Stylos, M. A. Chirigos, V. Papademetriou, and L. Lauer, *J. Immunopharmacol.*, *2*:113-132 (1980).
39. R. N. Buick, S. E. Fry, and S. E. Salmon, *Cancer, 45*:1238-1242 (1980).

40. S. E. Salmon and R. N. Buick, *Cancer Res.*, *39*:1133-1136 (1979).
41. S. Ladisch, G. H. Reaman, and D. G. Poplack, *Cancer Res.*, *39*/2544-2546 (1979).
42. L. Steel and M. Kaliner, *J. Biol. Chem.*, *256*:12692-12698 (1981).
43. M. A. Chirigos, A. Bartocci, and E. Read, in *Mediation of Cellular Immunity in Cancer by Immune Modifiers* (M. A. Chirigos, M. Mitchell, M. J. Mastrangelo, and M. Krim, eds.), Raven Press, New York, 1981, pp. 77-88.
44. R. B. Herberman, in *Mediation of Cellular Immunity in Cancer by Immune Modifiers* (M. A. Chirigos, M. Mitchell, M. J. Mastrangelo, and M. Krim, eds.), Raven Press, New York, 1981, pp. 261-267.
45. A. Bartocci, E. L. Read, R. D. Welker, E. Schlick, V. Papademetriou, and M. A. Chirigos, *Cancer Res.*, *43*:3514-3518 (1982).
46. E. Ribi, J. Cantrell, S. Schwartzman, and R. Parker, in *Augmenting Agents in Cancer Therapy* (E. M. Hersh, M. A. Chirigos, and M. J. Mastrangelo, eds.), Raven Press, New York, 1981, pp. 15-33.
47. R. L. Tuttle and J. Cantrell, in *Augmenting Agents in Cancer Therapy* (E. M. Hersh, M. A. Chirigos, and M. J. Mastrangelo, eds.), Raven Press, New York, 1981, pp. 91-100.
48. L. M. Wahl, S. M. Wahl, S. E. Mergenhagen, and G. R. Martin, *Proc. Natl. Acad. Sci. USA*, *71*:3598-3601 (1974).
49. J. B. Weinberg, H. A. Chapman, and J. B. Hibbs, *J. Immunol.*, *121*:72-80 (1978).
50. R. N. Apte, C. F. Hertogs, and D. H. Pluznik, *J. Immunol.*, *124*:1223-1229 (1980).
51. N. Maehara and M. Ho, *Infect. Immun.*, *15*:78-83 (1977).
52. G. Renoux and M. Renoux, *J. Immunopharmacol.*, *1*:247-267 (1979).
53. G. Renoux and M. Renoux, in *Augmenting Agents in Cancer Therapy* (E. M. Hersh, M. A. Chirigos, and M. J. Mastrangelo, eds.), Raven Press, New York, 1981, pp. 427-440.
54. M. A. Chirigos, E. Schlick, M. Piccoli, E. Read, K. Hartung, and A. Bartocci, in *Advances in Immunopharmacology*, Pergamon Press, New York, in press.
55. D. Metcalf and M. A. S. Moore, in *Hemopoietic Cells*, North Holland, Amsterdam, 1971.
56. J. Kurland and M. A. S. Moore, *Exp. Hematol.*, *5*:357-373 (1977).
57. F. W. Ruscetti and P. A. Chervenick, *J. Lab. Clin. Med.*, *83*:64-72 (1974).
58. A. Mangalik and W. A. Robinson, *Proc. Soc. Exp. Biol. Med.*, *158*:151-155 (1978).
59. E. R. Stanley and L. J. Guilbert, *J. Immunol. Meth.*, *42*:253-284 (1981).
60. M. A. Chirigos, V. Papademetriou, A. Bartocci, E. Read, and H. B. Levy, *Int. J. Immunopharmacol.*, *3*:329-337 (1981).
61. L. M. Pelus, H. E. Broxmeyer, M. DeSousa, and M. A. S. Moore, *J. Immunol.*, *126*: 1016-1021 (1981).
62. S. Motomura and T. M. Dexter, *Exp. Hematol.*, *8*:298-303 (1980).
63. P. Ralph and J. Nakoinz, *Cancer Res.*, *37*:546-550 (1977).
64. P. Ralph, H. E. Broxmeyer, and J. Nakoinz, *J. Exp. Med.*, *146*:611-616 (1977).
65. M. Maeda and Y. Ichikawa, *J. Cell. Physiol.*, *105*:323-331 (1980).
66. M. Maeda, Y. Ichikawa, and J. Azuma, *J. Cell. Physiol.*, *105*:33-38 (1980).
67. J. I. Kurland, L. M. Peuls, P. Ralph, R. S. Bockman, and M. A. S. Moore, *Proc. Natl. Acad. Sci. USA*, 76:2326-2330 (1979).

Section D

Endocrine Regulation of Immunity

26

Endocrine Regulation of Host Immunity

The Role of Steroids and Thymosin

Nicholas R. Hall and Allan L. Goldstein The George Washington University School of Medicine and Health Sciences, Washington, D.C.

I. INTRODUCTION

Differences in the ability of males and females to resist disease have been documented since the early part of the twentieth century. Mobius in 1903 (1) reported that females were less disposed than males to contract a variety of diseases including meningitis, pneumonia, syphilis, and typhoid fever. That this difference might be associated with the functioning of the thymus was suggested by Hammar (2) when he found that gonadectomy could result in hypertrophy of this gland. Since these early discoveries, it has subsequently been confirmed that not only are females generally less prone to infections, but that they are able to produce higher antibody titers than are males (3-8).

Stress has also been found to exert profound effects upon immunological mechanisms. As early as the second century A.D., Galen noted that melancholy women were more susceptible to cancer than were sanguine women. It is now known that activation of the pituitary-adrenal axis is responsible for many of the adverse consequences of stress upon an individual's ability to resist disease, a subject that has recently been reviewed (9,10).

It has been established that the generally enhanced state of immunity in females is due in part to the actions of gonadal steroids acting upon various parameters of immunity. Stress effects are mediated in part by the action of adrenal corticosteroids. Furthermore, recent evidence indicates that thymic hormones are able to influence the production of both gonadal and adrenal steroids. Nonsteroid hormones, such as somatotropin, thyroxin, and insulin as well as others, have also been found to influence the course of immunogenesis and to interact with thymic hormones. However, because of the large amount of evidence implicating steroids in the control of immunogenesis, this review will be restricted to this particular class of hormone. The one exception will be a discussion of the effects of adrenal catecholamines upon immunological measures since this is an important class of hormones released during the course of stress.

The emphasis upon steroids should not be interpreted as reflecting our belief that this class of hormone exerts a predominant influence upon immunity. To the contrary, somatotropin and thyroxine in particular have been shown to have profound effects upon immunity (11,12). It is only in the interest of continuity and space that the steroids have been selected for extensive review. Furthermore, there is recent evidence that thymosin peptides interact with the reproductive and stress circuits at the level of the hypothalamic-hypophyseal axis.

The artificial division of the immune system into reticuloendothelial, cellular, and humoral compartments has some advantages in academic and empirical settings. However, it is most disadvantageous when attempting to ask mechanistic questions because of the interactions that occur between these compartments. For example, detection of antibody titers to a complex T-dependent antigen requires viable macrophages, T lymphocytes, and B lymphocytes. Evidence to be cited in this review indicates that each of these cell populations can be influenced by manipulation of the endocrine system. Therefore, while a particular assay may be used to detect antibody production by plasma cells, a change in titer following hormonal manipulation might very well be the consequence of an effect upon the thymus or reticuloendothelial system—not necessarily the plasma cell. Nonetheless, for the purpose of formulating a working hypothesis of the underlying mechanism(s) by which steroids interact with the immune system, studies will be grouped on the basis of whether the measured index was a phagocytic response, a T-cell response, or a B-cell response.

One final note of caution before delving into a review of this subject should be heeded: all of the steroid hormones to be discussed, with the possible exception of the thymic-derived group, have established roles in regulating a variety of physiological functions, functions that when interfered with can have far-reaching effects upon the entire homeostatic milieu of the organism. Therefore, correlating the manipulation of a particular hormone with an altered state of immunity does not necessarily establish that hormone as a specific immunological response modifier. The measured changes may well be due to altered glucose metabolism, blood flow, or ionic balance and so forth, which in turn could have an adverse or beneficial effect upon many systems, not just host defense.

II. RETICULOENDOTHELIAL SYSTEM

Macrophages play an important role in both the initiation and regulation of the immune response (13). For optimal production of antibody to some antigens, cooperation between macrophages, T cells, and B cells is necessary (14,15). Macrophages are also necessary for optimal differentiation of T lymphocytes by mitogens (16). But under some conditions, such as high density, macrophages can be inhibitory (17,18). Macrophages have also been shown to have inhibitory effects in animals challenged with *Corynebacterium parvum* (19), in animals undergoing graft-versus-host reactions (20), and in animals with some virally induced tumors (21). Therefore, it is important to consider this population of cells in any discussion of hormonal effects upon immunity.

A. Catecholamines

Catecholamines produced by the adrenal gland have been implicated in altering the function of macrophages. α- and β-adrenergic receptors are present on the surface of phagocytic cells and, when stimulated, can result in elevated levels of intracellular cyclic GMP (cGMP) or cyclic AMP (cAMP) (22-29). That the catecholamines may be capable of interfering with the biological functions of these cells is suggested by the evidence that elevated cAMP is able to decrease the release of lysosomal hydrolases (30). While the catecholamines have been implicated in influencing phagocytic cells, it is difficult to discern whether all of these influences occur via endocrine pathways or whether autonomic pathways might be involved. Evidence of autonomic involvement has been reviewed elsewhere (9).

B. Adrenal Corticosteroids

Most of the adrenal influences upon the phagocytic cells appear to be via corticosteroids produced by the adrenal cortex. It has also been widely regarded that this influence is of an inhibitory nature based upon a number of studies correlating various forms of stress with depressed functioning of the reticuloendothelial system (31-36). Depression is certainly an effect that corticosteroids are able to exert upon macrophages. But under some conditions, enhanced phagocytic activity has also been described.

Measuring the uptake of ^{51}Cr-labeled human red blood cells in mice subjected to sublethal mechanical or thermal trauma, Schildt (37) reported biphasic changes. The ability of macrophages to engulf the labeled cells was indeed reduced during the early posttrauma days, but within 6 days, uptake was considered to be at normal levels while at 16 days posttrauma uptake was significantly elevated. Similar biphasic changes have been reported in humans subjected to sleep deprivation (38) and following surgical trauma (39). However, in the latter study, the changes occurred within hours instead of days. Recovery was noted at 2.5 hr after surgery with enhanced phagocytic activity by 3-4 hr. If these observations were due to activation of the hypothalamic-hypophyseal-adrenal axis, then experimental elevation of glucocorticoids would be expected to duplicate the effects of generalized stress. This expected duplication appears to occur, at least in some studies. Depressed phagocytic activity of human leukocytes has been reported following administration of adrenocorticotropic hormone (ACTH) or corticosteroids and following ACTH administration (40-41). But polymorphonuclear leukocytes from rabbits have been found to be unaffected by administration of large doses of cortisone for up to 11 days (42). The general morphology as well as intracellular levels of lysozyme, phagocytin, and histone were found not to differ from control cells.

Before discussing a possible mechanism by which these effects might be mediated, it is important to consider the assays that are commonly used to assess the viability of macrophages. Most of the conclusions of hormonal influences upon phagocytosis have been based upon changes in the uptake of finely divided carbon particles, of chromium phosphate, or of cells labeled with radioactive markers. Others are based upon the rate of uptake by macrophages of intravenously administered trypan-blue. While it is true that these techniques probably provide a reliable index of phagocytosis, it must be emphasized that these experimental approaches do not reveal the ability of the cell to destroy the foreign substance after engulfment has occurred.

The necessity to distinguish between the ability of a cell to phagocytize a particle versus the ability to subsequently destroy it has been documented. Chretien and Garagusi (43) found that polymorphonuclear leukocytes from patients treated with corticosteroids were able to phagocytize latex particles in a normal manner. However, reduction of nitroblue tetrazolium was found to be impaired in these cells. Consequently, it was concluded that while corticosteroids do not alter engulfment, they are able to inhibit intracellular killing. A similar conclusion was arrived at by Shilotri and Prasad (41). Bactericidal and hexosemonophosphate shunt activity of human leukocytes were found to be depressed when the donor was treated with ACTH. However, glycolytic activity was found to be normal. Since glycolytic activity is necessary for the uptake of particles by leukocytes, it was concluded that elevated levels of plasma cortisol impaired the ability of these cells to destroy the phagocytized bacteria but not to engulf them.

Determining the effects of hormones only upon phagocytic indices also fails to reveal whether the hormonal effect is direct or upon some factor capable of influencing phagocytosis. While Hirsch and Church (42) reported no effect of large doses of cortisone upon serum opsonic activity in rabbits, Saba (39) found correlations between serum opsonic activity and stress-induced suppression of the RES in humans. The correlation of RES activity and serum opsonins might be due to stress-induced changes in complement proteins with opsonic activity. This possibility is supported by an early observation (44) that ACTH administration to tuberculous patients could result in elevated complement activity. Thus, an increase in serum opsonins would be expected to increase the ability of macrophages to engulf a foreign configuration without necessarily affecting the lytic activity of the cell. If corticosteroids alter the ability of the macrophage to lyse particles, but by an independent mechanism can also bring about changes in serum opsonins, this would provide an explanation for some of the apparent contradictions reported in the literature.

In addition to modulating the ability of macrophages to phagocytize and subsequently to lyse foreign substances, there is evidence that corticosteroids can influence the ability of macrophages to regulate antibody production by lymphocytes. It has been shown that there is a correlation between depressed serum corticosteriod levels and the ability of mouse mononuclear phagocytes to influence the antibody response to sheep red blood cells (SRBCs) (45). Reduced serum corticosterone did not affect antibody production when 2×10^8 SRBCs were injected, but when 2×10^9 cells were administered a twofold increase in antibody titer was measured. It was also found that the number of monocytes increased when serum corticosterone was reduced, suggesting that the elevated number of monocytes was able to circumvent the proposed high-dose tolerance resulting from the large amount of administered antigen.

C. Gonadal Steroids

In general, the most potent stimulants of phagocytosis are the estrogenic hormones. The influence of this group of hormones on the phagocytic activity of the reticuloendothelial system appears to bear a direct relationship to their known estrogenic activity (46). It may be noted that although the androgen testosterone has little or no effect on the rate of phagocytosis, it, as well as thyroxine, will potentiate the activity of the estrogen when administered together with the latter. This particular property of testosterone is unexpected since the actions of this steroid generally are antagonistic to the biological response of the estrogens. These data may reflect the possibility that the estrogen molecule has two biological activities, one acting on the reticuloendothelial system and the other on the reproductive tract, and that these actions may be manifested independently (47).

A detailed study was described of the influence of the estrous cycle, pregnancy, and ovariectomy on reticuloendothelial activity (48). This was based on previous observations (49) that the administration of estrogenic hormones stimulated the appearance and activity of phagocytic cells in the endometrium of the uterine horns of the guinea pig. Other studies from the same laboratory had indicated that substances possessing estrogenic activity were among the most potent stimulators of reticuloendothelial cell activity (46). Utilizing a standard carbon clearance technique, two peaks of reticuloendothelial activity have been observed in the rat and mouse during the estrus cycle; one during the follicular phase and the other during the luteal phase at the time of endometrial degeneration (48). Two peaks of activity were also noted during pregnancy; one at the time of implantation and the other approaching the end of pregnancy prior to parturition. After ovariectomy, reticuloendothelial activity declined.

These studies establish catecholamines, adrenal corticosteroids, and gonadal steroids as potential regulatory hormones upon normal functioning of the reticuloendothelial system. In addition to their effects upon this important population of cells, they also have profound effects upon T- and B-lymphocyte measures.

III. CELLULAR IMMUNITY

A. Corticosteroids

It is widely accepted that activation of the hypophyseal-adrenal axis by a variety of stressors results in deleterious effects upon the ability of the organism to mount a successful defense against infectious agents. But when the effects of corticosteroids upon the thymus and T lymphocytes are examined using different experimental protocols, it becomes apparent that the mechanism underlying this overall suppression may be extremely complex. Hormones released by activation of the adrenal cortex have been found to alter thymocytes and thymic epithelial cells, as well as blood flow through this important gland.

A number of investigations have revealed the presence of receptors capable of binding cortiocosteroids associated with T lymphocytes. These receptors are primarily associated with the immature thymocytes that reside in the thymic cortex (50-51). Treatment of mice with hydrocortisone acetate has been found to destroy approximately 95% of these cells within a very short period of time (52). That this killing is due to corticosteroids acting upon the receptors is suggested by evidence that steroid-resistant mouse lymphoma cells have fewer receptors or else do not translocate the steroid-receptor complex into the nucleus (53-55). However, others have suggested that the suppressive effects of corticosteroids may not necessarily be due to the presence of specific receptors (56-57).

The suppressive effect of corticosteroids is also supported by early reports of histological changes in thymic tissues from corticosteroid-treated animals. Within a few hours after steroid administration, nuclear pyknosis and lymphocytolysis were associated with the thymic cortex (58-62). In addition, there are reports that corticosteroids are able to inhibit protein synthesis as well as the mitotic activity of thymocytes (60,63-65). Many studies since these investigations document the fact that lysis of cells within the cortex can indeed occur (10).

In addition, there is evidence that following the administration of corticosteroids, there is a migration of thymocytes to other immunological compartments. Some investigators have suggested that the thymocytes are not destroyed, but instead are redistributed to the bone marrow (66-71). This hypothesis is supported by the observation that there is enhanced responsivity by bone marrow cells when tested in several T-cell assays. These include assays for mitogenic stimulation, T-helper function, and graft versus host reactions (72-74). Nonetheless, there is the alternative interpretation that corticosteroids might induce some of these responses directly.

In guinea pigs, a species in which migration is supposed to occur (67), it has been reported that repeated injections of ACTH does result in increased cellularity of bone marrow (75). However, the increases were of myeloid and erythroid cells with no detectable change in bone marrow lymphocytes. The mechanism by which cells could rapidly leave the thymus might involve a change in blood flow through this gland. After a single injection of prednisolone, blood flow through the guinea pig thymus has been found to increase by twofold within 3 hr. Maximum flow occurred at 6 hr after injection with a return to normal starting after 24 hr (69). Blood flow through the submandibular gland was measured for control purposes, but no change was reported following steroid treatment. Using autoradiographic techniques, it was shown by the same author that the percentage of thymocytes in the thymic vein and carotid artery blood was also increased at 3 and 6 hr (70).

Regardless of whether lysis or migration predominates, the mouse thymic cortex becomes repopulated over a period of 7-14 days (76). This is also consistent with observations made by Larsson (70) that by 6 days, there is a net import of cells into the thymus of steroid-treated guinea pigs. These similarities between the mouse and guinea pig are important because guinea pigs are considered to be less sensitive to the immunosuppressive effects of corticosteroids than are mice (10).

Not all investigators have reported simply inhibition of the response being measured. Just as biphasic effects of stress and steroids were reported in studies of macrophages, similar results have been reported with respect to lymphocytes. Concanavalin A (ConA) stimulation of mouse lymphocytes has been found to be depressed up to 15 days after sound stress, but elevated after 25 days. In addition, there is evidence that different types of stress can differentially affect the immune response. Acute stress has been found to be inhibitory while prolonged or chronic stress can be stimulatory (77).

These effects were probably mediated by corticosteroids since treatment with this class of hormones has been reported to produce similar changes. It has been found that prednisolone, when administered to human patients, can result in a decrease in E-rosette-forming lymphocytes and phytohemagglutinin (PHA) responsiveness at 4-6 hr with a reversal to supranormal levels by 24 hr (78). Mouse spleen cells also show an elevated response to PHA at certain times after hydrocortisone acetate treatment (79).

Some of these biphasic effects of corticosteroids on T cells appeared to be dose dependent. In an in vitro study of embryonic mouse thymocyte development, Ritter (80) reported varied effects of corticosterone, depending upon the dose used. It was found that levels of corticosterone approximating physiological levels had an enhancing effect resulting in higher numbers of Thy 1.2 cells, while supranormal doses had an inhibitory effect. At the higher doses, the small lymphocytes appeared to be selectively killed while medium and large cells were left intact. Others have reported dose-dependent changes in electrokinetic properties and mitogen responsiveness of thymocytes from mice treated with steroids in vivo (81). Treatment with hydrocortisone decreased the spontaneous synthesis of DNA after 24 hr of incubation which coincided with the disappearance of cells of medium electrophoretic mobility. However, mitogenic responsiveness varied depending upon the dose of hydrocortisone. Lower doses enhanced thymocyte differentiation in response to PHA and ConA while higher doses were inhibitory. ConA responsiveness was affected most by the higher steroid doses, an observation consistent with the fact that the less mature, more steroid-sensitive thymocytes are most responsive to ConA stimulation (82).

In addition to differential responses of thymocytes depending upon the dose of corticosteroids, there is also evidence that there are differential effects depending upon the age of the animal (83). Newborn cells were found to be more susceptible to killing by cortisol than were thymocytes from older animals, and thymocytes from 6-day-old mice were more sensitive than were cells from 30-day-old animals.

Manipulating corticosteroids by treatment with amino glutethimide phosphate (AGP) or by adrenalectomy has also been found to alter T-cell function as well as distribution (84). Adrenalectomy or AGP treatment at any age resulted in enhanced delayed hypersensitivity to SRBCs. Furthermore, adrenalectomy at 3 weeks of age or continuous AGP resulted in an enlarged thymus, as well as a decrease in the cellularity of lymph nodes and an increase in the number of blood leukocytes. These changes were reversed with restoration of adrenal function. But after AGP administration at less than 3 weeks of age, changes in delayed hypersensitivity responsivity were not restored upon recovery of adrenal function. These data were cited as evidence for a role of corticosteroids in the ontogeny of the immune response.

An important function of some T cells is the production and release of a variety of substances that have biological influences upon various aspects of immunity. One such lymphokine is interferon. Since stress and elevated corticosteroids have been found to alter the number and distribution of T lymphocytes, it follows that interferon production might also be affected. Furhtermore, it would not be inconsistent with the previously cited observations if the effects were found to be biphasic.

While facilitative and inhibitory effects of corticosteroids upon interferon levels have not been reported in the same study, each effect has been documented separately. Generalized stress in humans has been found to be associated with elevated interferon production (38). A similar increase has been observed in mice exposed to electric shock (85). But in the latter study, elevations were seen only when stress preceded the administration of Newcastle disease virus by 5 hr. Electric shock was found to have no effect when applied during interferon production. While Solomon et al. (85) reported no effect of exogenous ACTH or corticosteroid administration upon interferon, they did observe that adrenalectomized mice had elevated interferon levels.

In contrast to these studies, others have reported that both psychological stress and corticosteroid administration affected interferon levels in mice (86). However, instead of an increase, 5 mg of cortisone 6-24 hr prior to intravenous administration of Newcastle disease virus resulted in depressed interferon responses in both serum and spleen. Chang and Rasmussen (87) also reported decreased interferon production in mice following high-intensity sound stress. While these discrepancies might well be regarded as glaring inconsistencies, they are quite consistent with some of the previously discussed biphasic effects of corticosteroids upon other aspects of immunity.

In addition to lymphocytes, epithelial cells are found within the thymus and are an integral part of the endocrine role played by this gland (88). Very little is known of the direct influence that the pituitary-adrenal axis has upon these cells, although there is evidence that ACTH is capable of inhibiting them (89). Tentative data have also been reported suggesting that there may be direct effects of glucocorticoids upon thymic hormone production. Comsa et al. (90), using a spectrophotometric assay, reported that corticosterone and desoxycorticosterone, when given to adrenalectomized rats, resulted in above-normal thymic hormone levels in the thymus. However, since tissues were pooled only one data point was given for each group, precluding statistical interpretation of the data.

B. Gonadal Steroids

In contrast to the apparent facilitative effect of physiological levels of estrogen upon phagocytic activity, high doses of estrogen appear to suppress DNA synthesis in the thymus and in thymic-dependent tissues (91,92). Indeed, extremely high doses have been found to be thymolytic, inducing wasting syndrome in neonatal mice (93-97). These thymolytic effects appear to be independent of adrenal activation since estrogen-induced thymic involution has been demonstrated in adrenalectomized rats (98). Furthermore, if anything, estradiol infusion into the adrenal circulation has been found to inhibit corticosteroid secretion (73). In one such study newborn mice were injected three times weekly with 0.05 mg of estradiol. At 3 weeks, there was a reduction in thymus size, as well as disruption of cortical and medullary cellularity. By 5 weeks, the thymus gland remained small, although there were no longer signs of thymic necrosis and the corticomedullary ratios had returned toward normal (95).

The effects of estrogen upon mitogenic activity and normal functioning of cellular immunity appear to parallel those of corticosteroids. Low concentrations of estrogen have been found to stimulate mitosis in immunocompetent cells, while high concentrations appear to be inhibitory (100). High doses have also been reported to decrease the PHA responsiveness of peripheral blood leukocytes and to block DNA synthesis of T lymphocytes (93,100-102). Consistent with the inhibitory effects of estradiol upon thymus growth and cellularity are reports that high doses of estrogen can delay graft rejection (103,104) and inhibit delayed hypersensitivity.

Another type of lymphocyte susceptible to the effects of estrogen is the natural killer cell (NKC). These cells are not only derived from bone marrow but also require it for continued generation (106). Continuous administration of estradiol, starting at 4 weeks of age, has been reported to result in decreased NKC activity in spleens from both male and female mice (107). Surprisingly, neither overiectomy nor castration was found to alter NKC activity. The inhibitory effects of estradiol were reversible, athough recovery required an 8-week period. While much of the evidence suggests that estrogen effects upon immunity are mediated by the thymus, neonatal thymectomy was found to have no effect upon the inhibitory influence of estradiol upon NKC activity. Because natural killer cells are bone marrow dependent (106), the possibility that the reported changes merely reflected a decrease in bone marrow volume had to be considered. But in a subsequent study, it was reported that the changes in NKC activity proceeded more rapidly than did changes in the bone marrow volume (107). This latter observation suggests a more direct and specific effect of estrogen upon this population of cells.

IV. HUMORAL IMMUNITY

A. Corticosteroids

Effects of stress and corticosteroids upon B-lymphocyte function have been well documented. In many instances, the effects upon B-cell assays have been found to be biphasic just as corticosteroid effects upon T-cell and macrophage assays were. At high concentrations, corticosteroids have been shown to have inhibitory effects upon antibody formation and mitogen responsiveness (10). However, at physiological concentrations, not only do corticosteroids exert stimulatory effects, but when evaluated in some paradigms are necessary for antibody formation to occur. Normally, serum is necessary when inducing antibody production using cultured lymphocytes. But in the absence of serum, 0.01-1 μM of hydrocortisone as a media supplement can support in vitro antibody production (119).

Evidence that adrenal hormones are able to exert facilitative effects upon immunoglobulin production has been reported for almost four decades. In one of the earliest studies it was found that adrenal cortical extract, given either in conjunction with antigens (120) or after immunization (121) could increase circulating antibody titers. Later Roberts et al. (122,123) examined the extent of production and release of antibody in vitro by tissues obtained from immunized rats and mice. The data demonstrated that the relative degree of antibody production among various tissues was related to the schedule and route of administration of antigen and that adrenalectomy prior to immunization delayed and depressed the production and release of immunoglobulins by lymphoid tissues.

These initial reports of the ability of adrenal cortical hormones to augment antibody production have been confirmed in some laboratories (119,124-127) but not in others (128-131). A possible explanation of these discrepant results is provided by the studies of Halpern et al. (126,127). These investigators were able to demonstrate both effects of cortisone (i.e, an augmentation and a depression of circulating antibody titers in rabbits). The animals were immunized with egg albumin; when significant quantities of antibody were present in the serum, the rabbits received another injection of the antigen in an amount adequate to reduce almost to zero the antibody titers. The animals were then divided into two groups: one received a single injection of cortisone and the other served as controls. Within 24-48 hr, the cortisone-injected animals exhibited a significant level of serum antibody, while antibody titers in the control rabbits were negligible. However, after the third day, the antibody levels in the steroid-treated rabbits began to drop to levels below that of the control group. When the latter had recovered completely their original level of antibody, generally after the fifth day following antigen administration, the animals treated with steroid had a lower precipitin level than the control rabbits. The increase in the serum antibody levels observed in the first 48 hr in the cortisone-injected animals was attributed to the lysis of lymphocytes which might have contained antibody (132) since the rise in antibody titers in the serum and the decrease in the number of lymphocytes in the blood and tissues paralleled one another. There might also have occurred a stimulatory effect of the steroid upon antibody production.

Experiments of the type just described emphasize the importance of the relationships of the schedules of administration of corticosteroids and of antigen in influencing the rate of antibody production. These variables may afford a possible explanation for the conflicting findings of authors who have observed an early acute increase in antibodies in the blood as a result of adrenal steroid treatment of previously immunized animals and, on the other hand, of those investigators who have reported a depressing effect of the steroid hormone on the production of antibody when administered during the sensitization period.

It may be of experimental significance in resolving certain of these discrepancies of the immunogenic influence of adrenal steroids to give consideration not only to schedule of administration and dose of antigen and of steroid, but also to the ratio of these two agents. Perhaps yet another factor may be the evidence that the ratio of lymphoid cells that undergo differentiation to antibody-producing cells are influenced not only by the dose of antigen but also by its properties (133). Regardless, the possibility that adrenal cortical hormones may, under specific conditions, enhance immunogenicity has been overshadowed by the more dramatic consequences of severe immunosuppression following the use of pharmacological doses of adrenal steroids.

Corticosteroids have also been found to influence immediate hypersensitivity reactions. Bogdanova and Kopytovskaya (134) reported that adrenalectomy increased the susceptibility of mice to anaphylaxis and that this increase could be reversed with exogenous cortisol. This finding could have been due to any of several known actions of corticosteroids on histamine, including inhibition of its synthesis, release, and/or binding to receptors (135-137).

In a subsequent experiment, it was found that surgical or pharmacological adrenalectomy (using metopirone) counteracted the anaphylactic shock-inhibiting effect of tuber cinereum lesions in the hypothalamus (138). It was concluded that the shock-inhibiting effect of tuberal lesions was due in part to hyperplasia and hyperfunction of the adrenal cortex.

B. Gonadal Steroids

Evidence has already been discussed suggesting that estrogens are able to influence macrophages and T lymphocytes. But, in addition, direct effects of estrogen upon antibody-producing cells also appear to occur.

In one series of experiments estradiol was administered at varying times relative to antigen administration (100). Significant increases in splenic PFCs were observed following a single injection of 2.5 μg of estradiol from 1 day prior to antigen until 3.5 days afterwards. Animals were sacrificed on day 4. Although administration of the steroid 1 day prior to or 1 day after the antigen injection resulted in the highest numbers of antibody-producing cells, the fact that an influence was observed long after the antigen had been phagocytosed suggested a nonphagocytic influence upon antibody production. This hypothesis was further supported by in vitro studies in which physiological amounts of estradiol were able to alter the proliferation of antibody-forming cells long after antigen processing.

But the type of influence depended at least in part upon the concentration of estradiol that was administered. Concentrations of 50-5000 pg/ml resulted in significant increases of PFCs. While not significant, a decrease was observed with concentrations of 20 ng/ml. Similar findings were reported when uptake of tritiated thymidine was examined. Increased uptake was observed in both thymic and splenic lymphocytes after 24 hr of incubation with 500 pg/ml.

Other investigators have reported enhancing effects of estrogen upon serum immunoglobulins (100,139-141). Increased IgA and IgG in rat uterine tissue have been reported at stages of the estrus cycle when endogenous estrogen levels are at maximum levels (142). IgG levels have been found to be highest at proestrus but hardly detectable at other times and following ovariectomy. IgA is also highest at proestrus but unlike IgG remains elevated at estrus. Both classes of immunoglobulins were elevated in uterine secretions after estradiol administration, although not in serum. The effects of estradiol were specific since progesterone, cortisol, and dihydrotestosterone were ineffective in stimulating uterine levels of IgA and IgG.

Suppressive effects of estrogen upon immunoglobulin production have been reported by several investigators (93,143), although as discussed in a previous section, these effects are probably mediated by the thymus. It should be noted, however, that some of the reported "facilitative" effects of estradiol may not be inconsistent with those data revealing inhibitory effects upon antibody production. In assessing serum antibody titers to an antigen, elevated levels could occur in one of two ways: increased production or decreased decay. Correlations between estrogen and increases in serum immunoglobulin levels may be due to inhibition of titer decay (144). It was found that although estradiol administration to female guinea pigs decreased the rate of attainment as well as the magnitude of the antibody response, it also decreased the rate of titer decay. Thus, at 7 weeks antibody titers were reduced in estrogen-treated animals relative to oil-injected controls. But at 8 and 9 weeks the titers were higher than controls. The possibility that a reduction of T-suppressor cells allowed for sustained antibody production in the decay phase of the immune response was suggested by the authors. However, a more generalized mechanism also should be considered, especially since hepatic necrosis has been reported in mice receiving exogenous estrogen (145).

C. Catecholamines

Catecholamines produced by both the sympathetic nervous system and by chromaffin cells in the adrenal medulla have been implicated in the modulation of immunity. Chemical sympathectomy, using the drug 6-hydroxydopamine (6-OHDA), has been found to have profound effects upon the immune system. Administration of 10-300 mg/kg of 6-OHDA to mice resulted in a significant depression of antibody to sheep red blood cells (SRBCs) (146). Antibodies against this T-cell-dependent antigen were measured by a plaque-forming cell assay and by determination of the hemagglutination titer. This inhibition was transitory with treated animals having antibody levels no different from control animals 14 days after the drug treatment. The return to normal of antibody production corresponded to the return to normal of norepinephrine content in the spleen. Our own investigations have revealed a similar depression of antibody formation in 6-OHDA-treated mice (147). Decreased numbers of PFCs and hemagglutination titers to SRBCs were found after a single sensitization with SRBCs. Mice were treated with either two injections of 50 mg/kg 6-OHDA or a single injection of 100 mg/kg. Since the antibody response to SRBCs depends upon an interaction of T and B cells, additional parameters of immunity were examined in order to determine if one or both populations of cells had been affected.

Evaluation of thymocyte levels of the enzyme terminal deoxynucleotidyl transferase and serum levels of thymosin α_1 revealed changes that were consistent with both a catecholaminergic and a corticosteroid mechanism. It was concluded that activation of phenethanolaminergic-N-methyltransferase by corticosterone could have resulted in increased serum levels of epinephrine. Therefore, corticosterone acting upon glucocorticoid receptors and elevated epinephrine acting upon supersensitive adrenergic receptors might both have contributed to the observed changes. In support of this hypothesis, 6-OHDA was found to be ineffective in adrenalectomized mice (147).

Other investigators have evaluated the effects of 6-OHDA after repeated injections to newborn rodents. Using this paradigm, either no effect (148) or a significant increase in PFCs has been reported (149). The discrepancy between the newborn and adult paradigms may involve the programming of neuroendocrine systems by the immune system at early stages of development.

Other types of evidence implicate catecholamines in playing a role during the course of immunogenesis. β-Adrenergic receptors do not appear on B lymphocytes unless the cells are actively producing antibody. This conclusion was reached when it was found that up to two-thirds of sensitized splenic leukocytes could be retained by chromatographic columns of insolubilized isoproterenol, a β-adrenergic agonist (150). Similar studies using unsensitized cells that were passed over a column and were subsequently used to reconstitute lethally-irradiated mice also suggested that the receptors do not appear until after sensitization (151). Recipient animals were able to mount an immunological response upon injection of SRBCs. Had the precursor cells had β-adrenergic receptors on their surfaces, they would have been retained by the column, diminishing the antibody reaction.

In contrast to the evidence that antibody-producing cells do not develop β-adrenergic receptors until after sensitization has occurred, T lymphocytes appear to possess these receptors at an earlier state of differentiation (152). Thymic stem cells were found to be responsive to both cAMP and isoproterenol with respect to the induction of the Thy1 alloantigen. In a subsequent study, Singh et al. (153) examined the effects of isoproterenol stimulation upon fetal and adult thymocytes. cAMP was found to be elevated in both populations following treatment with this β-adrenergic stimulator. Propranolol, a β-adrenergic antagonist, selectively blocked this rise. However, it was found that although both fetal and adult thymocytes were able to respond to β-adrenergic stimulation, the cAMP rise in fetal thymocytes was of a greater magnitude than that in adult cells.

These data would suggest a role for β-adrenergic stimulation during the maturation sequence of lymphocytes. They also implicate cAMP as an intracellular agent responsible for the effects of β-adrenergic stimulation. It would appear that the system is balanced by at least two mechanisms capable of causing a rise in intracellular cGMP. Stimulation of α-adrenergic receptors using phenylephrine and of cholinergic receptors using acetylcholine has been found to cause an elevation of this cycle nucleotide (153).

It is always necessary to consider the possibility that in vitro manipulation of lymphocytes may not necessarily reflect the manner by which these cells are modulated in vivo. However, in view of the changes found in TdT levels in thymocytes from 6-OHDA-treated mice, one has to consider the possibility that the catecholamine-depleting drug might exert its effects by interrupting the normal maturation sequence.

V. MECHANISM OF ACTION

A. Adrenal Steroids

The interpretation of data from experiments in which glucocorticoids were manipulated must take into account the chemical characteristics of the steroid. Certain properties are prerequisites for glucocorticoids to possess thymolytic activity. These include an unsaturated A ring, a ketone at position 3 and either an O or OH function at position 11 (154,155). Thus, cortisol, which meets all of these criteria, has the greatest thymolytic activity in mice, followed by cortisone, corticosterone, and dehydroxycorticosterone (155). (It is the relatively greater thymolytic activity associated with cortisol and cortisone that has resulted in the frequent use of these particular forms in both human and rodent studies. This is despite the fact that these forms represent the primary corticosteroid produced in man, not in rodents. Mice and rats synthesize corticosterone.) It is apparent when comparing the structures of various steroid hormones that all of the thymolytic forms have either an OH or O at the 11 position. Naturally occurring hormones lacking in one of these functions also appear to have less thymolytic activity (155).

Not all lymphoid tissues respond in the same way or extent to these different steroids. For example, lymph nodes undergo the greatest amount of involution following treatment with cortisol. Cortisone, corticosterone, and 11-dehydroxycorticosterone are equally effective in contrast to their action upon thymocytes (155).

Part of the difference between the effectiveness of corticosteroids upon thymocyte versus lymphoid cells may be due to the ability of these tissues to catabolize glucocorticoids. In mice, lymph node cells have a greater capacity to oxidize cortisol than do thymic cells, while the murine thymus has a greater capacity for reduction (155). Nonetheless, evidence has been reported showing that the capacity to catabolize steroids can be acquired by lymphocytes by giving the appropriate hormone over a period of time. After 9 days of cortisol administration, the ability of the mouse thymus to oxidize the steroids has been shown to increase (156). It has been suggested that an altered capacity to catabolize corticosteroids may be a form of lymphocyte growth regulation since oxidation of the 11 position or reduction of the 20 position renders the steroid ineffective in suppressing lymphocytes (154).

This has been demonstrated by blocking the interconversion of cortisol and cortisone by a 2-methyl group (155). 2-Methyl cortisol is able to cause involution of lymphoid tissue while 2-methyl cortisone does not. These data were cited as evidence that cortisone is able to affect lymphocytes only when reduced to cortisol. Since these studies were carried out in mice, it is difficult to propose a mechanism involving cortisol and cortisone whereby lymphocytes might regulate their own maturation. However, the possibility that interconversion from biologically active to inactive forms applies to those steroids found in rodents has to be considered. Such interconversion could be part of the mechanism by which corticosteroids might bring about the maturation of lymphocytes—a possibility suggested by Dougherty et al. (155) and supported by previously discussed studies demonstrating a requirement for glucocorticoids for in vitro antibody formation.

Several theories as to the intracellular mechanism of glucocorticoid inhibition of lymphoid cells have been argued in the literature. Nonetheless, the one that has the most supportive data proposes that glucocorticoids inhibit glucose transport (157,159). Significant inhibition of glucose uptake occurs within 20 min after the addition of corticosteroid to thymocytes (160). This in turn results in depressed adenosine triphosphate (ATP) concentrations within the tissue (157). These changes do not appear to be caused by the direct action of the glucocorticoid, however. Following the formation of a nuclear-glucocorticoid-receptor complex, there is evidence that an intermediate protein is formed (159). It is this intermediary protein which subsequently inhibits glucose transport.

B. Gonadal Steroids

The mechanism by which estrogen exerts its effects upon the immune system appears to involve the blockage of calcium stabilization of the cell membrane. This conclusion is based upon evidence demonstrating that estradiol is able to inhibit calcium-induced mitotic activity in thymic lymphocytes (161-163) as well as in bone marrow (164). In the latter study, male and female rats were injected with either $CaCl_2$ or $MgCl_2$. The magnesium salt was effective in both sexes in stimulating mitosis in both bone marrow and thymus. Calcium, however, was ineffective in the female rats unless the animals had previously undergone ovariectomy. Similarly, estrogen administration to ovariectomized rats prevented calcium-induced mitosis. This effect has not been observed with progesterone therapy (160) or with testosterone. In a related study assessing the effects of estrogen upon calcium-induced hyperpolarization of the plasma membrane, it was found that the structure of the steroid was correlated with its ability to induce hypopolarization and to inhibit calcium-induced mitogenic activity (161). Only 18-carbon steroids were found to be effective in inhibiting Ca-induced proliferation; 19-carbon androgens as well as 21-carbon progestins were ineffective.

Most of the available evidence suggests that the effects of estrogen occur at a very early stage of calcium-induced blastogenesis. cAMP has been described as a prerequisite for the mitogenic action of calcium (163). But estradiol had no effect upon cAMP-induced changes, or upon epinephrine- and caffeine-induced elevations of cAMP. Estradiol did inhibit the mitogenic action of parathyroid hormone, however, suggesting that estrogens may act by blocking the influx of calcium into the cell.

The mechanism by which progesterone exerts its inhibitory effects upon immunity does not appear to involve a classic steroid receptor mechanism (165). It has been reported that progesterone is able to inhibit the cellular response to both mitogenic and allogenic stimulation, but this inhibition was found to be reversible and apparently did not involve intracellular enzyme systems participating in DNA synthesis. Consequently, it was suggested that progesterone was exerting its apparent inhibitory effects by blocking the entry of [^{3}H] TdR into the cells. It is also important that the effective dose of 1-20 μg/ml of progesterone approximates the levels found in the human placenta (166). It was concluded by Clemens et al. (165) that instead of acting via a classic steroid receptor, progesterone probably exerts a more generalized effect upon the cell membranes. Thus, it would be able to impede the initial activation of a cellular or inflammatory response in close proximity to the progesterone-producing trophoblast. At the same time, the systemic maternal immune system would remain intact.

A precedent for such a mechanism was discussed by the authors. It was observed that progesterone can lead to hyperpolarization of myometrial cells (167), inhibit the binding of prostaglandin to membrane receptors in the corpus luteum (168), and interact with the oocyte membrane to stimulate *Xenopus* oocyte maturation (169). As is true of corticosteroids and of the estrogenic steroids, biological activity of various progesterone analogs appears to be related to the chemical structure. DiSorbo et al. (170) compared the effectiveness of progesterone and several analogs in competing with [^{3}H] triamcinolone acetonide (TA) for glucocorticoid receptors in thymus and liver tissue. It was found that 11^3-hydroxyl, 6α-methyl, 6α-16α-dimethyl, and 6α-methyl-17α-hydroxyl analogs were able to effectively compete with TA binding in vitro and to induce thymic involution when injected into adrenalectomized rats. On the other hand, progesterone, 16α-methyl-17α-hydroxyprogesterone, and 17α-hydroxyprogesterone were able to compete with TA binding, but were ineffective in causing thymic involution.

It was suggested by the authors that substitution of progesterone with a 6α-methyl group confers the steroid with its immunosuppressive properties just as the 11β-hydroxyl group is necessary for the immunosuppressive properties of glucocorticoids. It was further suggested that since progesterone lacks both the 11β-hydroxyl and 6α-methyl groups, yet can bind to glucocorticoid receptors, it should act as an antiglucocorticoid, The fact that it does not in vivo has been attributed to its rapid metabolism. Perhaps contributing to the metabolism of progesterone in immune tissue is the enzyme 20-α-hydroxy-steroid dehydrogenase (20α-SDH). 20α-SDH is a T-lymphocyte-associated enzyme found in thymocytes, lymph node, and splenic T cells (171-172). This enzyme reduces progesterone to 20α-dihydroprogesterone which lacks immunosuppressive activity (172). It has also been reported that orchidectomy, but not ovariectomy, causes a significant decrease in thymocyte 20α-SDH activity (173).

In addition to its reported direct effects upon cellular immunity, progesterone has also been found to act synergistically with estrogen in causing thymic involution. Sobhon and Jirasattham (174) reported that although progesterone alone was able to bring about a relative decrease of thymus weight, it was effective only at a very high dose. But when administered with estrogen and at a dose which alone was found to be ineffective, the decrease in thymus weight was considerably greater than the inhibition observed following estrogen alone. The decrease in weight following either testosterone, estrogen, or estrogen plus progesterone was correlated with a decrease in the size of the thymic lobules and width of the thymic cortex. There was also a decrease in the number of lymphocytes and an increase in the number of reticular cells in the cortex. In contrast, the number of lymphocytes and reticular cells in the thymic medulla was no different from control values.

The possibility was considered that the effects of the estrogen and progesterone were mediated by elevated levels of glucocorticoids. Evidence was discussed that estrogen can result in elevated ACTH and hypertrophy of the adrenal glands in ovariectomized rats (175). However, not all of the inhibitory effects reported could be attributed to pituitary-adrenal activation since the same effects were demonstrated in adrenalectomized animals (174).

It is curious that some interesting parallels exist between the effects of estrogen and progesterone upon immunological parameters and their effects upon reproductive physiology and behavior. For example, estrogen alone can result in thymic involution, but only when given in very high concentrations. High concentrations of estrogen alone can also stimulate sexual receptivity in ovariectomized female rodents. However, both phenomena can be induced using subthreshold doses of estrogen, provided that progesterone is also administered. Thus, there is synergism between these two hormones with respect to both immunological and behavioral measures. In the context of immunity, stimulation (100,139) and inhibition (93) of immune measures have been reported. It may be more than coincidence that progesterone has both stimulatory and inhibitory effects upon reproductive behavior as well as upon arousal thresholds. An initial injection of progesterone following estrogen priming of ovariectomized rats has been shown to facilitate sexual receptivity. But if a second injection of progesterone is given on the day after the first, it will result in inhibition (176).

Arousal thresholds as measured by changes in the EEG following electrical stimulation of the brain have also been correlated with the levels of the sex steroids (177). Progesterone treatment was found to result in an initial lowering of the threshold by as much as 30%, but then it rose to a point above the initial level and in 24 hr was two to three times as high. The thresholds for arousal measured in this manner were much the same regardless of whether the midbrain reticular formation, the caudate nucleus, or the dorsomedial thalamic nucleus was stimulated. Pregnancy or artifically prolonged progesterone treatment via injections was found to maintain the thresholds at elevated levels.

These data suggest that the effects of estrogen and progesterone upon immunity may be of a more generalized nature. It is also possible that estrogen has an enhancing effect upon the immune system by enabling other factors to exert their direct effects. A precedence for such a role can be found not only in the literature concerned with reproductive physiology but also in the literature concerned with sensory physiology. For example, Komisaruk (178) reported that estrogen treatment of ovariectomized rats increased significantly the area of both the genital and clitoral sensory field. It was suggested by the authors that this increased sensory field might assist the female in orienting to the thrusting of the male. Estrogen has also been shown to decrease the electroshock seizure threshold in female rats (179) and to increase the pituitary responsiveness of luteinizing hormone releasing factor (LHRF) (180). Furthermore estrogen priming has been found to facilitate progesterone uptake in uterine tissue and the nuclear uptake of progesterone in guinea pigs (181).

This discussion by itself could be regarded as mere coincidence and deemed irrelevant in the context of immunity. However, a more tolerant consideration of the parallels between reproductive function and immunity is warranted by the evidence that both can be affected by the major histocompatibility complex (MHC) genotype (182).

The MHC is associated with genetic control of the immune response as well as with allograft rejection. It is also associated with plasma testosterone levels (183), weights of steroid-sensitive organs (184), the binding of hormones to cell membranes (185,186), and mating preference (187). An excellent discussion of these associations has been published elsewhere (182). They are mentioned here because of their possible relevance to the previously discussed parallels between reproductive and immune phenomena, two systems that involve a high degree of recognition.

VI. THYMUS INTERACTION WITH STEROIDS

The evidence thus far reviewed documents profound influences of steroid hormones upon the various parameters of immunity. There is also evidence suggesting that steroid interactions with immunity are not one-sided but are reciprocal. Most of the evidence implicates the thymus gland in exerting a modulatory influence upon steroid hormones and their function.

One of the earliest studies reporting an influence of thymectomy upon steroid function was published by Paton in 1905 (188). This investigator found that thymectomized guinea pigs that were sacrificed when weighing less than 200 g had testes weighing 27% more than control tissues. However, no differences were observed in large animals. Other studies conducted during the early part of this century were not always consistent in their revelations. In a critical review of this subject, Andersen (189) concluded that any effects of thymectomy upon reproductive function were more likely the consequence of the surgical procedure rather than of a specific action of the thymus upon reproductive physiology.

In more recent years, however, it appears that the detection of thymic influences upon reproductive function may require additional or more sensitive assays than simply the weighing of gonadal tissue. Evaluation of the effects of thymectomy upon the growth of secondary reproductive structures in rats has revealed that the procedure results in significantly heavier ventral prostate glands and seminal vesicles (190). These changes were not pronounced in rats that were thymectomized at 6 to 6.5 weeks of age. In subsequent studies, it was found that thymectomy can alter the enzymatic activity of accessory reproductive structures in pubertal rats (190,191) and can influence the effects of gonadotropins upon the prostate gland (192). In the latter study, it was found that follicle-stimulating hormone (FSH) enhanced the stimulatory effects of thymectomy upon ventral and lateral prostate gland weights. The lateral, but not the ventral, prostate weight of thymectomized rats was enhanced by luteinizing hormone (LH) administration. The possibility that the differences in lateral versus ventral prostate weight following LH administration were due to the differential responsiveness of these tissues to hormones was discussed by the authors.

In addition to the effects of the thymus upon the male reproductive system, there is also evidence of a modulatory influence upon the female reproductive system. Athymic female mice have been found to have several deficiencies involving the reproductive system. The first ovulation is delayed, the ovarian tissue is diminished in size and lacks large follicles, and the animals display an abnormal estrus cycle (193-194). Similar changes have been reported in female mice that have undergone neonatal thymectomy (195). It has also been found that treatment with gonadotropin hormone can prevent some of the histological changes in the ovary that result from neonatal thymectomy (196).

In a subsequent study, Weinstein (197) measured levels of gonadotropin hormones in serum and pituitary tissue from congenitally athymic female mice. There were no significant differences in these hormones when compared with control animals. Nor was there any difference in the hypothalamic content of gonadotropin-releasing hormone. But differences were observed in the ability of the animals to respond to manipulation of the hormonal feedback mechanisms. By day 6 after ovariectomy, serum LH levels in normal mice were almost 10 times higher than in nonovariectomized animals. However, no increase was observed when the congenitally athymic mice were ovariectomized. Although not as great as in the control animals, serum levels of LH did increase by almost sixfold when the athymic mice were injected with gonadotropin-releasing hormone. Consequently, it was concluded that the aberrant cycling and lack of normal feedback following ovariectomy were indicative of a dysfunction involving the central nervous system (197). Since athymic mice implanted with thymic tissue at birth exhibited a normal elevation of LH following ovariectomy, a relationship between the thymus gland and normal functioning of neuroendocrine control systems is evident.

A. Effects of Thymic Extracts upon Steroids

Interest in thymic hormone research has intensified during the past two decades. As more sophisticated methods have been applied to evaluate the chemical and biological properties of thymic extracts, it has become apparent that they are comprised of a variety of biologically active polypeptides. This discussion will focus upon the biological effects of purified thymic peptides and the interactions of the thymic preparations with steroid hormones.

Attempts to measure the effects of thymic extracts upon the endocrine physiology of animals have been reported since as early as 1912 when Gudernatsch (see 189) reported delayed metamorphosis in tadpoles that had been fed thymic extracts. While some early investigators reported a retarding effect upon reproductive function in rodents fed thymic extracts, subsequent studies revealed that these observations could be attributed to nutritional deficiencies rather than an inhibitory substance within the tissue (189). When animals were fed thymic extracts supplemented with vitamins, the effects were not observed (198).

The injection of crude thymic extracts has been carred out over the decades as a means of studying the effects of the thymus upon the reproductive system. While not conclusive, there are claims reported in the literature that cryptorchidism can be cured by the injection of crude thymus extract (199-201). There is also evidence of synergism between thymic extracts and ovarian hormones, although apparently not specific to the thymus gland since muscle extracts were also found to be effective (302).

Research, using thymic preparations, has continued using increasingly more sophisticated procedures to process the extracts. In 1971, it was reported that gonadal degeneration occurred in thymectomized guinea pigs, but that this degeneration could be prevented by the administration of a thymic extract (203). Deschaux et al. (204) have extended this observation by comparing the effects of two thymic extracts upon a variety of endocrine systems. Extracts were prepared by the method of Bernardi and Comsa (205) or by the method of Goldstein et al. (206). Rats were thymectomized within 24 hr of birth and were treated with either homeostatic thymic hormone or thymosin. Animals were sacrificed at various ages, and serum levels of testosterone, corticosterone, LH, and ACTH were measured. Both thymic extracts were found to restore the decreased body, adrenal, and testes weight that followed thymectomy. Plasma corticosterone was decreased through 60 days in neonatally thymectomized rats, while ACTH showed biphasic changes. This peptide hormone was lower compared with controls at 15, 30, and 45 days, higher at

60 days, and normal by 90 days. These hormonal changes were not observed in thymectomized animals treated with either of the thymic extracts. Muscle extract was used as a control substance and was without effect. A similar, though opposite, biphasic pattern was exhibited by testosterone and LH. Elevations were observed at 30 days, a significant decrease at 60 days, and no difference at 90 days. Administration of thymic extracts was found to reduce the extent of these changes.

The mechanism(s) by which these changes occurred appeared to differ, depending upon the hormone. An influence at the level of the pituitary gland was suggested for the testosterone changes since the thymic extracts failed to prevent them when given to thymectomized-hypophysectomized rats. However, the extracts prevented the corticosterone changes regardless of whether the pituitary was present. It is also possible that the thymic extracts were having an influence at the level of the central nervous system with respect to the LH and testosterone changes. Such a mechanism is consistent with the hypothesis that thymic factors act at the level of the CNS to influence LH cyclicity and control in the female mouse (197). This conclusion is further supported by the observations that thymosin fraction 5 can stimulate LH release following superinfusion into hypothalamic tissue in vitro (207).

Thymosin fraction 5 is comprised of 40-50 peptide components with molecular weights ranging from 1000 to 15,000. While 20 of the peptides have been purified to homogeneity or near homogeneity, two have been characterized, sequenced, and evaluated in neuroendocrine protocols. These are thymosin α_1 and thymosin β_4.

Thus får, both peptides have been implicated in modulating adrenal or gonadal steroidogenesis at the level of the hypothalamic-hypophyseal axis. Thymosin α_1, when injected into the lateral ventricle of unanesthetized mice, has been found to stimulate a significant increase in serum corticosterone levels (208). However, this peptide is ineffective when cultured in vitro with isolated adrenal fasciculata cells (209). In contrast, thymosin β_4 has been found to stimulate LH release both in vivo following infusion into the lateral ventricle (210) as well as after infusion into isolated median eminence-pituitary cultures (207). Thymosin α_1 does not stimulate LH and β_4 does not stimulate corticosterone suggesting that their influences upon the respective neuroendocrine systems is relatively specific (210). Thus, these data support the conclusions of Deschaux et al. (204) and Weinstein (197) that thymic factors might modulate the reproductive and adrenal systems via the hypothalamus.

If thymus peptides are part of a physiological mechanism that regulates various neuroendocrine systems, it should be possible to detect them within the CNS. Results from our laboratory, as well as from other laboratories, indicate that they are and that they are at highest concentrations in regions involved in hormonal regulation. Belokrylov et al. (211) have reported the presence of low molecular weight polypeptides (mol wt $<$ 10,000) in extracted bovine cerebral cortex and white matter. Injection of this extract into rodents was found to significantly enhance antibody production against sheep red blood cells. A low molecular weight peptidelike substance with thymocyte-stimulating properties has also been extracted from the anterior pituitary gland (212). This substance was found to cause a significant elevation in $[^3H]$TdR uptake in thymocytes.

Using a radioimmunoassay developed to measure the purified peptide thymosin α_1, we conducted a preliminary analysis, using guinea pigs, of gross brain regions in order to assess whether this particular peptide is present in discrete brain regions. Tissue was dissected grossly into discrete regions and extracted using the procedure of Miller et al. (213). Thymosin α_1-like cross reactivity was found to be highest in the diencephalon and lowest in the cortex. Mesencephalon and brainstem contained intermediate levels.

Table 1 Distribution of Thymosin α_1-Like Immunoreactivity in Discrete Brain Regions of the Rat

Brain region	Peptide concentration[a] (pg/μg protein)
Hypothalamus	
Median eminence	6.33 ± 0.24
Arcuate n.	6.53 ± 0.54
Periventricular n.	3.33 ± 0.24
Paraventricular n.	3.18 ± 0.24
Supraoptic n.	3.52 ± 0.48
Ventralmedial n.	3.68 ± 0.26
Dorsomedial n.	3.36 ± 0.23
Anterior hypothalamic n.	2.68 ± 0.37
Posterior hypothalamic n.	3.32 ± 0.08
Medial preoptic n.	2.40 ± 0.12
Thalamus	
Periventricular n.	4.36 ± 0.16
Septal area	
N. accumbens	3.59 ± 0.91
Lateral septum	2.30 ± 0.51
Anterior septum	3.55 ± 0.68
Midbrain	
Central gray	3.08 ± 0.21
Substantia nigra	3.10 ± 0.22
Cortex	
Cingulate cortex	1.37 ± 0.28
Striatum	1.01 ± 0.29

[a]Each value represents the mean SEM of four determinations.
Source: The data in this table are from the Ph.D. thesis of E. Palaszynski, 1982.

These same relative differences have also been found in discrete regions of rat brain with highest levels of α_1 cross reactivity in the hypothalamus and pituitary gland and lowest levels in the cortex and spinal cord (214,210). A more extensive evaluation of thymosin α_1 content within the CNS was carried out by Palaszynski (215). The results of this study are summarized in Table 1.

Highest concentrations of thymosin α_1-like immuno-cross reactivity were found in the median eminence and arcuate nucleus. The next highest concentration was found in the ventromedial nucleus which is where neurons exhibit a significant increase in firing rate at the time of peak antibody formation (216).

In all brain regions assayed, one major peak of immunoreactivity was present which had a molecular weight similar to that of thymosin α_1. The thymosin α_1 antisera had less than 0.01% cross reactivity with the following peptides: bombesin, bradykinin, β-endorphin, enkephalin, α-melanocyte-stimulating hormone, neurotensin, substance P, thyrotropin releasing factor, and vasoactive intestinal polypeptide. Also, the antiserum did not appreciably cross react ($<$ 0.02%) with the following animo acids: aspartate, glutamine, lysin, and tyrosine.

Although these data do not constitute conclusive evidence that thymic peptides can modulate immunity at the level of the central nervous system, they are highly suggestive. Especially since thymosin peptides have been found to influence some of the same immunological parameters that can be altered by gonadal and adrenal steroids. Evidence also suggests that just as individual thymosin peptides influence differentially the neuroendocrine systems regulating gonadal and adrenal function, they also exert differential effects upon thymocyte differentiation.

VII. THYMOSIN PEPTIDES: BIOLOGY AND CHEMISTRY

A. Thymosin α_1

Thymosin α_1 is active in amplifying T-cell immunity (217,218), as well as in modulating the expression of terminal deoxynucleotidyl transferase (TdT) (219). Thymosin α_1 was isolated from fraction 5 by ion-exchange chromatography on CM-cellulose and DEAE-cellulose, as well as by gel filtration on Sephadex G-75. The yield of thymosin α_1 from fraction 5 varies depending upon the particular preparations and the assay system used. Thymosin α_1 is a polypeptide with a molecular weight of 3108 consisting of 28 amino acid residues and a pI of 4.2. The complete amino acid sequence of this peptide is shown in Fig. 1. The amino terminus of thymosin α_1 is blocked by an acetyl group.

Comparison of the sequence of thymosin α_1 with the published sequence of other thymic factors, such as thymopoietin II (220) and facteur thymique serique (FTS) (221), reveals no homology. Computer analysis of the sequence of α_1 has established that α_1 contains very little homology with any of the protein sequences that have been published to date.

Studies by Freire et al. (222) suggest that thymosin α_1 is produced in the thymus as part of a larger protein. These investigators have translated messenger RNA isolated from

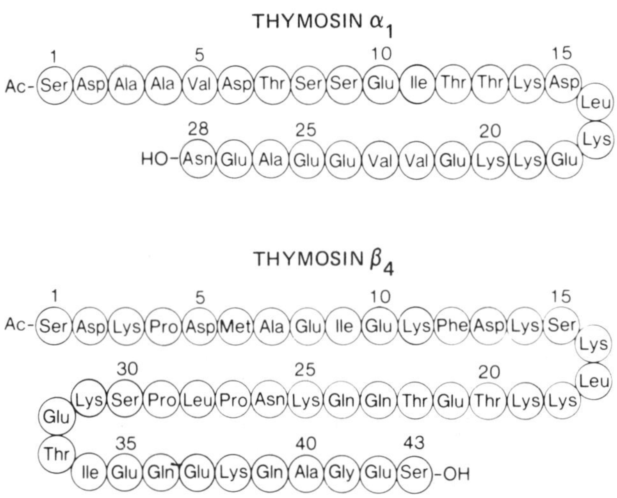

Figure 1 Amino acid sequence of thymosin α_1 and thymosin β_4.

calf thymus and carried out synthesis studies in a cell-free wheat germ system. Radioactive products that were immunoprecipitable with antisera against thymosin fractions were analyzed and found to be identical to those expected for tryptic peptides from thymosin α_1. More recently Freire et al. (222) purified the mRNA fraction from calf thymus polysomes by preparative polyacrylamide disc electrophoresis. The results of these studies suggest that thymosin α_1 is synthesized in the thymus as a longer peptide chain of 16,000 daltons and may be further processed (or degraded) to form the peptide detected in preparation isolated from the thymus. This concept is further supported by the observation that tissue thymosin α_1 concentration increases at elevated temperatures (223).

Others have reported the isolation and complete chemical characterization of a N^α-desacetyl thymosin α_1 utilizing recombinant DNA procedures (224). In this important development, the gene for thymosin α_1 was synthesized, inserted into a plasmid, and cloned in a strain of *Escherichia coli*. The primary nucleotide sequence required for the gene was constructed using prepared prokaryotic codons with elimination of codons of multiple specificities and minimization of AT- and GC-rich regions. In cloning the α_1 gene, the gene was inserted under lac operon control into the plasmid and expressed as part of a β-galactosidase chimeric protein. The structure of the N^α-desacetyl thymosin α_1 was confirmed by sequence analysis, and the molecule was found to be as biologically active in vitro as the chemically synthesized thymosin α_1.

B. Thymosin β_4

Thymosin β_4 is the first of the biologically active polypeptides from the β region of thymosin fraction 5 to be completely characterized (225). Thymosin β_4 was isolated by ion-exchange chromatography on a column of carboxymethyl-cellulose (M-52) in 10 mM NaOAC, 1 mN 2-mercaptoethanol, pH 5.0. Two stepwise linear gradients of 0-0.5 M NaCl and 0.5-1.0 M NaCl were used for the elution. Thymosin β_4 was derived from the second retained peak of the carboxymethyl-cellulose column. It was further purified by gel filtration of Sephadex G-50 in 6 M guanidinium HCl. The third protein peak was pooled and desalted on a Sephadex G-10 column in sterile water. The purified sample so obtained is identified as thymosin β_4. The complete sequence of β_4 is shown in Fig. 1. Thymosin β_4 is composed of 43 amino acid residues and has a molecular weight of 4982 and a pI of 5.1. The N-terminal end of the peptide is blocked by an acetyl group.

Thymosin β_4 induced TdT expression in TdT-negative murine bone marrow cells in vivo and in vitro. It also increases TdT activity in thymocytes from hydrocortisone-immunosuppressed mice in vitro (219). Thus, it appears that thymosin β_4 is acting on lymphoid stem cells and may influence the early stages of the maturation process of thymus-dependent lymphocytes.

A computer search for possible sequence homology between the sequence of thymosin β_4 and other published protein sequences has been conducted (personal communication through the National Biomedical Research Foundation, Georgetown University Medical Center, Washington, D.C.). The results do not indicate a statistically significant relationship of thymosin β_4 to any other sequence protein currently stored in the data bank. However, there is an interesting internal duplication between residues 18 and 30 and 31-43, as illustrated. Although thymosin β_4 was first isolated from the thymus gland, it has recently been reported that it is also a product of macrophages (226). Therefore, as is true of many peptides, thymosin β_4 may have different sources as well as different functions.

C. Thymosin β_3

Thymosin β_3 is isolated from fraction 5 and 5A by ion-exchange chromatography and gel filtration. Like β_4, it induces the expression of TdT-positive cells in several different model systems. Thymosin β_3 has an isoelectric point of 5.2 and a molecular weight of approximately 5500. Thymosin β_3 shares an identical sequence with β_4 through most of its amino-terminal portion and differs only at the carboxyl-terminal ends. Its complete sequence has not been determined.

D. Thymosin α_7

Thymosin α_7 has been isolated from fraction 5 by ion-exchange chromatography on CM-cellulose and DEAE-cellulose and by gel filtration on Sephadex G-75. It is highly acidic with an isoelectric point around 3.5 and is free of carbohydrate and lipid. Thymosin α_7 has a molecular weight of approximately 2200. The peptide has been found to be a potent inducer of suppressor cells (S. Horowitz, personal communication) and is also active in inducing T-cell markers (218).

E. Other Thymic Factors

The thymus appears to synthesize and secrete several biochemically distinct peptides. In addition to the thymosins, a number of factors with thymic hormonelike activity have been isolated from thymus tissue and blood. These preparations are in various stages of characterization. Four of the thymic hormones that have been sequenced to date (thymosin α_1, mol wt 3108; thymosin β_4, mol wt 4982; thymopoietin II, mol wt 5562; and FTS, mol wt 857) appear to be chemically unrelated.

VIII. DISCUSSION

Numerous reports of steroid interactions with immunological parameters can be found in the literature. But many of these investigations have utilized either pharmacological doses of the hormone under study or analogs not normally found in the animal model being utilized (e.g., the testing of hydrocortisone in rodents). Therefore, of paramount importance is the physiological significance of the reported changes.

An intriguing hypothesis explaining the biological significance of glucocorticoid inhibition of immune functioning has been discussed by Besedovsky and Sorkin (216). Data were presented demonstrating that at the time of maximum antibody production, there occurs a concurrent increase in serum corticosterone levels. It was suggested that this increase in a potentially inhibitory hormone plays an important role in immunospecificity. This hypothesis is based upon the following evidence.

Non-antigen-stimulated thymocytes residing in the thymic cortex are very susceptible to the inhibitory effects of steroids. Following immunogenic stimulation, the cells become more resistant to these inhibitory effects. Consequently, the elevated steroid would primarily inhibit the less responsive lymphocytes with either low or no affinity for the antigen. This would provide a regulatory influence preventing the proliferation of cells that might otherwise be activated by soluble factors produced by either leukocytes or thymic epithelial cells. It was noted by the authors that such a model is not inconsistent with lateral or afferent inhibition of neurons in order to reduce nonspecific signals.

It was predicted that if the above hypothesis were valid, then the injection of a second immunogen at the time of elevated corticosteroid levels would result in a lower titer of antibody. The predicted inhibition was observed. When SRBCs were injected into rats that had previously been immunized with TNP-horse red blood cells, there was a marked depression of the PFC response to the SRBCs. This depression was not observed in rats that had been adrenalectomized prior to the first immunization.

Thus, the corticosteroids could be regarded as fine tuning the immune response by suppressing the clonal expansion of cells that lack high affinity for the inducing immunogen. Such a hypothesis is consistent with some of the apparent contradictions in the literature as to whether corticosteroids are inhibitory or facilitative. Through the inhibition of certain cells, the net result might be an augmentation of the host's ability to respond to immunogenic challenge. As suggested by the authors, such a mechanism would also serve to reduce the probability of autoimmune disease, a concent that is supported by a number of clinical studies (227).

It has also been proposed that the thymus gland may regulate the adrenal cortex by acting as an antistressor (228). This hypothesis is consistent with the previously discussed evidence that thymic extracts are able to prevent the rise in ACTH and corticosterone that follows thymectomy (204). A regulatory influence of the thymus upon glucocorticoid effects is further supported by the observation that thymosin administration to steroid-treated mice either increased the ConA response of spleen cells if it were low, or decreased the response if it were elevated (229). There is additional evidence that thymic factors may interfere with the binding of corticosteroids and in this way perhaps suppress their activity. Bach et al. (230) reported that FTS was able to bring about a 60-70% inhibition of steroid binding when thymocyte cytosol preparations were incubated in the presence of the purified serum factor. In addition to the effects of steroids and thymic factors upon host defense, there is evidence that the neuroendocrine and immune systems are interdependent during ontogeny and that each is necessary for the subsequent functioning of the other (231-235).

It has also been demonstrated that within 1-2 hr following the injection of allogeneic cells, there occurs a rapid increase in serum LH levels (236). This would suggest that the previously discussed observations regarding the effects of gonadal hormones upon immunity may indeed reflect events that normally occur during the course of host defense. Furthermore, some of the changes involving gonadal hormones might well play a role in the protection of paternal alloantigens from maternal rejection, as discussed previously.

It was suggested by Pierpaoli and Maestroni (236) that the rise in LH might have been due to release of lymphokines from immunoreactive lymphocytes. While previously discussed studies suggest a role for thymic hormones acting at the level of the brain or pituitary to stimulate gonadotropin release, the possibility that lymphokines may also play a role cannot be discounted.

While none of the above hypotheses have been conclusively substantiated, there is sufficient evidence to suggest that the endocrine thymus is regulated in much the same way as are other endocrine tissues. A brief summary of the major evidence in support of this hypothesis follows.

1. Manipulation of the central nervous system can result in alterations in thymic-dependent immune functioning (237,238).
2. Hormones under CNS control are affected by neonatal thymectomy or by genetic absence of the thymus. Many of these hormonal aberrations can be corrected by early implantation of thymic tissue (233,234,239).

3. Injection of thymosin peptides directly into the brain can result in both endocrine and immunological changes (210).
4. Thymosin α_1 has been localized in hypothalamic tissue by the use of RIA (210,215).
5. During the course of immunity, electrical, morphological, and neurochemical changes can be detected in the CNS (216,238).

Consequently, it is proposed that the endocrine thymus is part of a neuroendocrine axis ultimately influencing its own functioning via peptides produced by thymic epithelial cells. A diagrammatic representation of how this axis might function is illustrated in Fig. 2.

While the evidence is in strong support of this model, an additional possibility which accounts for nearly all of the evidence cited has to be considered. Thymic hormones and lymphokines may simply act upon cells in the brain that are involved with defense against neurological disease. These might include supraependymal cells, which have many of the characteristics of macrophages (240), and certain glial cells, which can be induced to proliferate in the presence of supernatant from ConA-stimulated lymphocytes (24,). Furthermore, it has been shown that immunosuppression can be correlated with suppression of trauma-induced proliferation of glial cells (242).

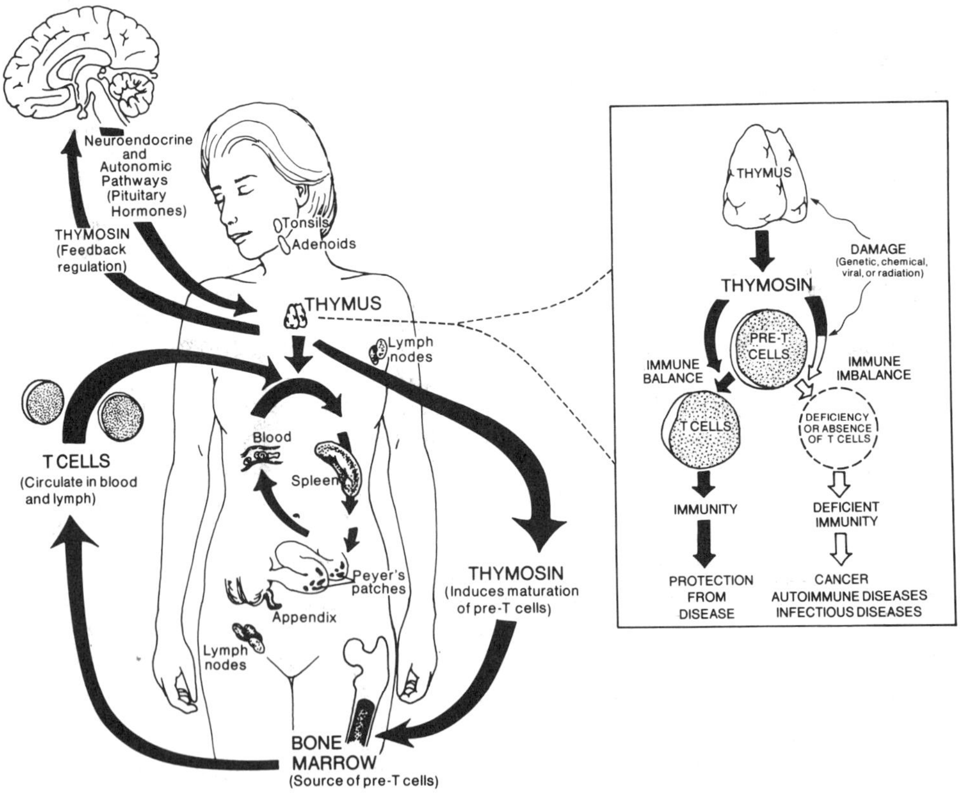

Figure 2 Proposed model illustrating the role of thymosin peptides in a CNS-thymus gland axis.

Macrophages have been found to synthesize and secrete prostaglandins (243). If such release were to occur from lymphokine or thymic peptide-activated macrophages in the brain, it might account for some of the hormonal changes that have been correlated with host defense. PGE_2 has been shown to cause the release of corticotropin-releasing factor (CRF) and LHRF in brain tissue (244,245) and to mimic some of the biological effects of LHRF when injected into the brain (246,247). This latter hypothesis does not necessarily contradict the model proposed in Fig. 2. To the contrary, it suggests a mechanism by which some of the observed hormonal changes might be brought about during the course of the immune response.

REFERENCES

1. P. J. Mobius, *Geschlecht and Krankeit, Beitr. Lehre Geschlects Unterschieden., vol. 1,* Verlag Carl Marhold, Halle, Germany, 1903, p. 39.
2. J. A. Hammar, *Die normal-morphologische thymus forschung*, Barth, Leipzig, 1936.
3. F. C. Goble and F. A. Konopka, *Trans. N. Y. Acad. Sci., 35*:325 (1973).
4. R. H. Michaels and K. D. Rogers, *Pediatrics, 47*:120 (1971).
5. G. Terres, S. L. Morrison, and G. S. Habicht, *Proc. Soc. Exp. Biol. Med., 127*:664 (1968).
6. D. W. F. Wheater and E. W. Hurst, *J. Pathol. Bacteriol., 82*:117 (1961).
7. D. S. Willoughby and D. W. Watson, *J. Bacteriol., 87*:1457 (1964).
8. U. Krzych, G. B. Thurman, A. L. Goldstein, J. P. Bressler, and H. R. Strausser, *J. Immunol., 123*:2568 (1979).
9. N. R. Hall and A. L. Goldstein, in *Psychoneuroimmunology* (R. Ader, ed.), Academic Press, New York, 1981, pp. 521-543.
10. A. A. Monjan, in *Psychoneuroimmunology* (R. Ader, ed.), Academic Press, New York, 1981, pp. 185-228.
11. N. Fabris, W. Pierpaoli, and E. Sorkin, *Clin. Exp. Immunol., 9*:227 (1971).
12. A. White and A. L. Goldstein, in *Immunogenicity* (F. Borek, ed.), North Holland Publishing Co., Amsterdam, 1972, pp. 334-364.
13. E. R. Unanue, *Adv. Immunol., 15*:95 (1972).
14. M. Feldman and G. J. U. Nossal, *Transplant. Res., 13*:3 (1972).
15. D. H. Katz and E. R. Unanue, *J. Exp. Med., 137*:967 (1973).
16. D. L. Rosenstreich, J. J. Farrar, and S. Dougherty, *J. Immunol., 116*:131 (1976).
17. R. M. E. Parkhouse and R. W. J. Duttin, *J. Immunol., 97*:663 (1966).
18. E. Perkins and T. Makinodan, *J. Immunol., 94*:765 (1965).
19. M. T. Scott, *Cell Immunol., 5*:469 (1972).
20. O. Sjoberg, *Clin. Exp. Immunol., 12*:365 (1972).
21. H. Kirchner, T. M. Chused, R. Herberman, H. T. Holden, and D. H. Lavrin, *J. Exp. Med., 139*:1473 (1974).
22. R. B. Zurier, G. Weissman, S. Hoffstein, S. Kammerman, and H. H. Tai, *J. Clin. Invest., 53*:297 (1974).
23. L. J. Ignarro and W. J. George, *Proc. Natl. Acad. Sci. USA, 71*:2027 (1974).
24. L. J. Ignarro, T. F. Lint, and W. J. George, *J. Exp. Med., 139*:1395 (1974).
25. I. Rivkin, J. Rosenblatt, and E. L. Becker, *J. Immunol., 115*:1126 (1975).
26. H. E. Schmidt-Gayk, K. H. Jakobs, and E. Hackenthal, *J. Reticuloendoth. Soc., 17*:251 (1975).
27. T. J. Higgins and J. R. David, *Cell Immunol., 27*:1 (1976).
28. H. D. Welscher and A. Cruchaud, *J. Reticuloendoth. Soc., 20*:405 (1976).
29. H. D. Welscher and A. Cruchaud, *Eur. J. Immunol., 8*:180 (1978).
30. H. R. Bourne, L. M. Lichtenstein, K. L. Melmon, C. S. Henney, Y. Weinstein, and G. M. Shearer, *Science, 184*:19 (1974).

31. B. Benacerraf, E. Kivy-Rosenberg, M. M. Sebestyen, and B. W. Zweifach, *J. Exp. Med., 110*:49 (1959).
32. G. Carteny, *Il Policlinico, 72*:228 (1965).
33. G. D'Amico and S. Cambria, *Giorn. It. Chirurg., 19*:501 (1963).
34. L. Lee, P. H. Prose, and M. Cohen, *Thromb. Diath. Haemorrh.* (Suppl.), *20*:87 (1966).
35. M. S. Rittenbury and L. D. Hanback, *J. Trauma, 7*:523 (1967).
36. L. L. Smith and U. P. Veragut, *Prog. Surg., 4*:55 (1964).
37. B. E. Schildt, *Acta Chir. Scand., 136*:359 (1970).
38. J. Palmblad, K. Cantell, H. Strander, J. Froberg, C-G. Karlsson, L. Levi, M. Granstrom, and P. Unger, *J. Psychosom. Res., 20*:193 (1976).
39. T. M. Saba, *Proc. Soc. Exp. Biol. Med., 133*:1132 (1970).
40. S. B. Crepea, G. M. Magnin, and C. V. Seastone, *Proc. Soc. Exp. Biol. Med., 77*:704 (1951).
41. P. G. Shilotri and J. S. Prasad, *Horm. Metab. Res., 8*:67 (1976).
42. J. G. Hirsch and A. B. Church, *J. Clin. Invest., 40*:794 (1961).
43. J. H. Chretien and V. F. Garagusi, *J. Reticuloendothel. Soc.* 11:358 (1972).
44. G. Pitner, L. C. Smith, and C. A. Calwell, *Bact. Proc., 22*:88 (1951) (Abstr.).
45. H. Van Dijk, J. Testerink, and I. Noordegraff, *Cell Immunol., 25*:8 (1976).
46. T. Nicol and D. L. J. Bilbey, in *Reticuloendothelial Structure and Function* (J. H. Heller, ed.), Ronald Press, New York, 1960, pp. 301-320.
47. T. Nicol and B. Vernon-Roberts, *J. Reticuloendothel. Soc., 2*:351 (1965).
48. T. Nicol and B. Vernon-Roberts, *J. Reticuloendothel. Soc., 2*:15 (1965).
49. T. Nicol, *Trans. Roy. Soc. Edinburgh, 58*:449 (1935).
50. H. Blomgren and B. Anderson, *Exp. Cell Res., 57*:185 (1969).
51. M. Ishidate and D. Metcalf, *Aust. J. Exp. Biol. Med. Sci., 41*:637 (1963).
52. J. J. Cohen and H. N. Claman, *Nature, 229*:274 (1971).
53. K. R. Yamamoto, M. R. Stampfer, and G. M. Tomkins, *Proc. Soc. Nat. Acad. Sci. USA, 71*:390 (1974).
54. C. H. Sibley and G. M. Tomkins, *Cell, 2*:213 (1974).
55. C. H. Sibley and G. M. Tomkins, *Cell, 2*:221 (1974).
56. K. A. Smith, G. R. Crabtree, S. J. Kennedy, and A. Munck, *Nature* (*Lond.*), *267*: 523 (1977).
57. Z. Werb, R. Foley, and A. Munck, *J. Exp. Med., 147*:1684 (1978).
58. T. F. Dougherty and A. White, *Science, 98*:367 (1943).
59. T. F. Dougherty and A. White, *Endocrinology, 35*:1 (1944).
60. T. F. Dougherty and A. White, *Am. J. Anat., 77*:81 (1945).
61. R. Schrek, *Endocrinol., 45*:317 (1949).
62. W. E. Ehrich and J. Seifter, in *The Effects of ACTH and Cortisone Upon Infection and Resistance* (G. Schwartzman, ed.), Columbia University Press, New York, 1953.
63. J. F. Bach, D. Duval, M. Dardenne, J. C. Solomon, T. Tursz, and C. Fournier, *Transplant. Proc., 7*:25 (1975).
64. M. Ishidate and D. Metcalf, *Aust. J. Exp. Biol. Med. Sci., 41*:637 (1963).
65. D. Bellamy, P. A. Janssens, and R. A. Leonard, *J. Endocrinol., 35*:19 (1966).
66. D. T. Y. Yu, P. T. Clements, H. E. Paulos, J. B. Peter, J. Levy, and E. V. Barnett, *J. Clin. Invest. 53*:565 (1974).
67. A. S. Fauci, *Immunology, 28*:669 (1975).
68. U. Ernstrom and B. Larsson, *Acta Path. Microbiol. Scand., 70*:371 (1967).
69. B. Larsson, *Acta Path. Microbiol. Scand., 70*:385 (1967).
70. B. Larsson, *Acta Path. Microbiol. Scand., 70*:390 (1967).
71. M. M. Zatz, *Israel J. Med. Sci., 11*:1368 (1975).
72. M. A. Levine and H. N. Claman, *Science, 167*:1515 (1970).
73. J. J. Cohen, *J. Immunol., 107*:841 (1972).
74. J. J. Cohen, M. Fischbach, and H. N. Claman, *J. Immunol., 105*:1146 (1970).

75. G. Hudson, G. Herdan, and J. M. Yoffey, *Br. Med. J.*, *1*:999 (1952).
76. H. Blomgren and B. Andersson, *Cell Immunol.*, *1*:545 (1970).
77. A. A. Monjan and M. I. Collector, *Science, 196*:307 (1977).
78. D. A. Cooper, V. Petts, E. Luckhurst, and R. Penny, *Clin. Exp. Immunol., 28*: 467 (1977).
79. M. J. Doenhoff and E. Leuchards, *Int. Arch. Allergy Appl. Immunol., 53*:505 (1977).
80. M. A. Ritter, *Immunology, 33*:241 (1977).
81. F. Dumont and F. Robert, *Int. Arch. Allergy Appl. Immunol., 51*:482 (1976).
82. J. D. Stobo, *Transplant. Rev., 11*:60 (1972).
83. M. H. Claesson and U. Tjell, *Acta Pathol. Microbiol. Scand., 84*:185 (1976).
84. H. Van Dijk and H. E. Jacobse-Geels, *Immunology, 35*:637 (1978).
85. G. F. Solomon, I. Merigan, and S. Levin, *Proc. Soc. Exp. Biol. Med., 126*:74 (1967).
86. M. W. Rytel and E. D. Kibourne, *J. Exp. Med., 123*:767 (1966).
87. S. S. Chang and A. F. Rasmussen, Jr., *Nature, 205*:623 (1965).
88. A. L. Goldstein, T. L. K. Low, G. B. Thurman, M. M. Zatz, N. R. Hall, C-P. Chen, S. K. Hu, P. B. Naylor, and J. E. McClure, *Rec. Prog. Herm. Res., 37*:369 (1981).
89. G. Morel, P. Deschaux, and R. Fontanges, *Experientia, 33*:544 (1977).
90. J. Comsa, H. Leonhardt, and K. Ozminski, *Thymus*, 1:81 (1979).
91. T. F. Dougherty, *Physiol. Rev., 32*:379 (1952).
92. J. R. Batchelor and B. A. Chapman, *Immunol., 9*:553 (1965).
93. J. S. Thompson, C. D. Severson, and R. W. Reilly, *Radiat. Res., 40*:46 (1969).
94. J. S. Thompson, M. D. Crawford, R. W. Reilly, and C. D. Severson, *J. Immunol. 98*:331 (1967).
95. R. W. Reilly, J. S. Thompson, R. K. Bielski, and C. D. Severson, *J. Immunol., 98*: 321 (1967).
96. G. Pincus, in *The Hormones*, Vol. 3 (G. Pincus, ed.), 1955, p. 668.
97. L. M. Heim and P. S. Timiras, *Endocrinology, 72*:598 (1963).
98. J. Schacher, J. S. L. Browne, and H. Selye, *Proc. Soc. Exp. Biol. Med., 36*:488 (1937).
99. P. Cushman, M. A. Pulido, and J. G. Hilton, *Acta Endocrinol., 48*:225 (1965).
100. J. F. Kenny, P. C. Pangburn, and G. Trail, *Infect. Immun., 13*:448 (1976).
101. R. J. Ablin, *Can. Med. Assoc. J., 115*:1082 (1976).
102. R. J. Ablin, P. D. Guinan, G. R. Bruns, H. I. Al Sheik, N. Sadoughi, and I. M. Bush, *Urol. Int., 3*:383 (1976).
103. R. W. Heslop, P. L. Krohn, and F. M. Sparrow, *J. Endocrinol., 10*:325 (1954).
104. S. R. Waltman, R. M. Burde, and J. Berrios, *Transplant, 11*:194 (1971).
105. V. S. Sljivic and G. W. Warr, *Br. J. Exp. Pathol., 54*:69 (1973).
106. O. Haller, R. Kiessling, A. Orn, and H. Wigzell, *J. Exp. Med., 145*:1411 (1977).
107. W. E. Seaman, M. A. Blackman, T. D. Gindhart, J. R. Roubinian, J. M. Loeb, and N. Talal, *J. Immunol., 121*:2193 (1978).
108. S. Leikin, in *Proceedings of the VIth Leukocyte Culture Conference* (M. R. Schwartz, ed.), Academic Press, New York, 1972, pp. 725-740.
109. S. Kasakura, in *Proceedings of the VIth Leukocyte Culture Conference* (M. R. Schwartz, ed.), Academic Press, New York, 1972, pp. 711-721.
110. N. Fabris, L. Piantanelli, and M. Muzzioli, *Clin. Exp. Immunol., 28*:306 (1977).
111. E. W. Adcock, F. Teasdale, C. S. August, S. Cox, G. Meschia, F. C. Battaglia, and M. Naughton, *Science, 181*:845 (1973).
112. F. Teasdale, E. W. Adcock, C. S. August, S. Cox, F. C. Battaglia, and M. A. Naughton, *Gynecol. Invest., 4*:263 (1973).
113. S. P. Chambers and A. G. Clarke, *J. Reprod. Fertil., 55*:309 (1979).

114. J. F. Hulka, K. Mohr, and M. W. Lieberman, *Endocrinology, 77*:897 (1965).
115. J. G. Turcotte, R. F. Haines, G. L. Bordy, T. J. Meyer, and S. A. Schwartz, *Transplant., 6*:248 (1968).
116. P. K. Siiteri, F. Febres, L. E. Clemens, R. J. Chang, B. Gondos, and D. Stiters, *Ann. N. Y. Acad. Sci., 286*:384 (1977).
117. N. Kaiser, R. J. Milholland, R. W. Turnelli, and F. Rosen, *Biochem. Biophys. Res. Commun., 49*:516 (1972).
118. N. Kaiser, A. J. Solo, R. J. Milholland, and F. Rosen, *J. Steroid Biochem., 5*:348 (1974).
119. C. T. Ambrose, *J. Exp. Med., 119*:1027 (1964).
120. J. H. Chase, A. White, and T. F. Doughtery, *J. Immunol., 52*:101 (1946).
121. T. F. Dougherty, A. White, and J. H. Chase, *Proc. Soc. Exp. Biol. Med., 59*:172 (1945).
122. S. Roberts, E. Adams, and A. White, *J. Biol. Chem., 174*:379 (1948).
123. S. Roberts, E. Adams, and A. White, *J. Immunol., 62*:155 (1949).
124. C. A. Fox and R. W. Whitehead, *J. Immunol., 30*:51 (1936).
125. C. W. Hammond, and M. Novak, *Proc. Soc. Exp. Biol. Med., 74*:155 (1950).
126. B. Halpern, G. Mauric, A. Holtzer, and M. Briot, *Acta Allergol., 4*:207 (1951).
127. B. Halpern, G. Mauric, A. Holtzer, and M. Briot, *J. Allergy, 23*:303 (1952).
128. H. N. Eisen, M. M. Mayer, D. H. Moore, R. Tarr, and H. C. Stoerk, *Proc. Soc. Exp. Biol. Med., 65*:301 (1947).
129. P. D. McMaster, in *The Significance of the Antibody Response* (A. M. Pappenheimer, Jr., ed.), Columbia University Press, New York, 1953, pp. 13-45.
130. T. F. Dougherty, *Prog. Allergy, 4*:319 (1955).
131. A. E. Gabrielsen and R. A. Good, *Advan. Immunol., 6*:91 (1967).
132. T. F. Dougherty, H. H. Chase, and A. White, *Proc. Soc. Exp. Biol. Med., 58*:135 (1945).
133. B. Benacerraf, in *Immunological Tolerance* (M. Landy and W. Braun, eds.), Academic Press, New York, 1969, pp. 3-11.
134. M. A. Bogdanova and L. P. Kopytovskaya, *Bull. Exp. Biol. Med., 69*:128 (1970).
135. R. W. Schayer, J. K. Davis, and R. L. Smiley, *Am. J. Physiol., 182*:54 (1955).
136. H. Yamasaki and T. Yamamoto, *Jpn. J. Pharmacol., 13*:223 (1963).
137. W. Schmutzler and G. P. Freundt, *Int. Arch. Allergy Appl. Immunol., 49*:209 (1975).
138. G. Filipp and B. Mess, *Ann. Allergy, 27*:607 (1969).
139. A. W. J. Broome and G. E. Lamming, *J. Endocrinol., 18*:229 (1959).
140. K. Stern and I. Davidson, *J. Immunol., 74*:479 (1955).
141. S. N. Tsao, *Proc. Soc. Exp. Biol. Med., 48*:38 (1941).
142. C. R. Wira and C. P. Sandoe, *Nature, 268*:534 (1977).
143. E. Von Haam and I. Rosenfeld, *J. Infect. Dis., 70*:243 (1942).
144. G. A. Feigen, R. C. Fraser, and N. S. Peterson, *Int. Arch. Allergy Appl. Immunol., 57*:488 (1978).
145. H. Selye, *Can. Med. Assoc. J., 41*:48 (1939).
146. K. Kasahara, S. Tanaka, T. Ito, and Y. Hamashima, *Res. Commun. Chem. Pathol. Pharmacol., 16*:687 (1977).
147. N. R. Hall, J. E. McClure, S.-K. Hu, N. T. Tick, C. M. Seals, and A. L. Goldstein, *Soc. Neurosci. (Abst.), 26*:4 (1980).
148. H. Besedovsky, A. Del Rey, E. Sorkin, M. Da Prada, and H. Keller, *Cell. Immunol., 48*:346 (1979).
149. J. M. Williams, R. G. Peterson, P. A. Shea, J. F. Schmedtje, D. C. Bauer, and P. L. Felton, *Brain Res. Bull., 6*(1):83 (1979).
150. K. L. Melmon, H. R. Bourne, Y. Weinstein, and M. Sela, *Science, 177*:707 (1972).

151. G. M. Shearer, K. L. Melmon, Y. Weinstein, and M. Sela, *J. Exp. Med., 136*:1302 (1972).
152. U. Singh and J. J. T. Owen, *Eur. J. Immunol., 6*:59 (1976).
153. U. Singh, D. S. Millson, P. A. Smith, and J. J. T. Owen, *Eur. J. Immunol., 9*:31 (1979).
154. D. L. Berliner and T. F. Dougherty, *Pharmacol. Rev., 13*:329 (1961).
155. T. F. Dougherty, M. L. Berliner, and D. L. Berliner, in *Progress in Hematology*, Vol. 3 (L. M. Tocantins, ed.), Greun and Stratton, New York, 1962, p. 155.
156. T. F. Dougherty, M. L. Berliner, and D. L. Berliner, *Endocrinology, 66*:550 (1960).
157. A. Munck, *Perspect. Biol. Med., 14*:265 (1971).
158. K. M. Mosher, D. A. Young, and A. Munck, *J. Biol. Chem., 245*:2074 (1971).
159. W. D. Wicks, in *Biochemistry of Hormones*, Vol. 8 (H. V. Rickenberg, ed.), 1974, pp. 211-241.
160. A. Munck, *J. Biol. Chem., 243*:1039 (1968).
161. J. I. Morgan, J. S. Bramhall, A. Z. Britten, and A. D. Perris, *Biochem. Biophys. Res. Commun., 72*:633 (1976).
162. J. I. Morgan, J. S. Bramhall, A. Z. Britten, and A. D. Perris, *J. Endocrinol., 69*:P29 (1976).
163. J. I. Morgan and A. D. Perris, *J. Endocrinol., 61*:LXXVII (1974).
164. G. R. Smith, M. L. Gurson, A. J. Ridell, and A. D. Perris, *J. Endocrinol., 65*:45 (1975).
165. L. E. Clemens, P. K. Siiteri, and D. P. Stites, *J. Immunol., 122*:1978 (1979).
166. D. Kumar, R. S. Azoury, and A. C. Barnes, *Am. J. Obstet. Gynecol., 87*:126 (1963).
167. D. G. Porter and H. R. Behrman, *Nature, 232*:627 (1971).
168. Ch. V. Rao, *Steroids, 27*:831 (1976).
169. R. Schrek, *Endocrinol., 45*:317 (1949).
170. D. DiSorbo, F. Rosen, R. P. McPartland, and R. J. Milholland, *Ann. N. Y. Acad. Sci., 286*:355 (1977).
171. Y. Weinstein, H. R. Lindner, and B. Eckstein, *Nature, 266*:632 (1977).
172. Y. Weinstein, *J. Immunol., 119*:1223 (1977).
173. A. S. Fuks and Y. Weinstein, *J. Immunol., 123*:1266 (1979).
174. P. Sobhon and C. Jirasattham, *Acta Anat., 89*:211 (1974).
175. J. I. Kitay, *Endocrinology, 73*:253 (1963).
176. R. D. Lisk, *Am. J. Physiol., 203*:493 (1962).
177. E. Terasawa and P. S. Timiras, *Brain Res., 14*:189 (1969).
178. B. R. Komisaruk, in *Reproductive Behavior* (W. Montagne, and W. A. Sadler, eds.), Plenum Press, New York, 1974, p. 97.
179. D. E. Wooley and P. S. Timiral, *Endocrinology, 70*:196 (1962).
180. J. A. Vilchez-Martinez, A. Arimura, and A. V. Schally, *Proc. Soc. Exp. Biol. Med., 146*:859 (1974).
181. M. Sar and W. E. Stumpf, *Science, 183*:1266 (1973).
182. D. Meruelo and M. Edidin, in *Contemporary Topics in Immunobiology*, Vol. 9, (H. J. Marchalonis and N. Cohen, eds.), Plenum Press, New York, 1980, pp. 231-252.
183. P. Ivanyi, R. Hampl, L. Starka, and M. Mickova, *Nature* (*New Biol.*), *283*:280 (1972).
184. P. Ivanyi, S. Gregorova, and M. Mickova, *Folia Biol., 18*:81 (1972).
185. D. Meruelo and M. Edidin, *Fed. Am. Soc. Exp. Biol. Proc. 34*:979 (1975).
186. W. Lafuse and M. Edidin, *Fed. Am. Soc. Exp. Biol. Proc., 37*:1600 (1978).
187. P. W. Andrews and E. A. Boyse, *Immunogenetics, 6*:265 (1978).
188. D. N. Paton, *J. Physiol., 32*:28 (1905).

189. D. H. Andersen, *Physiol. Rev., 12*:1 (1932).
190. C. R. Martin, *Am. J. Physiol., 206*:193 (1964).
191. L. Miller and C. R. Martin, *Fed. Amer. Soc. Exp. Biol. Proc. (Abst.), 28*:774 (1979).
192. B. Rosoff and C. R. Martin, *Gen. Comp. Endocrinol., 16*:484 (1971).
193. H. O. Besedovsky and E. Sorkin, *Nature, 249*:356 (1974).
194. S. Linter-Moore and E. M. Pantelouris, *Mech. Aging Dev., 4*:385 (1975).
195. Y. Nishizuka and T. Sakakura, *Endocrinology, 89*:886 (1971).
196. S. Lintern-Moore and E. M. Pantelouris, *Mech. Aging Dev., 5*:33 (1976).
197. Y. Weinstein, *Mech. Aging Dev., 8*:63 (1978).
198. B. Romeis, *Klin. Wochenschr., 5*:955 (1926).
199. J. Camus and J. J. Gournay, *Comp. Rend. Acad. D. Sci. CLXXVIII*:673 (1924).
200. P. Leveboullet and J. J. Gournay, *Bull. Soc. Pediatr. Paris, XXV*:341 (1927).
201. M. Mandelstamm, *Contribution a l'etude du rale physiologique du thymus*, Paris, 403, 47, p. 8
202. P. Deuticke and E. Graff, *Arch. F. Exper. Path. Pharm. CXLV:359* (1929).
203. J. Comsa, *Hormones, 2*:226 (1971).
204. P. Deschaux, B. Massengo, and R. Fontanges, *Thymus, 1*:95 (1979).
205. G. Bernardi and J. Comsa, *Experientia, 21*:416 (1965).
206. A. L. Goldstein, A. Guha, M. M. Zatz, and A. White, *Proc. Natl. Acad. Sci. USA, 69*:1800 (1972).
207. R. W. Rebar, A. Miyake, T. L. K. Low, and A. L. Goldstein, *Science, 214*:669 (1981).
208. J. P. McGillis, T. Feith, E. Kyeynne-Nyombi, G. V. Vahouny, N. R. Hall, and A. L. Goldstein, *Fed. Proc., 41*:4918 (1982).
209. G. V. Vahouny, E. Kyeyune-Nyombi, J. P. McGillis, N. S. Tare, K-Y. Huang, R. Tombes, A. L. Goldstein, and N. R. Hall, *J. Immunol., 30*:79 (1983).
210. N. R. Hall, J. P. McGillis, B. Spangelo, E. Palaszynski, T. Moody, and A. L. Goldstein, in *Current Concepts in Human Immunology* (B. Serrou, C. Rosenfeld, J. C. Daniels, and J. P. Saunders, eds.), Elsevier, New York, 1982, pp. 653-660.
211. G. A. Belokrylov, V. G. Morozov, and R. H. Khavinson, *Bull. Exp. Biol. Med., 86*:1631-1632 (1979).
212. R. K. Saxena and G. P. Talwar, *Nature, 268*:57-58 (1977).
213. E. Straus, J. E. Muller, H-S. Choi, F. Paronetto, and R. S. Yalow, *Proc. Nat. Acad. Sci., 74*:3033-3034 (1977).
214. N. R. Hall, E. W. Palaszynski, T. W. Moody, and A. L. Goldstein, *Soc. Neurosci.* (Abst.), (1981).
215. E. Palaszynski, Ph.D. dissertation, George Washington University, 1982.
216. H. O. Besedovsky and E. Sorkin, *Clin. Exp. Immunol., 27*:1-12 (1977).
217. T. L. K. Low, G. B. Thurman, M. McAdoo, J. E. McClure, J. L. Rossio, P. H. Naylor, and A. L. Goldstein, *J. Biol. Chem., 254*:981 (1979).
218. A. Ahmed, D. M. Wong, G. B. Thurman, T. L. K. Low, A. L. Goldstein, S. J. Sharkis, and I. Goldschneider, *Ann. N. Y. Acad. Sci., 332*:81 (1979).
219. S-K. Hu, G. B. Thurman, T. L. K. Low, J. McClure, and A. L. Goldstein, *New Trends Immunol. Cancer Ther.* (in press).
220. D. H. Schlesinger and G. Goldstein, *Cell., 5*:361 (1975).
221. J. M. Pleau, M. Dardenne, Y. Bouquit, and J. F. Bach, *J. Biol. Chem., 252*:8045 (1977).
222. M. Freire, E. Hannappel, M. Rey, J. M. Freire, H. Kido, and B. L. Horecker, *Proc. Nat. Acad. Sci., USA, 78*:192 (1981).
223. E. Hannappel, S. Davoust, and B. L. Horecker, *Biochem. Biophysical. Res. Commun., 104*:266 (1982).
224. R. Wetzel, H. L. Heyneker, D. V. Goeddel, P. Jhurani, J. Shapiro, R. Crea, T. L. K. Low, J. E. McClure, A. L. Goldstein, *Biochem., 19*:6096 (1980).

225. A. L. Golstein, T. L. K. Low, G. B. Thurman, M. M. Zatz, N. R. Mall, J. Chen, S-K. Hu, P. B. Naylor, and J. E. McClure, *Rec. Prog. Hor. Res., 37*:369–415 (1981).
226. E. Hannappel, G-J. Xu, J. Morgan, J. Hempstead, and B. L. Horecker, *Proc. Nat. Acad. Sci. USA, 79*:2172 (1982).
227. C. G. Craddock, *Ann. Int. Med., 88*:564 (1978).
228. C. R. Martin, *Am. J. Physiol., 206*:193 (1964).
229. G. B. Thurman, J. L. Rossio, and A. L. Goldstein, *Transplant. Proc., 9*:1201 (1977).
230. J. F. Bach, D. Duval, M. Dardenne, J. C. Salomon, T. Tursz, and C. Fournier, *Transplant. Proc., 7*:25 (1975).
231. W. Pierpaoli, N. Fabris, and E. Sorkin, in *Homrones and the Immune Response, Ciba Foundation Study Group. No. 36* (G. E. W. Wolstenholme and J. Knight, eds.), London, Churchill, 1970, pp. 126-143.
232. W. Pierpaoli, N. Fabris, and E. Sorkin, in *Cellular Interactions in the Immune Responses* (S. Cohen, G. Cudkowicz, and R. T. McCluikey, eds.), Darger, Basel, 1971, p. 25.
233. W. Pierpaoli and E. Sorkin, *Experientia, 28*:1385 (1972).
234. W. Pierpaoli and E. Sorkin, *Nature* (*New Biol.*), *238*:282 (1972).
235. W. Pierpaoli and H. O. Besedovsky, *Clin. Exp. Immunol., 20*:323 (1975).
236. W. Pierpaoli and G. J. M. Maestroni, *Cell. Immunol., 31*:355 (1977).
237. N. R. Hall and A. L. Goldstein, in *Psychoneuroimmunology* (R. Ader, ed.), Academic Press, New York, 1981, pp. 521-543.
238. N. R. Hall, in *Peptides, Hormones, and Behavior* (C. B. Nemeroff and A. J. Dunn, eds.), Spectrum, New York, 1984, pp. 913-938.
239. W. Pierpaoli, H. G. Kopp, and E. Bianchi, *Clin. Exp. Immunol., 24*:501 (1976).
240. R. Bleier and R. Albrecht, *J. Comp. Neurol., 192*:489 (1980).
241. A. Fontana, A. Grieder, S. T. Arrenbrecht, P. Grob, *J. Neurol. Sci., 46*:55 (1980).
242. M. L. Billingsley, N. R. Hall, and H. G. Mandel, *Immunopharmacology 5*:95 (1982).
243. M. J. Stadecker and E. R. Unanue, *Ann. N. Y. Acad. Sci., 332*:550 (1979).
244. P. G. Harms, S. R. Ojeda, and S. M. McCann, *Science, 181*:760 (1973).
245. G. A. Hedge, *Prostaglandins, 11*:293 (1976).
246. N. R. Hall and W. G. Luttge, *Brain Res. Bull., 2*:203 (1977).
247. N. R. Hall, W. G. Luttge, and R. B. Berry, *Prostaglandins, 10*:177 (1975).

27

Human Lymphocyte Studies Can Predict Responses to Thymic Factor Therapy

Nigel A. Byrom and John R. Hobbs Westminster Medical School, London, England

I. INTRODUCTION

The capacity of mature T lymphocytes to form spontaneous rosettes with sheep erythrocytes (E rosettes) has been used for over a decade to assess cellular immunocompetence in humans. Total peripheral blood T-lymphocyte levels (1) are determined under optimal rosetting conditions, whereas active or early T lymphocytes are determined under suboptimal conditions (2).

In normal children most peripheral blood T lymphocytes form active rosettes and few null (non-T, non-B) lymphocytes are detected. With increasing age, and particularly in cases of primary or secondary cellular immunodeficiency, levels of functional T lymphocytes tend to decline while levels of thymic hormone-inducible (immature or blocked ?) T lymphocytes (T_i-cells) tend to increase (3).

Thymic hormone extracts [e.g., Thymosin fraction 5 (Hoffmann-LaRoche) and Thymostimulin (TP-1 of Serono Laboratories)] have been shown by many authors to induce null cells of T lineage to form E rosettes both in vitro and in vivo in a very wide range of immunodeficiency situations. Similarly, thymic hormone activity has been demonstrated in human and in animal sera, and especially in fetal sera such as fetal calf serum (FCS) (5). Since many human disease states are associated with T-lymphocyte deficiency, and since T-lymphocyte levels tend to correlate with clinical conditions and prognosis (2,6-8,63,84-87,105,107,111), many studies are in progress to identify which diseases are likely to respond to modulation of immune status by thymic factor therapy.

Since 1975 we have been using the E-rosette test to assess baseline T-lymphocyte levels in over 1000 normal individuals and patients with a very wide range of immunodeficiencies, and here we summarize our findings for the main groups of subjects studied.

During this time we have worked with Thymosin fraction 5 (1975-1979) and with Thymostimulin (1979 to date), and both preparations have been studied over a wide (logarithmic) dilution range in order to determine the optimum concentration for E-rosette formation for each individual subject.

Early studies indicated that fetal calf serum, as used by many authors in lymphocyte separation, enumeration, and culture procedures, mimics the effect of thymic hormone extracts and may spuriously increase the apparent levels of E-rosette-forming cells (E-RFC) in immunodeficient subjects though usually not in normal individuals or in patients with normal T-lymphocyte numbers (3). Consequently, the incidence of T lymphopenia may have been underestimated in many studies and misleading conclusions have been obtained from many thousands of experiments.

In recent months, we have used monoclonal (mouse antihuman) antisera to identify T-lymphocyte subsets in some of the disease groups under study, often in addition to the E-rosette test. Although it has been known for almost 10 years that patients with atopic conditions such as atopic eczema frequently have a T lymphopenia (3,35-41), only recently has there been confirmation that these patients have a relative deficiency of cytotoxic/suppressor T cells (9,122). Until the monoclonal lymphocyte phenotyping antisera have been fully evaluated and accepted, however, we continue to use them in parallel with the established E-rosette test.

In the sections that follow, the results have been listed disease by disease. Three disease groups have been selected by us for in vivo study, and controlled clinical trials of Thymostimulin are currently in progress at Westminster Hospital and associated hospitals in (a) atopic eczema (adults), (b) malignant melanoma (newly diagnosed poor-prognosis patients undergoing surgery), and (c) recurrent genital herpes.

II. MATERIALS AND METHODS

A. Isolation of Lymphocytes

Peripheral blood, taken by venepuncture, was collected in heparinized tubes. Lymphocytes were isolated on Lymphoprep (Nyegaard, Oslo), washed in serum-free RPMI 1640 medium, and adjusted to a concentration of 5×10^6/ml.

B. Preparation of Sheep Red Blood Cells (SRBCs)

Sheep erythrocytes, always taken from the same sheep, were stored in Alsever's solution for not more than 1 week prior to use. When required, they were washed three times in phosphate-buffered saline (PBS) and resuspended at a concentration of approximately 1.0×10^7/ml in serum-free medium.

C. Total E-Rosette Test

One-tenth of a milliliter of lymphocyte suspension was incubated with an equal volume of (a) Thymosin fraction 5 (Hoffmann-LaRoche, Nutley, New Jersey) or Thymostimulin (TP-1; Serono Laboratories U.K. Ltd., Welwyn Garden City, England), diluted in log steps from 0.04 to 4000 μg/ml, or (b) heat-inactivated, SRBC-absorbed fetal calf serum (FCS) (Gibco-BioCult, Glasgow, Scotland, or Sera-Lab, Sussex, England), and incubated in plastic tubes at 37°C for 10 min. The same batches of thymic hormone preparations and of fetal calf serum were used throughout each individual study. One-fifth of a milliliter of the erythrocyte suspension was added to each tube with thorough mixing. Final thymic hormone concentrations ranged from 0.01 to 1000 μg/ml, and the final fetal calf serum concentration was 25%. Tubes were centrifuged gently at 150 X g for 5 min to bring the cells into contact, then incubated at 37°C for 15 min and at 4°C overnight. The next day, cell pellets were gently resuspended and E rosettes (lymphocytes binding three or more erythrocytes) were scored under a phase-contrast microscope.

D. Active E-Rosette Test

The active E-rosette test was conducted as for the total rosette test but incubating at 4°C only, and for only 3 hr.

E. T-lymphocyte Subset Analysis

The standard procedure for the Ortho-Mune mouse monoclonal antihuman T-lymphocyte (OKT) antibody tests was used (Ortho Diagnostics, High Wycombe, England), except that the recommended fetal calf serum was either omitted entirely throughout or tested in parallel with serum-free control medium.

An indirect immunofluorescent assay was employed, with fluoresceintagged goat antimouse antiserum (Cappel Laboratories, Cochranville, Pennsylvania) as the second antibody. Results were scored optically using a Leitz Orthoplan microscope (Leitz Instruments Ltd., Luton, England) fitted with an HBO 200-mercury vapor lamp and a fluorescence vertical illuminator.

Lymphocyte samples with very low percentages of cells reacting with the respective OKT reagents were incubated with Thymostimulin at 100 μg/ml for not less than 1 hr, and the OKT test was repeated.

III. SUBJECTS, RESULTS, AND DISCUSSION

A. Normal Control Subjects

1. Children

Normal healthy children (30 total; 19 male, 11 female) with ages ranging from 5 to 16 (mean 10 ± 3) years were the children of hospital staff or were inpatients admitted presurgery; parental consent was obtained before taking blood samples from any child. No child receiving treatment that was likely to affect immune parameters was included, and none had any history or family history of atopic disease.

2. Adults

Over 200 apparently healthy normal adults were tested in all, in batches concurrent with the various patient groups studied. These adults, whose ages ranged from 16 to 73 years, were hospital staff or blood donors or tissue-typed prospective bone marrow donors. As far as possible, subjects with histories or family histories of atopy, immunodeficiency, malignant or chronic disease, or who had received medication during the previous 2 weeks were excluded. Sex-matching of the patients and controls was not considered necessary, as we know of no published work showing significant sex dependence of T-lymphocyte levels. Age-matching was attempted, wherever possible, since T-lymphocyte levels have been shown to be age-related (3,10,11).

T-lymphocyte levels, as determined by total E-rosette formation, were significantly higher in our present study than in normal adults (Table 1), as reported by other authors. However, T-lymphocyte percentages were similar in both groups. The higher absolute T-lymphocyte counts of the children were found to reflect merely the higher overall lymphocyte counts of children.

Lymphocytes from most of the children failed to respond to in vitro Thymosin, whereas many samples from adults contained lymphocytes that were Thymosin-inducible (sometimes highly so). In adult subjects, the mean level of Thymosin-inducible lymphocytes (T_i cells) was 14.9%, considerably higher than the 4.7% reported by Wara et al. (12); these latter authors included FCS in their assay system, and thymic or other factors in the serum may have resulted in underestimation of the T_i-cell levels (5,13).

The finding of higher levels of Thymosin-responsive lymphocytes in adults than in children is consistent with reports of higher blood thymic hormone levels in children than adults (4). Percentage of Thymosin-inducible T lymphocytes (T_i) was directly proportional to age ($p < 0.008$; Fig. 1).

Rosette formation by lymphocytes from almost 75% of children was frankly inhibited by in vitro Thymosin at all concentrations, inferring that the circulating levels of thymic hormones in children are, indeed, already high. As found previously (12,14,15), Thymosin failed to increase T-lymphocyte percentages of normal subjects with high baseline values. In therapeutic practice this is, in fact, the case; for example, cancer patients only show significant increases in T lymphocytes where the pretreatment baseline value is low (89). Reports in normal and malignant situations all indicate that thymic factor therapy should be restricted to those patients with T lymphopenia; excessive doses of thymic factors could even prove immunosuppressive (13) and at best would represent wastage of valuable thymic extract material.

The results from our normal child group support the concept (16) that thymus-dependent immunity undergoes a senescence. Following birth, the thymus gland atrophies and blood thymic hormone levels fall; meanwhile, the diseases of aging (cancer and autoimmune and infectious diseases) are found to increase. It seems likely that much age-

Table 1 Levels of T Lymphocytes and Thymosin-Inducible T-Lymphocytes in Normal Adults and Children

		Total lymphocytes	T lymphocytes in medium alone	Maximum T lymphocytes with Thymosin	Thymosin-inducible T lymphocytes
Normal adults (N = 50)	Percent	–	47.7	62.6	14.9
	Per mm^3 [a]	2424	1155	1525	369
Normal children (N = 30)	Percent	–	52.2 (NS)[b,c]	52.7 (0.0004)	0.5 (0.0009)
	Per mm^3	3506 (0.00005)	1718 (0.0003)	1816 (0.04)	67 (0.006)

[a]Absolute numbers of lymphocytes per cubic millimeter of peripheral blood.
[b]NS, not significant.
[c]P values (in parentheses) were obtained by the Mann-Whitney U test.

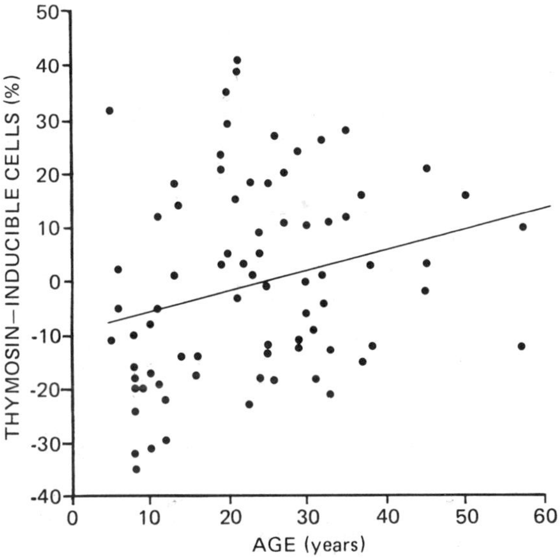

Figure 1 Increase in peripheral blood Thymosin-inducible null cell levels in direct proportion to increasing age in 80 normal control subjects. Correlation coefficient, $p = 0.30$. P (Wilcoxon paired test) < 0.008.

related disease is secondary to the decline in T-lymphocyte levels and the increase in null cell levels. However, there is often also an age-related decline in total lymphocyte levels (3), and this may be due in part to declining stem cell production by the bone marrow. Declining lymphopoiesis may also be the result of declining thymic hormone levels, since these hormones have been shown to enhance lymphocyte production (17,18). Thus, the prophylactic treatment of geriatrics by thymic factor therapy may significantly reduce morbidity and mortality.

Earlier studies from this laboratory (19) indicated that normal adults with the HLA antigens A1, B8 tended to have above-normal levels of (apparent) B lymphocytes in the peripheral blood. It was therefore of interest to determine whether T-lymphocyte levels correlated with tissue type. Using the total E-rosette test, 30 normal adults having HLA B8 were compared with 30 age-matched adults who did not have this antigen.

A strong correlation has been reported between HLA B8 and a wide range of diseases (21) with apparent involvement of cellular immunity (e.g., systemic lupus erythematosus and myasthenia gravis). Many of these diseases have an autoimmune component, often associated with loss of depletion of the suppressor T lymphocytes. Thymic deficiency could result in a deficit of suppressor cells (16). In our present study (Table 2), HLA B8+ subjects were found to have a high level of Thymosin-inducible cells, suggesting that there may be a low circulating thymic hormone level and defective T-lymphocyte maturation which could in turn result in autoantibody production. HLA B8– individuals, on the other hand, have no Thymosin-inducible T lymphocytes; indeed, added Thymosin actually inhibited E-rosette formation in some samples. Thus it would appear that, at the optimum Thymosin concentration of 20 μg/ml, HLA B8+ individuals tend to have a relative Thymosin deficiency, and this may be relevant to the link between this haplotype and autoimmune and/or atopic disease (see section on atopic eczema). It will be of interest to determine

Table 2 Thymosin Inducibility of HLA B8+ But Not of HLA B8– Lymphocytes[a]

	Total lymphocytes	T-lymphocytes (total E-rosette test) With medium alone	With fetal calf serum	With Thymosin (20 μg/ml)	Thymosin-inducible T-lymphocytes (T_i-cells)
HLA B8+ subjects (N = 30)	2350	1270 (54%)	1410 (60%)	1480 (63%)	220 (9%)
HLA B8– subjects (N = 30)	2400	1350 (57%)	1200 (52%)	1320 (55%)	0 (0%)

[a]Results are in cells/mm³ of peripheral blood (percentages in parentheses).
Source: Ref. 20.

levels of cytotoxic/suppressor (OKT8+) lymphocytes in the presence and absence of B8, with and without prior Thymosin induction.

The presence of fetal calf serum in the E-rosette test produced differential results in the two populations in Table 2, with serum producing a similar effect to that of Thymosin.

B. Children with Wiskott-Aldrich Syndrome

A total of 4 boys were studied: a 5-year-old; a boy of 6 months of age; two brothers aged 2 years and 8 months, respectively. The mean age of the patients was 26 months, and it was not found possible to match these for age with the control group of 30 children whose mean age was 9.9 years.

1. In Vitro Studies

The mean T-lymphocyte percentage (Table 3) in the patients was significantly lower than that in the control group, although the difference could be abolished by Thymosin in vitro as reported elsewhere (12).

2. In Vivo Study

The 5-year-old-boy (see details above) was given Thymosin therapy at age 7 years when he had severe atopic eczema involving his entire skin surface and failing to respond to dietary or corticosteroid measures. Pretherapy results had averaged: T lymphocytes, 350/mm^3 of peripheral blood; Thymosin-inducible (T_i) lymphocytes, 1200/mm^3; eosinophils, 900/mm^3; total serum IgE, 7000 IU/ml. He received 2 mg Thymosin fraction 5/kg body weight daily for 14 days, by which time complete clearing of his skin had occurred except for a few lesions in the antecubital fossae. Posttherapy results averaged: T lymphocytes, 1750/mm^3; T_i cells, 400/mm^3; eosinophils, 300/mm^3; total serum IgE, 200 IU/ml. Concanavalin A (ConA) induced suppression of the autologous mixed-lymphocyte reaction (MLR), originally zero, improved to give a 55% reduction. After a break of 4 days without treatment, a skin test of neat Thymosin produced an immediate reaction with pseudopodia so no further Thymosin therapy was given in case of anaphlyl-axis. His skin remained excellent for 6 months, motivating us to initiate a clinical trail of thymic hormone therapy in adult patients with lifelong atopic eczema (see below).

Although thymic hormone therapy may prove useful in reconstituting cellular immunity in Wiskott-Aldrich patients, it cannot, of course, overcome the main problem

Table 3 T-Lymphocyte Levels (Total E-Rosette Test) and Thymosin Inducibility of Normal Children and of Children with Wiskott-Aldrich Syndrome

		Total lymphocytes	T lymphocytes in medium alone	Maximum T lymphocytes with Thymosin	Thymosin-inducible T lymphocytes (T_i)
Normal children (N = 30)	Percent	–	52.2	52.7	0.5
	Per mm^3 [a]	3505	1718	1816	67
Wiskott-Aldrich children (N = 4)	Percent	–	11.5 (0.004) [b]	36.0 (NS)	23.3 (0.04)
	Per mm^3	3858 (NS)	355 (<0.004)	728 (<0.01)	482 (NS)

[a]Absolute number of lymphocytes per cubic millimeter of peripheral blood.
[b]P values (in parentheses) obtained by Mann-Whitney U test.
[c]NS, not significant.
Source: Ref. 3.

of thrombocytopenia which can only be corrected by bone marrow transplantation. Indeed, enhancement of the immune response in these patients, although it may improve the eczema and lessen the incidence of infections, may exacerbate graft-versus-host disease if the patient receives a bone marrow graft subsequently. Our patient had a very rare tissue type and no sibling marrow donor, and eventually died from his thrombocytopenia before a compatible unrelated marrow donor could be selected from the panel on our computer.

C. Children with Atopic Asthma

A total of 30 asthmatic children (15 male, 15 female) had ages ranging from 8 to 17 (mean 11 ± 3) years. They were all undoubted asthmatics in whom immediate hypersensitivity had been well documented. Every patient had had a plasma total IgE level in excess of 1000 IU/ml at some time in the previous 2 years. No patient was receiving corticosteroids or adrenocorticotropic hormone testing. Some had mild, some moderate, and some severe asthma symptoms.

As a group, the asthmatics (Table 4) had a significantly lower T-lymphocyte mean than the normal group, as has been reported previously (24-26). The difference was, however, abolished if the lymphocytes were preincubated with Thymosin at optimum concentration before adding the sheep erythrocytes for the E-rosette test. It was noted that if fetal calf serum was present in the assay system when baseline E-rosette levels were determined then no T-lymphocyte deficit was observed. Thymosin-like activity of fetal calf serum may have been responsible for the failure of some authors to detect T lymphopenia in asthma patients (27).

The T lymphopenia detected in the asthmatics may underly the known increased incidence or severity of infections and defective cellular reactivity already reported in such patients (25). The observed Thymosin-inducibility of lymphocytes, taken together with the finding of low circulating thymic hormone levels (28), elevated levels of autoantibodies (29), and excessive procuction of IgE (23,25,30-33), suggests that asthma

Table 4 T-Lymphocyte Levels (Total E-Rosette Test) and Thymosin Inducibility of Normal Children and Children with Atopic Asthma

		Total lymphocytes	T lymphocytes in medium alone	Maximum T lymphocytes with Thymosin	Thymosin-inducible T lymphocytes (T_i)	T lymphocytes in medium plus fetal calf serum (FCS)
Normal children (N = 30)	Percent	--	52.2	52.7	0.5	45.3
	Per mm^3 [a]	3506	1718	1816	67	1555
Asthma children (N = 30)	Percent	–	31.5 (0.0008)[b]	53.1 (NS)	20.8 (0.0006)	50.9 (NS)
	Per mm^3	3501 (NS)	1043 (0.0008)	1770 (NS)	693 (0.0006)	1695 (NS)

[a]Absolute numbers of lymphocytes per cubic millimeter of peripheral blood.
[b]P values (in parentheses) were obtained by the Mann-Whitney U test.
[c]NS, not significant.
Source: Ref. 23.

may result from a defective maturation of suppressor T-lymphocyte mechanisms as described in atopic eczema and in atopy in general (9,34). Thymic hormone therapy may enhance suppressor mechanisms and bring IgE production under control with concomitant clinical benefit.

D. Patients with Atopic Eczema

1. Children

A total of 30 children (16 male, 14 female) had ages ranging from 1 to 14 (mean 9 ± 4) years. All had undoubted eczema, with the age of onset ranging from 0 to 11 years. At least 75% of the patients had a family history of atopy; all were referred to an out-patient clinic with active disease.

A total of 16 patients had eczema alone, 5 had eczema + allergic rhinitis, 5 had eczema + asthma, and 4 had eczema + asthma + allergic rhinitis. Two had overt infection at the time of testing. None had received systemic cotticosteroids or ACTH during the previous year. A total of 5 had mild symptoms, 8 had moderate symptoms, and 17 had severe disease.

As in the child asthma group (above), the eczema group had a significantly lower T-lymphocyte mean than did the normal group (Table 5), as has been reported (36-41).

This T lymphopenia apparently underlies a defect in cellular immunity, consistent with the known incidence and/or severity of infection and the defective cellular reactivity reported in patients with atopic eczema (37,41-43).

The use of fetal calf serum in the E-rosette assay system results in spurious overestimation of levels of E-RFC in the eczema population (for a review, see Ref. 44). Similarly, FCS has been found to normalize the depressed in vitro responses of eczema patients' lymphocytes to the mitogen, phytohemagglutinin (PHA) (39,45).

Preincubation of lymphocytes with Thymosin at optimum dilution resulted in normalization of E-rosette formation (Table 5) in the eczema group, as in the asthma

Table 5 T-Lymphocyte Levels (Total E-Rosette Test) and Thymosin Inducibility of Normal Children and Children with Atopic Eczema

		Total lympho-cytes	T-lympho cytes in medium alone	Maximum T lympho-cytes with Thymosin	Thymosin-inducible T cells (T_i)	T lympho-cytes in medium plus fetal calf serum (FCS)
Normal children (N = 30)	Percent	–	52.2	52.7	0.5	45.3
	Per mm^3 [a]	3506	1718	1816	67	1555
Eczema children (N = 30)	Percent	–	35.3 (0.005)[b]	56.4 (NS)	20.9 (0.0004)	61.3 (NS)
	Per mm^3	3456 (NS)	1214 (0.008)	1936 (NS)	713 (0.0008)	1757 (NS)

[a]Absolute numbers of lymphocytes per cubic milliliter of peripheral blood.
[b]P values (in parentheses) were obtained by the Mann-Whitney U test.
[c]NS, not significant.
Source: Ref. 35.

group (Table 4). Significantly high levels of Thymosin-inducible (immature T ?) lymphocytes apparently circulate in the peripheral blood of eczema patients, and it appears that eczema patients fail to produce enough of at least one of the thymic hormones as has been demonstrated for asthmatic children (28).

In an earlier paper (22), we reported a strong correlation between the levels of Thymosin-inducible T cells (T_i) and total plasma IgE levels. It is possible that the T_i cells are increased at the expense of a more mature T-lymphocyte population capable of suppressing IgE levels. We could find no evidence that sera containing high levels of IgE could themselves lead to an increase in T_i-cell levels or otherwise inhibit E-rosetting, although it remains a possibility that histamine could block rosette formation. It appears likely that the presence of excess T_i cells precedes lack of control of IgE production. In animals it has been shown that reaginic antibody formation is influenced by T lymphocytes (46), and studies in rats (47-49) revealed a T-lymphocyte subpopulation capable of suppressing reaginic antibody formation. Moretta et al. (50) have detected a T-lymphocyte subpopulation ($T\gamma$) capable of suppressing immunoglobulin production, and this subpopulation has been found to be deficient in atopic patients (34,51,52). In later studies (see below) we used monoclonal antisera to characterize T-lymphocyte subsets in adult atopic eczema patients.

2. Adults

First Study. A total of 30 adults (14 male, 16 female) had ages ranging from 17 to 55 (mean, 27) years. All had undoubted atopic eczema and had been referred to an outpatient clinic with active disease. None had overt infection at the time of investigation, and none had recently been treated with systemic corticosteroids. Age distributions for eczema and normal adults were not significantly different.

In percentage terms, though not in absolute numbers, the T-lymphocyte depletion was more marked in the child eczema patients than in the adult patients (Table 6), in view

Table 6 T-Lymphocyte Levels (Total E-Rosette Test) and Thymosin Inducibility of Normal Adults and Adults with Atopic Eczema

		Total lympho-cytes	T lympho-cytes in medium alone	Maximum T lympho-cytes with Thymosin	Thymosin-inducible T cells (T_i)	T lympho-cytes in medium plus fetal calf serum (FCS)
Normal adults (N = 50)	Percent	–	47.7	62.6	14.9	49.2
	Per mm^3 [a]	2424	1155	1525	369	1226
Eczema adults (N = 30)	Percent	–	40.0 (0.003)[b]	60.4 (NS)[c]	20.4 (NS)	50.3 (NS)
	Per mm^3	2349 (NS)	892 (NS)	1416 (NS)	524 (NS)	50.3 (NS)

[a]Absolute numbers of lymphocytes per cubic millimeter of peripheral blood.
[b]P values (in parentheses) obtained by Mann-Whitney U test.
[c]NS, not significant.

of the age-related decline in T-lymphocyte levels and the reciprocal increase in T_i-cell levels (Fig. 1). Levels of T_i cells were comparable in the normal and eczema adult populations, although there may still be qualitative differences.

Once more, Thymosin and fetal calf serum abolished the quantitative T-lymphocyte discrepancy between the groups in Table 6.

Second Study. With the advent of monoclonal antisera against T-lymphocyte subgroups (Ortho-Mune, OKT series), the study was repeated using further populations of 20 normal adults and 20 patients with undoubted atopic eczema.

For this study, T lymphocytes were detected by the active E-rosette test performed using medium alone, medium containing Thymostimulin at optimum concentration, and medium containing 25% fetal calf serum. The following T-lymphocyte subsets were tested for: total T lymphocytes (OKT3+), helper/inducer (OKT4+), and cytotoxic/suppressor (OKT8+). Since previous studies had suggested that suppressor cells are in deficit in eczema patients, the OKT8 test was performed in the absence of serum, in the presence of FCS (as recommended by Ortho), and in the presence of Thymostimulin (see Materials and Methods section).

In this (second) adult eczema study the source of sheep erythrocytes differed from that used in the first study, and the rosetting procedure also differed. Nevertheless, the eczema group showed the usual deficit (Table 7) of E-RFC but only when Thymostimulin and fetal calf serum were omitted from the test. The active rosette test is generally considered to be a more accurate test of T-lymphocyte status than the total E-rosette test (6,53).

Referring to Table 8, the results of the OKT3 (pan-T) test indicate that both groups of subjects have identical levels of T lymphocytes overall, so presumably eczema patients have higher levels of immature or blocked T lymphocytes or perhaps a lower E-receptor density or inferior SRBC-binding affinity; indeed, defective E-rosetting by eczema patients' lymphocytes may simply be the result of the lymphocytes having a low intracellular cyclic GMP (cGMP) level (4).

Table 7 T-Lymphocyte Levels (Active E-Rosette Test) and Thymostimulin Inducibility of Normal Adults and Patients with Atopic Eczema

	T lymphocytes in medium alone (%)	Maximum T lymphocytes with Thymostimulin (%)	Thymostimulin-inducible T lymphocytes (%) (T_i)	T lymphocytes in medium plus fetal calf serum (%)
Normal Adults (N = 20)	44	49	5	52
Eczema adults	35 (<0.04)[a]	54 (NS)[b]	19 (<0.01)	60 (NS)

[a]P values (in parentheses) were obtained by the Mann-Whitney U test.
[b]NS, not significant.

As previously reported (9,51,54) this present study reveals an imbalance of T-lymphocyte subsets in atopic eczema, with helper/inducer cells slightly increased in proportion and cytotoxic/suppressor cells proportionately decreased. The net result is a grossly abnormal ratio of OKT4+/OKT8+ lymphocytes. Other authors note an inverse relationship between cytotoxic/suppressor lymphocyte levels and eczema severity (51, 52), even in the same patient studied longitudinally, with normalization of the levels of these cells concomitant with clinical remission following specific hyposensitization (51). Another paper (54) reports that the helper/suppressor cell ratio and the total serum IgE level are directly proportional to one another. It is still unclear whether excessive IgE production in atopics is the result of enhanced helper activity, reduced suppressor activity, or both, or indeed neither.

The results in Table 8 also indicate that Thymostimulin induction can normalize the levels of OKT8+ lymphocytes in eczema lymphocyte populations studied in vitro while normal lymphocytes fail to respond. This suggests that eczema patients may be failing to produce significant thymic factors presumed necessary for suppressor cell

Table 8 T Lymphocyte Subsets (Ortho-mune OKT Test) and Thymostimulin (TP-1)[a] Inducibility of Normal Adults and Patients with Atopic Eczema[b]

	T lymphocytes overall (OKT3+) (%)	Helper/inducer cells (OKT4+) (%)	Cytotoxic/suppressor (OKT8+) cells in medium (%)			OKT4+/ OKT8+ (Ratio)
			Alone	+TP-1	+FCS	
Normal Adults (N = 20)	74	44	20	25	27	1.74
Eczema Adults (N = 20)	74 (NS)	47 (NS)	20 (<0.02)	25 (NS)	25 (NS)	2.63 (<0.01)

[a]TP-1, Thymostimulin.
[b]All values are given as percentages of the total lymphocyte population.
[c]NS, not significant.
[d]P values (in parentheses) obtained by the Mann-Whitney U test.

maturation; alternatively, elevated histamine levels may be blocking otherwise mature and functional lymphocytes. Preliminary results from our double-bind clinical trial of Thymostimulin in eczema indicate that some OKT8– lymphocytes can be induced to become OKT8+ in vivo too.

Finally, fetal calf serum was found to result in spurious overestimation of levels of OKT8+ lymphocytes, and we recommend that the use of this serum (as recommended by the manufacturers of Ortho-Mune reagents) should be discontinued. Our studies in normal individuals indicate that serum is not a necessary ingredient in the medium for the performance of the OKT tests; phosphate-buffered saline (PBS) appears to substitute for medium plus serum in a satisfactory manner. We understand that the manufacturers have withdrawn or will withdraw the recommendation to use fetal calf serum in their test procedures.

In Vivo Study, using Thymosin. Patient M.D., a 29-year-old male, had had asthma and atopic eczema throughout childhood and as an adult still suffered from severe atopic eczema which failed to respond to dietary or corticosteroid therapy. He had confluent eczema, covering the entire cutaneous surface apart from one small area of normal skin on one ankle which was used for skin testing (negative). Three blood samples pretherapy gave average results of: T lymphocytes, 170/mm^3; T_i cells, 600/mm^3; eosinophils, 2800/mm^3; total serum IgE, 4700 IU/ml. He received 1 mg Thymosin/kg body weight repeated at 3-day intervals to a total of four doses, as an inpatient. By 14 days his skin was the best he could remember in 18 years, with a 50% reduction of the skin surface area involved in the eczema. Four posttherapy blood samples averaged: T lymphocytes, 1450/mm^3; T_i cells, 240/mm^3, eosinophils, 1800/mm^3; total serum IgE level, 3200 IU/ml. ConA-induced suppression of his mixed-lymphocyte reaction (MLR) against mitomycin-treated stimulator cells from a pool of five donors showed pretherapy an average reduction by 20%; following therapy this average was 70%; a highly significant increase in T-suppresor function. It was unclear, however, from this study whether some of the obvious beneficial clinical effects of the thymic factor therapy may have been due to placebo effect (e.g., the relief of stress resulting from the patient's absence from work and from his hospitilization).

Another male patient with several intractable atopic eczema, 23-year-old M.W., also had virtually total skin involvement. This had been complicated during the previous six months by outbreaks of *Herpes simplex* over the upper half of his body. This lasted about 5 days and recurred at 10-20 day intervals. Pretherapy results averaged: T lymphocytes, 1300/mm^3; T_i cells, 650/mm^3; eosinophils, 800/mm^3; total serum IgE, 1100 IU/ml. To a skin test dose of undiluted Thymosin he produced an immediate reaction with pseudopodia. Instead of Thymosin, he received Levamisole (Janssen) 150 mg on alternate days for 8 weeks, with weekly granulocyte monitoring. He considered his eczema improved, but no less extensive. The herpes outbreaks had improved, being less frequent (20-30 days between attacks), less extensive, and clearing within 2 days of onset. Posttherapy results averaged: T lymphocytes, 2100/mm^3; T_i cells, 150/mm^3; eosinophils, 300/mm^3; total serum IgE level, 300 IU/ml. ConA-induced suppression of the MLR improved marginally from 10 to 38%.

Both of these adult eczema patients showed pretherapy in vitro evidence of impaired T-lymphocyte function and benefitted considerably within 2 weeks of commencing immunoreconstitution therapy. As predicted from in vitro studies, the defects were corrected by therapy: T-lymphocyte levels increased (as detected by the total E-rosette test);

T_i-cell levels, eosinophils, and total serum IgE levels were reduced; and suppressor T-lymphocyte activity was increased.

The positive skin test to Thymosin in patient M. W. may have been due to using the drug neat for this intradermal challenge. It appears that many normal subjects produce a flare and even a wheal with undiluted thymic extract, and that the skin test material should be diluted at least 1 in 100 (de Weck, personal communication). Subsequent atopic eczema and other patients were skin tested with a 1% solution of Thymostimulin (Thymosin being unavailable to us at the time).

In Vivo Study Using Thymostimulin (Preliminary Results). Six adult male patients (ages 24-43 years), each with a lifelong history of intractable atopic eczema but no other significant atopic manifestations, were treated with a course of Thymostimulin in a double-blind placebo-controlled clinical trial with cross-over. Male patients were selected as we were anxious to avoid treating women of childbearing age until preliminary clinical studies had indicated that it was safe to do so. Treatment consisted of 2 weeks of low dose Thymostimulin or placebo (randomly and blindly allocated; dose 0.75 mg/kg twice weekly by the intramuscular route), followed by 2 weeks of the same material at double this dose. After an interval of 2 weeks, during which no medication was administered but monitoring (for late effects of therapy or for effects of withdrawal of therapy) was continued, the treatment regime was repeated for the other preparations (placebo or Thymostimulin, respectively). Both preparations (Thymostimulin and placebo) were coded by a pharmacist not involved with the trial as A or B. Some patients, of course, started with Thymostimulin therapy and finished with placebo; others started with placebo and finished with Thymostimulin.

The trial was monitored clinically by scoring blind such features as erythema, excoriation, lichenification, vesiculation, edema, crusting, pigmentation, itch, and loss of sleep, together with assessment of the total skin surface area involved in the eczema. At least two experienced dermatologists independently assessed each of the clinical parameters on a graded scale and subsequently arrived at average numerical scores for each of the parameters studied. Skin condition was assessed twice weekly.

Total lymphocyte and eosinophil counts (peripheral blood) were determined once weekly, together with T-lymphocyte levels (active E-rosette test plus OKT3 positively, in parallel), and levels of cytotoxic/suppressor T lymphocytes (OKT8+) and helper/inducer T lymphocytes (OKT4+). Total serum IgE levels were also determined weekly throughout the 10 weeks of the trial and during the posttrial follow-up period.

At the end of each patient's treatment the drug codings were broken and changes in clinical and laboratory parameters were compared with time elapsing since the start of Thymostimulin therapy. To date, no significant changes in total lymphocyte or eosinophil levels or in total T-lymphocyte levels have been noted as a result of Thymostimulin therapy in our patients. Similarly, total IgE levels, difficult to quantitate by radioimmunoassay at very high concentrations, showed little change as a result of Thymostimulin therapy, with mean levels of 20,000 IU/ml (range, 14,000-82,000, depending on the patient) throughout the trial. Assessment of skin condition parameters revealed only very minor reductions in severity gradings due to Thymostimulin therapy, although all patients remarked that they felt much better and their skin texture was noted to be glossy and smooth after about 3 weeks of Thymostimulin therapy though not at any time on placebo therapy (when skin tended to be dry, scaly, and rough).

However, levels of OKT8+ (cytotoxic/suppressor) T lymphocytes, initially low, were found to increase to normal levels on Thymostimulin therapy though not on placebo therapy. Mean pretreatment level of OKT8+ lymphocytes was 19% (410/mm^3) compared with normal control-group mean levels of 25% or 625/mm^3. After 1 week of TP-1 therapy (low dose, 0.75 mg/kg) the mean level of OKT8+ lymphocytes had increased to 23% (437/mm^3), and there was no further increase following the second week of low-dose Thymostimulin therapy. After the third week of Thymostimulin (first week of high dose, 1.5 mg/kg), the OKT8+ lymphocyte mean had risen to the normal control mean percentage of 25% (though still only 530/mm^3 in absolute numbers) with no further increase during the fourth week of therapy. The normalization of OKT8+ lymphocyte levels as a result of TP-1 therapy had been predicted by pretherapy in vitro studies; the largest increases in these lymphocytes were seen in those patients with the lowest pretreatment baseline levels.

We conclude that thymic hormone therapy may prove of value in the treatment of atopic eczema and other forms of atopy, but that the dose level of Thymostimulin at least may have to be increased to a level still higher than we have used so far (e.g., to more than 2 mg/kg).

E. Patients with Solid Tumors (Preliminary Studies)

A total of 30 adult patients with solid tumors comprised of 17 with hypernephroma, 4 with breast cancer, and 9 with malignant melanoma were studied. [See Refs. 3 and 13 for the results of the melanoma patients, now superseded by the results of a much larger melanoma group (see below)].

All patients with carcinoma of the kidney had histologically the clear cell variety of the disease, and all were investigated in the postnephrectomy period. Only 3 were disease-free at the time of investigation; the remaining 14 patients had advanced metastatic disease. Mean age was around 60 years. All patients had received radiotherapy or chemotherapy.

The mean age of the breast cancer patients was around 40 years. One had disseminated disease, while the other had no obvious metastases. All patients had received radiotherapy.

Patients with advancing malignant neoplasms are known to have depressed cell-mediated immunity (55-60) and markedly depressed peripheral blood T-lymphocyte levels (3,6,8,13,61-65). In this present study, T-lymphocyte percentages and absolute numbers were again found to be significantly lower than normal; overall lymphocyte counts were depressed in both groups of cancer patients (Table 9).

Cell-mediated immunity in cancer patients may, however, be further impaired by conventional treatments such as chemotherapy (66) and/or radiotherapy (67-70). It is not clear how much of the T-lymphocyte depression in these patients was the result of the disease (87) and how much was iatrogenic. Although radiotherapy may result in a T lymphopenia lasting for a period of years (70-75), the immunosuppressive effects of surgery are only temporary (76-79), and all of our subsequent studies (in vitro and in vivo) were on patients treated by surgery alone (Sect. III. F).

Nevertheless, even in these patients who had received immunosuppression as a side effect of aggressive antitumor therapy, in vitro Thymosin incubation restored E-rosette formation to normal in lymphocyte populations from both types of tumor patient. These results provided the justification for more detailed laboratory studies and, ultimately, clinical studies (see below) using thymic factor therapy.

Table 9 T-Lymphocyte Levels (Total E-Rosette Test) and Thymosin Inducibility of Normal Adults and Patients with Hypernephroma or Breast Cancer

		Total lympho-cytes	T lymphocytes in medium alone	T lymphocytes with Thymosin	Thymosin-inducible T cells (T_i)
Normal adults (N = 18)	Percent	–	51	57	6
	Per mm^3 [a]	2416	1232	1377	137
Hypernephroma patients (N = 17)	Percent	–	37 (0.02)[b]	59 (NS)	22 (0.0001)
	Per mm^3	2058 (0.0003)	761 (0.0008)	1214 (NS)	453 (0.0003)

[a]Absolute numbers of lymphocytes per cubic millimeter of peripheral blood.
[b]P values (in parentheses) obtained by the Mann-Whitney U test.
[c]NS, not significant.
Source: Refs. 3 and 13.

F. Patients with Malignant Melanoma

1. In Vitro Studies

A total of 85 patients (54 women and 31 men) with histologically proven malignant melanoma were studied. The classification of Lewis et al. (80) was used to assign 42 patients to stage I, 9 to stage IIa, 14 to stage IIb, 5 to stage IIab, and 15 to stage III. The overall age range of the patients was 13-80 (mean, 49) years. Approximately half the patients were symptom-free and half had active disease at the time of the study. No patient had received radiotherapy or chemotherapy at any time or had received surgery within 2 weeks of investigation.

A total of 50 healthy normal control subjects whose age range was 18-50 (mean, 29) years were blood donors or members of the hospital staff. They were not matched for age and sex with the patients, but their ages were not significantly different from those of the patients.

The results are summarized in Table 10. The mean level of T lymphocytes (total E-rosette test) in the normal control group was 48%, significantly higher than the mean levels in the patient groups: stage I, 38%; stage II, 32%; stage III, 27%; all stages, 34%. In addition to this stage-related decline in T-lymphocyte percentages, a significant stage-related decline in total lymphocytes was detected. As a result, absolute numbers of T lymphocytes per cubic millimeter of peripheral blood demonstrated a particularly marked and stage-related decline. The finding of a T-lymphocyte deficit has been reported for melanoma previously, in both percentage and absolute terms (3,6,13,63,64). Indeed, Bourgoin et al. (63) also found T-lymphocyte depletion to be stage-related.

Depressed T-lymphocyte levels in the patients are apparently disease-related and not the result of prior treatment, since untreated stage I patients showed some T-lymphocyte depletion. No patient had received radiotherapy or chemotherapy, both of which (see Sect. III. E) result in low T-lymphocyte numbers and may facilitate tumor progression and nullify therapeutic benefits (70). Follow-up studies on some of the stage I melanoma

Table 10 T-Lymphocyte Levels (Total E-Rosette Test) and Thymosin Inducibility of Normal Adults and of Staged Malignant Melanoma Patients[a]

	Total lympho-cytes	T lymphocytes in medium alone	T lymphocytes in medium plus Thymosin	Thymosin inducible T-lymphocytes (T_i)	T lymphocytes in medium plus fetal calf serum (FCS)
Normal adults (N = 50)	2424	1155	1525	369	1226
Melanoma stage I (N = 41)	2151 (NS)[b,c]	818 (NS)	1288 (NS)	482 (NS)	1025 (NS)
Stage II (N = 22)	1937 (<0.001)	556 (0.0006)	1117 (<0.05)	483 (NS)	858 (NS)
Stage III (N = 11)	1889 (0.004)	619 (<0.002)	1241 (0.02)	591 (NS)	936 (NS)
All stages (N = 74)	2042 (<0.0005)	694 (<0.00001)	1209 (NS)	484 (NS)	945 (0.0001)

[a]All values are in absolute numbers of lymphocytes per cubic millimeter of peripheral blood.
[b]NS, not significant.
[c]P values (in parentheses) were obtained by the Mann-Whitney U test.
Source: Refs. 3 and 81.

patients after surgery showed no significant suppression of immunological parameters; as mentioned in Sect. III. E, the immunosuppressive effect of surgery has been found to be only temporary and unlikely to influence prognosis adversely.

The finding of T-lymphocyte depletion in melanoma patients correlates with other evidence of depressed cell-mediated immunity. Lymphocyte-mediated cytotoxicity (82), skin test sensitivity (63), and lymphocyte transformation to allogeneic lymphocytes (60), for example, are often impaired or even absent in melanoma.

In view of the important role of T lymphocytes in immunosurveillance, any qualitative or quantitative T-lymphocyte depletion might be expected to result in the emergence and metastasis of malignant cell clones. Normal T-lymphocyte levels have been reported in stage I melanoma patients, but matastasis tended to be preceded by a fall in T-lymphocyte levels (6). T-lymphocyte levels were found by other authors (62,83) to be depressed in advanced or recurring melanoma but normal in cured patients (62). Wybran and Fudenberg (2) found that three-quarters of newly diagnosed or untreated cancer patients undergoing relapse were T lymphopenic, whereas only 5% of normal control subjects and only 3% of cancer patients in remission had depressed T-lymphocyte levels. Symptom-free bronchogenic cancer patients had higher T-lymphocyte levels than patients with active disease (84). Normal T-lymphocyte levels were found in cured patients with adenocarcinoma of the lung (84) and in patients with breast cancer (85). Conversely, T-lymphocyte levels tend to be depressed in patients with advancing or recurring tumors other than melanoma [e.g., cancer of undefined type (2) and in bronchongenic cancer (8,86)]. A strong correlation was found between immunocompetence levels assessed by a battery of of in vitro and in vivo tests and the observed course of breast cancer disease (87). The importance of maintaining normal levels of T lymphocytes is evident.

In agreement with the results of virtually every study of lymphocytes from cancer patients, a marked increase in null (non-T, non-B) lymphocytes was detected in this study (3,13,64,81,85). Incubation of melanoma lymphocytes with Thymosin at optimum concentration abolished the T-lymphocyte deficit (Table 10) as reported previously for melanoma (3,13,64,81,88,89) and for other types of cancer (3,89,90) following induction with thymic factors. Thymosin-like induction of E rosettes to normal levels also followed incubation of melanoma lymphocytes with fetal calf serum (Table 10), as described for melanoma (3,5,13,81), for breast cancer (3,13,85), and for Hodgkin's disease (91,92). Evidence is mounting that T lymphocytes in patients with cancer become blocked with lipoprotein, immune complexes, antilymphocyte antibodies, or other extraneous material which inhibits E-rosette formation and possibly also T-lymphocyte function, and this blocking may enhance tumor development. Such blocking factors may be removed by treatment of lymphocytes with proteolytic enzymes (85,93), by extensive washing (94), or by incubation with fetal calf serum or thymic factors or Levamisole (95). Reincubation of lymphocytes from breast cancer patients (85), from Hodgkin patients (91), or melanoma patients (3) with autologous plasma after restoration of E-rosette formation leads to redepression of rosetting; this suggests that T-lymphocyte blocking factors circulate in cancer patients, and thymic factor therapy may abrogate their effects and enhance tumor immunity. It is, however, still unclear whether the low T-lymphocyte percentages detected in cancer patients are the result of blocking of mature T lymphocytes or defective maturation of precursor (T_0?) cells as a result of a shortfall of thymic hormone production.

Apart from the stage-related decline in T-lymphocyte percentages in the melanoma patient group, a stage-related decline in total lymphocyte levels was observed in accordance with published findings (63). Similar results have been described in patients with bronchial carcinoma (77,86). Thymic factors are known to stimulate lymphopoiesis (17,18), and the lymphocyte depletion in this and other series of cancer patients may be due to thymic insufficiency or, of course, to immunological exhaustion. The triple action of thymic hormones (stimulation of lymphocyte production, enhancement of T-lymphocyte maturation, and modulation of T-lymphocyte function) (16) makes this a logical form of therapy in cancer. Metastatic melanoma patients who maintain a normal lymphocyte level have a significantly improved prognosis (96). Lymphocytic infiltration of the tumor is also a good prognostic sign.

Impaired cell-mediated immunity has been correlated with poor prognosis in cancer (98,99). Breast cancer patients with intact cellular immunity had disease-free periods of at least 2-3 years' duration, whereas most immunoincompetent patients had recurrences within the first year (87). Dubois and Serrou (100) found that intact cell-mediated immunity in metastatic patients correlated with longer survival time.

2. In Vivo Studies

Preliminary studies had indicated that total lymphocyte counts and T-lymphocyte counts were reduced, in a stage-related manner, in melanoma patients. Thymostimulin, like Thymosin, is known to have lymphopoietic activity and to increase T-lymphocyte levels in malignant melanoma (64), and we used it to treat newly diagnosed stage I malignant melanoma patients concurrently with radical surgical excision of their primary lesions. In a pilot study, two patients with advanced metastatic disease were also studied for comparison purposes, although Thymostimulin therapy was not commenced until surgical excision of the remaining melanoma deposits from the regional lymph nodes had already been completed.

Of the eight patients currently on Thymostimulin therapy, seven are males, since the vast majority of reports have shown that males have a significantly worse survival rate than females. The poor survival rate may, however, reflect the fact that males have a high frequency of axial primaries and prognosis is significantly worse in patients with axial primaries; females, on the other hand, have a higher incidence of peripheral primaries, which carry a better prognosis (reviewed in Ref. 101). We therefore select male patients with truncal primaries for treatment since they represent the worst prognostic group (5-year survival rate ranges from about 10% to a maximum of about 50%) and will be expected to give a reliable indication of the efficacy of this therapeutic modality in melanoma (based upon survival) in 2-3 years in a multicenter national trial.

The most important prognostic indicator in stage I cutaneous malignant melanoma is, of course, the depth of the primary lesion, with tumors exceeding 2 mm in thickness being associated with a poor prognosis (121). Male patients with truncal primaries of thickness exceeding 2 mm would appear to have an exceptionally bad prognosis.

No patient who has received immunosuppressive therapy (e.g., chemotherapy) is accepted for treatment. In view of the low/zero toxicity of Thymostimulin and the extremely poor prognosis of this group of patients, it appears unethical to have a placebo control group or an untreated group. Instead, one might use a computer to match currently treated patients with historical untreated patients, matching essentially by sex, site of primary lesion, depth of primary lesion, stage of disease, and age of patient. In the event, however, to achieve an acceptable clinical trial design, both historical and concurrent (untreated) controls will be used.

Only very preliminary results are available at present, since no patient has received Thymostimulin therapy for longer than 7 months. To the best of our knowledge, no patient undergoing treatment has shown any indication whatsoever of recurrence or metastasis of their tumors; this is even the case for the two pilot study patients who had widespread lymph node involvement.

Thymostimulin therapy commences prior to surgical excision of the primary melanoma and consists of 50 mg injected intramuscularly twice week for the 2 weeks of hospitalization. Thereafter maintenance therapy will consist of 25 mg Thymostimulin once weekly to 6 months (minimum). Individual case histories follow.

*Case 1.** Case 1 is a 54-year-old woman with a 3-year history of primary malignant melanoma on the thigh, who commenced Thymostimulin therapy (pilot study) following surgical removal of all known cutaneous and distant lymph node secondaries at Lewis stage III. Pretherapy values were: total lymphocytes, 1890/mm^3; total T lymphocytes (OKT3+), 38% or 720/mm^3; helper/inducer T lymphocytes (OKT4+), 10% or 190/mm^3; cytotoxic/suppressor T lymphocytes (OKT8+), 26% or 490/mm^3. After 4 weeks of Thymostimulin therapy the values had increased: total lymphocytes, 2800/mm^3; total T, 75% or 2130/mm^3; helper T, 46% or 1235^3; suppressor T, 25% or 700/mm^3.

*Case 2.** Case 2 is a 15-year-old boy with a 2-year history, presenting with a junctional naevus on the cheek in 1980. After an excision in 1981, there was a local recurrence which was again excised. By February 1982, a computer-assisted tomography

---

*Pilot study.

(CAT) scan showed an ipsilateral parotid mass but no distant metastases. In March 1982, an exploratory operation showed huge amounts of metastatic melanoma deposits throughout the parotid area and the cervical lymph node chain. With this evidence of gross metastasis, it was thought inappropriate to carry out a severely mutilating operation although all accessible melanoma deposits were removed immediately prior to the start of Thymostimulin therapy that same month.

Prior to commencement of Thymostimulin therapy, the lymphocyte parameters were: total lymphocytes, 2300/mm^3; total T, 84% or 1935/mm^3; helper T, 53% or 1220/mm^3; suppressor T, 21% or 480/mm^3 (subnormal). After 3 months of Thymostimulin therapy, however, there was no improvement in these values although no improvement is expected where baseline values are already normal (89).

Case 3. (First patient for the clinical trial proper.) Case 3 is a 57-year-old man who underwent a wide surgical excision of a nodular malignant melanoma (Clark level V), invading to a depth of over 1 cm on his back. There was no evidence of lymph node involvement (Lewis stage I). Chest x-ray, hematology, and blood chemistry were normal.

Lymphocyte results in absolute numbers per cubic milliliter of blood (percentages in parentheses) were as follows:

Weeks of Thymostimulin therapy	Total lymphocytes	Total T (OKT3+)	Helper T (OKT4+)	Suppressor T (OKT8+)
0	↓ 1515[a]	↓ 1150 (76%↑)	↓ 770 (51%↑)	↓ 320 (21%↑)
2	↑ 2940	—	—	—
12	↑ 3700	↑ 3070 (83%↑)	↑ 2145 (58%↑)	↑ 1145 (31%↑)

[a]Arrow denotes departures from normal levels.

After 3 months of Thymostimulin therapy, as predicted by pretherapy in vitro tests, the percentage of suppressor T lymphocytes became normal; the percentages of the other T-lymphocyte subsets were already normal pretherapy. The total lymphocyte count, at the low end of our normal range (1200-3500/mm^3) prior to Thymostimulin therapy, had doubled by 2 weeks of therapy and tripled by 3 months.

Case 4. (Trial patient No. 2.) Case 4 is a 49-year-old man with a nodular malignant melanoma in the scapular area arising from a preexisting mole. Pretherapy results were: total lymphocytes, 2700/mm^3; total T, 75% or 2030/mm^3; helper T, 36% or 975/mm^3; suppressor T, 18% or 490/mm^3 (slight deficits of both helper and suppressor T lymphocytes). After 2 weeks of Thymostimulin therapy, the total lymphocyte count had increased to 3145/mm^3, total T increased slightly to 2139/mm^3, although the percentage, already normal pretherapy, did not increase. Helper T increased considerably to 55% or 1730/mm^3 (normal level 46% or 1150/mm^3) while suppressor T failed to increase (16% or 500/mm^3). No further results available as yet.

Case 5. (Trial patient No. 2). Case 5 is a male patient aged 21 years with a malignant melanoma of the chest wall. There is no evidence of lymph node involvement or metastasis. Lymphocyte results in absolute numbers (percentages in parentheses) were:

Weeks of Thymostimulin therapy	Total lymphocytes	Total T (OKT3+)	Helper T (OKT4+)	Suppressor T (OKT8+)
0	2445	↓1440 (59%↓)	↓780 (32%↓)	↓465 (19%↓)
1	↑2640[a]	↑1930 (73%)	↑1215 (46%)	↑370 (14%↓)
2	2560	↑1900 (74%)	↑1280 (50%↑)	↑820 (32%↑)
3	↓1950	↓1230 (63%↓)	↓1035 (53%↑)	↓↓156 (8%↓↓)
4	↓↓1310	↓↓770 (59%↓)	↓↓600 (46%)	↓↓235 (18%↓)

[a]Arrows denote departures from normal levels.

This patient's total lymphocyte count was normal prior to therapy, and showed little increase as a result of therapy. Although T-lymphocyte percentages in the respective subsets were all low pretherapy, normal percentages had been achieved after 2 weeks of treatment. Subsequent to this all lymphocyte subpopulations declined, although the reason is unclear.

Case 6. (Trial patient No. 4.) Case 6 is a 38-year-old male with a melanoma which presented 6 months prior to surgery. The pigmented lesion, arising from a preexisting mole on the flank, proved to be a nodular malignant melanoma penetrating the dermis to a depth of 3-4 mm (Clark level V). Malignant cells were clearly seen in the lymphatics at the base of the lesion, indicating that a rapid progression from Lewis stage I could normally be expected. Thorough examination at that stage, however, indicated: normal respiratory and cardiovascular systems; normal chest x-ray; normal liver function tests and other blood chemistry; no palpable evidence of lymph node involvement.

The lesion was removed initially by the general practitioner but in the knowledge of the histology results was reexcised with a wider margin, by a plastic surgeon, and Thymostimulin therapy was started.

Lymphocyte results in absolute numbers per cubic millimeter of peripheral blood (percentages in parentheses) were:

Weeks of Thymo-stimulin therapy	Total lymphocytes	Total T (OKT3+)	Helper T (OKT4+)	Suppressor T (OKT8+)	E-receptor bearing (OKT11+)
-1	↓↓1275[a]	–	–	–	–
0	–	– (56%↓)	–(46%)	– (19%↓)	– (55%↓)
1	↓1700	↓1050 (62%↓)	710 (42%↓)	375 (22%↓)	1070 (63%↓)

[a]Arrows denote departures from normal levels.

The results indicate a general improvement to date but are, of course, only very preliminary.

Case 7. (Trial patient No. 5.) Case 7 is a male patients aged 39 years with a superficial spreading malignant melanoma of the trunk, adjacent to a preexisting benign nevus. Part of the tumor, however, penetrated to the reticular dermis (Clark level IV). (Lymphocyte results are not yet available.)

Case 8. (Trial patient No. 6.) Case 8 is a male patient aged 56 years with a poorly differentiated malignant melanoma of the superficial spreading type arising de novo as a darkly pgimented raised lesion just below the axilla. There is no evidence of axillary, supraclavicular or groin lymphadenopathy. Chest x-ray is clear, and liver function tests are normal.

Lymphocyte results in absolute numbers (percentages in parentheses) were:

Weeks of Thymo-stimulin therapy	Total lymphocytes	Total T (OKT3+)	Helper T (OKT4+)	Suppressor T (OKT8+)	E-receptor bearing (OKT11+)
2 (pre surgery)	↓↓1275[a]	–	–	–	–
4	2635	↓1515 (64% ↓)	↓970 (41%↓)	↓ 520 (22%↓)	1585 (67%)
6	↑2555	↓1278 (50%↓)	↓945 (37%↓)	↓ 435 (17%↓)	–

[a]Arrows denote departures from normal levels.

Discussion (All Cases). All patients whose results are so far available had pre-Thymostimulin total lymphocyte counts within our normal range of 1200-2500/mm^3. Nevertheless, in cases 3, 6, and 8 the total lymphocyte counts started at the low end of this normal range; interestingly, cases 3 and 6 had tumor invasion to Clark level V, and case 8 had invasion to Clark level IV. All three patients would normally be expected to have a very poor prognosis indeed. The ability of Thymostimulin therapy to increase the total lymphocyte counts in all of these patients to normal or even above-normal levels is remarkable, since metastatic melanoma patients who maintain normal lymphocyte levels have a significantly improved prognosis (96). Those patients with normal total lymphocyte counts pretherapy tended to show only small increases (e.g., only a 16% improvement in case 4 and 8% in case 5). Thymostimulin therapy, provided it was inducing genuine lymphopoiesis and not merely causing redistribution of lymphocytes from one body compartment to another, would therefore be expected to be most beneficial for patients with low pretherapy total lymphocyte counts. The mean pretherapy total lymphocyte count for the patients as a group was 1915/mm^3, increasing to a mean maximum value of 2755/mm^3 on therapy (a 44% increase).

The mean pretherapy percentage of T-lymphocytes (OKT3 test) was 75%, while the mean on therapy was 79% (our normal adult mean is 74%). Thymostimulin therapy restored all subnormal T-lymphocyte percentages to normal levels, but had little effect in those cases where levels were already normal. The largest increase was in case 1 (advanced metastatic disease), from 38% pretherapy to 76% on therapy (a 50% increase). As predicted by in vitro studies (using E-rosette tests and OKT3 tests), Thymostimulin therapy appears to hold promise for immunoreconstitution in melanoma patients, especially where pretherapy T-lymphocyte percentages and absolute numbers are low. Added to this is the low/zero toxicity of Thymostimulin in comparison with other less powerful immunostimulants such as Levamisole and BCG, both of which have unacceptable side effects in some patients.

Having shown that Thymostimulin in vitro and in vivo restores total T-lymphocyte percentages to normal in the melanoma situation it was of interest to determine whether both of the main T-lymphocyte subsets (helper/inducer or cytotoxic/suppressor) were being increased by this drug. In most of the cases presented here, it is the cells with the helper/inducer phenotype which increase as a result of therapy, while the levels of cytotoxic/suppressor cells tended to remain unchanged. The mean level of helper/inducer lymphocytes at the outset was 38% while the mean on Thymostimulin therapy was 45% (our normal control mean is 46%); the means for cytotoxic/suppressor cells were 21 and 30%, respectively (normal control mean, 25%). It may be significant that it appears to be the helper/inducer cells which are deficient in these cancer patients (an immunologically hyporeactive group ?), whereas it is the cytotoxic/suppressor cells which were deficient in the atopic eczema patients (a hyperreactive group ?).

Our pilot study of two patients (cases 1 and 2) who had advanced disease gave valuable information concerning dose rates for Thymostimulin and confirmed the finding of other investigators that there are no apparent side effects in patients treated with this material [see *Thymus, Thymic Hormones and T Lymphocytes* (F. Aiuti and H. Wigzell, eds.), Academic Press, London, 1980.] The two pilot study patients received 1 mg of Thymostimulin/kg body weight twice a week for the first 2 weeks (induction regime), followed by 1 mg/kg once a week (maintenance regime) up to 1 year. For the formal trial of Thymostimulin in newly diagnosed stage I male patients with truncal primary malignant melanoma we were able to decrease the dosage to 25 mg per patient (flat rate) twice a week for 2 weeks (starting presurgery for the induction), followed by 25 mg per patient once a week for at least 6 months. This modified protocol results in considerable economies in the amounts of the drug required, and the shorter time period for the course of treatment improves patient compliance and motivation and simplifies treatment protocols for the various plastic surgery centers and individual general practitioners administering the weekly injections.

It is hoped to treat 100 patients in this trial, and the results to date will be presented at the International Symposium on Thymic Factor Therapy in London in April 1983. The most important evidence for efficacy of this treatment, the 2-year survival data, will not, however, be available for some considerable time yet.

G. Patients with Mycosis Fungoides

A total of 30 patients had mycosis fungoides (19 males, 11 females). Most were in clinical stage II or III and have active disease. All patients were studied prior to active therapy which in most cases was by PUVA (psoralen activated by UV-A light).

The total lymphocyte count (Table 11) was significantly lower in the mycosis fungoides (MF) group than in the normal control group, although most authors have reported no difference (101) or only a slight but insignificant reduction in MF (102-103). However, Cyr et al. (104) reported that 126 of 165 patients (76%) had an overall lymphopenia, while Fuks et al. (105) found that 21% of their series of MF patients had a lymphocyte count below $1000/mm^3$. The discrepancy between these sets of results may relate to stage or activity of disease, since one paper reports that only 5% of the patients with erythematous disease, but 45% of patients with tumor stage disease, were lymphopenic (105). In our own study, most patients had advanced and/or progressive disease and would be expected to have low lymphocyte counts since lymphopenia is associated with poor prognosis (105). One group failed to detect lymphopenia in their MF patient population, possibly because their normal control group was itself lymphopenic by most standards (101).

The mean level of T lymphocytes in the MF patients in this present study was significantly lower than the control group mean, in accordance with the results of the great majority of studies (102,103,106-108), although others have reported normal levels (101,109,110). This discordance may be the result of technical differences in T-lymphocyte enumeration procedures, or differences in disease activity in the patients; for example,

Table 11 T-Lymphocyte Levels (Total E-Rosette Test) and Thymosin Inducibility of Normal Adults and of Patients with Mycosis Fungoides

		Total lymphocytes	T lymphocytes in medium alone	Maximum T lymphocytes with Thymosin	Thymosin-inducible T lymphocytes (T_i)
Normal adults (N = 30)	Percent	–	47.7	62.6	14.9
	Per mm^3 [a]	2424	1155	1525	369
Mycosis fungoides patients	Percent	–	37.2 (0.02)[b]	59.8 (NS)	19.7 (NS)
	Per mm^3	1637 (<0.00001)	561 (<0.00001)	888 (<0.00001)	288 (NS)

[a]Of peripheral blood.
[b]P values (in parentheses) were obtained by the Mann-Whitney U test.
[c]NS, not significant.

patients with advanced disease tend to have lower T-lymphocyte percentages (107) or lower total lymphocyte counts (105) than patients with early stage disease. Similarly, patients in remission tend to have normal T-lymphocyte levels (107). In our study, most patients had advanced/progressive disease, consistent with low T-lymphocyte levels.

Mycosis fungoides patients with low T-lymphocyte levels are reported as having reciprocally elevated levels of null cells (102,107), and this has been our own experience. The mean null cell level in the MF patient group was 50% (755/mm^3), significantly higher than the control group mean (39% or 950/mm^3; p = 0.03). This difference could be abolished if the lymphocyte were preincubated with Thymosin prior to performing the E-rosette test; in other words the MF patients had elevated levels of Thymosin-inducible (immature or blocked ?) T lymphocytes, as had the melanoma, hypernephroma, and breast cancer patients described earlier in this chapter.

Ultrastructural studies (reviewed in Ref. 107) have indicated that MF cells, like Sézary cells, bind sheep erythrocytes in the manner of T lymphocytes. Some MF cells, as a result of malignant transformation, may have absent or defective E-rosetting capacity, possibly leading to an increase in the level of null cells. Alternatively, blocking factors may be produced secondary to the disease process, and these may block normal T lymphocytes and inhibit E-rosetting as well as T-lymphocyte function. The finding of above-normal levels of Thymosin-inducible null cells of T lineage in the MF samples suggests that at least some T lymphocytes are blocked with serum factors. The ability of thymic hormone preparations to reverse this blocking (103) suggests that thymic factor therapy may be of value in the treatment of MF, with the added advantage that lymphopoiesis may be enhanced in the process.

H. Patients with Acute Anterior Uveitis

Uveitis patients initially attended an eye hospital or an eye clinic with acute symptoms, No patient on systemic therapy was included in the study, although most patients were on topical therapy. A total of 53 patients had uveitis alone, with no evidence of rheumatic or other disease; in 39 it was the first attack, and in the remaining 14 it was a recurrence. Blood samples were taken upon referral to the rheumatology department (mean 15 days after the onset of acute symptoms), 1 month later (mean 50 days postonset), and not less than 3 months later (mean 245 days postonset).

A total of 75 normal, healthy control subjects (mostly hospital staff with similar age and sex distributions to the patient group) were also investigated.

In Table 12, the 19 patients tested at 101 days to 1 year are included among the 34 patients tested at 31-100 days and these, in turn, are included among the 46 patients tested at 0-30 days after the onset of symptoms.

In these uveitis patients who were all apparently free from rheumatic disease there was a significant T lymphopenia and a transitory overall lymphopenia. The T lymphopenia was persistent, being present many months after clinical recovery. Autologous plasma did not inhibit E-rosette formation, suggesting a lack of T-lymphocyte blocking factors of the type described in breast cancer (85) or in Hodgkin disease (91,92). In vitro Thymosin increased E rosettes in both the control and the uveitis groups, abolishing the T lymphopenia in most cases. The histocompatibility antigen HLA B27 is strongly associated with uveitis (112), but levels of T lymphocytes and of T_i-cells were similar in both B27+ and B27− uveitis patients.

In patients experiencing their first attack of uveitis, the mean T-lymphocyte levels was not significantly subnormal until some 20 days after the onset of clinical symptoms.

Table 12 T-Lymphocyte Levels (Total E-Rosette Test) and Thymosin Inducibility of Normal Adults and of Patients with Acute Anterior Uveitis

		Total lymphocytes	T lymphocytes in medium alone	Maximum T lymphocytes with Thymosin	Thymosin-inducible T lymphocytes (T_i)
Normal controls (N = 70)	Percent	–	46.0	62.7	16.7
	Per mm^3 [a]	2445	1125	1533	408
0-30 days (N = 46)	Percent	–	39.8	54.0	14.2
	Per mm^3	2282 (<0.05)[b]	909 (<0.01)	1233 (<0.01)	324 (NS)
31-100 days (N = 34)	Percent	–	39.4	60.8	21.4
	Per mm^3	1959 (<0.01)	771 (<0.001)	1191 (<0.01)	420 (NS)
101 days to 1 year (N = 19)	Percent	–	36.1	40.5	4.4
	Per mm^3	2013 (NS)	727 (<0.01)	815 (<0.01)	88 (<0.01)

[a]Of peripheral blood.
[b]P values (in parentheses) were obtained by the Mann-Whitney U test.
[c]NS, not significant.
Source: Ref. 111.

In patients having a recurrence of uveitis, however, the mean level of T lymphocytes was already subnormal by about 2 weeks after clinical onset. After an attack of uveitis, T-lymphocyte levels often failed to return to normal levels as long as 1 year after clinical remission (Table 12).

In the household contacts of uveitis patients there was also a significant T lymphopenia, but in these subjects depressed T-lymphocyte levels tended to be transient and were only seen up to about 3 months after onset of symptoms. No clinical symptoms were reported in any of the household contacts during their T lymphopenia. T lymphopenia was a feature of sexual and nonsexual contacts alike, and of first-degree and other relatives alike. Normal T-lymphocyte levels were restored in the lymphocytes of the contacts after in vitro incubation with Thymosin (3,111).

To sum up, uveitis patients showed an overall depletion of total lymphocytes; T lymphocytes were significantly reduced, while null and B lymphocytes were increased. A similar depletion of total lymphocytes was seen in the contact group, but without a significant increase in B lymphocytes. The presence of T lymphopenia in the uveitis contact group for about 3 months after an onset of uveitis suggests involvement of one or more infective agents, at least one of which may be widespread and not necessarily sexually transmitted or confined to relatives. The presumptive infective agents might not cause overt disease in the majority of individuals with T lymphopenia, presumably because these people are not genetically predisposed. Perhaps the inheritance of HLA B27 linked immune response (Ir) genes renders certain individuals vulnerable to clinical symptoms while other individuals exposed to the same infectious agents but lacking the genetic predisposition remain healthy.

These lymphopenia and T-lymphopenia results can, of course, be interpreted in several ways. Nevertheless, infection remains a strong possibility, especially as asymptomatic controls as well as patients had low counts of these lymphocytes. Transient lymphopenia has been recorded in certain viral infections (113). Wybran and Fudenberg (114) found T lymphopenia in all of 21 patients with viral upper respiratory disease and in none of the 20 patients with bacterial infections. Indeed, thymus-dependent immunity has been shown to be depressed by viral infections in animals as well as humans (115). In controlled experimental infections of human volunteers with wild-type or attenuated influenza virus (7), there was a transient T lymphopenia which could be abolished in vitro by incubation with Thymosin; T-cell levels returned to normal upon clinical recovery. In clinical trials of Thymostimulin in eight children with T-lymphocyte deficiency and severe viral infections (hemorrhagic chickenpox, interstitial pneumonia, *Herpes simplex* stomatitis), T-lymphocyte levels increased significantly in all patients, and all made a rapid clinical recovery; in most cases, in vitro pretherapy studies accurately predicted the outcome of therapy (116).

Since T-lymphocyte levels in first-attack uveitis patients were normal until about 3 weeks after the onset of clinical symptoms, it seems likely that the T lymphopenia in the uveitis patients is secondary to the disease process itself. But chronic T lymphopenia after the first attack may predispose to further attacks.

The ability of Thymosin to normalize rosette formation by lymphocytes from uveitis patients implies that many of the null cells were, in fact, cells of the T lineage (possibly immature, blocked, or just less active). The in vitro abolition of the T lymphopenia of the uveitis patients recalls the abolition by Thymosin of the T lymphopenia of volunteers infected experimentally with influenza virus (7). A clinical trial of thymic hormone therapy in patients with uveitis therefore appears justified in order to restore

T-lymphocyte levels to normal with the objective of: (a) hastening clinical remission (duration of symptoms is normally around 8 weeks) and (b) lengthening the interval between disease episodes. In fact, our clinical trial of Thymostimulin therapy in uveitis patients has been arranged and commenced at the end of 1982.

I. Conclusions

Our 8-year experience of the E-rosette test in a very wide range of clinical disease situations and in many hundreds of normal subjects suggests that this is a reliable and perhaps underestimated indicator of cellular immune status. We have shown on numerous occassions that the practice of adding fetal calf serum to the E-rosette assay system is not only unnecessary but downright misleading, since factors (thymic or other hormones ?) in the serum may give rise to highly artifactual and misleading results. While fetal calf serum may have little effect on E-rosette formation by lymphocytes from most normal subjects (especially children), it may enhance rosette formation by patients' lymphocytes in vitro to levels very much ligher than those existing in vivo. Thus, the use of fetal calf serum may lead to gross underestimation of the extent of T lymphopenia in humans.

Fetal calf serum might also explain the difference between the low levels of rosette-forming cells detected by the active or early E-rosette test (where only existing, active, nonblocked T lymphocytes can make rosettes under the suboptimal conditions pertaining) and the total rosette test, where immature, inactive, or blocked T lymphocytes too are able to generate or regenerate E receptors during overnight incubation with thymic-like factors under optimal conditions (late rosettes). It follows, therefore,that the active or early rosette test is only useful in the assessment of cellular immune status and that the total rosette test is largely irrelevant except for the assessment of immunomodulators (as in the studies reported in this chapter).

In most cases, the E-rosette test probably underestimates the true percentage of T lymphocytes under suboptimal conditions, since one tends to set an arbitrary threshold of positivity (e.g., ignoring all those lymphocytes which are probably T lymphocytes but which under the conditions of the test happen to have bound only one or two lymphocytes). In a survey (3) of 45 publications listing a mean T-lymphocyte percentage in normal subjects, the grand mean T-lymphocyte level was 54% or 1435/mm^3; the true level of T lymphocytes as determined by more sensitive monoclonal antibody techniques is probably around 70% or 1700/mm^3 (Byrom, et al., in preparation).

We confirm earlier findings that T lymphocytes decline with increasing age, and that thymic hormone-inducible (T_i) null cell levels increase with increasing age, as has been demonstrated previously (4).

The results support the concept of a T-lymphocyte deficit in atopic patients. More specifically, we have shown that at least in our adult eczema patients there is a deficit of cytotoxic/suppressor (OKT8+) lymphocytes while the helper/inducer (OKT4+) cells are, if anything, increased. Our preliminary results indicate that eczema patients may have only about 75% of the normal level of cytotoxic/suppressor lymphocytes, but that the level may be restored to normal after Thymostimulin therapy, as predicted by pretreatment studies in vitro. Normalization of the OKT8+ lymphocyte levels did not, apparently, have any effect on total serum IgE levels (at least in the short term), although some striking improvements were seen clinically on Thymostimulin therapy. A further clinical trial is envisaged in atopic eczema using a higher dose than was used initially (e.g., 1.5-2 mg/kg) and continuing with this dose rate for more than the 2 weeks being used at present. With the advent of more highly purified or synthetic suppressor peptides (e.g., the Suppressin of Dr. Michael Osband in Boston, Massachusetts) it is hoped that more marked clinical remissions will be achieved in patients with atopic conditions.

In patients with cancer, the importance of maintaining normal levels of total lymphocytes and of T lymphocytes in particular is now being acknowledged. In our own studies, pretreatment in vitro experiments are accurately predicting which melanoma patients are likely to respond best (from an immunological point of view, at least) to Thymostimulin therapy. As invariably shown by other authors, those melanoma patients who responded best to Thymostimulin therapy were those with the lowest T-lymphocyte levels as determined in vitro pretherapy. We conclude that thymic factor therapy holds great promise in the treatment of cancer, provided it is commenced at the time of tumor debulking after early intervention in stage I and providing antagonistic cytotoxic treatments are not used. All our stage I melanoma patients on Thymostimulin therapy are maintaining normal total and T-lymphocyte counts, and all are apparently in clinical remission.

There is now strong evidence of T-lymphocyte blocking factors in the plasma of cancer patients, resulting in considerable T-lymphocyte energy. Chisari and Edgington (117) isolated an inhibitory factor (a low-density β-lipoprotein, which they termed *rosette-inhibiting factor* or RIF) which blocks E-rosetting lymphocytes (nonactive type ?) and renders them null. It is apparently these nonactive lymphocytes which can be induced by thymic factors and by fetal calf serum to form E rosettes. It is plausible that rosette-inhibiting factors produced in patients with certain types of cancers and even certain viral infections can bind to receptors on the T-lymphocyte surface (122) and either directly or indirectly increase intracellular cAMP levels. The cAMP, in turn, is known to inhibit not only E-rosetting (118,119) but also lymphocyte proliferation, antibody production, T-lymphocyte cytotoxicity, and numerous other immunological parameters (reviewed in Ref. 120). On the other hand, Thymosin and possibly other thymic factors increase intracellular cGMP levels, antagonizing all the above-mentioned immunoinhibitory activities of cAMP; Thymosin is not known to stimulate cAMP levels (4). As a consequence of all this, the immune status of the patient may represent a balance between factors (including RIF ?) which increase lymphocyte cAMP levels and factors (e.g., thymic factors) which increase cGMP levels.

In the light of several years of experience of working with each of the major thymic factor preparations (Thymosin and Thymostimulin) in vitro we are not aware of any major differences in terms of effect on E-rosette formation. Both materials were potent inducers of E-rosette formation at the microgram level. We have used both materials in human therapy for periods of up to 6 or 7 months in individual patients without any (apparent) side effects, and patient compliance has been excellent.

We always skin test in advance intended recipients of thymic factor therapy and we find that a 1% (v/v) solution of the thymic extract is a satisfactory skin test dilution. All patients, irrespective of diagnosis, who were lymphopenic pretherapy have shown a rapid increase in their total lymphocyte counts to normal levels, and thymic factor therapy clearly has an important role in correcting lymphopenia in immunodeficiency diseases of virtually every kind. Thymic factor therapy promises to be a potent and nontoxic therapeutic modality for the treatment of both primary and secondary immunodeficiency during the 1980s.

ACKNOWLEDGMENTS

We acknowledge with great gratitude the important contributions of a very large number of our clinical and scientific colleagues over the past 5 years. Drs. K. Hugh-Jones,

P. W. M. Copeman, R. C. D. Staughton, S. Retsas, D. C. Bodenham, R. W. Hiles, R. W. Norris, P. Samman, and Prof. D. A. Brewerton kindly allowed us to study patients under their care. Drs. J. Harper, M. Webley, M. Mobayen, R. Griffiths, C. Reid, C. Volkers, and M. Stodell were all deeply involved in the assessment and/or treatment of patients in this study. Drs. A. Perez and F. Caballero (visiting scientists from Venezuela) made major contributions to the laboratory assessment and the clinical management of the atopic patients. Dr. D. C. O. James kindly supplied lymphocytes from tissue-typed prospective bone marrow donors to use as normal control lymphocytes.

Ms. Mary Ann Campbell and Miss Nita Nagvekar performed vast numbers of lymphocyte surface marker studies by E-rosette and OKT methods, respectively. Hematological studies were performed by Mr. Tony Lane and Mr. Alan Dean. Serum IgE determinations were made by Mr. David Perry, Mr. Martin Gibbs, or Mr. Michael Chooi. All data analysis was by Dr. David Timlin, by kind permission of Dr. T. D. Preston.

REFERENCES

1. M. Jondal, G. Holm, and H. Wigzell, *J. Exp. Med.*, *136*:207 (1972).
2. J. Wybran and H. H. Fudenberg, *J. Clin. Invest.*, *53*:1026 (1973).
3. N. A. Byrom, in *Thymic Factors in Relation to Lymphocyte Surface Markers*, Ph.D. thesis of the University of London, 1978.
4. A. L. Goldstein, T. L. K. Low, G. B. Thurman, M. M. Zatz, N. Hall, J. Chen, S.-K. Hu, P. B. Naylor, and J. E. McClure, *Rec. Prog. Horm. Res.*, *37*:369 (1981).
5. N. A. Byrom, M. A. Campbell, R. C. D. Staughton, and D. M. Timlin, *Lancet*, *ii*:1132 (1977).
6. M. G. Bernengo, G. Capella, M. Peruccio, and G. Zina, *Br. J. Derm.*, *98*:655 (1978).
7. M. A. Scheinberg, N. R. Blacklow, A. L. Goldstein, T. A. Parrino, F. B. Rose, and E. S. Cathcart, *N. Engl. J. Med.*, *294*:1208 (1976).
8. H. M. Anthony, J. A. Kirk, K. E. Madsen, M. K. Mason, and G. H. Templeman, *Clin. Exp. Immunol.*, *20*:29 (1975).
9. C. B. Zachary and D. M. MacDonald, *Br. J. Derm.*, *107* (Suppl. 22):14 (1982).
10. N. Matsaniotis, N. A. Mantalenaki, M. Apostolou, and P. Liakopoulou, *Br. Med. J.*, *3*:743 (1974).
11. C. Alexopoulos and P. Babitis, *Lancet*, *i*:426 (1976).
12. D. W. Wara, A. L. Goldstein, N. E. Doyle, and A. J. Ammann, *N. Engl. J. Med.*, *292*:70 (1975).
13. N. A. Byrom, S. Retsas, A. J. Dean, and J. R. Hobbs, *Clin. Oncol.*, *4*:25 (1978).
14. H. Moutsopoulos, K. H. Fye, S. Sawada, M. J. Becker, A. Goldstein, and N. Talal, *Clin. Exp. Immunol.*, *26*:563 (1976).
15. M. P. Scheid, M. K. Hoffmann, K. Komoro, U. Hammerling, J. Abbott, E. A. Boyse, G. H. Cohen, J. A. Hooper, R. S. Schulof, and A. L. Goldstein, *J. Exp. Med.*, *138*:1027 (1973).
16. A. L. Goldstein, G. B. Thurman, G. H. Cohen, and J. A. Hooper, in *Biological Activity of Thymic Hormones* (D. W. Van Bekkum, ed.), Kooyker, Rotterdam, 1975, p. 173.
17. D. M. Metcalf, *Br. J. Cancer*, *10*:442 (1956).
18. A. L. Goldstein, F. D. Slater, and A. White, *Proc. Natl. Acad. Sci. USA*, *56*:1010 (1966).
19. N. A. Byrom, M. A. Campbell, A. J. Dean, D. C. O. James, D. Timlin, and J. R. Hobbs, *Lancet*, *i*:1149 (1977).
20. J. R. Hobbs, S. Malka, and N. A. Byrom, *Prot. Biol. Fluids*, *25*:605 (1977).
21. L. P. Ryder and A. Svejgaard, in *Association Between HLA and Disease*, HLA and Disease Registry, Copenhagen, 1976.

22. J. R. Hobbs, N. A. Byrom, M. A. Campbell, P. W. M. Copeman, M. Gibbs, A. M. Lane, A. Perez, R. C. D. Staughton, and D. M. Timlin, in *Thymus, Thymic Hormones and T Lymphocytes* (F. Aiuti and H. Wigzell, eds.), Academic Press, London, 1980, p. 143.
23. N. A. Byrom, F. Caballero, M. A. Campbell, M. Chooi, A. M. Lane, K. Hugh-Jones, D. M. Timlin, and J. R. Hobbs, *Clin. Exp. Immunol.*, *31*:490 (1978).
24. S. Gupta, R. Frenkel, M. Rosenstein, and M. H. Grieco, *Clin. Exp. Immunol.*, *22*: 438 (1975).
25. D. I. Grove, T. O. Burston, M. L. Wellby, R. M. Ford, and I. J. Forbes, *J. Allergy*, *55*:152 (1975).
26. S. Ghazanshahi, R. Townley, E. Chaperone, and G. Villacorte, *Ann. Allergy*, *36*:324 (1976).
27. K.-H. Hsieh, *Ann. Allergy*, *37*:383 (1976).
28. E. Garaci, V. Del Gobbo, C. Favalli, M. G. Promrov, L. Santucci, and F. Titti, in *Thymus, Thymic Hormones and T Lymphocytes* (F. Aiuti and H. Wigzell, eds.), Academic Press, London, 1980, p. 269.
29. U. Serafini, G. Torrigiani, and C. Masala, *Transactions of the World Asthma Conference*, Eastbourne, March 23-26, 1965, organized by the Chest and Heart Association, London, 1965, p. 79.
30. S. G. O. Johansson, *Proc. Roy. Soc., B*, *63*:975 (1969).
31. T. Berg and S. G. O. Johansson, *Int. Arch. Allergy*, *36*:219 (1969).
32. L. Kumar, R. W. Newcomb, K. Ishizaka, and E. Middleton, Jr., *Pediatrics*, *47*:848 (1971).
33. K. Saha, D. D. Kulpati, R. Padmini, D. N. Shivpuri, and P. L. Shali, *Clin. Allergy*, *5*:339 (1975).
34. S. Romagnani, R. Biagotti, E. Maggi, A. Amadori, M. G. Giudizi, and M. Ricci, in *Developments in Clinical Immunology* (M. Ricci, A. S. Fauci, P. Arcangeli, and P. Torzuoli, eds.), Academic Press, London, 1978, p. 185.
35. N. A. Byrom, R. C. D. Staughton, M. A. Campbell, D. M. Timlin, M. Chooi, A. M. Lane, P. W. M. Copeman, and J. R. Hobbs, *Br. J. Derm.*, *100*:499 (1979).
36. J. Palacios, E. W. Fuller, and W. K. Blaylock, *J. Invest. Derm.*, *47*:484 (1966).
37. W. C. Lobitz, J. F. Honeyman, and N. W. Winkler, *Br. J. Derm.*, *86*:317 (1972).
38. J. R. Luckasen, A. Sabat, R. W. Goltz, and J. H. Kersey, *Arch. Derm.*, *110*:375 (1974).
39. J. M. Andersen and N. Hjorth, *Acta Dermatovener.* (*Stockh.*), *55*:345 (1975).
40. K. Thestrup-Pedersen, J. Ellegaard, H. Thulin, and H. Zachariae, *Clin. Exp. Immunol.*, *27*:118 (1977).
41. A. Hovmark, *Acta Dermatovener.* (*Stockh.*), *57*:237 (1977).
42. S. J. McGeady and R. H. Buckley, *J. Allergy. Clin. Immunol.*, *56*:393 (1975).
43. A. Hovmark, *Acta Dermatovener.* (*Stockh.*), *55*:181 (1975).
44. N. A. Byrom and D. M. Timlin, *Br. J. Derm.*, *100*:491 (1979).
45. D. I. Grove, J. G. Reid, and I. J. Forbes, *Br. J. Derm.*, *92*:611 (1975).
46. K. Ishizaka and H. Okudaira, *J. Immunol.*, *110*:1067 (1973).
47. K. Okumura and T. Tada, *J. Immunol.*, *106*:1019 (1971).
48. K. Okumura and T. Tada, *J. Immunol.*, *107*:1682 (1971).
49. M. Taniguchi and T. Tada, *J. Immunol.*, *107*:579 (1971).
50. L. Moretta, S. R. Webb, C. E. Grossi, P. M. Lydyard, and M. D. Cooper, *J. Exp. Med.*, *146*:184 (1977).
51. G. W. Canonica, M. C. Mingari, G. Melioli, M. Colombatti, and L. Moretta, *J. Immunol.*, *123*:2669 (1979).
52. D. L. Schuster, B. A. Bongiovanni, D. L. Pierson, J. F. Barbaro, D. T. O. Wong, and A. I. Levinson, *J. Immunol.*, *124*:1662 (1980).

53. H. H. Fudenberg, J. Wybran, and D. Robbins, *N. Engl. J. Med.*, *27*:475 (1975).
54. L. Perelmutter and L. Potvin, *Ann. Allergy, 45*:18 (1980).
55. M. Al-Sarraf, S. Sardesai, and V. K. Vaitkevicius, *Cancer, 27*:1426 (1971).
56. T. Han and H. Takita, *N. Engl. J. Med.*, *286*:605 (1972).
57. N. Suciu-Foca, J. Buda, J. McManus, T. Thiem, and K. Reemtsma, *Cancer Res.*, *33*:2373 (1973).
58. W. J. Catalona and P. B. Chretien, *Cancer, 31*:353 (1973).
59. W. J. Catalona, W. F. Sample, and P. B. Chretien, *Cancer, 31*:65 (1973).
60. C. Butterworth, C. J. Oon, G. Westbury, and J. R. Hobbs, *Eur. J. Cancer, 10*:639 (1974).
61. D. Catovsky, E. Miliani, A. Okos, and D. A. G. Galton, *Lancet, ii*:751 (1974).
62. C. Potvin, J. I, Tarpley, and P. B. Chretien, *Clin. Immunol. Immunopathol.*, *3*:476 (1975).
63. J. J. Bourgoin, M. Vitris, J. Rifa, and J. Geneve, *Behring Inst. Mitt.*, *56*:263 (1975).
64. M. G. Bernengo, G. Capella, A. De Matteis, P. A. Tovo, and G. Zina, *Clin. Exp. Immunol.*, *36*:279 (1979).
65. M. F. Martelli, A. Velardi, P. Rambotti, C. Cernetti, A. M. Bracaglia, E. Ballatori, and S. Davis, *Cancer, 49*:245 (1982).
66. A. R. Cheema and A. M. Hersh, *Cancer, 28*:851 (1971).
67. J. W. Thomas, P. Coy, H. S. Lewis, and A. Yuen, *Cancer, 27*:1046 (1971).
68. A. C. Campbell, P. Hersey, I. C. M. MacLennan, H. E. M. Kay, and M. C. Pike, *Br. Med. J.*, *2*:385 (1973).
69. A. B. Cosimi, F. Brunstetter, W. T. Kemmerer, and R. N. Miller, *Arch. Surg.*, *107*:531 (1973).
70. J. L. Tarpley, C. Potvin, and P. B. Chretien, *Cancer, 35*:644 (1975).
71. J. Stjernsward, M. Jondal, F. Vansky, and R. Sealy, *Lancet, i*:1352 (1972).
72. H. I. Heier, I. Christensen, S. S. Fröland, and A. Engeset, *Lymphology, 8*:69 (1975).
73. J. M. Anderson, J. B. Campbell, S. E. Wood, J. E. Boyd, and F. Kelly, *Clin. Oncol.*, *1*:201 (1975).
74. A. C. Campbell, G. Wiernik, J. Wood, P. Hersey, C. A. Waller, and I. C. M. MacLennan, *Clin. Exp. Immunol.*, *23*:200 (1976).
75. B. Petrini, J. Wasserman, H. Blomgren, and E. Baral, *Clin. Exp. Immunol.*, *29*:36 (1977).
76. J. Goodman, W. Schaffner, H. Collins, E. Battersby, and M. Koenig, *N. Engl. J. Med.*, *278*:117 (1968).
77. M. J. Krant, G. Manskopf, C. S. Brandrup, and M. A. Madoff, *Cancer, 21*:623 (1968).
78. S. Kumar and G. Taylor, *Lancet, ii*:564 (1974).
79. S. K. Park, J. I. Brody, H. A. Wallace, and W. S. Blackmore, *Lancet, i*:53 (1971).
80. M. G. Lewis, R. L. Ikonopisov, R. C. Nairn, T. M. Phillips, G. Hamilton-Fairley, D. C. Bodenham, and P. Alexander, *Br. Med. J.*, *iii*:547 (1969).
81. N. A. Byrom, M. A. Campbell, A. J. Dean, D. M. Timlin, C. Volkers, D. C. Bodenham, and J. R. Hobbs, *Cancer Treat. Rep.*, *62*:1769 (1978).
82. G. A. Currie and C. Basham, *Br. J. Cancer, 26*:427 (1972).
83. A. Claudy, N. Fouad-Wassef, and N. Pelletier, *Annales de Dermatologie et de Syphiligraphie*, *102*:69 (1975).
84. A. L. Dellon, C. Potvin, and P. B. Chretien, *Cancer, 35*:687 (1975).
85. R. H. Whitehead, J. Thatcher, C. Teasdale, G. P. Roberts, and L. E. Hughes, *Lancet, i*:330 (1976).
86. H. M. Anthony, J. A. Kirk, K. E. Madsen, M. K. Mason, and G. H. Templeman, *Clin. Exp. Immunol.*, *20*:41 (1975).
87. A. Adler, J. A. Stein, and S. Ben Efraim, in *Tumour-Associated Antigens and their Specific Immune Response* (F. Spreafico and R. Arnon, eds.), Academic Press, London, 1979, p. 325.

88. M. G. Bernengo, C. Barbera, A. De Matteis, M. Meregalli, and G. Zina, in *Thymus, Thymic Hormones and T Lymphocytes* (F. Aiuti and H. Wigzell, eds.), Academic Press, London, 1979, p. 325.
89. D. E. Kenady, C. Potvin, and P. B. Chretien, in *Immune Modulation and Control of Neoplasia by Adjuvant Therapy* (M. A. Chirigos, ed.), Raven Press, New York, 1978, p. 347.
90. J. Shoham, in *Thymus, Thymic Hormones and T Lymphocytes* (F. Aiuti and H. Wigzell, eds.), Academic Press, London, 1980, p. 273.
91. Z. Fuks, S. Stober, and H. S. Kaplan, *N. Engl. J. Med.*, *295*:1273 (1976).
92. Z. Fuks, S. Strober, D. P. King, and H. S. Kaplan, *J. Immunol.*, *117*:1331 (1976).
93. P. D. J. Holland, O. Browne, and R. D. Thorne, *Br. J. Cancer*, *31*:164 (1975).
94. C. Rugarli, R. Scorza, and M. G. Sabbadini, *Lancet*, *i*:1297 (1975).
95. G. S. Del Giaco, in *Developments in Clinical Immunology* (M. Ricci, A. S. Fauci, P. Arcangeli, and P. Torzuoli, eds.), Academic Press, London, 1978, p. 129.
96. J. Wagstaff, K. Phadke, N. Adam, N. Thatcher, and D. Crowther, *Cancer*, *49*:439 (1982).
97. V. J. McGovern, M. C. Mihm, C. Bailly, J. C. Booth, W. H. Clark, A. J. Cochran, E. G. Hardy, J. D. Hicks, A. Levene, M. G. Lewis, J. H. Little, and G. W. Milton, *Cancer*, *32*:1446 (1973).
98. F. R. Eilber and D. L. Morton, *Cancer*, *25*:362 (1970).
99. P. B. Chretien, W. L. Crowder, H. R. Gertner, W. F. Sample, and W. J. Catalona, *Surg. Gynecol. Obstetr.*, *136*:380 (1973).
100. J. B. Dubois and B. Serrou, *Br. J. Surg.*, *61*:326 (1974).
101. P. A. Cooperider and H. H. Roenigk, *Arch. Dermatol.*, *114*:207 (1978).
102. R. MacKie, F. R. Sless, R. Cochran, and M. De Sousa, *Br. J. Derm.*, *94*:173 (1976).
103. M. David, B. Shohat, N. Trainin, and E. Feuerman, *Cancer*, *46*:41 (1980).
104. D. Cyr, C. M. Geokas, and G. H. Worsley, *Arch. Dermatol.*, *94*:558 (1966).
105. Z. Y. Fuks, M. A. Bagshaw, and E. M. Farber, *Cancer*, *32*:1385 (1973).
106. N. F. Mendes, C. C. Mussati, and E. A. Tolnai, *Int. Arch. Allergy Appl. Immunol.*, *46*:695 (1974).
107. C. B. Nordqvist and P. J. Kinney, *Cancer*, *37*:714 (1976).
108. H. Zachariae, J. Ellegaard, E. Grunnet, H. Sogaard, and H. Thulin, *Acta Dermatovener.*, *55*:466 (1975).
109. D. Zucker-Franklin and W. J. Melton, *Proc. Natl. Acad. Sci USA*, *71*:1887 (1974).
110. R. Braylan, D. Variakojis, and S. Yachnin, *Clin. Res.* (Abstr.), *21*:870 (1973).
111. N. A. Byrom, M. A. Campbell, J. R. Hobbs, A. J. Dean, D. M. Timlin, M. Webley, and D. A. Brewerton, *Lancet*, *ii*:601 (1979).
112. D. A Brewerton, M. Caffrey, A. Nicholls, D. Walters, and D. C. O. James, *Lancet*, *ii*:994 (1973).
113. J. F. Woodruff and J. J. Woodruff, *Cell. Immunol.*, *1*:333 (1970).
114. J. Wybran and H. H. Fudenberg, *J. Clin. Invest.*, *52*:1026 (1973).
115. A. I. Notkins, S. E. Mergenhagen, and R. J. Howard, *Ann. Rev. Microbiol.*, *24*: 525 (1970).
116. L. Businco, P. Rossi, I. Quinti, and R. Perlini, in *Thymus, Thymic Hormones and T Lymphocytes* (F. Aiuti and H. Wigzell, eds.), Academic Press, London, 1980, p. 295.
117. F. V. Chisari and T. S. Edgington, *J. Exp. Med.*, *142*:1092 (1975).
118. M. H. Grieco, I. Siegel, and Z. Goel, *J. Allergy Clin. Immunol.*, *50*:148 (1976).
119. F. V. Chisari and T. S. Edgington, *J. Exp. Med.*, *140*:512 (1974).
120. H. M. Ögmundsdottir and D. M. Weir, *Clin. Exp. Immunol.*, *40*:223 (1980).
121. E. P. Van Der Esch, N. Cascinelli, F. Preda, A. Morabito, and R. Bufalino, *Cancer*, *48*:1668 (1981).
122. J. R. Hobbs, N. Byrom, P. Elliott, C.-J. Oon, and S. Retsas, *Exp. Hematol.*, *5* (Suppl.):95 (1977).

28

Immunosuppressive Effects of Human Chorionic Gonadotropin on Delayed-Type Hypersensitivity in Mice

Anna Bartocci, Roy D. Welker, Mario Piccoli,* Erich Schlick, Vasilios Papademetriou, Klaus Hartung,† and Michael A. Chirigos National Cancer Institute-Frederick Cancer Research Facility, Frederick, Maryland

Bruce C. Nisula National Institute of Child Health and Human Development, National Institutes of Health, Bethesda, Maryland

I. INTRODUCTION

Pregnancy as well as malignancy represents an immunological state whereby a primarily competent immune system permits the survival of antigenic tissue within the host. Many theories have been proposed to explain the tolerance in both conditions, and there are many common denominators between pregnancy and malignancy. Of special interest among these is the potential role of human chorionic gonadotropin (hCG). hCG is a glycoprotein tropic hormone consisting of two subunits, hCGα and hCGβ (1,2). The hormone is normally synthesized by the cyto- and syncytiotrophoblast of the human placenta (2-4). In addition, synthesis of hCG and its subunits has been demonstrated in trophoblastic neoplasias, in a large fraction of ovarian and testicular tumors (5), and in many nontrophoblastic, nongonadal tumors (6-8).

Several investigators have proposed that hCG is an immunosuppressive agent that contributes to diminished tissue rejection in both pregnancy and malignancy. This hypothesis derives from the reports that hCG preparations cause appreciable inhibition of immune responses in mice, rats, and humans (9-13). Recently, the ability of the hCG molecule to decrease cellular immunity has been challenged, since purified preparations of hCG failed to inhibit some in vitro immune responses (14-17). Rather, the results of these studies suggested that many batches of commercial hCG possess a potent, nontoxic contaminant responsible for the immunosuppression attributed to hCG. In vitro immune responses, however, are intrinsically limited with respect to the number of

---

Current affiliations:
*Institute of General Pathology, State University of Rome, Rome, Italy.
†Bundeswehrkrankenhaus, Klinische Medizin, Labor, Koblenz, Federal Republic of Germany.

facets of the immune system they can evaluate; in vivo immune responses offer a more general, albeit more complex, test system for evaluating potential immunological effects. Accordingly, to investigate a possible immunosuppressive role of the hCG molecule in vivo, we designed studies to examine its effects on delayed-type hypersensitivity (DTH) to sheep red blood cells (SRBCs) in mice. In this report, we show that significant DTH suppression is exerted by both commercially available and purified preparations of hCG, and we suggest a role for prostaglandins in mediating the immunosuppressive activity.

II. MATERIALS AND METHODS

A. Mice

Male and female CD_2F_1 (BALB/cCr X DBA/2Cr) ($H\text{-}2^d/H\text{-}2^d$) mice, 8-10 weeks old, were supplied by the Mammalian Genetics and Animal Production Section, Division of Cancer Treatment, National Cancer Institute, NIH, Bethesda, Maryland.

B. Reagents

Commercial preparations of crude hCG (c. hCG) (2570-3230 IU/mg protein) were purchased from Sigma Chemical Co., St. Louis, Missouri and from Organon, West Orange, New Jersey (∿2850 IU/mg protein). Extensively purified hCG (∿14,000 IU/mg) (p.hCG), hCGα and hCGβ subunits, and neuraminidase desialylated hCG (asialo hCG) were prepared by Drs. S. Briken and R. E. Canfield (4,17-19) and supplied by the Center for Population Research of the National Institute of Child Health and Human Development of the National Institutes of Health. All hCG preparations were stored at $-20°C$ until used.

Sheep red blood cells (SRBCs) were purchased from Flow Laboratory, McLean, Virginia. Indomethacin (INDO) (Sigma Chemicals Co., St. Louis, Missouri) was dissolved in absolute ethanol and diluted in PBS. Aspirin (ASP) was dissolved in 70% ethyl alcohol and diluted in PBS. The injected solutions of indomethacin and ASP contained less than 0.8 and 0.1% ethanol, respectively. These concentrations of alcohol were added to control solutions (indomethacin- or ASP-free) and had no effects on DTH responses (data not shown).

C. DTH Reaction

Delayed-type hypersensitivity (DTH) was studied in CD_2F_1 mice ($H\text{-}2^d/H\text{-}2^d$) 8-10 weeks old of both sexes. SRBCs were washed three times with sterile PBS and brought to a concentration of 2.0×10^9 cells/ml. Animals were sensitized on day 0 with 1×10^8 SRBCs injected intradermally (ID) into the left hind footpad. On day 4, 1×10^8 SRBCs were injected ID into the right hind footpad. Twenty-four hours later, mice were sacrificed, and the thickness of both footpads was measured with a gravity-sensitive calibrated device. The interval between the sensitizing and challenging doses as well as the concentration of SRBCs used had been determined to be optimal in preliminary studies. The extent of the DTH reaction of the individual groups was determined as follows: the thickness of both hind footpads was measured three times and the average difference between the left (control) and right (sensitized) foot pad was recorded individually for each mouse. Experimental groups received various hCG preparations or vehicle intraperitoneally (IP) daily for 4 days prior to or after the sensitizing SRBC administration. In a separate set of experiments, experimental groups received different doses of INDO or

ASP simultaneously with p. hCG for 4 days. The mean value ± standard error of the mean (SEM) for each group of 10 mice was calculated and statistical analysis of the results was performed using the two-tailed Student's t-test.

III. RESULTS

Injections of either crude or purified hCG into male CD_2F_1 mice before sensitization (see Material and Methods) resulted in a strong suppression of DTH response (Table 1). Significant inhibition of the DTH response was obtained with both crude commercial hCG preparations, and both batches of purified hCG (CR 121 and CR 123). Injection of bovine serum albumin as a foreign protein control failed to modify the DTH response (data not shown). In order to determine whether the immunosuppressive activity of hCG could be in some way modified by the sex of the animal, we compared the activity of p. hCG in male and female mice. Using the same experimental methodology (four injections of 100 IU of hCG prior to the SRBC sensitization), we demonstrated no significant differences in the reactivity of male and female mice to the hormone (Table 2). To study the effect of timing of the hCG exposure related to sensitization on the DTH response, we gave the same dose of p. hCG (100 IU per mouse) before and after primary sensitization. No suppression of the DTH response was observed when hCG was given after sensitization (Fig. 1), indicating that the mechanism involved in the suppression is not effective after antigen presentation. Asialo hCG and the α and β subunits of hCG were tested with the same experimental model (Fig. 2). Neither the subunits nor the asialo hCG given in a dosage similar to hCG produced any inhibition of the DTH response, suggesting that a structural integrity of the hCG molecule is required for the suppressive effect. We next analyzed the activity of different doses of p. hCG on the DTH response (Fig. 3). The suppressive effect of the hormone was dose dependent and significant to an hCG dose of 10 IU per mouse. Although the inhibition was not significant at the 1 IU per mouse dose level, in other experiments dosages as low as 0.8 IU per mouse have produced significant inhibition of footpad swelling. Figure 4 shows the percent of maximal suppression obtained with different doses of p. hCG, ranging from 1 to 100 IU per mouse

Table 1 Effect of Crude hCG (c. hCG) and Purified hCG (p. hCG) on Delayed-Type Hypersensitivity to SRBCs in CD_2F_1 Mice

Group	Increase in footpad swelling (MM)	p value[c]
Saline	0.01	—
SRBCs	0.20 ± 0.01[d]	—
SRBCs + c. hCG (Sigma)[a]	0.16 ± 0.04	NS[e]
SRBCs + c. hCG (Sigma)[b]	0.12 ± 0.04	0.05
SRBCs ± c. hCG (Organon)[a]	0.12 ± 0.02	0.05
SRBCs + c. hCG (Organon)[b]	0.12 ± 0.03	0.05
SRBCs + p. hCG (CR 121)[b]	0.10 ± 0.03	0.01
SRBCs + p. hCG (CR 123)[b]	0.13 ± 0.03	0.05

[a]1000 IU/mouse IP for 4 days.
[b]100 IU/mouse IP for 4 days.
[c]P value for the comparison of the experimental group to the sensitized (SRBCs) group
[d]Values shown are mean ± SEM with at least 10 mice in each group.
[e]NS, not significant.

Table 2 Effect of Purified hCG (p. hCG) on Delayed-Type Hypersensitivity to SRBCs in Females and Males

Group	Increase in footpad swelling (MM)	p value[b]
Females		
Saline	0.01	–
SRBCs	0.20 ± 0.01	–
SRBCs + p. hCG[a]	0.10 ± 0.01	$p < 0.01$
Males		
Saline	0.01	–
SRBCs	0.21 ± 0.02	–
SRBCs + p. hCG[a]	0.10 ± 0.03	$p < 0.01$

[a]100 IU/mouse IP for 4 days; batch CR 121 was used.
[b]P value for the comparison of the experimental group to the sensitized (SRBCs) group.

of hCG. The ED_{50} was between 10 and 20 IU per mouse. The minimal effective dose was between 0.5 and 5 IU per mouse based on the data obtained from several experiments. The simultaneous administration of indomethacin (2 mg/kg) or aspirin (0.4 mg/kg) with purified hCG completely abrogated the suppressive effect of the hormone (Table 3), suggesting a vital role for prostaglandins in the induction of the suppressive activity. The possibility of an unrelated stimulation of the DTH response can be eliminated since aspiring and indomethacin themselves failed to increase DTH readings beyond control levels (Table 3).

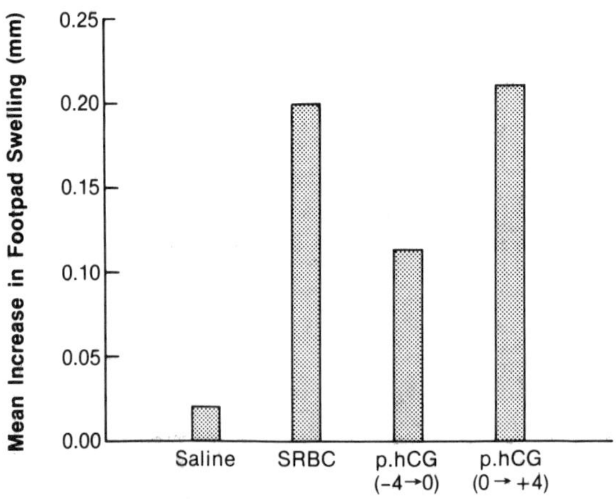

Figure 1 Effect of timing of administration of purified hCG (p. hCG), on delayed-type hypersensitivity to SRBCs in CD_2F_1 mice. The preparations were administered IP for 4 days before (–4→0) or after (0→+4) the SRBC sensitization (day 0).

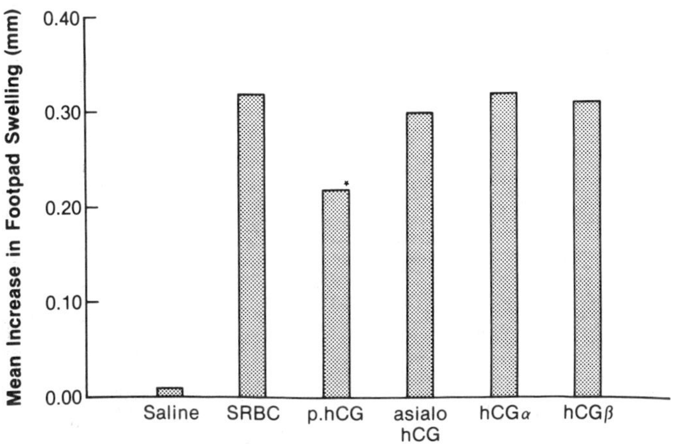

Figure 2 Effect of p. hCG, asialo-hCG, α-subunit (hCGα) and β-subunit (hCGβ) on delayed-type hypersensitivity response in CD_2F_1 mice. The preparations were administered IP at a dose of 10 μg per mouse (10 μg p. hCG ∿ 150 IU per mouse) for 4 days before the SRBCs. P value reflects the comparison of the experimental groups with the immunized (SRBCs) control group. *$p < 0.001$.

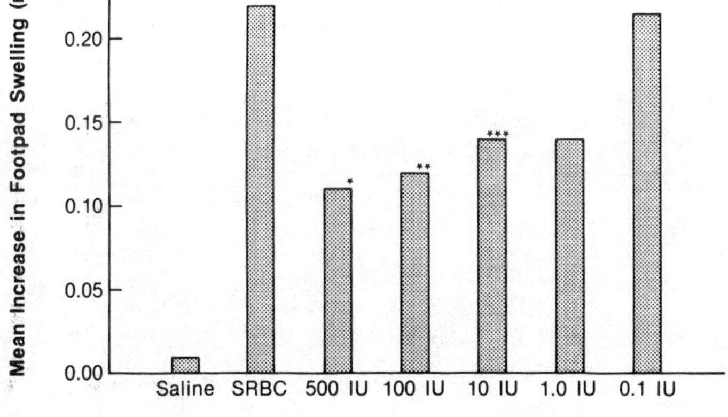

Figure 3 Effect of varying doses of p. hCG on delayed-type hypersensitivity response in CD_2F_1 mice. p. hCG was given IP in daily dosage as indicated, for 4 days before the SRBCs. The p value reflects comparison of the experimental group with the immunized (SRBC) control group. *$p < 0.001$. **$p < 0.01$. *** $p < 0.05$.

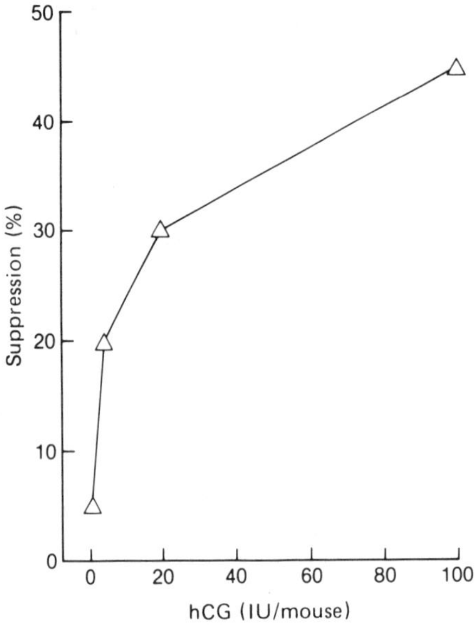

Figure 4 DTH suppressing activity by hCG expressed as percent decrease in footpad swelling compared with the immunized SRBC control group. P. hCG was given IP in daily dosage as indicated for 4 days, before the SRBCs.

IV. DISCUSSION

These investigations clearly demonstrate a suppressive role of hCG on the delayed-type hypersensitivity (DTH) response in vivo. Some investigators have failed to demonstrate in vitro immunosuppressive activity with purified hCG (14-17) and have suggested the presence of active contaminants in crude commercial hCG preparations (12,17). However, we have previously reported in vivo DTH suppression by both crude and purified

Table 3 Effect of Inhibitors of Prostaglandin Synthesis on the Immunosuppressive Activity of p. hCG (Delayed-Type Hypersensitivity in CD_2F_1 Mice)

Group	Increase in footpad swelling (mm)	P value[c]
Saline	0.01	–
SRBC	0.22 ± 0.02[d]	0.001
SRBCs + p. hCG[a]	0.08 ± 0.01	NS[e]
SRBCs + p. hCG[a] + INDO[b]	0.24 ± 0.06	NS
SRBCs + p. hCG[a] + ASP[b]	0.19 ± 0.03	NS
SRBCs + INDO[b]	0.23 ± 0.04	NS
SRBCs + ASP[b]	0.21 ± 0.02	NS

[a]100 IU/mouse IP for 4 days (p. hCG/CR 121).
[b]INDO 2 mg/kg for 4 days; ASP 0.4 mg/kg for 4 days.
[c]P value for the comparison of the experimental groups with the sensitized (SRBCs) control
[d]Values shown are mean ± SEM with at least 10 mice in each group.
[e]NS, not significant.

hCG preparations (18). In the present report, we confirm and extend these findings by including a comparison of two highly purified and two crude commercial hCG preparations for in vivo DTH suppressive activity. Significant suppression was observed with both the purified preparations, as well as both commercial preparations. These data strongly indicate that the hCG molecule itself is responsible for the DTH suppressing activity. Although some reports show inconsistent results with differing dose levels (20) of p. hCG, we can demonstrate a dose-response relationship of the hormone. The minimal effective dosage was about 1 IU per mouse, a dose level not far from that at which the gonadotropic effect of hCG is manifest in this species (21). There are several possible explanations for the disparity in our results and those previously reported. The discrepancy between the effects of c. hCG and p. hCG in vitro could be due to a contaminant present in the crude hormone. It is well known that numerous hCG preparations contain pregnancy-correlated factors inhibiting (14,15) or stimulating (22) the reactivity of the lymphocytes in vitro. Further, the failure of p. hCG to induce an immunosuppression in vitro could be explained by the inability of the cells present in the culture to react with the hormone. From our study of the effects of p. hCG on DTH, as in vivo test, we can conclude that hCG has a strong immunosuppressive activity. Ruling out the possibility of a direct role of hCG on those aspects of the immune system evaluated by the in vitro experiments, we would hypothesize that a cofactor such as a steroidal product or prostaglandins, possible released by the gonads, is responsible for the observed suppression in vivo. Obviously, the cofactor is absent in vitro. Studies are under way to evaluate the identity of the cofactor and the mechanism of action.

Investigators have found free α and β hCG subunits in urine during pregnancy (23,24), and free forms of both subunits are probably present in serum during pregnancy (23,24). Both subunits are also produced in large amounts by some neoplasms (25). There have been studies concerning the importance of the sialic acid content of hCG that indicate that its reduced biological activity following desialylation is attributable to enhanced clearance of the molecule (26). Although there have been differing reports on hCG subunit intrinsic activity (27), results from our studies show that the α and β subunit preparations, and the asialo-hCG preparation manifest no significant DTH suppression; we can therefore assert that the structural integrity of the hCG molecule is essential for its DTH-suppressing activity.

Our data offer insight into the mechanism of action of the immunosuppressive effect of the hCG molecule. Two known prostaglandin (PG) inhibitors, aspirin and indomethacin, given simultaneously with hCG completely blocked the effects of hCG, supporting a role for PG in the observed DTH suppression by hCG. The immune-inhibiting activity of PG of the E series is well known (28,29) and has been related to the presence of an adherent PG–producing suppressor cell (30,31). PGE seems to act by increasing intracellular cyclic AMP (cAMP) and inducing nonspecific T suppressor activity (32).

Although a role for PG in hCG-induced DTH suppression seems clear, the exact mechanism which leads to PG production has not been elucidated. It has been shown that the hCG molecule can activate adenylcyclase in gonadal and thyroid tissue (33,34). However, thyroidal mediation of the hCG effect can be excluded since dosages 100-fold larger than those employed herein would be required (21). On the other hand, it is conceivable that gonadal stimulation is involved. The fact that the subunits and asialo-hCG were inactive would be consistent with this possibility. Regardless of the anticedent hormonal mechanisms by which hCG elicits its effect, we would speculate that the release of PG in vivo is the step that results in the generation of T lymphocytes with suppressor activity.

There has been much speculation about the mechanism of escape of the human fetus and placental trophoblast cells from maternal immune surveillance since these cells are of an allogeneic nature. Neoplastic cells can be compared with trophoblastic cells in their invasive nature, membrane constituents, tendency to secrete fetal proteins such as hCG, and regression to fetal phenotype (35), as well as in their ability to escape immune surveillance. Trophoblast cells and neoplastic cells may share another characteristic, in that hCG has been shown to be an integral part of human trophoblast plasma membranes (35), and ectopic production of hCG by a variety of nontrophoblastic tumors has been observed (6-8). It has been shown that daily hCG injections prolong skin allograft survival in animals (35), and our results show considerable depression of DTH function in mice. Since we have shown significant DTH suppression by highly purified hCG, the possibility of a role for hCG in the escape of trophoblastic and neoplastic cells from immune surveillance by hCG secretion becomes more probable.

REFERENCES

1. F. C. Morgan and R. E. Canfield, *Endocrinology, 88*:1045 (1971).
2. S. Birken and R. E. Canfield, in *Chorionic Gonadotropin* (S. J. Segal, ed), Plenum Press, New York, 1980, pp. 65-88.
3. Y. Yoshimoto, A. R. Wolfson, and W. D. Odell, *Science, 197*:575 (1977).
4. A. R. Midgley, Jr. and G. B. Pierce, *J. Exp. Med., 115*:289 (1962).
5. K. D. Bagshawe, *Choriocarcinoma: The Clinical Biology of the Trophoblast and its Tumors,* The Williams and Wilkins Co., Baltimore, 1969.
6. G. D. Braunstein, J. L. Vaitukaitis, P. P. Carbone, and G. T. Ross, *Ann. Intern. Med., 78*:39 (1973).
7. D. W. Golde, M. Schambelan, B. D. Weintraub, and S. W. Rosen, *Cancer, 33*:1048 (1974).
8. D. O. Goldenstein, T. S. Kesese, and A. T. Serim, *Surg. Gynecol. Obstet., 138*:747 (1974).
9. M. D. Kaye and W. R. Jones, *Am. J. Obstet. Gynecol., 109*:1029 (1971).
10. E. W. Adcock, F. Teasdale, C. S. August, S. Cox, G. Meschia, F. C. Battaglia, and M. A. Naughton, *Science, 181*:845 (1973).
11. S. F. Contractor and H. Davies, *Nature (New Biol.), 243*:284 (1973).
12. T. Han, *Immunology, 29*:509 (1975).
13. F. M. Clarke, H. Morton, and G. J. Clume, *Clin. Exp. Immunol., 32*:318 (1978).
14. A. V. Muchmore and R. M. Blaese, *J. Immunol., 118*:881 (1977).
15. J. L. Caldwell, D. P. Stites, and H. H. Fudenberg, *J. Immunol., 115*:1249 (1975).
16. D. Gundert, W. E. Merz, V. Hilgenfeldt, and R. Brossmer, *FEBS Lett., 539*:309 (1975).
17. J. H. Morse, G. Stearns, J. Arden, G. Agosto, and R. E. Canfield, *Cell. Immunol., 25*:178 (1976).
18. A. Bartocci, V. Papdemetriou, E. Schlick, B. C. Nisula, and M. A. Chirigos, *Cell. Immunol., 71*:326 (1982).
19. G. S. Taliadouros, S. Amr, P. Louvet, S. Birken, R. E. Canfield, and B. C. Nisula, *J. Clin. Endocrinol. Metab., 54*:1002 (1982).
20. D. Beck, H. Gimsberg, and Y. Naot, *Am. J. Obstet. Gynecol., 129*:14 (1977).
21. B. C. Nisula, G. S. Taliadouros, and P. Carayon, in *Human Chorionic Gonadotropin* (S. Segal, ed.), Plenum Press, New York, 1980, p. 17.
22. J. Morse, P. Ehrlich, and R. Canfield, *J. Immunol., 128*:2187 (1982).
23. G. Taliadouros, S. Anur, J. Lovet, S. Bisken, R. Canfield, and B. Nisula, *J. Clin. Endocrinol. Metab., 54*:1002 (1982).

24. P. Franchimont and A. Reuter, in *Structure-Activity Relationships of Protein and Polypeptide Hormones* (M. Margoulies and F. C. Greenwood, eds.), Excerpta Medica, Amsterdam, 1972, pp. 381-387.
25. B. D. Weintraub, G. K. Krauth, S. W. Rose, and A. S. Rabson, *J. Clin. Invest.*, *56*: 1043 (1975).
26. G. A. Morell, G. Gregoriadis, H. Scheinberg, J. Hickman, and G. Ashwell, *J. Biol. Chem.*, *246*:1461 (1971).
27. S. Ramakrishnan and G. P. Talwar, in *Human Chorionic Gonadotropin* (S. Segal, ed.), Plenum Press, New York, 1979, pp. 213.
28. X. Murata, M. Kawamura, and I. Morite, *Biochem Biophys. Acta*, *528*:507 (1978).
29. G. D. Stockman and D. M. Mumford, *Exp. Hemat.*, *2*:65 (1974).
30. J. S. Goodwin, A. D. Beukhurst, and R. P. Messner, *J. Exp. Med.*, *146*:1719 (1977).
31. Z. Metzger, J. Hoffeld, and J. J. Oppenheim, *J. Immunol.*, *124*:983 (1980).
32. A. M. Fulton and J. Levy, *Cell. Immunol.*, *59*:54 (1981).
33. C. A. Villee and S. G. Gabbe, in *Gonadotropins* (B. B. Saxens, C. G. Beling, and H. M. Gandy, eds.), Wily Interscience Publications, New York, 1972, pp. 312.
34. P. Carayon, G. Lefort and B. C. Nisula, *Endocrinology*, *106*:1907 (1980).
35. Y. W. Loke, in *Immunology and Immunopathology of the Human Fetal-Maternal Interaction*, North Holland, Amsterdam, 1978.

29

The Mode of Action of Imuthiol (Sodium Diethyldithiocarbamate)

A New Role for the Brain Neocortex and the Endocrine Liver in the Regulation of the T-Cell Linage

Gerard Renoux Laboratoire d'Immunologie, Faculté de Médecine, Tours, France

I. INTRODUCTION

Cancers, autoimmune diseases, infectious diseases, and allergies are all disease states associated with immune impairment or dysfunction, and the defect is frequently aggravated by conventional therapies. Thus, it was assumed that an agent active on the immune system would be successful, particularly in cancer patients. Unfortunately, clinical trials have yielded conflicting results, unfairly accentuated by attempts of immunotherapy in very advanced cases unresponsive to any other known treatment. Much experimental and clinical testing has been conducted without a firm biological base, and important guidelines were not taken into account, sometimes because they were only partially known a few years ago. They include the influence of malignancy on the components of the immune network; the role of host factors on the pharmacokinetics of the drug thus modifying its potential; the host-parasite relationship; and the influence of associated therapies that could modify the expression of tumor antigens, the function of immunocompetent cells, and the response of tumor cells to the host immunological system. These pitfalls were exaggerated by a blind reliance on the pertinence of laboratory data based on test models in animals artificially chosen among ancient lines of tumor cell which may retain little resemblance to neoplasia in the human being (1). In addition, and until recently little attention was directed to the pharmacological features and mode of action of biological response modifiers (BRMs) to ascertain their real efficacy. Meanwhile, many agents came into use before their composition was known, and the extent of their toxicity, deleterious and adverse effects, and even carcinogenicity, was appreciated. Consequently, there has ensued a rather ambiguous interpretation of the value of agents intended to modify the immune machinery. Despite the problems that beset its development, immunomodulation remains a fascinating approach to the treatment, and even prevention, of the diseases where immunological disturbances have been demonstrated. Furthermore, the immune system is generally considered as a self-monitoring and autoregulated system. Accordingly, assays to determine the possible effectiveness of an agent that is supposedly a biological response modifier (BRM) were, and still are, frequently based on in vitro tests which generated exaggerated expectations, for the simple reason a test tube is neither a human or a mouse.

The usefulness of in vitro assays is in essence to endeavor for the understanding of the discrepancies that may arise between in vivo and in vitro tests. The pathways that conducted from levamisole to sodium diethyldithiocarbamate (imuthiol)* may well serve to illustrate the paramount importance of comparing the data from the two sets of assays. This comparison leads to a clarity concerning the background of the ambivalent effects of levamisole and to the development of imuthiol, a nonantigenic, nontoxic, and noncarcinogenic compound, specifically active on the T-cell lineage.

The available data thus far show that imuthiol fulfills safety requirements and exerts a unique influence on the T-cell lineage. Furthermore, and most significantly, studies on the mode of action of imuthiol provide new and unsuspected insights into the relationships between the immune system in its most elaborate arm (the T-cell lineage) and other regulatory systems, namely the endocrine liver and the brain.

II. STUDIES ON THE AMBIVALENT EFFICACY OF LEVAMISOLE CONDUCTED TO SODIUM DIETHYLDITHIOCARBAMATE

Both the time of administration and the dose are critical in modifying the effectiveness of levamisole, as well as the animal strain or the age and the sex of recipients (2-4). Levamisole shows also a time- and dose-dependent efficacy in syngeneic skin graft rejection (5), and against a variety of animal tumors (3,6). In addition, pretreatment with levamisole for 7 days before immunization markedly inhibits the number of specific plaque-forming cells (PFCs) in a kinetic study of 7-day postantigenic stimulus with sheep red blood cells (SRBCs) (2). Chronic administration of levamisole, three times a week for 4 weeks, abrogates the lymphoproliferative responses to mitogens and even the background DNA incorporation, and inhibits IgM and IgG spleen cell-antibody responses tested 4 days after the arrest of the treatment, as summarized by Fig. 1.

The findings imply a warning against the indiscriminate use of a standard dose of levamisole in a variety of clinical situations: random and uncritical use of the agent has, indeed, produced inconsistent results. They also led us to studies in an attempt to explain the ambivalent influence of levamisole.

Levamisole possesses an imidazole moiety. As is shown in Table 1, administration of imidazole does not modify the magnitude of IgM or IgG spleen cell responses to SRBCs. However, a dose of 0.05 mg/kg would classify immunized mice as nonresponders not affected by imidazole and as responders evidencing a significant increase in the number of PFCs. The very similar result in mice treated with 5 mg/kg levamisole (2) could not be purely coincidental, as levamisole hydrochloride salt contains 27.8% imidazole.

A treatment with imidazole decreases the magnitude of delayed hypersensitivity to SRBCs, does not evoke the production of serum factors enhancing the immune responsiveness of recipients, and is unable to promote in vivo prothymocyte differentiation,

*The term *imuthiol* is now replacing the previous abbreviation DTC, as the latter could be easily confused with the chemotherapeutic agent, DTIC.

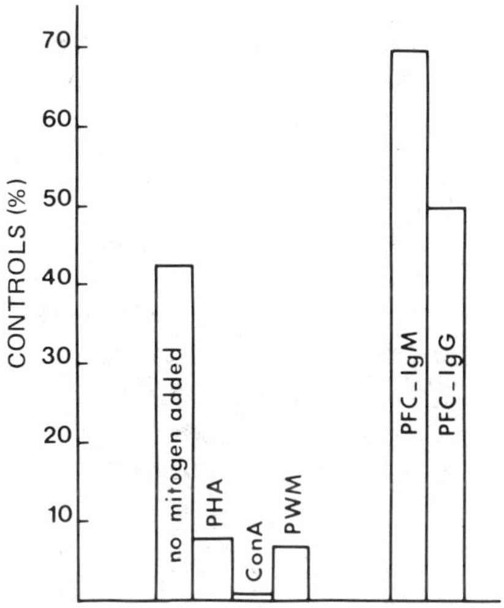

Figure 1 Influences of chronic administration (25 mg/kg, three times a week for 4 weeks) of levamisole on BALB/c immune responsiveness. Data are expressed in percents of control values (eight mice per group): no mitogen added (background) = 2215 ± 1897; PHA = 68,470 ± 7120; ConA = 97,814 ± 970; PWM = 34,100 ± 174, expressed as cpm ± SE of triplicate cultures of 5 X 10^5 lymphocytes per well. Direct (IgM) and indirect (IgG) antibody-forming spleen cells (PFC) were enumerated 2 days after immunization with 10^8 SRBCs: IgM = 350 ± 220; IgG = 75 ± 21.

in contrast to the positive influences of levamisole (3,7-9). In vitro induction assays for Thy 1^+ are consistently negative with levamisole (3,8,9), as well as in the presence of imidazole (8) in a range of doses which includes the concentration at which imidazole's known action is to decrease cellular cyclic AMP (cAMP) and increase cyclic GMP (cGPM) (10).

Another assay suggests also that the in vitro influence of levamisole is associated with the imidazole nucleus. The effects of both agents on the ability of immunized B cells to excrete specific antibodies were compared in an in vitro test which reasonably

Table 1 Influence of Imidazole and Levamisole on Direct (IgM) or Indirect (IgG) Plaque-Forming Spleen Cell Responses to Immunization with 1 X 10^8 SRBCs

Treatment (mg/kg)		PFC/10^8 spleen cells[a]	
		IgM	IgG
Imidazole	0.05	1164 ± 564[b]	42 ± 22[b]
	2.5	670 ± 118	38 ± 11
Levamisole	2.5	2440 ± 370	178 ± 51
	25	906 ± 120	201 ± 91
Controls		610 ± 63	37 ± 8

[a]Tested 2 days after immunization and treatment (2).
[b]A wide SEM evidencing a "dispersing" effect of levamisole (see text).

excludes cooperation of B cells with other immunocompetent cells (8). Figure 2 summarizes a representative experiment where spleen cell suspensions from 10 mice were individually tested in triplicate in the presence of the drugs added to agar medium. Stimulation or inhibition of IgG-antibody excretion by levamisole parallels those of imidazole, and remarkably at the concentrations of imidazole which increase responses to alloantigens or phytohemagglutinin (PHA) and decrease cAMP levels (10,11). The findings uncover an as yet unexplained influence of imidazole on protein release at the surface of B cells.

Theophylline, an agent which inhibits phosphodierestases, stabilizes the levels of intracellular cAMP (12), in contrast to imidazole which activates phosphodierestases. Theophylline, which at the concentration administered (approximately 200 μg per mouse) has no measurable effect on the mouse responsiveness to SRBCs, enhances the activity of a 0.625-mg/kg suboptimal dose of imuthiol but has no influence to modify the depressed response induced by the same amount of levamisole (Table 2).

All in all, the data affirm that the in vitro activities of levamisole are related to imidazole's cholinergiclike action. It is indeed well-documented that agents lowering the ratio of cAMP to cGMP inhibit differentiation and favor proliferation of lymphocytes (10). A similar mechanism could explain the in vivo inhibiting effect of levamisole: increased cGMP levels (or a decrease in cAMP) will prevent cell differentiation which is triggered by increased cAMP/cGMP ratio (13,14).

A concept thus emerged that the in vivo efficacy of a single levamisole administration is likely linked to its sulfur region. A large series of sulfur-containing agents were tested (15) in a search to obviate the ambivalent effect of levamisole. All drugs known as toxic or as sensitizing agents, due to their thiazole or benzol ring structures (16), were

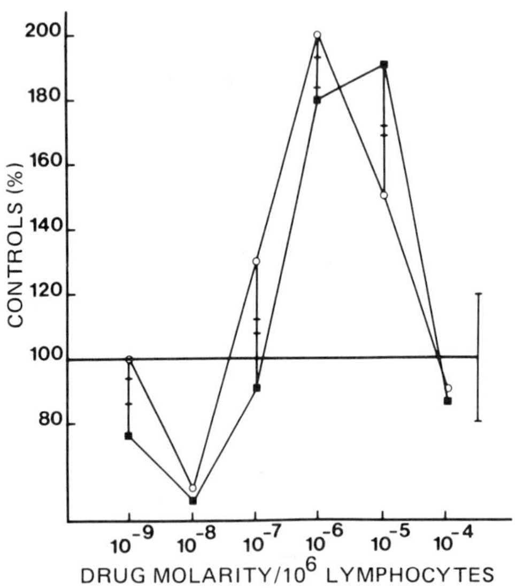

Figure 2 Influences of levamisole (■) or imidazole (○) in modifying the in vitro B-cell expression of IgG-specific antibody response by spleen cells sampled 4 days after immunization with 10^8 SRBCs. Ten C3H/He mice per group; triplicate assays per dose. Controls values (no drug added) were 40,380 ± 8500/10^6 spleen cells. Vertical bars indicate SEM.

Table 2 Influences of Theophylline on the In Vivo Stimulation Induced by Levamisole or Imuthiol in Response to SRBCs

Treatment (mg/kg)	Levamisole	Imuthiol
None (controls)	766 ± 58	825 ± 105
0.625	344 ± 38[a]	844 ± 48
0.625 + 10 Theophylline	438 ± 62[b]	2003 ± 91[c]

[a]Significant inhibition ($p < 0.01$) in comparison with untreated and immunized mice.
[b]Not significantly different ($p > 0.05$) from animals treated with levamisole alone.
[c]Significant increased ($p < 0.01$) above imuthiol alone. Mice (N = five per group) were sacrificed 2 days after IV immunization with 10^8 SRBCs and simultaneous SC treatment.

discarded. Sodium diethyldithiocarbamate (imuthiol) was selected (17) as best fitting the above requirements and the specifications for a BRM, such as low toxicity, absence of carcinogenicity and tumor-promoting influence, and known activities on defined sets of immunocompetent cells.

III. PHARMACOLOGY AND IMMUNOPHARMACOLOGY: A SUMMARY

A. Pharmacology

Imuthiol is likely to be the BRM the characteristics of which have been best studied. From a recent review (18), one could abstract the main data and lay stress on pharmacological features that could strengthen the immunopotentiating and immunoregulating activities of imuthiol.

It is a lipophilic and chelating compound which possess detoxifying activities against chemical carcinogens and against agents toxic for the liver,through its influence on metalloenzymes, or as a free radical scavenger. Its anticancer effect could likely be extended by direct effects on some malignant tumors, as it has been shown that imuthiol was cytotoxic for spindle cell carcinoma cells (19) and for melanoma cells (20). An imuthiol-induced reduction of the tumor burden, if confirmed in experimental and clinical testing, would provide additional chances for cancer cures. Its effects against drug-induced damage could justify its use in associated chemoimmunotherapies to reduce to toxicity of cytolytic agents, for example of cis-platinum (21-23), or to increase their activity, for example of bleomycin (24); these effects are all the most interesting that imuthiol can restore immune responsiveness abrogated by chemotherapies (25). Protection against the lethal effects of ionizing radiations could similarly facilitate their therapeutic use.

The antibiotic efficacy of imuthiol, at doses which do not alter normal cells, could help in controlling severe infections that resist antibiotics alone. It might also partially account for immunorestoration in such patients. Imuthiol can also protect against the wasting disease induced by a bacterial endotoxin, and evidences an anabolizing effect in emaciated mice (17), which effects might be useful in some clinical situations.

Administration of imuthiol is safe as clearly shown by a National Cancer Institute study where mice and rats were treated with either 17.5 or 140 g/kg daily for at least 100 consecutive weeks without any other changes from controls than a prolonged survival of female mice and a reduction in the incidence of spontaneously arising tumors (26).

The data are confirmed by current studies showing the beneficial influence of imuthiol on aged BALB/c mice (Bruley-Rosset, personal communication) and on NZB mice where imuthiol prevents against lymphomas (M. Renoux).

Imuthiol has an antistress activity through regulation of dopamine-β-hydroxylase, and its influence on superoxide dismutase levels strongly suggests an anti-inflammatory activity.

B. Immunopharmacology

Imuthiol induces in vivo distinctive properties in recruitment and activation of T cells and natural killer (NK) cells. It induces T cells to generate enhanced levels of cytotoxic activities and responses to mitogens and alloantigens. Resting T cells are induced by imuthiol to develop suppressive activities, B cells to secrete antibodies of the IgG class, and monocytes and macrophages to participate in delayed-type hypersensitivity phenomena. In contrast, it has no direct effect on B cells and macrophages, or on unspecific polyclonal activities (1,3,8,9,15-18,25,27-32). This unique influence on the T-cell lineage is obtained equally by systemic or oral administration. In contrast with the immunodepression afforded by long-term treatment with most other BRMs, chronic administration of imuthiol stimulates the host to increased T-cell-associated responses (25). Its influences on NK activity are evident at time periods differing from those where interferon or interferon inducers are known to be active, and are not associated with changes in interferon levels (32).

Similar data are observed in concurrent clinical trials. Imuthiol is neither a mitogen nor a polyclonal activator in humans; it regulates the activities of T cells without apparent, direct effects on B cells.

These features clearly distinguish imuthiol from other thiols, such as 2-mercaptoethanol or levamisole, the activities of which are mediated by a mitogenic, active both on T and B cells, general lymphocyte activator (33).

Other features that distinguish imuthiol from most BRMs are that imuthiol is inactive in vitro, is virtually nontoxic, does not give rise to sensitization, and does not induce an expansion of the reticuloendothelial system that might trigger lymphoid disorders.

IV. MODE OF ACTION OF IMUTHIOL

The constituents and the dimer of imuthiol are inactive. Imuthiol is prepared by reacting diethylamine with carbon disulfide in the presence of sodium hydroxide and is the first metabolite of disulfuram. It was therefore necessary to determine whether related compounds also influence mouse immune responsiveness. Female C3H/He mice, 6-8 weeks of age, were immunized intravenously with 10^8 SRBCs and treated with either 8 mg/kg carbon disulfide alone, 17 mg/kg diethylamine alone, or both agents separately administered via the subcutaneous route. These doses correspond to the relative amounts of each compound contained in 25 mg/kg imuthiol, a quantity which increases the number of PFCs specific for SRBCs (17,25,29). A dose of 25 mg/kg disulfuram was given SC as this agent splits into two molecules of imuthiol. Table 3 summarizes a representative experiment and shows that neither the constituents nor the dimeric form of imuthiol are able to modify the functional activation of mouse spleen cells in respond to immunization with SRBCs. The lack of influence of disulfuram may be attributable to insolubility, in that the organism could readily metabolize slowly liberated and slight amounts

Table 3 Comparison of Carbon Disulfide, Diethylamine, and Disulfuram on Mouse Spleen Cell Responses to SRBCs

Treatment (mg/kg)	PFC/spleen[a]	
	IgM	IgG
Saline	14,810 ± 1650	7650 ± 980
CS[b]	14,340 ± 1520	7240 ± 1725
A[b]	14,415 ± 1690	8330 ± 1000
CS and A[b]	15,020 ± 2555	8415 ± 670
Disulfuram, 25	15,110 ± 995	8217 ± 530

[a]Mean ± SE of direct (IgM) or indirect (IgG) antibody-forming spleen cells evaluated 4 days after IV immunization with 10^8 SRBCs and concomitant SC treatment. Five or ten mice per group.
[b]CS: 8 mg/kg of carbon disulfide; A: 17 mg/kg of diethylamine; CS and A: 8 mg/kg CS subcutaneously injected in the left flank, simultaneously to injection of 17 mg/kg A in the right flank.

of dithiocarbamate to inactive compounds (34). The ineffectiveness of carbon disulfide alone implies that there occurs no recombination of the sulfur with any naturally occurring amine.

Imuthiol acts through the increased production of specific factor(s). Low concentrations of imuthiol (10^{-9} to 2 X 10^{-6}M) increase survival and viability of lymphocytes and polymorphonuclears (35), yet these concentrations are inactive in vitro on immune responses (28). Imuthiol is not a polyclonal activator as it has no other influence on PWM-induced response than a slight but consistent inhibition (8,17,29), and as it suppresses the nonspecific response to horse red cells in SRBC-immunized mice (Table 4). As is shown in Table 5, the agent is not a mitogen augmenting the background thymidine incorporation. Since, in contrast imuthiol increase lymphoproliferative responses to T-cell mitogens (8,17,29.30,31), the data suggested an indirect influence on T cell-mediated events. Indeed, the serum of imuthiol-treated mice transfers to recipient mice the ability for enhanced T-cell responses (28).

Figure 3 depicts a representative experiment: as little as 0.1 ml per mouse of serum from C3H/He mice obtained 2 days after treatment with 25 mg/kg imuthiol suffices to increase significantly ($p < 0.01$) the response of C57B1/6 to immunization with SRBCs

Table 4 Imuthiol-Stimulated Responses Are Not Polyclonal Responses[a]

Treatment	IgM-PFC to	
	SRBC	HRBC
Saline-treated controls	580 ± 75	15 ± 4
2.5 mg/kg Imuthiol	1276 ± 93	0
25 mg/kg Imuthiol	1250 ± 48	0
50 g/kg *E. coli* LPS	1260 ± 108	36 ± 6

[a]Antibody-forming spleen cells (PFC) against sheep red cells (specific SRBC responses) and against horse red cells (nonspecific HRBC responses) were evaluated on female C3H/He mice (N = five per group) 2 days after IV immunization with 1.10^8 SRBCs and concomitant SC treatment. *E. coli* LPS served as a control of polyclonal activation.

Table 5 Influence of Imuthiol on Spontaneous Lymphocyte DNA Synthesis[a]

Time	Humans[b]	C3H/He[c]	BALB/c[c]
0	638 ± 504	8587 ± 2420	2215 ± 1897
1 hr	NT	8768 ± 2603	2728 ± 1178
1 day	737 ± 541	9809 ± 1265	2025 ± 1101
2 day	482 ± 343	9353 ± 2004	1768 ± 119
7 day	554 ± 400	8294 ± 791	1348 ± 309

[a]Results are rexpressed as the mean cpm ± SE of individual triplicate assays.
[b]Seventy-eight patients treated with either 5 or 10 mg/kg.
[c]Four mice per strain and time of evaluation.

or lymphoproliferation in the presence of PHA or concanavalin A (ConA); PWM-induced responses are not affected. The plasma half-life of imuthiol is less than 20 min (36; our current study). The observed effect is therefore due to the in vivo increased production of enhancing factor(s) through the influence of imuthiol, not necessarily directly acting on the cells of the immune system.

Imuthiol is active on congenitally thymusless mice. It seemed important, at this stage of experimentation, to ascertain whether imuthiol was also active on nu/nu mice, as such data would indicate whether the thymus was a direct target for the agent.

Imuthiol does indeed induce the in vivo acquisition of specific T-cell markers by precommitted and undifferentiated precursor spleen cells without modifying the percentage of B cells, and is inactive in vitro (8,9,29,30,31). The imuthiol-induced maturation stimulus is accompanied, as is shown in Fig. 4, by acquisition of functional activity. Imuthiol-treated nu/nu mice respond to immunization with SRBCs by the de novo

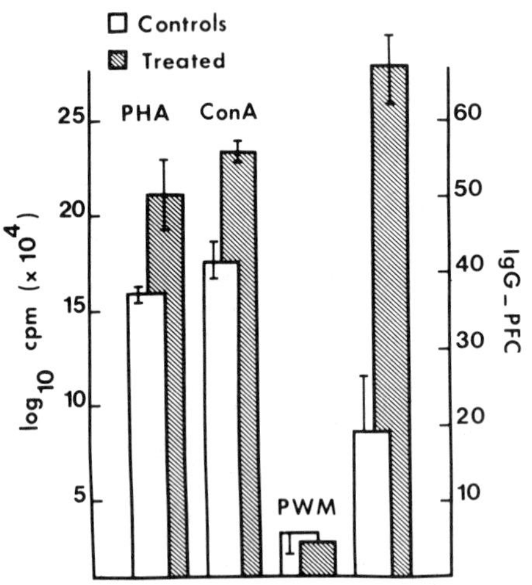

Figure 3 Effect of the serum of imuthiol-treated C3H/He mice on immune responsiveness of C57B1/6 mice. Female C57B1/6 mice are nonresponders to levamisole (4) and low responders to imuthiol (17). They were treated with 0.1 ml of normal mouse serum as controls or 0.1 ml of C3H/He serum sampled 48 hr after a treatment with 25 mg/kg imuthiol. N = five mice per group. Vertical bars indicate SEM.

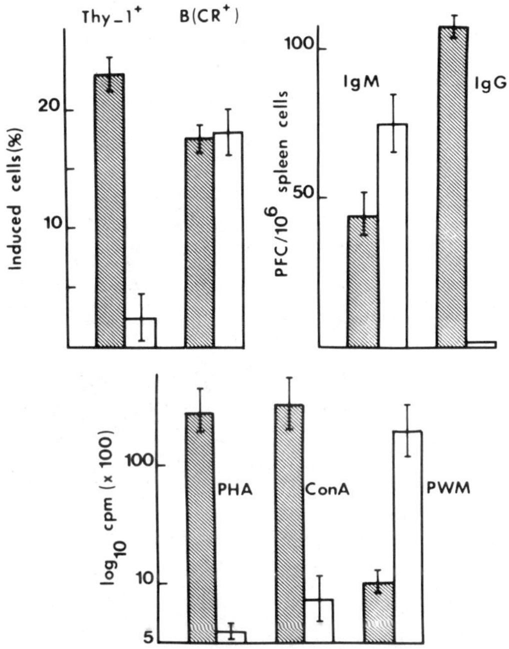

Figure 4 Imuthiol induces functionally active T cells in congenitally athymic mice. Five nu/nu (C57B1/6 background) mice per group were treated SC with 25 mg/kg imuthiol (shaded columns) or pyrogen-free saline as controls. Spleen T (Thy 1^+) and B(CR^+) cell percentages were evaluated 24 hr after treatment, as well as responses to mitogens. Sheep red cells (10^8) were injected IV, 1 day after treatment, and the numbers of specific direct (IgM) and indirect (IgG) antibody-plaque-forming spleen cells (PFC) evaluated 4 days later. Vertical bars indicate SEM.

appearance of an appreciable number of specific IgG antibody-forming spleen cells, a T-cell mediated event, associated with a significant ($p < 0.01$) decrease in the number of IgM-PFCs. Similarly, lymphoproliferative responses to the T-cell mitogens, PHA and ConA, are evoked de novo in spleen cells from imuthiol-treated nu/nu mice, whereas the treatment significantly reduces the response to PWM, a B-cell mitogen in mice (Fig. 4). Under similar experimental conditions, none of the known thymic hormones are able to increase above background values the percent of Thy 1^+ cells, a feature attributed to the short half-life of small polypeptides (37).

The data confirm that the influence of imuthiol is specifically directed on the T-cell lineage. They cannot be ascribed to the stimulation by imuthiol of remnants of the thymus in nu/nu mice, as it has been shown that the so-called thymuslike organs of adult nu/nu mice have the structure of parathymic lymph nodes (38,39).

Hepatosin is a specific T-cell inducer. The finding that imuthiol triggers in nu/nu mice thymocyte differentiation led us to postulate that extrathymic molecules also play a part in the endocrine regulation of the immune system. Spleen, liver, kidney, and lymph nodes were therefore examined for their capacity to produce the inducer in vitro, spontaneously or in the presence of imuthiol. Spleen, kidney, or lymph node cells cultured for 24 hr, and even in the presence of imuthiol (from 10^{-3} to 10^{-10} mM/ml) do not release in the supernatant a fraction able to alter the spontaneous percentage (4 + 3) of Thy 1$^+$ cells in induction assays. In contrast, liver cells synthesize, and particularly when cocultured with imuthiol, a heat-resistant, endotoxin-free peptide, mol wt approximately 5 Kd. This novel factor is designated hepatosin for convenience and to identify its origin (40,41).

The results, as summarized in Table 6, show that hepatosin manifests the properties already present in the serum of either euthymic or athymic imuthiol-treated mice: that is, in vivo induction of functionally active T cells after a single treatment and nonconcomitant appreciable influence on the B-cell lineage. Propanolol, a β-adrenergic blocking agent which ablates induction by ubiquitin (42), does not prevent the induction of Thy 1$^+$ cells by hepatosin (40). Imuthiol increases the production of this factor in liver cultures.

Concurrent studies already show (a) that hepatosin reduces spleen weight and increases specific IgG responses in NZB mice (M. Renoux); (b) that hepatosin increases the mean survival time and immune responses in syngeneic fibrosarcoma-bearing C57B1/6 mice (L. Simon, personal communication); and (c) induces HTLA$^+$ cells from human null cells (J. L. Touraine, personal communication). Taken together, the findings are viewed as suggesting that hepatosin evinces a hormonelike behavior, having a specific effect both in vitro and in vivo (following a single administration) and across the species barrier.

T-cell activities and the influence of imuthiol thereon are controlled by the brain neocortex. In the process of our studies, the influence of imuthiol on the T-cell lineage through the synthesis of specific serum factors and its anabolizing effect against endotoxin-induced wasting disease suggested to us the operation of a central control (17). We postulated that the best approach could be to intervene first on upper brain areas and thereafter to follow the pathways among other regions of the central nervous system.

As summarized in Table 7, the partial ablation of the *left* cerebral neocortex does, indeed, inhibit T-cell-mediated responses and NK activity; in contrast, a similar lesion in the *right* neocortex has no effect other than a small but reproducible increase in these activities; the number and activities of B cells remained unchanged (43-47). Separate

Table 6 Properties of Hepatosin, a Heat-Stable Factor Synthetized by the Liver, in the Presence of Imuthiol

Mol wt	Approximately 5000 daltons
O.D.	max. 250 nm, no reading at 320-340
In vitro	
Thy 1$^+$ conversion,[a] 3.5-hr assay	0.001 ng/ml
B (CR$^+$) conversion,[a] 18-hr assay	None, even at 10 μg/ml
In vivo	
T1a$^+$, Thy 1$^+$ conversion	1 ng per mouse[b]
Responses (de novo) to PHA and ConA	1 ng per mouse[b]
IgG-PFCs de novo	1 ng per mouse[b]
Enhancement of responses in nonresponder mice	10 ng per mouse[c]
B(CR$^+$) conversion	None, even at 15 μg per mouse

[a]Nu/nu spleen cells or bone-marrow cells from a variety of mice.
[b]Evaluation between 12 hr and 4 days after a single treatment of nu/nu mice.
[c]C57B1/6 mice are nonresponders to levamisole (4).

Table 7 Effects of Partial Brain Neocortex Ablation on Mouse Immune Responsiveness[a]

Test	Controls	Right decorticates	Left decorticates
Spleen T cells (%)	31 ± 1.5	36 ± 3	19 ± 1.7[b]
Spleen B cells (%)	33 ± 2	35 ± 2.8	33 ± 2.8
IgM-PFC	14,953 ± 2608	23,065 ± 8695	15,435 ± 1807
IgG-PFC	6848 ± 1802	9426 ± 623[b]	3200 ± 870[b]
PHA	90,741 ± 9249	130,555 ± 12,035[b]	62,036 ± 9260[b]
ConA	149,816 ± 16,766	172,145 ± 13,890[b]	107,407 ± 11,056[b]
NK, lytic units (10^7 cells)	50	42	25[b]

[a]Tests were performed 10 weeks postsurgery on female C3H/He mice, then 16-17 weeks old.
[b]Significantly ($p < 0.05$) different from controls.

assays show that ablating the left neocortex depresses considerably the activity of the serum factor that induces the acquisition of the Thy 1 phenotype, which activity is increased after a lesion of the right neocortex (48). Taken together, the data strongly suggest that the brain neocortex modulates recruitment and activities of the cells in the T-cell lineage. The brain lesions did not affect antibody-dependent cell-mediated cytotoxicity toward chicken erythrocytes (44), indicating that the frontoparietal neocortex does not control macrophages, as these cells have been proposed as bearing the predominant cytotoxic activity with erythrocytes as targets (49).

The impact of the cerebral neocortex on T cells is all the more interesting in that the ablation involved approximately one-third of the total right or left cortex, that mice with a unilateral lesion served as controls for symmetrically lesioned mice, and that the responses were evaluated 10 weeks after surgery at a time when a possibility exists for readaptation of cortical activities, yet when the consequences of anesthetic and surgical stress are minimal.

A concurrent study shows that lesioning the cerebral neocortex markedly affects the tempo of the MLC response to MHC-incompatible stimulator cells. The response in cultures of cells from mice lacking a part of the left neocortex is delayed in comparison with control cultures, suggesting an initial lack in a T-cell subset; in contrast, the MLC response of spleen cells from right-lesioned mice shows maximal thymidine incorporation at a time (day 7) when control cells have become unresponsive (50). This study gives evidence also that imuthiol increases the responses of left-decorticated animals to mitogens and heteroantigens and is inactive on these parameters when administered to right decorticates; in contrast, imuthiol enhances the NK activity and the MLC response of mice lacking the right neocortex but not of mice without a left neocortex.

The findings suggest that the brain neocortex exerts an influence at early stages of T-cell differentiation and that there could be a balanced brain assymetry in which the right hemisphere may control the inductive influence of signals emitted by the left hemisphere. They confirm that imuthiol does not act directly to differentiate T cells but, through a stimulation controlled by the central nervous system network, influences the endocrinological network for the synthesis of a hormone specific for the T-cell lineage.

Imuthiol and the Qa-1 antigenic system: Imuthiol increases the amount of Thy 1 antigen and recruits Thy 1^+ cells from precommitted precursor cells, and preliminary assays suggest that the impact of brain lesion on MLC responses and the influence of imuthiol thereon could be related to modifications in the amount of MHC-coded cell-surface antigens.

The Qa-1$^+$ cells compose part of the Lyt 1 and Lyt 123 sets; they are essential for responses to PHA and required for optimal responses to ConA. In vitro assays reveal that the ConA-induced suppression of the α-SRBC PFC response is reduced by elimination of the Qa-1$^+$ cells, and the participation of Qa-1$^+$ cells in the regulation of the SRBC antibody response is an important feature of the Qa-1 system (51).

Dr. E. A. Boyse kindly supplied us with B6TL(+) (the Qa-1$^+$ strain) and B6-H-2$^{\underline{k}}$ (the Qa-1$^-$ strain) mice congenic in the region spanning the *TLa* locus, and with α-Qa-1 serum, (B6 X A-*TLa*^{b}) anti-A strain leukemia ASLI.

To evaluate the influence of imuthiol on the Qa-1 phenotypes involved in proliferative responses to mitogens, mice of either strains were treated with 25 mg/kg imuthiol 2 days prior to tests. The proliferative responses of spleen cells preselected with α-Qa-1 plus complement (the Qa-1$^-$ population) were compared with the responses of unselected spleen cells treated with normal mouse serum +C (52). Figure 5 depicts the assay; responses to LPS are not represented, as they were not affected by imuthiol treatment or by α-Qa-1 preselection. Obviously, the increased proliferative responses induced by imuthiol in B6-TL(+) mice are associated with enhanced amounts of Qa-1 antigen, as shown by a ConA response of cells from treated mice significantly reduced ($p < 0.01$) in

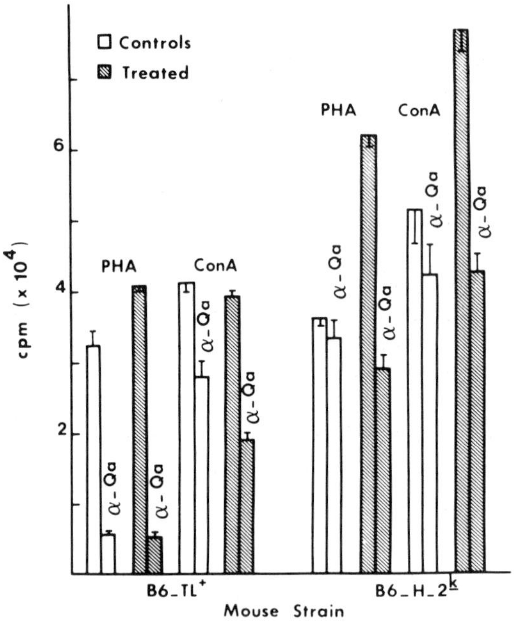

Figure 5 Influence of imuthiol on the Qa-1 phenotype involved in the proliferative responses to mitogens. Tests for [^{3}H] thymidine incorporation by spleen cells were performed 2 days after SC administration of 25 mg/kg or saline in controls. Cells were preselected by cytolysis with α-Qa-1 (at the 1:25 dilution) or normal mouse serum and complement, and after treatment the numbers of remaining viable cells were equalized to 1 X 10^6/ml and cultured in the presence of either 2 μg/ml concanavalin A, 1 μg/ml PHA-P, or 50 μg lipopolysaccharide (LPS). Mean data ± SEM of triplicate tests for three mice. Data not shown: proliferation in the presence of LPS as nor imuthiol neither preselection with α-Qa-1 modified the responses.

comparison with controls, after preselection with α-Qa-1. Furthermore, imuthiol induces in B6-H-2^k mice the appearance of a highly significant number ($p < 0.01$) of Qa-1^+ cells that is not revealed by α-Qa-1 preselection in untreated mice. Thus, imuthiol increases the expression of Qa-1^a anitgen as it does induce TLA^+ and Thy 1^+ cells in nu/nu mice. The data suggest that imuthiol might have revealed the low dose of Qa-1 antigen already present at the surface of B6-H-2^k cells, by increasing its amount or, alternatively that the expression of an as yet unidentified antigen of the ASLI leukemic cells (used to prepare the α-Qa serum) present in low amount on B6-H-2^k cells is increased by imuthiol.

The participation of Qa-1^+ cells in the in vivo stimulation of α-SRBC responses afforded by imuthiol was evaluated on mice of either congenic strains immunized IV with 10^8 SRBCs and concomitantly treated with 25 mg/kg imuthiol, SC administered. Figure 6 shows that the primary IgM α-SRBC PFC responses are strikingly reduced both in B6-TL(+) and in B6-H-2^k mice treated with imuthiol, while the primary IgG PFC responses are increased in treated mice. Since untreated B6-TL(+) mice, Qa-1^+, are low responders to immunization with SRBCs, one could infer that Qa-1^+ cells contribute to T-suppressive activity. However, a comparison of the data summarized in Fig. 5 with those of Fig. 6 would suggest that at least a subpopulation of Qa-1^+ cells (the one evoked by imuthiol in B6-H-2^k mice) may limit its suppressor effect to IgM antibody production and intervene in the switch from IgM to IgG—an hypothesis which fits to previous data showing an early production of IgG antibodies in imuthiol-treated animals (17). The data strongly suggest that imuthiol can either increase the amount (synthesis) of cell-surface antigens or, alternatively, can stabilize high-level surface expression, as it has been shown that "Qa-1 antigen is very unstable, so that subpopulations in which it was turned over more slowly might be the only one to score as Qa-1^+" (53).

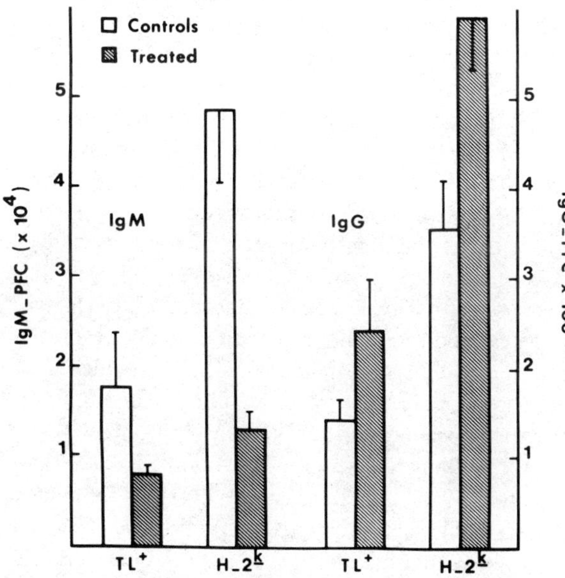

Figure 6 Influence of imuthiol on the primary antibody responses to SRBCs of mice from two strains congenic at the *TLA* locus. Direct (IgM) and indirect (IgG) plaque-forming spleen cells (PFCs) were enumerated on day 4 post-IV immunization with 10^8 SRBCs and simultaneous SC injection of 25 mg/kg imuthiol or saline as controls. Mean data ± SEM for five mice per group.

V. DISCUSSION

The findings reported herein reveal that the complexities of the biological activities underlying the clinical effectiveness of some agents proposed as BRMS could be linked to chemical structures. Most significantly, immunopharmacological studies comparing in vitro assays and in vivo testing of imuthiol led us to uncover yet unsuspected links between the immune system, the endocrine liver, and upper brain areas.

Attempts to elucidate the causes of the ambivalent effect of levamisole have shown the adverse effect was linked to the influence of the imidazole region. This is supported also by reports on immunosuppression induced in vivo by imidazole-containing compounds, such as niridazole (54-57), metrodinazole (58), methyl-mercapto-imidazole (59), or DTIC (60) and azathioprine (61,62), although some of these agents could in vitro enhance proliferative responses. This suggests that an imidazole-containing agent should be tested for long-term effects in animals before assuming it could be a BRM.

These studies on the mode of action of levamisole have contributed to the development of imuthiol. The unique influence of imuthiol on the T-cell lineage, associated with important biological activities and virtually no toxicity (18), may well deserve its use in clinical situations where a T-cell defect or impairment is associated with a disease. Imuthiol could be a basis for improved chemoimmunotherapies, and its administration could protect against the detrimental effects of radiation. Its antibioticlike effects support the clinical testing of imuthiol against infections, particularly in immunosuppressed patients. Available data from phase I and II studies (29,63) are already sufficient to suggest the use of imuthiol in the preoperative management of cancer patients and after radical surgery to prevent or reduce the risk of recurrences or metastases.

The imuthiol-induced increase in the Qa-1 antigenic system (as well as preliminary data on changes in the amounts of MHC-coded cell-surface antigens) questions whether the agent would act at a transcription level or whether it keeps intact labile surface antigens. However, our results thus far indicate that the distinctive influence on the T- cell lineage are not associated with concomitant appreciable effects on B cells or macrophages.

These unique features, and the pharmacological activities of imuthiol, clearly distinguish it from levamisole (Table 8) and also from other proposed agents. Immunopharmacological studies have therefore been undertaken seeking to comprehend these features. As imuthiol was found inactive in vitro, it was thus inferred it acts by indirect means. To evaluate the possible impact of imuthiol on thymic activities, assays were conducted on healthy nu/nu mice, devoid of thymus remnants. Thymectomized mice were deliberately not employed, as the percentage of Thy 1^+ cells is only reduced (64) and some T-cell activities can remain for weeks and eventually return to normal levels (65-67) after adult thymectomy, and as removal of the thymus in neonatal life is attended by significant impairments, but not suppression, in both cellular and humoral immunity (68).

Imuthiol triggers in nu/nu mice the appearance of functionally active T cells and the production of a specific T-cell factor, making it clear that extrathymic molecules also play a part in the endocrine regulation of the immune system: liver was found as the most probable nonthymic site. The heat-stable factor, hepatosin, has notable effects on T lymphocytes which effects make it evident that quantitative assays can be developed which, in turn, could support a program of fractionation, purification, and identification.

Hepatosin induces *only* T cells (imuthiol has a similar effectiveness), and its activity is not to be ascribed to the presence of nonspecific agents, since these agents induce in vitro both T and B cells (42), nor is latent viral infection, either of cultured cells or of recipient nu/nu mice, likely to account for our findings since spleen, lymph nodes, and

Table 8 Main Differences between Levamisole and Imuthiol

Test	Response	
	Levamisole	Imuthiol
Range of activity in vivo	Narrow, variable	Large
In vitro activities (imidazolelike)	Yes	No
Direct influence on B cells and macrophages	Yes	No
Acts through a general lymphocyte activator	Yes	No
Evidence for nonresponders	Yes	No
Inhibitory activities	Yes	No
Sensitization	Yes	No
Low dose toxicity	Yes	No
Antibiotic activity	No	Yes
Possible direct anticancer effect	No	Yes

kidney supernatants were ineffective, and controls for in vitro or in vivo induction manifested few Thy 1^+ cells, or none at all. Products of tissue breakdown remaining in supernatants would not account for the activity, since control supernatants were devoid of influence. Ubiquitin is not the active factor: hepatosin has no effect on the B-cell lineage, propanolol has no influence on the induction by hepatosin, and hepatosin induces T cells after only a single administration. Owing to similarities in inductive and differentiating effects, it could well be that hepatosin is the serum factor induced by imuthiol in nu/nu mice (8,9,28) and one of the serum factors evoked by imuthiol upon administration to normal mice (8,48).

That imuthiol is inactive in vitro and remarkably effective in vivo has therefore led to demonstrate a role for the endocrine liver in the development and function of T lymphocytes. That hepatosin supplies a specific signal for T-cell differentiation raises new questions regarding the conventional thoughts on an exclusive role of the thymus in this regard. Other reports show that sheep (69,70) or human (71,72) fetal lymphocytes demonstrate T-cell responses even before the appearance of an identifiable thymus, that pre-T cells disappear from the spleen of nu/nu mice early after engraftment of a neonatal thymus (73), and that a syngeneic thymus graft in C57B1/6 nu/nu mice impairs the inducing capability of imuthiol (74). A current study (A. Pompidou, personal communication) suggests that, in turn, hepatosin would induce thymic hyperactivity. Under such a context, hepatosin can be viewed as a nonthymic T-cell differentiating factor, contributing to the thymus independence of the pathway from pluripotential stem cells to the commitment of T cells. All in all, the findings suggest a distinctive role for the thymus to control, via feedback regulation, the extrathymic synthesis of a specific T-cell-differentiating hormone we designated hepatosin.

The indirect effectiveness of imuthiol has also led to investigating the role of brain areas on the immune system. Ablation of either the left or the right frontoparietal cortex is well tolerated and does not induce appreciable, gross behavioural changes in mice (43-48). The changes in T-cell numbers and responsiveness are certainly due to the influence of the ablated area as trauma- or stress-induced influences are eliminated by appropriate controls and the time interval between surgery and tests, as well as by assays repeated over a long period of time and on a large number of animals.

Partial ablation of the cerebral neocortex has no influence on B-cell activity and likely also on macrophage function; there are reports to show that the parasympathetic system intervenes on B cells (75,76), and the hypothalamus on macrophages (77). Removal of the left neocortex is attended by significant impairment in T-cell-associated responses and NK activity, whereas ablating the right neocortex induces a consistent increase in these responses (43-47). These influences of the brain neocortex are likely mediated through modulation of the endocrine network involved in the synthesis of T-cell-specific hormones, as ablation of the left neocortex suppresses the serum-recruiting ability which is increased in right neocortex-deprived mice; stimulation of this activity requires an intact right brain (48). In addition, a concurrent study shows that only an intact brain (but not a thymus) would permit imuthiol to be efficacious (50).

It could be therefore that the number and functional activity of cells from the T-cell lineage are modulated by a balanced brain assymetry in which the right hemisphere controls the inductive influence of signals emitted by the left hemisphere. It suggests that an essential role for the central nervous system could be to maintain body integrity in face of an adverse environment as it controls behavioural and psychic mechanisms.

Immunopharmacological studies on the mode of action of imuthiol, a T-cell-specific BRM inactive in vitro, add a new dimension to the detoxifying and protecting role of the liver. They give evidence that the brain neocortex modulates T-cell recruitment and function, and that lateralization for cognitive processes should be extended to immune recognition: the notion that the immune system is a self-monitoring, autoregulated system cannot stand any longer.

ACKNOWLEDGMENTS

This work was supported by grants in aid from Institut Mérieux and, in parts, by grants from INSERM, Ligue Nationale contre le Cancer, New York Cancer Research Institute, and Conseil Scientifique, Université de Tours. I am indebted to K. Bizière, J. M. Guillaumin, P. Bardos, and D. Degenne; particularly to my wife, Micheline, who participated enthusiastically. I thank Miss S. Guesdon for excellent typing and illustrations.

REFERENCES

1. G. Renoux, in *Immunopharmacology* (M. Rola-Pleszczinski and P. Sirois, eds.), Elsevier/North Holland, Amsterdam, 1982, pp. 289-316.
2. G. Renoux and M. Renoux, *J. Immunol.*, *113*:779 (1974).
3. G. Renoux, R. L. Kassel, M. Renoux, N. C. Fiore, J. M. Guillaumin, and A. Palat, in *Modulation of Host Resistance in the Prevention or Treatment of Induced Cancer* (M. A. Chirigos, ed.), Fogarthy International Center Proceedings No. 28, Washington, D.C., 1977, pp. 45-51.
4. G. Renoux, M. Renoux, and J. M. Guillaumin, *Int. J. Immunopharmacol.*, *1*:43 (1979).
5. G. Renoux, M. Renoux, M. N. Teller, I. M. Mountain, S. McMahon, and J. M. Guillaumin, *Clin. Exp. Immunol.*, *25*:288 (1975).
6. R. K. Johnson, D. P. Houchens, M. R. Gaston, and A. Goldin, *Cancer Chemother. Rep.*, *59*:697 (1975).
7. G. Renoux and M. Renoux, *Ann. Immunol. (Inst. Pasteur)*, *128C*:275 (1977).
8. G. Renoux and M. Renoux, in *Control of Neoplasia by Modulation of the Immune System* (M. A. Chirigos, ed.), Raven Press, New York, 1977, pp. 67-80.
9. G. Renoux and M. Renoux, *J. Exp. Med.*, *145*:466 (1977).
10. J. W. Hadden, R. G. Coffey, E. M. Hadden, E. Lopez-Coralles, and G. H. Sunshine, *Cell. Immunol.*, *20*:98 (1975).

11. T. B. Strom, C. B. Carpenter, M. R. Garovoy, K. F. Austen, J. P. Merril, and M. Kaliner, *J. Exp. Med.,,138*:381 (1973).
12. G. A. Robinson, R. W. Butcher, and E. W. Sutherland, *Ann. Rev. Biochem., 37*:149 (1968).
13. I. H. Pastan, J. S. Johnson, and W. B. Anderson, *Ann. Rev. Biochem., 44*:491 (1975).
14. J. Watson, *J. Exp. Med., 141*:97 (1975).
15. G. Renoux and M. Renoux, *C. R. Acad. Sci. Paris, 278D*:1139 (1974).
16. N. W. Blacow (ed.), *Martindale the Extra Pharmacopoiea, 26*th ed., The Pharmaceutical Press, London, 1972, *passim*.
17. G. Renoux and M. Renoux, *J. Immunopharmacol., 1*:247 (1979).
18. G. Renoux, *J. Pharmacol. (Paris), 13*:95 (1982).
19. A. K. Powell, *Br. J. Cancer, 8*:529 (1954).
20. P. Blagoeva and I. Stoichev, *Experientia, 35*:1389 (1979).
21. R. F. Borch and M. E. Pleasant, *Proc. Natl. Acad. Sci. USA, 76*:6611 (1979).
22. R. F. Borch, J. C. Katz, P. H. Lieder, and M. E. Pleasant, *Proc. Natl. Acad. Sci. USA, 77*:5441 (1980).
23. G. R. Gale and L. W. Atkins, *J. Clin. Hemat. Oncol., 11*:41 (1981).
24. P. S. Lin, L. Kwock, and N. T. Goodchild, *Cancer, 46*:2360 (1980).
25. G. Renoux and M. Renoux, *Clin. Immunol. Immunopathol., 15*:21 (1980).
26. National Cancer Institute, *Tech. Rep. Series, 172*: (1979).
27. P. J. Neveu, *Clin. Exp. Immunol., 32*:419 (1978).
28. G. Renoux, M. Renoux, J. M. Guillaumin, and C. Gouzien, *J. Immunopharmacol., 1*:145 (1979).
29. G. Renoux and M. Renoux, in *Augmenting Agents in Cancer Therapy* (E. M. Hersh, M. A. Chirigos, M. Mastrangelo, eds.), Raven Press, New York, 1981, pp. 427-440.
30. G. Renoux and M. Renoux, in *Immunomodulating Agents* (R. L. Fenichel, ed.), Marcel Dekker, New York, in press, 1982.
31. P. J. Neveu, D. Perdoux, and L. Lafleur, *Int. J. Pharmacol., 4*:9 (1982).
32. G. Renoux, M. Renoux, P. Bardos, D. Degenne, and A. Musset, in *Natural Cell-Mediated Immunity* (R. B. Herberman, ed.), Academic Press, New York, in press, 1982, pp. 442-448.
33. G. Hewlett, H-G. Opitz, and H. D. Schlumberger, in *Lymphokines 4* (E. Pick and M. Landy, eds.), Academic Press, New York, 1981, pp. 89-105.
34. J. H. Strömme and L. Eldjarn, *Biochem. Pharmacol., 15*:287 (1966).
35. D. A. Rigas, C. Eginitis-Rigas, and C. Head, *Biochem. Biophys. Res. Comm., 88*:373 (1979).
36. M. D. Fairman, D. E. Dodd, and R. F. Hanzlick, *Res. Comm. Chem. Path. Pharmacol., 21*:543 (1978).
37. G. Goldstein, M. P. Scheid, U. Hammerling, E. A. Boyse, D. H. Schlesinger, and H. D. Niall, *Proc. Natl. Acad. Sci. USA, 72*:11 (1975).
38. Ch. K. Hsu, R. A. Whitney, and C. T. Hansen, *Nature, 257*:681 (1975).
39. A. C. Cordier and S. M. Haumont, *Am. J. Anat., 157*:227 (1980).
40. G. Renoux and M. Renoux, *Abst. 8th Int. Congr. Pharmacol.*, 437 (1981).
41. G. Renoux and M. Renoux, *Int. J. Immunopharmacol., 4*:300 (1982).
42. M. P. Scheid, G. Goldstein, and E. A. Boyse, *J. Exp. Med., 147*:1727, 1978.
43. G. Renoux, K. Bizière, M. Renoux, and G. Renoux, *C. R. Acad. Sci. (Paris), 290D*: 71g (1980).
44. P. Bardos, D. Degenne, Y. Lebranchu, K. Bizière, and G. Renoux, *Scand. J. Immunol., 13*:609 (1981).
45. K. Bizière, M. Renoux, and G. Renoux, *Neuroscience*, 7:528 (1982).
46. G. Renoux, K. Bizière, and M. Renoux, *Bull. Acad. Med. (Paris), 166*:88 (1982).
47. G. Renoux, K. Bizière, P. Bardos, D. Degenne, and M. Renoux, in *Natural Cell-*

Mediated Immunity (R. B. Herberman, ed.), Academic Press, New York, 1982, pp. 639-643.
48. G. Renoux, K. Bizière, M. Renoux, and J. M. Guillaumin, *Scand. J. Immunol.*, *17*:45 (1983).
49. E. Ojo and H. Wigzell, *Scand. J. Immunol.*, *7*:297 (1978).
50. G. Renoux, M. Renoux, K. Bizière, J. M. Guillaumin, P. Bardos, and D. Degenne, *J. Neuroimmunol.*, *5*:227 (1983).
51. T. H. Stantor, C. E. Calkins, J. Jandinsly, D. J. Schendel, O. Stutman, H. Cantor, and E. A. Boyse, *J. Exp. Med.*, *148*:963 (1978).
52. G. Renoux and M. Renoux, *Abst. 4th Int. Congr. Immunol.*, 3.3.21, 1980.
53. E. Rothenberg and D. Triglia, *Immunogenetics*, *14*:455 (1981).
54. A. A. F. Mahmoud, M. A. Mandel, K. S. Warren, and L. T. Webster, *J. Immunol.*, *114*:279 (1975).
55. L. T. Webster, A. E. Butterworth, A. A. F. Mahmoud, E. N. Mugola, and K. S. Warren, *N. Engl. J. Med.*, *292*:1144 (1975).
56. J. R. Salaman, M. Bird, A. M. Godfrey, B. M. Jones, D. Millar and J. J. Miller, *Trnasplant. Proc.*, *9*:989 (1977).
57. B. M. Jones, M. Bird, P. J. A Griffin, P. R. Massey, D. Millar, J. J. Miller, S. C. Reeves, and J. R. Salaman, *J. Immunol.*, *123*:143 (1979).
58. D. I. Grove, A. A. F. Mahmoud, and K. S. Warren, *Int. Arch. Appl. Immunol.*, *54*: 422 (1977).
59. J. J. Miller and S. C. Reeves, *IRCS Med. Sci.*, *7*:310 (1979).
60. A. Vecchi, M. C. Fioretti, A. Mantovani, A. Barzi, and F. Spreafico, *Transplantation*, *22*:619 (1976).
61. E. W. Uyeki, *Biochem. Pharmacol.*, *16*:53 (1967).
62. J. L. Amiel, G. Mathé, M. Matsukura, A. M. Mery, G. Daguet, R. Tenenbaum, S. Garattini, C. Brezin, and V. Palma, *Immunology*, *7*:511 (1964).
63. G. Renoux, M. Renoux, J. Greco, J. Baudouin, M. Lavandier, and E. Lemarié, in *New Trends in Human Immunology and Cancer Immunotherapy* (B. Serrou and Cl. Rosenfeld, eds.), Doin, Paris, 1980, pp. 974-985.
64. H. Cantor, E. Simpson, V. L. Sato, C. G. Fathman, and L. A. Herzenberg, *Cell. Immunol.*, *15*:180 (1975).
65. L. C. Andersson, P. Häyry, M. A. Bach, and J. F. Bach, *Nature*, *252*:252 (1974).
66. J. W. Kappler, P. C. Hunter, D. Jacobs, and E. Lord, *J. Immunol.*, *113*:27 (1974).
67. C. A. Janeway, *J. Immunol.*, *114*:1408 (1975).
68. R. A. Good, A. P. Dalmasso, C. Martinez, O. K. Archer, J. C. Pierce, and B. W. Papermaster, *J. Exp. Med.*, *116*:733 (1962).
69. B. J. Bryant, in *Progress in Immunology* (L. Brent and J. Holborows, eds.), North-Holland, Amsterdam, 1974, pp. 5-14.
70. P. Toivanen, T. Asantila, and J. Vahala, in *Immuno-Aspects of the Spleen* (J. R. Battisto and J. W. Streilein, eds.), Elsevier/North Holland, Amsterdam, 1976, pp. 13-21.
71. M. C. Carr, E. Lieber, and H. H. Fudenberg, *Cell. Immunol.*, *1*:455 (1970).
72. C. H. L. Rieger, J. V. Lustig, R. Hirshhorn, and R. M. Rothberg, *J. Pediatr.*, *90*:707 (1977).
73. G. E. Roelants, K. S. Mayor, L. B. Hägg, and F. Loor, *Eur. J. Immunol.*, *6*:75 (1977).
74. G. Renoux and M. Renoux, *Thymus*, *2*:139 (1980).
75. H. O. Besedowsky, A. Del Rey, E. Sorkin, M. Da Prada, and H. H. Keller, *Cell. Immunol.*, *48*:346 (1979).
76. K. Miles, J. Qunitans, E. Chelnicka-Schorr, and B. G. W. Arrason, *J. Neuroimmunol.*, *1*:101 (1981).
77. T. L. Rozman, R. J. Cross, W. H. Brooks, and W. R. Markesbery, *Immunology*, *45*:737 (1982).

Section E

Role of Prostaglandins as Regulators of the Immune Response

30

Prostaglandins as Modulators of T- and B-Lymphocyte Function

Jan L. Ceuppens University of Leuven School of Medicine, Leuven, Belgium

James S. Goodwin University of New Mexico School of Medicine, Albuquerque, New Mexico

I. INTRODUCTION

This chapter reviews the literature linking prostaglandins to the regulation of the immune response. Prostaglandins (PGs) are local hormones with an important role in the regulation of cell functions and cell interactions. They are derivatives of the unsaturated fatty acid linoleic acid. Dihomo-γ-linolenic acid and arachidonic acid are incorporated in the phospholipids of the cell membranes and become the precursors of the prostaglandins of the 1 and 2 series, respectively. In Greenland, Eskimos and others with a high dietary intake of fish, linoleic acid in the diet is largely replaced by eicosapentaenoic acid. This fatty acid is present in high amounts in fish oils and gives rise to the 3 series of prostaglandins. These precursors can be released from phosopholipid stores in the cell membrane via phospholipase A, and they are then further metabolized by the enzymes cyclooxygenase or lipoxygenase or directly oxidized by superoxide radicals. The cyclooxygenase pathway leads to synthesis of endoperoxides, the stable prostaglandins (mainly E_2 and $F_{2\alpha}$), thromboxanes, and prostacyclines. The alternative lipoxygenase pathway (1) leads to synthesis of hydroperoxy eicosatetraenoic acids (HPETEs) and hydroxyeicosatetraenoic acids (HETEs). The 5-HETEs are precursors for the leukotrienes (e.g., slow-reacting substance of anaphylaxis) which are highly potent compounds with vasoactive and chemotactic properties. This review will concentrate on the role of prostaglandin E_2 (PGE_2).

PGE_2 is produced in every tissue examined except mature erythrocytes. The short half-life of this compound limits its activity to the site of production. Production in a given tissue is initiated by a stimulus in that tissue, and the PGE_2 then modifies further response to that stimulus. For example, vasopressin stimulates the production of PGE_2 in the distal nephron; PGE_2 in turn makes the collecting duct less sensitive to the action of vasopressin in increasing water permeability (2). The different prostaglandins have different, sometimes opposite, effects. All this makes them important for feedback regulation and homeostasis in a broad sense. PGE_2, for example, inhibits mast cell degranulation by increasing intracellular cyclic AMP (cAMP) (3), while $PGF_{2\alpha}$ makes the mast cell more susceptible to degranulating stimuli by increasing intracellular cyclic GMP (cGMP) (4). Another well-known example is the platelet-aggregating activity of thromboxane A_2, while prostacyclin I_2 (mainly produced in the endothelial cells of the vessel wall) inhibits platelet aggregation (5). Sometimes seemingly opposite functions can be carried by the same molecule. PGE_2 has important proinflammatory properties: it induces vasodilatation and enhances edema formation caused by other inflammatory stimuli like bradykinin and histamine (5). Prostaglandin synthesis inhibitors are potent anti-inflammatory agents (6). But, at the same time, PGE_2 is a feedback inhibitor of the immune response (7), and inhibits release of lysosomal enzymes from granulocytes, mast cell degranulation, and thrombocyte aggregation (5). These effects can be considered as anti-inflammatory, and are illustrated by the facts that PGE_1 inhibits adjuvant arthritis in rats (8) and that PGE_1 injections into NZB/NZW mice prevent immune complex-induced glomerulonephritis (9-14) and prolongs survival (14).

Several pharmacological agents can interfere with prostaglandin synthesis. Steroids inhibit the enzyme phospholipase, while most nonsteroidal anti-inflammatory agents like acetylsalicylic acid and indomethacin interfere with cyclooxygenase activity (6). Specific inhibitors of the thromboxane pathway [e.g., imidazole (15) and 9,11-azoprosta-5, 13-dienoic acid (16)] and of the prostacyclin pathway [e.g., tranylcypromine (17)] have been synthesized. It has to be emphasized that specific PG synthetase inhibitors have actions other than on PG synthesis. Even in submicromolar concentrations, indomethacin is not a specific PG synthetase inhibitor. At 10^{-8} M it inhibits cAMP dependent protein kinase (18), and at higher concentrations it inhibits phosphodiesterase (19). Recently, the stimulating effect of nitroglycerin (NTG) on prostacyclin synthesis by human endothelial cells was described, thereby providing a basis for the vasodilating effect of this drug (20).

II. PROSTAGLANDINS AND IMMUNE FUNCTION

That inhibition of immune function by endogenous prostaglandins represents a physiological feedback mechanism in vivo was first shown by Webb and Osheroff (21), who found that injection of mice with sheep red blood cells (SRBCs) led to an 80-fold increase in intrasplenic $PGF_{2\alpha}$. Prior administration of a PG synthetase inhibitor prevented the $PGF_{2\alpha}$ increase and also resulted in a significantly increased number of plaque-forming spleen cells 3-5 days after sensitization. Thus, antigen challenge initiated prostaglandin production as a negative feedback mechanism.

We examined the effects of prostaglandins on mitogen-stimulated [^{3}H] thymidine incorporation in human peripheral blood mononuclear cells (PBMCs) (22). We found that PGE_1 or PGE_2, but not PGA, $PGF_{1\alpha}$ or $PGF_{2\alpha}$, inhibited [^{3}H] thymidine incorporation when added in small concentrations (10^{-9} - 10^{-6} M) to concanavalin A (Con A) or phytohemagglutinin (PHA)-stimulated cultures of PBMCs. PGE did not inhibit pokeweed mitogen (PWM) stimulation of PBMCs, but did inhibit PWM stimulation of purified T cells. Since PHA and ConA stimulate T cells, while PWM is primarily a B-cell mitogen, these data suggested that PGE inhibits T-cell but not B-cell mitogenesis. PGE_2 is produced in PHA-stimulated cultures of PBMCs in amounts that, when added exogen-

Table 1 Percentage Increase in [^{3}H] Thymidine Incorporation Caused by Indomethacin as a Function of Dose of Mitogen

PHA concentration (μg/ml)	Percentage increase	cpm[a]	
		Without indomethacin	With indomethacin
0.2	1059 ± 134	411 ± 213	4764 ± 3155
0.4	233 ± 86	4823 ± 1,566	16,069 ± 1724
1.0	101 ± 33	18,164 ± 3,410	35,533 ± 6281
2.0	70 ± 10	27,768 ± 5,569	47,205 ± 5591
4.0	71 ± 10	33,079 ± 5,876	56,630 ± 7378
8.0	40 ± 6	43,428 ± 8,923	60,777 ± 11,753
20.0	4 ± 3	52,111 ± 16,428	54,196 ± 17,197

[a]The data are expressed as mean ± SEM of cpm, and of percentage increase in [^{3}H] thymidine incorporation, in three experiments on different subjects.
Source: Ref. 26.

ously, cause significant inhibition of mitogen stimulation (7,22). Since PGE_2 is produced in sufficient quantities in PHA cultures to cause an inhibition of [^{3}H] thymidine incorporation in those cultures, one would expect that the addition of PG synthetase inhibitors to PHA cultures would result in increased [^{3}H] thymidine incorporation. This phenomenon is demonstrated in Table 1 at seven different concentrations of PHA. It is clear that addition of indomethacin enhanced [^{3}H] thymidine incorporation in PHA cultures, and that indomethacin caused a greater percentage increase in [^{3}H] thymidine incorporation as the dose of PHA was decreased. The percentage increase in [^{3}H] thymidine incorporation ranged from 1059 ± 134% at the lowest dose of PHA (0.2 μg/ml) to 4 ± 3% at the highest dose (20 μg/ml). Similar results were obtained with RO-20-5720, an experimental cyclooxygenase inhibitor which is chemically unrelated to indomethacin (23).

One possible explanation for this varying response to prostaglandin synthetase inhibitors might be that the PBMCs are more sensitive to the inhibiting effects of endogenous PGE_2 at lower concentrations of mitogen. This indeed appears to be the case. Figure 1 graphs the percentage inhibition caused by four concentrations of PGE_2 in [^{3}H] thymidine incorporation induced by different concentrations of mitogen. A family of curves is generated, cultures with the lowest concentrations of PHA showing the greatest sensitivity to exogenously added PGE_2. This would appear to be a general rule for all inhibitors: the lower the mitogen dose, the more sensitive the culture is to inhibition (24).

Physiological concentrations of PGE_2 (10^{-8} M or less) comparable with those found in inflammatory sites (25) have now been shown by several authors to suppress most in vitro manifestations of T-lymphocyte functions: mitogen responsiveness (7,26,27), antigenic stimulation (28), E-rosette formation (29,30), lymphokine production (including Interleukin 2 or TCGF) (31-33), the generation of cytotoxic cells in mixed lymphocyte culture (34,35), and T-cell cytotoxicity (36). Decreased TCGF or Interleukin 2 production contributes to the decreased T-cell proliferation caused by PGE_2 (33), but it is not the only mechanism; the proliferative response of TCGF-dependent cells to added TCGF is also inhibited by small concentrations (10^{-9} M) of PGE_2 (32). The cytotoxic activity of non-T lymphocytes, namely natural killer (NK) and antibody-dependent cytotoxic activity, are also inhibited by PGE_2 (36-41). However, it should be mentioned here, as

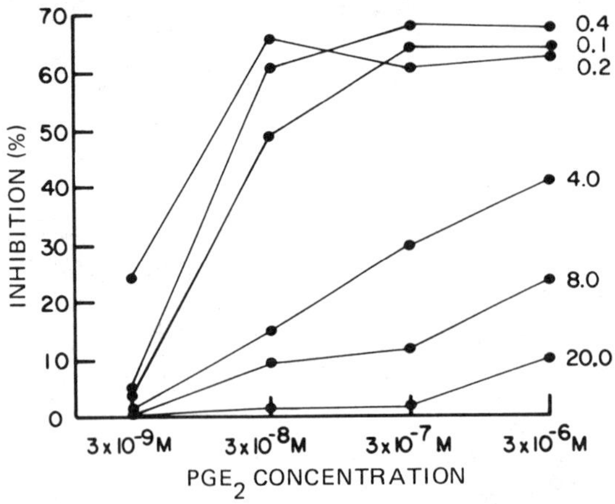

Figure 1 Percentage inhibition of [^{3}H] thymidine incorporation caused by PGE_2 at six concentrations of PHA. Data are from one experiment, and show that, at any given level of PGE_2, more inhibition is caused in PHA cultures as the concentration of the mitogen is decreased. In this experiment, the PHA concentration of 4.0 μg/ml gave optimal stimulation. (From Ref. 26.)

will be further discussed, that under certain experimental conditions PGE_2 can enhance NK activity (42,43).

The role of arachidonic acid derivatives other than PGE on the immune system is less clear. Prostacyclin analogs inhibit mitogen stimulation of human lymphocytes (44, 45). Pharmacological products selectively blocking the synthesis of thromboxane (Tx) or the lipoxygenase pathway also inhibit mitogenesis (46,47). These studies would suggest that TxA_2 and lipoxygenase metabolite products may promote lymphocyte function. It is also possible that these effects are secondary to increased PGE_2 production in the cultures when the other pathways are blocked.

III. THE PGE_2 PRODUCING SUPPRESSOR CELLS

In human peripheral blood, the cell responsible for PGE_2 production is a monocyte (22, 48,49), while there is evidence in mice that T cells also produce large amounts of PGs (50, 51). Monocytes exposed to mitogens (22,52), endotoxins (53), zymosan (54), antigen-antibody complexes (55), or Fc fragments of IgG (52) increase their PGE_2 production. Immune stimulation thus seems to induce a mechanism tempering the intensity of the response.

An increased activity of the prostaglandin-producing suppressor cell has been shown in several chronic inflammatory conditions, including coccidioidomycosis (56), *Brucella abortus* infections in cattle (57), multiple sclerosis (58), and sarcoidosis (59). It appears that at least part of the anergy seen in these conditions is due to the immunosuppressive activity of macrophages. Muscoplat's group has used in vitro prostaglandin blockade as a tool to distinguish cattle previously exposed to *Brucella abortus* but unresponsive to the antigen from nonexposed cattle (57). PBMCs from previously exposed but anergic cattle, as well as from nonexposed animals, will not respond to *Brucella* antigen in vitro. After addition of indomethacin to the cultures, PBMCs from the previously exposed anergic animals give a positive response to *Brucella* while PBMCs from the unexposed animals remain unresponsive. This would suggest that prostaglandins are involved in specific immunosuppression against *Brucella* in the anergic animals.

The depressed PHA response of PBMCs from patients with disseminated coccidioidomycosis can be reversed with indomethacin (56). It was not possible, however, to reverse the specific anergy to the infecting agent. Thus, PBMCs from subjects with disseminated coccidioidomycosis did not respond to coccidioidin in vitro even with indomethacin in the cultures. This is clearly different from the case with brucellosis in cattle described above. Prostaglandin-mediated suppression has also been studied in the depressed cellular immunity associated with sarcoidosis (59). The depressed PHA response of patients with sarcoidosis could be largely reversed by removing the glass-adherent cells but not by inhibition of prostaglandin synthesis. This finding supports the contention of Rice et al. that there are at least two monocyte suppressor mechanisms in human PBMCs, only one of which is dependent on prostaglandin synthesis (60). Plasma of patients with tuberculosis contains a factor (probably a mycobacterial wall antigen, alone or bound in immune complexes) that inhibits the proliferation of normal lymphocytes through enhancement of PG synthesis (61). Increased PG production by adherent cells is also observed during a graft-versus-host response and is responsible in part for GVH-induced immunosuppression (62). Efferent lymph from nodes of sheep challenged with antigen was found to suppress the in vitro transformation of peripheral blood lymphocytes to a variety of antigens, and the suppressor factor was shown to be prostaglandin E_2 (63).

IV. CHANGES IN SENSITIVITY OF LYMPHOCYTES TO PGE_2

Changes in the sensitivity of lymphocytes to PGE_2 have been observed in several instances.

1. Lymphocytes from normal individuals with the HLA-B12 haplotype have a decreased sensitivity to prostaglandins and histamine, and this could play a role in propensity for autoimmune disorders in these subjects (64).
2. Lymphocytes from patients with multiple sclerosis exhibit a defective response to PGE_2 in one assay system (65) but not in another (66). Further evidence for an actual role for PGE in this disease is provided by a study from Zurier's laboratory showing that lymphocytes from patients with multiple sclerosis have an increased adherence to measles-infected cells which could be reversed in vitro or in vivo by the administration of prostaglandin synthetase inhibitors (58,67).
3. Page and co-workers have reported that lymphocytes from patients with juvenile periodontitis are less sensitive to inhibition by PGE_2 (10^{-5} M) than are cells from patients with adult periodontitis or normal controls (68). They postulate that a defect in the response of lymphocytes to PGE_2 allows for the exuberant immune reactivity seen in subjects with juvenile periodontitis.
4. Lymphocytes from healthy subjects over age 70 are much more sensitive to inhibition by exogneous PGE_2 than are PBMCs from young adults (69-71). The amount of PGE_2 required to cause 50% inhibition of the PHA (4 μg/ml) response of healthy subjects over age 70 was approximately 10^{-8} M. This was more than two orders of magnitude lower than the amount required for 50% inhibition in 17 young adults ($>3 \times 10^{-6}$ M). This increased sensitivity to PGE would appear to account for some of the depression in cellular immune function found in healthy old people.

5. An increased sensitivity to PGE_2 was observed after surgery and in women in labor (72). Thus, it would appear that physical stress causes lymphocytes to become more sensitive to PGE_2, and the increased sensitivity to inhibition by this endogenous immunomodulator is responsible in part for the depressed cellular immune function following physical stress.
6. Lymphocytes from patients with rheumatoid arthritis also are more sensitive than normal to inhibition by exogenous PGE_2 (73). It may be that this increased sensitivity was secondary to the fact that all patients had been on long-term treatment with cyclooxygenase inhibitors for their disease.

V. EFFECT OF PG SYNTHETASE INHIBITORS ON CELLULAR IMMUNE FUNCTIONS IN VIVO

Cyclooxygenase inhibitors in vivo act as general immunostimulants, increasing cellular immune responses in humans and experimental animals (74-80). Muscoplat et al. studied the effect of indomethacin administration on delayed hypersensitivity skin responses in guinea pigs previously sensitized to *Mycobacterium bovis* (75). Oral administration of indomethacin simultaneous with intradermal injection of *Mycobacterium bovis* antigen resulted in a more than twofold increase in skin thickness compared with the guinea pigs not given indomethacin. Delayed skin test responses to picryl guinea pig albumin were also shown to be enhanced by indomethacin in guinea pigs (76).

Inhibition of endogenous prostaglandin biosynthesis by indomethacin shortened allograft survival, and this effect was completely abrogated by concurrent injections of a PGE_2 analog (77). Another in vivo correlate of the immunosuppressive activity of PGE_2 is that local injection of PGE_2 can cause reactivation of herpes simplex infection in the mouse ear (78). Natural killer (NK) cell activity is also enhanced in vivo by PG synthesis inhibitors. Brunda et al. have shown that in vivo administration of indomethacin or aspirin resulted in a marked restoration of NK activity in tumor-bearing animals (37). Tracey and Adkinson showed that the Bacillus Calmette-Guérin (BCG) augmentation of NK activity could be further potentiated by indomethacin in vivo (and in vitro) (79).

The effect of indomethacin administration in humans on delayed hypersensitivity skin testing has also been studied (74,80). Indomethacin administration (100 mg/day) for 5 days did not influence the amount of induration caused by a battery of three common antigens in 10 normal subjects (80). When indomethacin was administered to subjects with depressed cellular immunity there was an enhancement of delayed hypersensitivity (74). Two previously anergic patients with common variable immunodeficiency became reactive to skin tests while on indomethacin (100 mg/day) and became anergic again after the medication was stopped. The in vitro response of the patients' lymphocytes to PHA also rose while they were taking indomethacin (Fig. 2).

In summary, several in vivo studies confirm the in vitro experiments showing that PGE acts as a feedback inhibitor of cellular immune response and that these responses can be enhanced in vivo as well as in vitro by administration of cyclooxygenase inhibitors.

VI. CELLULAR ACTIVATION BY PGE_2

Until now we have discussed immunosuppressive activities of PGE_2 on immunocyte function. It is clear, however, that under certain experimental conditions PGE_2 can deliver

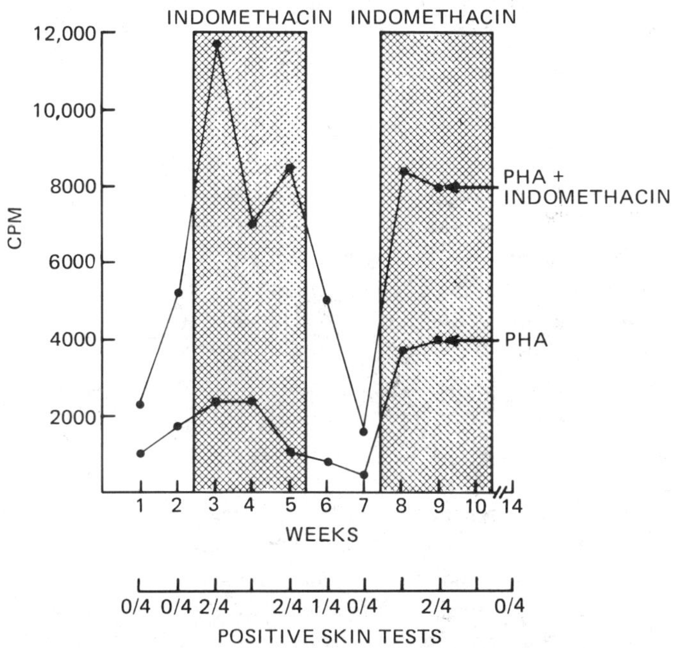

Figure 2 Effect of indomethacin administration in vivo on the response to PHA in vitro and on the response to skin testing in a patient with adult-acquired immunodeficiency. The two shaded areas represent the period of indomethacin administration (25 mg, q.i.d.). The in vitro response of the patients' peripheral blood mononuclear cells to an optimal concentration of PHA and to PHA plus indomethacin (1 μg/ml) is graphed. (From Ref. 74.)

activating signals. For example, PGE induces immature thymocytes to differentiate into mature T cells (81). Similar data have been obtained with B-cell differentiation (82). In multiple slcerosis patients an increased production of PGE_2 by the monocytes causes increased adherence of the lymphocytes to measles-infected cells (67) and an increased number of active E-rosette-forming lymphocytes (83). PGE also causes activation of suppressor cells in some assay systems. For example, Webb and co-workers showed that PGE_2 activates a glass wool-adherent suppressor T cell to release two peptides (84), which in turn suppress the response of nonadherent T cells to mitogens (50,51). The authors concluded that the inhibition of mitogenic lymphocyte stimulation was indirectly mediated by activation of suppressor cells. Fischer et al. have recently demonstrated that PGE_2 production is a necessary but not sufficient component of the generation of human ConA-activated suppressor cells that inhibit plasma cell differentiation of B cells (85), as well as T-cell responses to mitogens and alloantigens. Data from our laboratory suggest an analogous PGE requirement for the generation of another type of suppressor cell, the so-called $T\gamma$ cell (86).

Stobo and associates have shown that PGE_2 can increase the mitogenic reactivity of preincubated low-density T cells (87), while it decreases the reactivity of medium- and high-density T cells. The changes in cAMP in the three populations were very similar. It is unlikely that these cells correspond to the PGE_2-activated suppressor cell of Webb, since these low-density T cells had helper activity in functional assays (88). Stobo et al. concluded that PGE_2 should be considered as a regulator rather than as a universal suppressor for T-cell reactivity. More recently, we have shown that the suppressor-cytotoxic subset of T cells, as defined by monoclonal antibodies, has an increased mitogen-induced proliferation with exposure to PGE if the cells are first preincubated (89).

Dual effects (inhibition or activation) of PGE have been observed on B cells, natural killer (NK) cells, and macrophages. A short exposure of peripheral blood mononuclear cells to PGE_2 followed by a 24-hr incubation increases NK activity, while PGE_2 added during effector-target cell interaction inhibited NK activity (42). PGE_2 can both enhance and block NK activation by interferon (43). Interferon-induced and lipopolysaccharide (LPS) induced tumoricidal activity of monocytes is inhibited by high doses of PGE_2 (90,91), but indomethacin inhibits and PGE_2 restores endotoxin-induced tumoricidal activity of macrophages (92). Other authors have shown that PGE reduces the cytotoxic effect of BCG-activated macrophages but enhances the growth-inhibitory capacity of normal macrophages (93). The authors suggested that PGE may play a role in regulating macrophage function based on the level of activation of the macrophage. Phagocytosis by macrophages has been shown to be enhanced by PGE_2 by some authors and inhibited by others (94,95). Small concentrations of PGE_2 (10^{-9} M) cause suppression of macrophage spreading and adherence, while larger concentrations of PGE_2 (10^{-7} and 10^{-6} M) cause enhanced migration (96). Endotoxins and lymphokines induce collagenase production by macrophages, and this production is dependent on the rise in cAMP induced by PGE_2 (97). Collagenase production is blocked by indomethacin and restored by exogenous PGE_2.

It should be clear from these data that PGE cannot be considered as a universal cell inhibitor, and that its physiological role is very complex. PGE concentrations, activation and differentiation state of the target cell, and length of PGE-target cell interaction all seem to be important factors whose complete roles have not been fully delineated.

VII. MECHANISM OF ACTION OF PGE_2 ON THE CELLULAR LEVEL

Most attention has been focused on the effect of PGE_2 on intracellular cAMP. PGE_2 activates adenylate cyclase with a subsequent rise in cAMP (98). CAMP itself is an inhibitor of lymphocyte activation (98,99). We have addressed the possibility that cAMP is a second messenger for the action of PGE_2 in several studies. We have demonstrated the presence of receptors for PGE_2 on the lymphocyte surface, while there were no binding sites for PGA, $F_{1\alpha}$, or $F_{2\alpha}$ (100). The dissociation constand (Kd) for PGE_2 binding was 2×10^{-9} M and the B_{max} was 200 binding sites per cell, assuming uniform distribution. These binding sites for PGE_2 are lost during overnight incubation, which parallels the loss of inhibitory effect by PGE_2 on mitogenic stimulation of preincubated lymphocytes (26). PGE, but not PGF, caused increases in intracellular cAMP in lymphocytes, and this effect was also lost with preincubation (101). Thus, the functional effects (inhibition of mitogenesis), the cell surface receptors, and the cAMP response share a specificity for PGE over PGF. Webb et al. demonstrated by cAMP extraction and by direct fluorescence visualization an increase in intracellular cAMP in spleen cells after antigenic challenge with sheep red blood cells, which is dependent on a concomitant increase in prostaglandin levels (21,102).

It should be noted that the link between PGE effects and cAMP is not entirely established, and the possibility still exists that many of the effects of PGE on immune function are mediated in ways independent of adenylate cyclase stimulation.

VIII. EFFECT OF PROSTAGLANDINS ON THE HUMORAL IMMUNE RESPONSE

The influence of PGs on the humoral immune response can be mediated through direct effects on B cells, through effects on helper and suppressor T cells, or through effects on other accessory cells. Only pharmacological doses of PGE_2 inhibit immunoglobulin production by human B cells in vitro (103,104). Most effects at physiological doses seem to be mediated through the T-cell regulation of antibody production.

In our approach to this problem, we first studied the effect of PGE_2 on helper and suppressor T-cell populations. $T\gamma$ cells have been shown by Moretta et al. to be suppressive for PWM-driven B-cell differentiation into plasma cells (105). T cells bearing a receptor for the Fc portion of IgG ($T\gamma$ cells) had a 27-fold rise in cAMP after exposure to PGE_2, whereas the remaining T cells had a fourfold increase (106). Thus, suppressor T cells have a high density of PGE_2 receptors on their membrane relative to helper cells. As explained in the previous section, this rise in cAMP can be either an inhibition or an activation signal, depending on the cell type and state of activation. We have recently used an in vitro culture system of human peripheral blood mononuclear cells stimulated with PWM to evaluate the in vitro effect of prostaglandins and prostaglandin synthetase inhibitors on immunoglobulin production (104). Three different cyclooxygenase inhibitors (indomethacin, carprofen, and piroxicam) suppressed immunoglobulin synthesis by about 50%, without affecting cell viability. This inhibitory effect could be reversed by adding low doses of PGE_2 (3×10^{-8} - to 3×10^{-9} M). On the other hand, PGE_2 in concentrations of 3×10^{-9} - 3×10^{-8} M had no effect on purified B cells stimulated with T-cell-derived B-cell growth factors. Further experiments revealed that endogenous PGE_2 produced in the cultures inhibited a radiosensitive, mitomycin-sensitive suppressor T cell. Irradiation of T cells with 1000 rads prior to culture completely eliminated the effects of indomethacin and PGE_2. The same loss of effect was observed after mitomycin treatment of the T cells. Thus, suppressor cell control of polyclonal Ig production is itself under negative regulation by endogenous PGE_2. This suppressor cell is predominantly but not entirely recognized by OKT8, a monoclonal antibody reacting with T cells of the suppressor-cytotoxic subset. Indeed, PGE_2 almost completely inhibits the suppressive activity of OKT8(+) cells added to the culture of B + OKT4(+) helper T cells (Table 2). On the other hand, elimination of OKT8(+) cells reduced but did not entirely eliminate the enhancing effect of PGE_2 on immunoglobulin production.

We next extended these observations to autoantibody production in vitro. As a model for this we used rheumatoid factor (RF) production by PBMCs stimulated with PWM (107). This RF production is dependent on OKT4(+) T helper cells and is inhibited by OKT8(+) suppressor cells (108). We found that PG synthetase inhibitors suppressed RF production in PWM-stimulated cultures of lymphocytes from young controls, old persons (>70 years), and patients with rheumatoid arthritis (RA), and that this effect could be reversed by adding low doses of PGE_2 (Fig. 3). Again, irradiation of T cells prior to culture eliminated the effects of PGE_2 and indomethacin. Therefore, it would seem that endogenous PGE_2 can induce or increase autoantibody production through a tonic inhibition of suppressor cell activity. In this respect we should also

Table 2 The Target of Indogenous PGE_2 is an OKT8(+) T cell [a]

Cultures		IgM production (ng/ml) Exp. 1	Exp. 2	Exp. 3	Exp. 4
B+T	No drug	4000	–	–	1125
	Indomethacin	695	–	–	500
	Indo + PGE	3650	–	–	1675
$B+T_4(+)$	No drug	5400	1600	1300	2350
	Indo	5400	1490	1500	2200
	Indo + PGE	5780	1540	1450	2625
$B+T_4(+)$	No drug	2900	975	720	900
$+T_8(+)$	Indo	1150	510	540	425
	Indo + PGE	4950	1600	1400	2025

[a]Cultures of B+T cells, B+OKT4(+) T cells, and B+OKT4(+) + OKT8(+) T cells were established from four subjects. No drug, indomethacin (0.5 μg/ml), or indomethacin plus PGE_2 (3×10^{-8} M) were added. Indomethacin and PGE_2 had little effect on cultures of B+OKT4(+) T cells. The addition of PGE to cultures of B+OKT4(+) + OKT8(+) T cells appeared to eliminate the suppression caused by the addition of the OKT8(+) T cells.
Source: Ref. 104.

consider that PGE_2 accumulates at sites of inflammation (25), which may explain why rheumatoid factor is preferentially produced in rheumatoid joints, with the high concentrations of PGE_2 inhibiting the normal suppressor cell control of rheumatoid factor production. We have more recently found that PG synthetase inhibitors in vivo cause a reduction in serum RF levels in patients with rheumatoid arthritis to approximately 62% of the baseline level after 10 weeks treatment (187).

Aging has also been associated with increased autoantibody production and decreased suppressor cell function (109,110). As mentioned earlier, T cells of old persons are more sensitive to PGE_2 than T cells from young controls. This is also true for suppressor T cells. Indomethacin caused significantly greater inhibition of IgG (60 ± 7%) and IgM (58 ± 4%) production in PWM cultures of PBMCs from 12 subjects over 70 than of IgG (44 ± 5%) and IgM (47 ± 3%) production of PBMCs from 12 young controls (104). PGE_2 at different concentrations also induced a significantly greater enhancement of IgG production in lymphocyte cultures from old individuals than from young individuals. These data suggest that one reason for depressed suppressor cell function with age is an increased sensitivity to inhibition by PGE_2.

The data from our laboratory discussed in the last paragraph must be placed in the context of experimental results of other investigators; some of these data would appear to conflict with ours. Cook et al. studied the effect of PGE and PG synthesis inhibitors on in vitro secondary antibody responses to KLH in rabbits and obtained results similar to ours (111). On the other hand, Zimecki and Webb, studying the in vitro response of mouse splenocytes to the T-independent antigens polyvinyl pyrolidone and DNP-Ficoll found that addition of prostaglandin synthetase inhibitors caused a 50-300% increase in the number of plaque-forming cells produced (112). This enhancing effect of the PG synthetase inhibitors persisted in highly purified B-cell preparations with no T cells and less than 5% macrophages. They concluded from these findings that B cells may regulate their response to certain antigens by producing prostaglandins. Kurland et al. have found that excessive

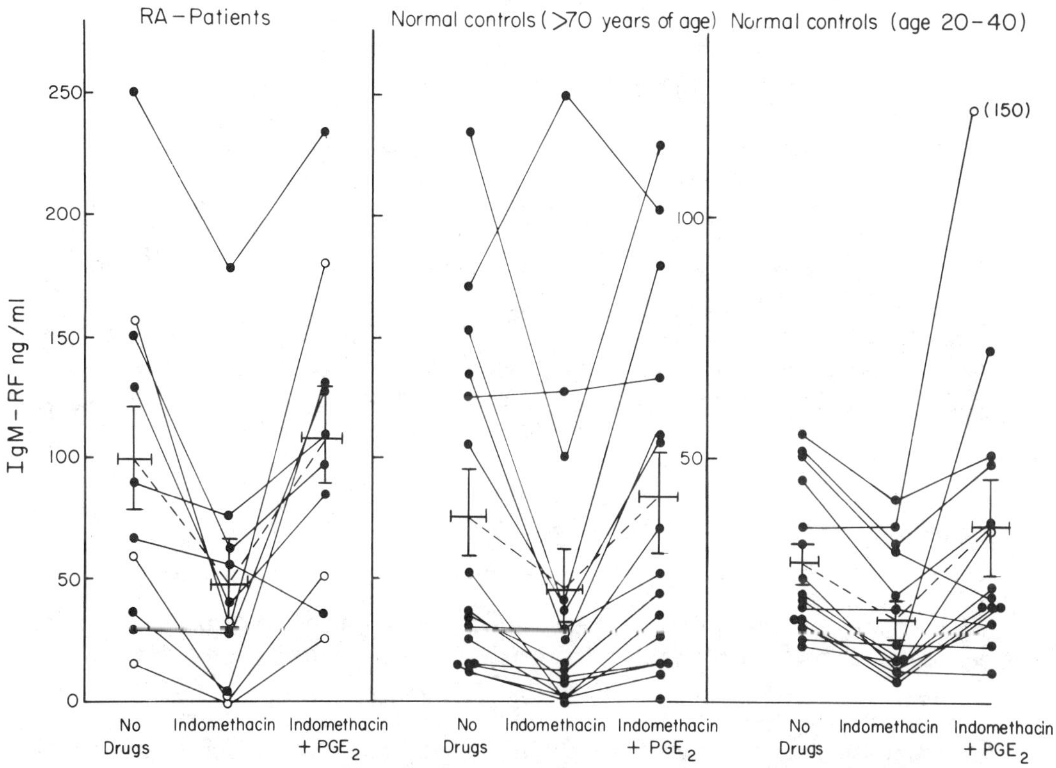

Figure 3 Effects of indomethacin (0.5 μg/ml) and PGE_2 (30 nM) on IgM-rheumatoid factor production. Lymphocytes from 10 patients with rheumatoid arthritis, 15 healthy controls aged over 70 years, and 14 healthy controls aged 20-40 years were cultured with pokeweed mitogen. Open circles = rheumatoid arthritis patients who received no medication for 7 days before blood was taken. In all three groups indomethacin caused a significant inhibition of IgM-RF production (p = 0.002 for RA patients; p = 0.02 for controls over 70 years of age; and p = 0.0001 for controls aged 20-40 years, by paired t-test). Addition of 30 nM PGE_2 caused a significant enhancement in IgM-RF production over the level with indomethacin (p = 0.003 for RA patients; p = 0.01 for controls over 70 years; and p = 0.02 for controls aged 20-40 years). (From Ref. 107.)

amounts of mouse macrophages inhibit B-cell proliferation in a semisolid agar culture system, and this inhibition is largely reversed by indomethacin (113). Monocytes can also suppress PWM-driven human B-cell differentiation when added in excessive amounts, but this suppressive activity is not PG mediated (114).

In several reports, blocking PG synthesis enhanced in vitro B-cell function, possibly through an effect on helper or suppressor cells (115,116). Fisher et al. have demonstrated that PGE_2 in doses of 3×10^{-7} M can activate human suppressor T cells that subsequently inhibit human B-cell differentiation into plasma cells (85). PGE_2 has also been shown in vitro to activate mouse suppressor lymphocytes that inhibit primary antibody responses to DNP-LPS (117). The role of thromboxanes in suppressor cell induction has been suggested by Orme and Shand (118) who showed that a thromboxane synthetase inhibitor can block suppressor cell generation in a plaque-forming cell assay. In vivo studies, although the number is restricted, have also shown an enhancement of humoral immune responses with indomethacin rather than an inhibition. As mentioned above, Webb showed that administration of indomethacin or RO-20-5720 to mice resulted in a greater number of direct splenic plaque-forming cells after injection of SRBSs (21). Kazimiera et al. repeated these experiments and showed that indomethacin-treated mice had an increased antibody titer to SRBCs (119).

We examined the effect of indomethacin administration on humoral immunity in humans by administering indomethacin (100 mg/day) to 15 normal subjects for 2 days before to 10 days after they received a bivalent influenza vaccine (80). Compared with 15 age- and sex-matched controls, the indomethacin-treated group had a significantly increased antibody titer to A-Victoria ($p < 0.025$). There was no difference in titer to A-New Jersey. Since 90% of the subjects had antibody titers to A-Victoria prior to vaccination, while none had prior titers to A-New Jersey, the results suggested that indomethacin administration enhanced the secondary but not the primary humoral immune response.

IX. PROSTAGLANDINS AND TUMOR GROWTH

A. Increased Activity of the PG-Producing Suppressor Cell During Tumor Growth

Tumors, just as other antigenic stimuli, lead to increased activity of the PG-producing suppressor cell. Pelus and Strausser (120) were the first to show that indomethacin can partly reverse the decreased mitogen response of spleen cells from tumor-bearing animals. More directly, Pelus and Bockman (121) showed that macrophages from tumor-bearing mice produced significantly more PGE than cells from normal littermates. The existence of indomethacin-sensitive adherent suppressor cells has also been shown by Glaser in tumor-bearing mice (122). Spleen cells of tumor-bearing mice inhibited the in vitro generation of secondary cytotoxic reactivity of spleen cells of tumor-free mice, sensitized in vitro with SV-40-induced tumor cells. The suppressor cells were shown to be macrophages, and indomethacin eliminated the suppressive activity. A possible mechanism for the systemic activation of monocytes in tumorous animals is an increase in circulating immune complexes (123).

Studies of patients with various types of cancer demonstrated overactivity of the PG-producing suppressor cell. We have investigated the role of the prostaglandin-producing suppressor cell in the hyporesponsiveness to PHA of PBMCs from patients with Hodgkin disease (124). Six patients with untreated Hodgkin disease, nodular sclerosing type, were studied. The mean response of the Hodgkin disease lymphocyte was 48% of the mean control response. This increased to 94% of normal with addition of indomethacin. Thus, indomethacin almost totally reversed the depressed PHA response in Hodgkin disease lymphocytes. The suppression of the PHA response in the patients with Hodgkin disease was also reversed by removal of glass-adherent cells prior to culture. This was expected, since the PG-producing suppressor cells are glass adherent (22).

PGE_2 production was then measured in mitogen cultures of PBMCs (500,000/ml) from three patients with Hodgkin disease and three age- and sex-matched controls. The mean PGE_2 production of the Hodgkin disease PBMCs was 20,600 ± 7620 pg/ml (6×10^{-8} M) in 48 hr versus 6368 ± 2944 pg/ml (1.6×10^{-8} M) for the controls (mean ± SD, $p < 0.02$). The amount of PGE_2 produced in the cultures of Hodgkin disease lymphocytes caused 65% inhibition when added exogenously to Hodgkin disease glass-nonadherent cells, while the amount of PGE_2 produced by the controls caused 35% inhibition when added to normal glass-nonadherent cells. Other studies have demonstrated the increased activity of the PG-producing suppressor cell in Hodgkin disease (125-127).

In other human cancers the evidence that overactivity of the normal PGE feedback inhibition is a major cause of T-cell dysfunction is less clear. In 10 anergic patients with a variety of metastatic solid tumors the enhancement of mitogen responses with indomethacin was only slightly greater than control (128). Vosixa and Thies, in a study of 24 cancer patients, found an increased activity of the PG-producing suppressor cell in 6 of 24 patients (129). In 24 patients with melanoma studied by Balch and Tilden, indomethacin induced a larger increase in the patients' mitogen responses than in the controls (130). However, in all of these studies the patients' responses remained quite depressed after indomethacin.

B. PGE Production by Tumor Cells

Apart from activation of the PG-producing suppressor cell, tumor cells themselves can produce immunodepressing PGE. The first data about PGE_2 production by tumors came from investigators interested in the mechanism of hypercalcemia associated with cancer not metastatic to bone. PGE_2 is a potent stimulator of bone resorption in vitro (131). Enhanced PGE production by naturally occurring or experimentally induced cancers has now been documented in several studies (131-141). Owen and co-workers, using a carcinogen-induced bladder tumor in Fisher rats, showed that direct contact between functionally active lymphocytes and tumor cells is necessary for increased tumor cell prostaglandin production to occur (142).

C. The Effect of Prostaglandin Synthetase Inhibitors on Tumor Growth In Vivo

If increased prostaglandin production by the tumor and by host macrophages is important in inhibiting the immune response of the host—especially in the immediate environment of the tumor—and in allowing the tumor to escape immunological rejection, then we would expect that administration of PG synthesis inhibitors in vivo to experimental tumor-bearing animals or cancer patients would result in (a) an improvement in immune function, and (b) retardation of tumor growth.

That this can occur in vivo was first shown by Plescia and co-workers (143,144). Administration of PG synthesis inhibitors to tumor-bearing mice resulted in restoration of the antibody response to sheep erythrocytes and in slowing of tumor growth. Several other laboratories have achieved similar results. Brunda et al. demonstrated that splenocytes from mice with Moloney virus-induced sarcomas had severely suppressed NK activity, and that this NK activity could be restored to normal by administration of aspirin or indomethacin in vivo (37). Hial et al. administered aspirin or indomethacin in mice that had received a mast cell ascites tumor or Lewis lung carcinoma (145). Both drugs in normal therapeutic doses caused a substantial slowing of the growth of both tumors. At higher indomethacin doses (5 mg/kg/day) there was elimination of the tumors in 50% of the cases, but there were also signs of gastric toxicity and weight loss in the mice. In these studies, as in the ones by Plescia, the PG synthetase inhibitors were started simultaneously with tumor inoculation. When there was a delay between tumor inoculation and drug administration, the antitumor effects were less pronounced. Lynch et al. (146) and Lynch and Salomon (147) reported that indomethacin and aspirin inhibited the growth of a methylcholanthrene-induced fibrosarcoma in mice. The drugs were not started until 7 days after tumor inoculation, when the tumor was already palpable. In approximately

20% of the indomethacin-treated mice the tumor completely regressed and did not reappear after cessation of the drug. Strausser and colleagues have reported that indomethacin will delay the onset and slow the growth of Moloney sarcoma virus-induced tumors in mice (148,149). If the drug is started at the same time as virus injection, no tumors develop. Bennett et al. reported that treatment with flurbiprofen (an inhibitor of PG synthesis) started before injection of mammary cancer cells reduced tumor growth and lengthened the survival time of mice (150). Indomethacin started 14 days after injection of the carcinogen reduced significantly the appearance of intestinal tumor in a study by Pollard and Luckert (151).

In most of these studies it is not clear that the inhibition of tumor growth is indeed induced by an effect on the immune system. Lynch et al., while confirming that the administration of PG synthetase inhibition does slow the growth of or eliminate many experimental tumors, dispute the claim that these drugs work via stimultion of the host's immune system (146). They showed that mice that had completely eliminated their tumors with indomethacin treatment were not immune to rechallenge with the same tumor. Augmentation of the immune response in tumor-bearing mice by indomethacin did not correlate with the antitumor effects of the drug. The data are, however, still consistent with the possibility that PG synthetase inhibition works via augmentation of NK activity and macrophage cytotoxicity, neither of which demonstrate immunological memory.

There are indications that inhibition of PG synthesis can inhibit tumor metastasis by mechanisms not related to the immune system. PGs may have a role in the establishment of bone metastases (152,153). PGE is indeed a powerful stimulus for bone resorption (131) and is necessary for the production of osteoclast-activating factor by leukocytes (154).

Finally, we should consider the effect of PGs and of PG synthetase inhibitors on carcinogenesis and on the tumor cells themselves. This effect can be different, according to the tumor type studied. The formation of squamous cell carcinoma was shown to be markedly enhanced by concomitant PGE_2 and $PGF_{2\alpha}$ administration to mice treated with 3-methylcholanthrene (MCA) for 2 months (155). Carcinogens such as TPA (a phorbol ester) or polycyclic aromatic hydrocarbons increase PGE production of the target cells (156-159). A positive correlation was found between carcinogenicity and stimulation of PG production (156). Cycloheximide inhibited the TPA-induced morphological changes and prostaglandin synthesis (158). It is therefore possible that prostaglandins are involved in the actions of these tumor promotors. Buick et al. studied the clonigenic activity of tumor cells obtained from malignant effusions from 31 patients with epithelial tumors (160). They found that host macrophages stimulated the growth of these cells in vitro and that PG synthetase inhibitors eliminated this stimulation. One possible interference from these data is that cyclooxygenase metabolites stimulate the growth of these cancer cells. There are also indications that breast cancers with high PGE production are more locally invasive and have a higher tendency for metastatic spread (132,134,139).

Not all the evidence, however, points to a beneficial effect of PG synthetase inhibitors to inhibit tumor growth. Some tumor cell lines are inhibited by PGE, while cyclooxygenase inhibitors stimulate their growth (161,162). Daily injection of a PGE analog into the site of a B16 melanoma tumor cell inoculation slowed the growth of these tumors by about 60% (161). The B16 melanoma studied is unusual in that its main arachidonic acid metabolite is PGD_2 (163). This same cell line was used in a study showing that PGE_2 administration can improve immune response and survival of tumor-bearing animals (164). Addition of indomethacin to cytotoxic drug regimens resulted in either no change or a decrease in the effectiveness of the chemotherapy against B16 melanoma (165). In another study using the B16 melanoma cell line, Stringfellow and Fitzpatrick showed that PGD_2 production by these tumor cells was inversely correlated with their metastatic potential (163). Exposure of the melanoma cells to indomethacin prior to inoculation resulted in a substantial increase in the rate of pulmonary metastases. PGE_2 added to cultures of erythroleukemia cells in the presence of the inducer DMSO produced 73% inhibition of cell growth (166). Jubiz et al. reported that daily injections of $PGF_{2\alpha}$ inhibited the growth of a hormone-dependent mammary tumor in mice (167). This effect was associated with a reduction in serum progesterone concentrations and was abolished by concomitant progesterone injection, suggesting that the $PGF_{2\alpha}$ worked in this system by inhibiting endogenous progesterone synthesis. The effect of PGs on tumor cell growth can also be dose dependent. Karmali et al. showed that the proliferation of Raji cells (a cell line derived from a Burkitt lymphoma) is enhanced by PGE_2 in a concentration of 10^{-12} - 10^{-11} while doses above 10^{-9} inhibit cell growth (168).

D. Suppressor Cell Activation by Nonspecific Immunostimulants

Disappointing results of clinical trials with nonspecific immune stimulation in cancer patients became more understandable in the light of recent work showing that *Corynebacterium parvum* and BCG, in addition to nonspecifically enhancing humoral and cellular immune responses (169), also induce the generation of suppressor cells in the host animals (170-175). The BCG-induced splenic suppressor cell in mice is adherent, phagocytic, and lacks the Thy 1 antigen (172). This macrophagelike cell inhibits NK cell activity, the generation of cytotoxic T cells, mitogen- or alloantigen-induced T-cell proliferation, and the plaque-forming response to antigens (170-175). A possible mechanism for such macrophagelike suppressor cells is via production of PGs. There are now some data suggesting that PGs may indeed be important in the function of these cells. First, both *C. parvum* and BCG induce macrophages to increase their PG production more than 50-fold (176,177). Second, BCG causes macrophages to produce factors that stimulate or inhibit NK activity (79). It remains to be seen whether in vivo indomethacin will prevent the late development of splenic suppressor cells and the concomitant late decrease in NK activity, T-cell cytotoxicity, and humoral immune responses.

This whole question was given more relevance by the finding that in vivo indomethacin substantially increased the antitumor activities of *C. parvum* and BCG (79,147). In one report the injection of 10^9 killed *C. parvum* organisms into fibrosarcoma tumors at 10 days and then again at 17 days after grafting resulted in elimination of the tumor by day 50 (147). However, if the *C. parvum* injections were given at days 17 and 24, when the tumor was substantially larger, there was no effect on subsequent tumor growth. The addition of indomethacin to this latter regimen resulted in elimination of the tumor in 50% of the cases. Similar findings were reported for BCG. When the *C. parvum* was given by intraperitoneal injection rather than intratumor, no effect on tumor growth was noted unless indomethacin was also administered, in which case the tumor regressed in 50% of the mice.

X. DISCUSSION

PGE_2 is produced by monocytes and macrophages, and its production is increased by membrane activation. The PGE_2 produced inhibits several lymphocyte functions: proliferation, lymphokine production, cytotoxic activity, and suppressor activity. However, there are also indications that certain cell types can be activated by PGE_2, including NK cells and some suppressor cells. Although it is beyond any doubt that prostaglandins have important immunoregulatory functions, the complexity of fine regulation awaits further elucidation. The latter is the more important since prostaglandin metabolism can be manipulated in vivo by drugs and by nutrition (178), allowing potential applications in the pharmacological and nutritional modulation of the immune system. In this respect we would like to discuss three major areas: autoimmunity, cancer, and immune deficiency.

A. Immune Deficiency

Information in this area is very limited. We reported enhancement of delayed hypersensitivity in two patients with common variable immunodeficiency with indomethacin administration (74). Indomethacin in vivo also restored in vitro lymphocyte reactivity in some patients with Hodgkin disease (126). However, no data on actual clinical improvement have been published. Both in vitro experiments and animal models make us expect that this might occur in certain forms of cellular deficiency, especially in anergy that is secondary to chronic inflammatory conditions.

B. Cancer

Much of the evidence presented so far suggests that treatment with PG synthetase inhibitors would probably be beneficial in cancer treatment. The arguments can be summarized as follows:

1. Tumor growth stimulates prostaglandin-producing suppressor cells (monocytes and macrophages).
2. Many tumors produce PGE.
3. PGE_2 is an immunosuppressive agent and inhibits T cells, NK cells, and macrophages in their cytotoxic activity.
4. The PGs produced by tumors could facilitate metastasis formation in bone tissue by their enhancing effect on bone resorption.
5. Immunotherapy with BCG or *C. parvum* enhances prostaglandin production by monocytes.
6. PG synthetase inhibitors interfere with platelet aggregation, and this could reduce intravascular tumor cell trapping.

There are, however, a great deal of conflicting data about the role of prostaglandins in cancer growth, and these have to be considered in the discussion about the usefulness of PG synthesis modulation in cancer patients.

1. The effect of prostaglandins on tumor cell growth is different—enhancement or inhibition—according to the tumor cell type. This leaves open the very important question of which type of experimental tumor if any, human cancers will most approximate, and therefore the question of what types of cancer should be the subject of a trial with PG synthetase inhibitors.
2. Virus-infected animals and those bearing various types of malignancies progressively lose their ability to respond to interferon inducers. Prostaglandins (A, E, and F) can restore this response (179). In addition, there is some evidence that prostaglandins may be necessary for the antiviral activity of interferon (180) and that PGA itself has antiviral activity (181).

3. Pretreatment of NK cells with PGE_2 followed by 24-hr incubation in medium actually increases NK activity (42). Under certain experimental conditions, PGE_2 also enhances macrophage tumoricidal activity (92,93).
4. Prostaglandins other than PGE_2 may have completely different functions on the immune system, and perhaps enhance the defense against tumors. The PG synthesis inhibitors available now, however, are nonspecific and do not inhibit selective pathways.

A survey of human cancers in which PG production was measured was done recently by Karmali (182). A systematic study of PG production by all types of human cancers is needed, as well as a careful quantitation of the types of PGs produced. Because of the work with B16 melanoma tumors in mice, one would certainly be wary of giving indomethacin to patients with tumors that produce large amounts of PGD_2, if indeed such tumors occur in humans. PGE production is one of the mechanisms by which tumors can escape immune surveillance. In vivo studies in experimental animals only can determine the relative importance of this particular escape mechanism among others.

C. Autoimmunity

Prostaglandin synthetase inhibitors are now currently used as anti-inflammatory agents in many immunological diseases such as rheumatoid arthritis (RA) and systemic lupus erythematosus (SLE). Although their anti-inflammatory activity is obvious, it is less clear what the effect is on the basic disease process. In SLE and probably also in RA, suppressor cell function is decreased (183). If our data that endogenous PGE_2 tonically inhibits a suppressor cell for immunoglobulin and autoantibody formation have relevance to the in vivo situation, then PG synthesis inhibitors would be expected to improve the basic disease process. However, if PGs or thromboxanes are involved in the generation of suppressor cells, as suggested by the studies of Webb et al., then PG synthesis inhibitors could further impair an already deficient suppressor cell system. Since PGE_2 also inhibits nonspecifically many lymphocyte effector functions, PG synthesis inhibition could further enhance cytodestructive mechanisms. We also have to consider the data that PGE_1 inhibits adjuvant arthritis in rats (8,184), immune complex-induced vasculitis (184-186), and that PGE_1 injections in NZB/NZW mice prevent glomerulonephritis (13) and prolong survival of NZB/NZW mice even when treatment is begun after nephritis has developed (13,185). These considerations are not intended to suggest that the use of PG synthetase inhibitors in the treatment of rheumatic diseases should be abandoned, but to increase efforts in elucidating the exact mechanisms of PGs in immune regulation. These studies should be directed toward a better understanding of the effects of different prostaglandins on different cell subpopulations of the immune system.

REFERENCES

1. C. W. Parker, *J. Allergy Clin. Immunol., 63*:1 (1979).
2. G. W. Lum, G. A. Alsenbrey, M. J. Dunn, T. Berl, R. W. Schrier, and K. M. McDonald, *J. Clin. Invest., 59*:8 (1977).
3. M. Kaliner and F. Austen, *J. Immunol., 112*:664 (1974).
4. M. Kaliner, *J. Allerg. Clin. Immunol., 60*:204 (1977).
5. L. E. Trang, *Sem. Arth. Rheum., 9*:153 (1980).
6. J. R. Vane, *Nature (New Biol.), 231*:232 (1971).
7. J. S. Goodwin and D. R. Webb, *Clin. Immunol. Immunopathol., 15*:106 (1980).

8. R. B. Zurier and F. Quagliata, *Nature, 234*:304 (1971).
9. E. R. Hurd, J. M. Johnston, J. R. Okita, P. C. MacDonald, M. Ziff, and J. N. Gilliam, *J. Clin. Invest., 67*:476, 1981.
10. S. Izui, V. E. Kelley, P. J. McConahey, and F. J. Dixon, *J. Exp. Med., 152*:1645 (1980).
11. V. E. Kelley and A. Winkelstein, *Clin. Immunol. Immunopathol., 16*:316 (1980).
12. K. R. McLeish, A. F. Gohara, W. T. Gunning, and D. Senitzer, *J. Lab. Clin. Med., 96*:470 (1980).
13. R. B. Zurier, I. Damjanov, D. M. Sayadoff, and N. F. Rothfield, *Arth. Rheum., 20*:1449 (1977).
14. R. B. Zurier, D. M. Sayadoff, S. B. Torrey, and N. F. Rothfield, *Arth. Rheum., 20*:723 (1977).
15. P. Needleman, A. Raz, J. A. Ferrendelli, and M. Minkes, *Proc. Natl. Acad. Sci. USA, 74*:1916 (1977).
16. R. R. Gorman, G. L. Bundy, D. C. Peterson, F. F. Sun, O. V. Miller, and F. A. Fitpatrick, *Proc. Natl. Acad. Sci. USA, 74*:4007 (1977).
17. R. J. Gryglewski, S. Bunting, S. Moncada, R. J. Flower, and J. R. Vane, *Prostaglandins, 12*:685 (1976).
18. H. S. Kantor and M. Hampton, *Nature (Lond.), 276*:841 (1978).
19. C. P. Ciosek, R. W. Ortel, N. M. Thanassi,, and D. S. Newcombe, *Nature (Lond.), 251*:148 (1974).
20. R. I. Levin, E. A. Jaffe, B. B. Weksler, and K. Tack-Goldman, *J. Clin. Invest., 67*:762 (1981).
21. D. R. Webb and P. L. Osheroff, *Proc. Natl. Acad. Sci. USA, 43*:1300 (1976).
22. J. S. Goodwin, A. D. Bankhurst, and R. P. Messner, *J. Exp. Med., 146*:1719 (1977).
23. V. H. Grant, H. Baruth, L. Randall, C. Ashley, and J. R. Paulsrud, *Prostaglandins, 10*:59 (1975).
24. J. S. Goodwin, R. P. Messner, and R. C. Williams, *Cell. Immunol., 45*:303 (1979).
25. D. R. Robinson and L. Levine, in *Prostaglandin Synthetase Inhibitors* (H. J. Robinson and J. R. Vane, eds.), Raven Press, New York, 1974.
26. J. S. Goodwin, R. P. Messner, and G. T. Peake, *J. Clin. Invest., 62*:753 (1978).
27. A. Novagrodsky, A. L. Rubin, and K. H. Stenzel, *J. Immunol., 1*:122 (1979).
28. C. C. Muscoplat, D. J. Klausner, C. J. Brunner, E. D. Sloane, and D. W. Johnson, *Infect. Immun., 26*:311 (1979).
29. U. Erten, T. Emre, A. O. Cavdar, and R. K. Turner, *Prostagl. Med., 5*:255 (1980).
30. D. Venza-Teti, A. Misefari, V. Sofo, V. Fimiani, and M. F. Lavia, *Immunopharmacology, 2*:165 (1980).
31. D. Gordon, M. Bray, and J. Morley, *Nature, 262*:401 (1976).
32. P. E. Baker, J. V. Fahey, and A. Munck, *Cell. Immunol., 61*:52 (1981).
33. R. S. Rappaport and G. R. Dogde, *J. Exp. Med., 155*:943 (1982).
34. T. L. Darrow and R. H. Tomar, *Cell. Immunol., 56*:177 (1980).
35. K. H. Leung and E. Mihich, *Nature, 288*:597 (1980).
36. R. M. Schultz, J. N. Stoychkov, N. Pavlidis, M. A. Chirigos, and Z. L. Olkowski, *J. Reticuloendo. Soc., 26*:93 (1979).
37. M. J. Brunda, R. B. Herberman, and H. T. Holden, *J. Immunol., 124*:2682 (1980).
38. J. D. Roder and M. Klein, *J. Immunol., 123*:1785 (1979).
39. M. R. Garovoy, T. B. Strom, M. Kaliner, and C. B. Carpenter, *Cell Immunol., 20*:197 (1975).
40. K. F. Trofatter and C. A. Daniels, *J. Immunol., 122*:1363 (1979).
41. M. J. Droller, M. U. Schneider, and P. Perlman, *Cell. Immunol., 39*:165 (1978).
42. R. Kendall and S. Targan, *J. Immunol., 125*:1770 (1980).
43. S. Targan, *J. Immunol., 127*:1424 (1981).

44. A. Kingston, J. E. Kay, and J. Ivanyi, *Int. J. Immunopharmacol., 2*:243 (1980).
45. D. Gordon, D. C. Henderson, and J. Westwick, *Br. J. Pharmacol., 67*:17 (1979).
46. J. P. Kelly, M. C. Johnson, and C. W. Parker, *J. Immunol., 122*:1556 (1979).
47. K. H. Leung and E. Mihich, *Int. J. Immunopharmacol., 2*:244 (1978).
48. M. S. Kennedy, J. D. Stobo, and M. E. Goldyne, *Prostaglandins, 20*:135 (1980).
49. J. I. Kurland and R. Bockman, *J. Exp. Med., 147*:952 (1978).
50. D. R. Webb and I.Nowowiejski, *Cell. Immunol., 41*:72 (1978).
51. D. R. Webb, R. J. Rogers, and I. Nowowiejski, *Proc. N.Y. Acad Sci., 332*:262 (1980).
52. J. H. Passwell, J. M. Dayer, and E. Merler, *J. Immunol., 123*:115 (1979).
53. J. L. Humes, R. J. Bonney, L. Pebes, M. E. Dahlgren, S. J. Sadowski, F. A. Kuehl, and P. Davies, *Nature, 269*:149 (1977).
54. J. J. Ellner and P. J. Spagnuolo, *J. Immunol., 123*:1689 (1979).
55. R. J. Bonney, P. P. Naruns, P. Davies, and J. L. Humes, *Prostaglandins, 18*:605 (1979).
56. Cantanzaro, *Cell. Immunol., 64*:235 (1981).
57. J. M. B. Kaneene, R. K. Anderson, D. W. Johnson, and C. C. Muscoplat, *Vet. Immunol. Immunopathol., 4*:375 (1983).
58. P. Dore-Duffy and R. B. Zurier, *Clin. Immunol. Immunopath., 19*:303 (1981).
59. J. S. Goodwin, R. DeHoratius, H. Israel, G. T. Peake, and R. P. Messner, *Ann. Intern. Med., 90*:169 (1979).
60. L. Rice, A. Laughter, and J. J. Twomey, *J. Immunol., 122*:991 (1979).
61. M. E. Kleinhenz, J. J. Ellner, P. J. Spagnuolo, and T. M. Daniel, *J. Clin. Invest., 68*: 153 (1981).
62. W. S. Lapp, M. Mendes, H. Kirchner, and D. Gemsa, *Cell. Immunol., 17*:353 (1980).
63. J. Hopkins, I. McConnell, and J. Raniwalla, *Immunology, 43*:205 (1981).
64. C. S. Staszak, J. S. Goodwin, G. M. Troup, D. R. Pathak, and R. C. Williams, *J. Immunol., 125*:181 (1980).
65. P. J. Kirbey, J. Morley, J. R. Ponsford, and W. I. MacDonald, *Prostaglandins, 11*: 621 (1976).
66. J. S. Goodwin and R. P. Messner, *Prostaglandins, 15*:281 (1978).
67. P. Dore-Duffy and R. B. Zurier, *J. Clin. Invest., 63*:154 (1979).
68. R. C. Page, J. A. Clagett, L. D. Engel, G. Wilde, and T. Sims, *Clin. Immunol. Immunopathol., 11*:77 (1978).
69. J. Goodwin and R. P. Messner, *J. Clin. Invest., 64*:434 (1979).
70. J. S. Goodwin, *Clin. Immunol. Immunopathol., 25*:243 (1982).
71. J. S. Goodwin, *Prostaglandin Med., 3*:395 (1979).
72. J. S. Goodwin, S. Bromberg, C. Staszak, P. A. Kaszubowski, R. P. Messner, and F. J. Neal, *J. Immunol., 127*:518 (1981).
73. S. Wolinsky, J. S. Goodwin, R. P. Messner, and R. C. Williams, Jr., *Clin. Immunol. Immunopathol., 17*:31 (1980).
74. J. S. Goodwin, S. Murphy, A. D. Bankhurst, D. S. Selinger, R. P. Messner, and R. C. Williams, Jr., *J. Clin. Lab. Immunol., 1*:197 (1978).
75. C. C. Muscoplat, P. M. Rakich, C. O. Theon, and P. W. Johnson, *Infect. Immun., 20*:627 (1978).
76. E. Lipsmeyer, *Transplantation, 33*:107 (1982).
77. C. B. Anderson, B. M. Jaffee, and R. J. Graff, *Transplantation, 23*:444 (1977).
78. W. A. Blyth, T. J. Hill, H. J. Field, and D. A. Harbour, *J. Gen. Virol., 33*:547 (1976).
79. D. E. Tracey and N. F. Adkinson, *J. Immunol., 125*:136 (1980).
80. J. S. Goodwin, D. S. Selinger, R. P. Messner, and W. P. Reed, *Infect. Immun., 19*:430 (1978).

81. M. A. Bach, C. Fournier, and J. F. Bach, *Ann. N.Y. Acad. Sci., 249*:316 (1975).
82. S. W. Burchiel and N. L. Warner, *J. Immunol., 124*:1016 (1980).
83. H. Offner, D. Danneskiold-Samse, and P. Dore-Duffy, *Clin. Immunol. Immunopath., 22*:159 (1982).
84. T. J. Rogers, I. Nowowiejski, and D. R. Webb, *Cell. Immunol., 50*:82 (1980).
85. A. Fischer, A. Durandy, and C. Griscelli, *J. Immunol., 126*:1452 (1981).
86. P. Kaszubowski and J. S. Goodwin, *Cell. Immunol., 68*:343 (1982).
87. J. D. Stobo, M. S. Kennedy, and M. E. Goldyne, *J. Clin. Invest., 64*:1188 (1979).
88. M. E. Goldyne and J. D. Stobo, *Crit. Rev. Immunol., 2*:189 (1981).
89. N. Gualde and J. S. Goodwin, *Cell. Immunol., 70*:373 (1982).
90. R. M. Schultz, N. A. Pavlidis, W. A. Stylos, and M. A. Chirigos, *Science, 202*:320 (1978).
91. S. Taffet and S. W. Russell, *J. Immunol., 126*:424 (1981).
92. B. Drysdale and H. S. Shin, *J. Immunol., 127*:760 (1981).
93. M. E. McCarthy and B. S. Zwilling, *Cell. Immunol., 60*:91 (1981).
94. J. Schnyder, B. Dewald, and M. Baggiolini, *Prostaglandins, 22*: (1979).
95. E. Razin, S. Bauminger, and A. Globerson, *J. Reticuloendoth. Soc., 23*:237 (1978).
96. W. D. Cantarow, H. T. Cheung, and G. Sundharadas, *Prostaglandins, 16*:39 (1978).
97. L. M. Wahl, C. E. Olsen, S. M. Wahl, J. B. McCarthy, A. L. Sanberg, and S. E. Mergenhagen, *Ann. N.Y. Acad. Sci., 332*:271 (1979).
98. J. W. Smith, A. L. Steiner, and C. W. Parker, *J. Clin. Invest., 50*:442 (1971).
99. K. L. Melmon, H. R. Bourne, Y. Weinstein, G. M. Shearer, J. Kram, and S. Bauminger, *J. Clin. Invest., 53*:13 (1974).
100. J. S. Goodwin, A. Wiik, M. Lewis, A. D. Bankhurst, and R. C. Williams, Jr., *Cell. Immunol., 43*:150 (1979).
101. J. S. Goodwin, S. Bromberg, and R. P. Messner, *Cell. Immunol., 60*:298 (1981).
102. D. R. Webb, T. J. Rogers, S. Ong, and A. Steiner, *Prostagl. Med., 5*:141 (1980).
103. T. Morito, A. D. Bankhurst, and R. C. Williams, *Prostaglandins, 20*:383 (1980).
104. J. L. Ceuppens and J. S. Goodwin, *Cell. Immunol., 70*:41 (1982).
105. L. Moretta, S. R. Webb, C. E. Grossi, P. M. Lydyard, and M. D. Cooper, *J. Exp. Med., 146*:194 (1977).
106. J. S. Goodwin, P. A. Kaszubowski, and R. C. Williams, Jr., *J. Exp. Med., 150*: 1260 (1979).
107. J. L. Ceuppens and J. S. Goodwin, *Lancet, 1*:528 (1982).
108. M. Rodriguez, J. Ceuppens, and J. S. Goodwin, *J. Immunol., 128*:2422 (1982).
109. H. M. Hallgren and E. J. Yunis, *J. Immunol., 118*:1004 (1977).
110. S. Kishimoto, S. Tomino, H. Mitsuya, and H. Fujiwara, *J. Immunol., 123*:1586 (1979).
111. R. Cook, *Cell. Immunol., 40*:128 (1978).
112. M. Zimecki and D. R. Webb, *J. Immunol., 117*:2158 (1976).
113. J. I. Kurland, P. W. Kincade, and M. A. S. Moore, *J. Exp. Med., 146*:1420 (1977).
114. F. Gmelig-Myerling and T. Waldmann, *J. Immunol., 126*:529 (1981).
115. J. A. Mattingly and J. D. Kemp, *Cell. Immunol., 48*:195 (1979).
116. D. R. Webb and I. Nowowiejski, *Cell. Immunol., 33*:1 (1977).
117. A. M. Fulton and J. G. Levy, *Cell. Immunol., 59*:54 (1981).
118. I. Orme and F. L. Shand, *Int. J. Immunopharmacol., 2*:245 (1980).
119. D. Kazimiera, K. D. Grinwich, and O. J. Plescia, *Prostaglandins, 14*:1175 (1977).
120. L. M. Pelus and H. R. Strausser, *Int. J. Cancer, 18*:653 (1976).
121. C. Pelus and R. Bockman, *J. Immunol., 123*:2118 (1979).
122. M. Glaser, *Eur. J. Immunol., 10*:489 (1980).
123. L. Poleshuck and H. Strausser, *Prost. Med., 4*:1363 (1980).
124. J. S. Goodwin, R. P. Messner, A. D. Bankhurst, G. T. Peake, J. H. Saiki, and R. C. Williams, Jr., *N. Engl. J. Med., 297*:263 (1977).

125. R. S. Bockman, *J. Clin. Invest., 66*:523 (1980).
126. R. P. DeShazo, *Clin. Immunol. Immunopathol., 17*:66 (1980).
127. W. L. Sibbitt, A. D. Bankhurst, and R. C. Williams, Jr., *J. Clin. Invest., 61*:55 (1978).
128. A. D. Bankhurst, G. Kauffman, J. S. Goodwin, and R. C. Williams, Jr., *J. Lab. Clin. Immunol., 3*:3 (1980).
129. G. Vosixa J. Thies, *Clin. Immunol. Immunopathol., 13*:30 (1979).
130. C. M. Balch and A. B. Tilden, *Surgery, 90*:77 (1981).
131. D. C. Klein and L. G. Raisl, *Endocrinology, 86*:1436 (1970).
132. A. Bennett, E. M. Charlier, A. M. McDonald, J. S. Simpson, I. F. Stamford, and T. Zebro, *Lancet, 2*:624 (1977).
133. A. Bennett, M. Del Tacca, I. F. Stamford, and T. Zebro, *Br. J. Cancer, 35*:881 (1977b).
134. A. Bennett, A. M. McDonald, J. S. Simpson, and I. F. Stamford, *Lancet, 1*:1218 (1975).
135. S. M. Burchiel, M. Rubin, J. Giorgi, G. T. Peake, and N. L. Warner, *The Importance of Tumor Markers in Clinical Medicine,* (P. Wolfe, ed.), Masson Corp., 1979.
136. K. B. Cummings and R. P. Robertson, *J. Urol., 118*:720 (1977).
137. G. Husby, R. G. Strickland, G. L. Rigler, G. T. Peake, and R. C. Williams, Jr., *Cancer, 40*:1629 (1977).
138. T. J. Powles, R. C. Coomes, A. M. Neville, H. T. Ford, J. C. Gazet, and L. Levine *Lancet, 2*:138 (1977).
139. P. H. Rolland, P. M. Martin, J. Jacquemier, A. M. Rolland, and M. Toga, *J. Natl. Cancer Inst., 64*:1061 (1980).
140. J. A. X. Sykes and J. S. Maddox, *Nature (New Biol.), 237*:59 (1972).
141. A. H. Tashjian, E. F. Voelkel, L. Levine, and P. Goldhaber, *J. Exp. Med., 136*: 1329 (1972).
142. K. Owen, D. Gomolka, and M. J. Droller, *Cell. Immunol., 55*:428 (1980).
143. O. J. Plescia, A. H. Smith, and K. Grinwich, *Proc. Natl. Acad. Sci. USA, 72*: 1848 (1975).
144. K. D. Grinwich and O. J. Plescia, *Prostaglandins, 14*:1175 (1977).
145. V. Hial, Z. Horokova, R. E. Shaff, and M. A. Beaven, *Eur. J. Pharmacol., 37*:367 (1976).
146. N. R. Lynch, M. Casatles, M. Astonin, and J. C. Salomon, *Br. J. Cancer, 38*:503 (1978).
147. N. R. Lynch and J. Salomon, *J. Natl. Cancer Inst., 62*:117 (1979).
148. J. L. Humes, J. Cupo, and H. R. Strausser, *Prostaglandins, 6*:463 (1974).
149. H. R. Strausser and J. L. Humes, *Int. J. Cancer, 15*:724 (1975).
150. A. Bennett, J. K. Houghton, D. J. Leaper, and I. F. Stanford, *Prostaglandins, 17*: 179 (1979).
151. M. Pollard and P. H. Luckert, *Science, 214*:558 (1981).
152. C. S. B. Galasko and A. Bennett, *Nature, 263*:508 (1976).
153. T. J. Powles, S. A. Clar, D. M. Easty, C. G. Easty, and A. M. Neville, *Br. J. Cancer, 28*:316 (1973).
154. T. Yoneda and G. R. Mundy, *J. Exp. Med., 149*:279 (1979).
155. A. Lupulescu, *J. Natl. Cancer Inst., 61*:97 (1978).
156. L. Levine, *Nature, 268*:447 (1977).
157. L. Levine and K. Ohucki, *Nature, 276*:274 (1978).
158. K. Ohuchi and L. Levine, *J. Biol. Chem., 253*:4783 (1978).
159. H. Yamasaki, R. A. Mufson, and I. B. Weinstein, *Biochim. Biophys. Res. Commun., 89*:1018 (1979).
160. R. Buick, S. Fry, and S. Salmon, *Br. J. Cancer, 41*:695 (1980).

161. M. G. Santoro, G. W. Philpott, and B. M. Jaffe, *Nature, 263*:777 (1976).
162. R. D. Thomas, G. W. Philpott, and B. M. Jaffe, *Exp. Cell. Res., 84*:40 (1974).
163. D. Stringfellow and F. Fitzpatrick, *Nature, 282*:76 (1979).
164. C. Favalli, E. Garaci, E. Etheredge, M. G. Santoro, and B. M. Jaffe, *J. Immunol., 125*:897 (1980).
165. D. Hofer, A. M. Dubitsky, P. Reilly, M. G. Santoro, and B. M. Jaffe, *Prostaglandins, 20*:1033 (1980).
166. M. G. Santoro and B. M. Jaffe, *Br. J. Cancer, 39*:408 (1979).
167. W. Jubiz, J. Frailey, and J. B. Smith, *Cancer Res., 39*:998 (1979).
168. R. A. Karmali, D. F. Horrobin, J. Menenzes, and P. Patel, *Pharmacol. Res. Commun., 11*:69 (1979).
169. J. W. Hadden, L. Delmonte, and H. F. Oettgen, in *Immunopharmacology* (J. W. Hadden, R. C. Coffey, and F. Spreafico, eds.), Plenum Press, New York, 1977, p. 279.
170. H. Korchner, M. Glaser, and R. B. Herberman, *Nature, 257*:396 (1975).
171. G. R. Klimpel, *Cell. Immunol., 47*:218 (1980).
172. G. Klimpel and C. S. Henney, *J. Immunol., 120*:563 (1978).
173. G. R. Klimpel, M. Okada, and C. S. Henney, *J. Immunol., 123*:350 (1979).
174. R. Neta and S. B. Salvin, *Infect. Immun., 23*:360 (1979).
175. C. A. Savary and E. Lotzova, *J. Immunol., 120*:239 (1978).
176. W. Grimm, M. Seitz, H. Kirchner, and D. Gemsa, *Cell. Immunol., 40*:419 (1978).
177. S. M. Wahl, L. M. Wahl, J. B. McCarthy, L. Chedid, and S. E. Mergenhagen, *J. Immunol., 122*:2226 (1979).
178. J. Ceuppens and J. Goodwin, in *Human Cancer Immunology,* vol. 4, North Holland, Amsterdam, in press, 1984.
179. D. A. Stringfellow, *Science, 201*:376 (1978).
180. K. Chandrabose, R. Pottathic, P. Cuatrelasas, and D. Lang, *Fed. Proc.* (Abstr.), *39*:325 (1980).
181. M. G. Santoro, A. Benedetto, C. Carruba, E. Garaci, and B. Jaffe, *Science, 209*: 1032 (1980).
182. R. A. Karmali, *Prostagland. Med., 5*:11 (1980).
183. N. Talal, *Transplant. Rev., 31*:240 (1976).
184. S. L. Kunkel, H. Ogawa, P. B. Conran, P. A. Ward, and R. B. Zurier, *Arth. Rheum., 24*:1151 (1981).
185. S. L. Kunkel, R. T. Thrall, R. G. Kunkel, P. A. Ward, and R. B. Zurier, *J. Clin. Invest., 64*:1525 (1979).
186. R. B. Zurier, I. Kamjanov, P. L. Miller, and B. F. Biewer, *J. Clin. Lab. Immunol., 1*:95 (1978).
187. J. S. Goodwin, J. L. Ceuppens, and M. A. Rodriguez, *J.A.M.A., 250*:2485 (1983).

31

Prostaglandins and Cyclooxygenase Inhibitors

Joseph Chang and Alan J. Lewis Wyeth Laboratories, Inc.,
Philadelphia, Pennsylvania

I. INTRODUCTION

In 1971, Vane and others (1-3) demonstrated that aspirinlike drugs (also referred to as nonsteroidal anti-inflammatories) inhibited the enzymatic synthesis of prostaglandins (PGs) from their fatty acid precursor, arachidonic acid (AA); furthermore, they suggested that this was the basis for the therapeutic action of these drugs. PGs were the first described of the biologically active products of AA produced by PG synthetase, or PG cyclooxygenase, as it is more precisely defined. Other intermediates that have subsequently been discovered during AA metabolism include PG endoperoxides, thromboxane (Tx), and prostacyclin (4). Peroxidation of AA to the leukotrienes, hydroperoxy, and hydroxy fatty acids by a series of lipoxygenases has attracted more recent attention (5).

The role of these 20-carbon metabolites, often referred to as eicosanoids, in physiological and pathological states is under intensive investigation. The PGs, in particular, play an important role in immunological regulation, and the use of PG cyclooxygenase inhibitors has greatly contributed to this development. The following account will focus on the role of PGs and other eicosanoids on immune surveillance and will emphasize the effects of PG cyclooxygenase inhibitors on host-tumor interaction.

II. CYCLOOXYGENASE INHIBITORS

These are a diverse group of chemical structures that consists of substrate analogs, aspirinlike drugs, and miscellaneous inhibitors, including antioxidants and metal ions (4,6). Much of this chapter will focus on the use of aspirinlike drugs (see Table 1) which, in general, possess important antiinflammatory, antipyretic, and analgesic actions. Brief mention will be made of inhibition of enzymes involved in the synthesis of the other eicosanoids

Table 1 Major Inhibitors of the Metabolism of Arachidonic Acid

Cyclooxygenase inhibitors	Lipoxygenase inhibitors[a]
Aspirin	BW 755C
Benorylate	Eicosatetraynoic acid (ETYA)
Diflunisal	Nordihydroguaiaretic acid (NDGA)
Fenbufen	Nafazatrom (Bay g 6575)[b]
Fenclofenac	Phenidone
Fentiazac	Timegadine
Flufenamic acid	
Flurbiprofen	Thromboxane synthetase inhibitors
Ibuprofen	
Indomethacin	Imidazole and analogs
Ketoprofen	L 8027
Meclofenamic acid	N-0164
Naproxen	U-51605
Phenylbutazone	U-54701
Piroxicam	U-54874
Ro-20-5720	
Sulindac	Phospholipase inhibitors
Tolmetin	
	Corcicosteroids
	Mepacrine
	p-Bromophenyacyl bromide
	Local anesthetics

[a]These compounds also inhibit cyclooxygenase to varying degrees.
[b]Also stimulates protacyclin synthesis (9)
Source: Refs. 4, 6-8.

(Table 1). On a cautionary note, virtually no drug exerts a single action and the cyclooxygenase inhibitors are no exception. They possess inhibitory effects on a variety of other enzymes including prostaglandin 15-dehydrogenase (10), phosphodiesterase (11), and cyclic AMP (cAMP) protein kinase (12), although at concentrations usually much higher than those reported for cyclooxygenase inhibition (6). In vitro responses obtained with these drugs do not correlate with equivalent in vivo responses; in addition, a number of in vitro studies with these drugs performed using concentrations exceeding those selective for cyclooxygenase require careful interpretation. It is insufficient to ascribe the effects that result from addition of a PG cyclooxygenase inhibitor to PGs unless evidence is available to show that addition of PGs reverses the effect of the inhibitor. Inhibition of the cyclooxygenase pathway may also result in increased substrate availability for conversion to products of the lipoxygenase pathways (13). Consequently, increased synthesis of the latter products may also contribute to the effects of cyclooxygenase inhibition. Finally, inhibitors of PG synthesis may alter immune reactivity indirectly by altering cells not primarily involved in the immune response.

What appears to be a homogeneous group of drugs with a defined mechanism of action therefore is clearly not so. Fortunately, many of the studies reported have used relatively few examples of this class of drug, namely, indomethacin, aspirin, and flubiprofen, allowing comparison among studies. The use of other PG cyclooxygenase inhibitors should also be considered since differences in the duration, site, and even mode of action of these drugs have been described (14).

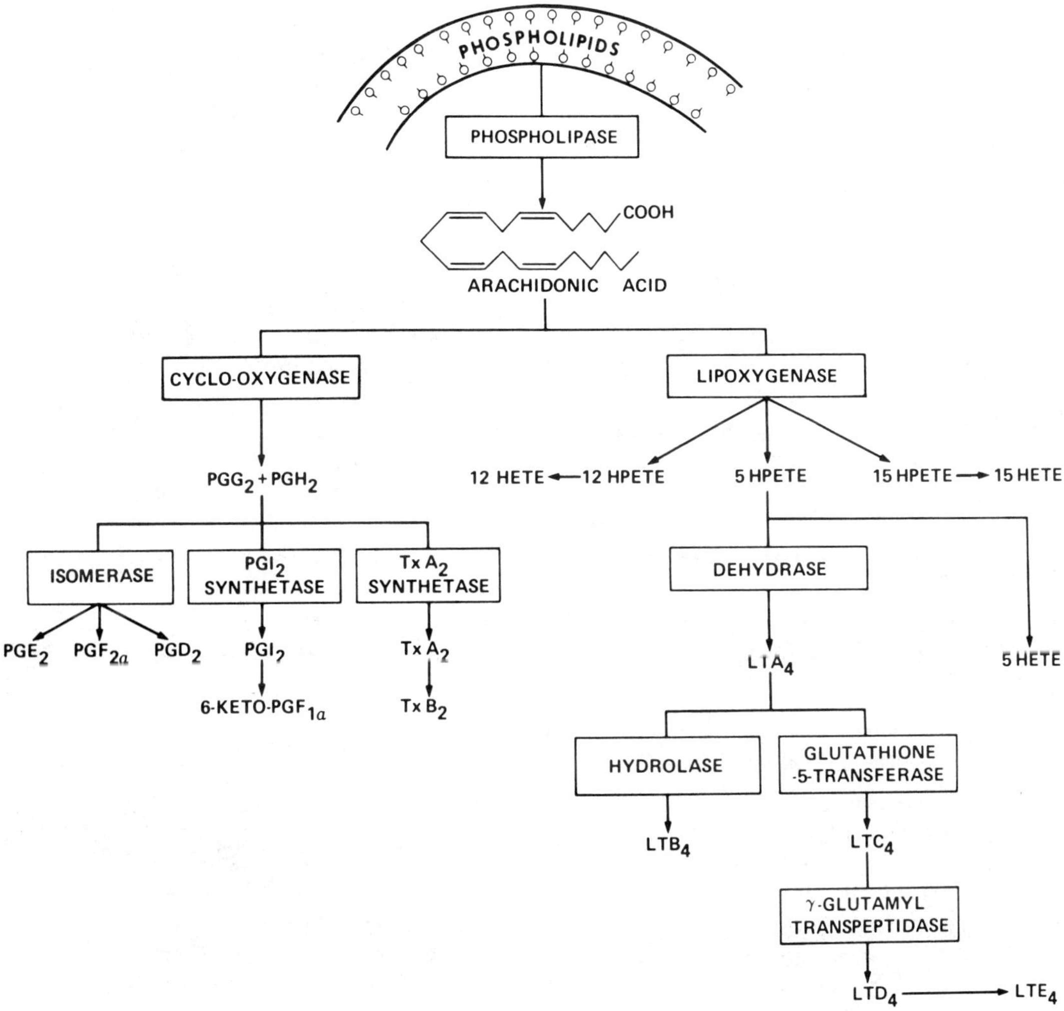

Figure 1 Pathways of AA metabolism.

III. AA METABOLISM

The pathways of AA metabolism are shown in Fig. 1. It is generally accepted that the principal source of AA is phospholipids which are structural components of cell membranes (15-17). The synthesis of PGs and leukotrienes is activated by the initial release of free AA from phospholipid stores (18,19). Recent evidence suggests that liberation of AA involves enzymatic methylation of phospholipids and the action of phospholipases (20, 21). The phospholipase which is clearly important in several tissues is phospholipase A_2 (15), which cleaves most AA-containing phospholipids at the 2-position. In addition, more recent evidence suggests that, especially in mast cells and platelets, the sequential action of a phosphatidyl inositol-specific phospholipase C and diglyceride lipase may lead to AA availability (22-24). The relative contribution of this pathway to the overall substrate availability is still unclear although it has been shown that the release of AA from diacylglycerol corresponds to the rate of synthesis of AA metabolites (24). Generation of free AA results in the triggering of PG (4) and leukotriene synthesis (5). The cyclooxygenase catalyzes the addition of molecular oxygen to the fatty acid and cyclizes it to the unstable intermediate, PGG_2. This is converted to PGH_2, which subsequently isomerizes enzymatically, or nonenzymatically, to the classic PGs, PGE_2, $PGF_{2\alpha}$, and PGD_2. Concurrently, malondialdehyde and 12-hydroxy 5,8,10, heptadecatrienoic acid (HHT) are also formed. In certain tissues, the endoperoxides are also transformed to TxA_2 and PGI_2 and, unlike PGE_2, $PGE_{2\alpha}$, and PGD_2, these products are rapidly degraded to TxB_2 and 6-keto-$PGF_{1\alpha}$.

In addition to the cyclooxygenase pathway, the existence of a second major pathway has been revealed by which lipoxygenases catalyze the transformation of AA (5). Lipoxygenases have been found to be present in platelets, leukocytes, leukemic basophils, and lung (25-27). Although chemical oxidation of AA can give rise to six possible isomers of hydroperoxy eicosatetraenoic acids (HPETEs), lipoxygenase enzyme-catalyzed reactions, depending on cell type, can only generate 5-, 12-, 15-, and 11-HPETE. The 5-HPETE isomer has been shown to be further metabolized to the recently characterized leukotrienes (29,30). The enzymatic conversion of 5-HPETE results in the unstable epoxide, LTA_4 (31). LTA_4 is either hydrated enzymatically to form 5,12 diHETE (LTB_4) (32), or through the action of glutathione-S-transferase, is linked to glutathione at the C-6 position to form 5-hydroxy-6-sulfido-glutathionyl-eicosetetraenoic acid (LTC_4), (33-35). Through the removal of glutamic acid, catalyzed by γ-glutamyl-transpeptidase, LTC_4 is converted to LTD_4 (36), which may undergo further degradation to yield LTE_4.

IV. PRODUCTION OF AA METABOLITES BY TUMOR CELLS, MACROPHAGES, AND LYMPHOCYTES

A. Tumors

Both human and animal solid and metastasizing tumors are capable of synthesizing large amounts of PGs, although the cellular origin is uncertain (37-39). Macrophages and other leukocytes have been implicated as major sources of PG production (see Sec. IV.B). The type of PG synthesized is also highly variable (40). In humans, elevated PGs (largely PGE_2 and $PGF_{2\alpha}$), or PG-like material have been reported for tumors of the large bowel (41,45,46), breast (42,43), lung, pancreas (44), thyroid (45,46), kidney (47), and squamous carcinomas of the head and neck (48). An increased level of PGE_2 production by human breast cancer has been correlated with metastasis to bone (42) suggesting that PGs play a role in tumor spreading. In contrast, PGD_2 and PGE_2 formation by malignant melanoma cells (38) and rat mammary carcinoma (49), respectively, correlates inversely with metastatic potential. Since adherence of platelets to circulating tumor cells has been suggested as a means to initiate a metastatic focus, the antimetastatic effects of PGs may be a result of their ability to inhibit platelet aggregation (also see Sec. VIII).

Elevated PG levels are not always found in human cancer (50). For example, PGE_2 equivalents correlated with the extent of inflammation and necrosis but not with tumor size, site, or degree of differentiation in human squamous carcinoma of the head and neck (48).

PG production by tumors is also implicated in increased bone resorption and hypercalcemia that are commonly associated with cancer. Bone resorption by PGs is well established (51-54), and elevated plasma PGE_2 levels have been demonstrated in hypercalcemic patients (55,56). However, PG production is not always observed in hypercalcemia (57), and tumor PG production is not always associated with hypercalcemia (58).

B. Macrophages and Lymphocytes

The synthesis of PG and related lipids by macrophages has been shown to occur extensively in a variety of macrophage populations and was recently reviewed by Goldyne and Stobo (59). The variety of different substances that stimulate AA metabolism in these cells include zymosan particles (60), immune complexes (61), tumor promoters [e.g., tetradecanoyl phorbol acetate (TPA)] (62), neutral proteases (63), Fc fragments (64), and endotoxin (65). The major PGs include PGE_2, PGI_2, and TxA_2. Despite the variety of factors capable of stimulating in vitro PG synthesis by macrophages, significant variations occur in the capacity of different populations of macrophages to synthesize PG (66). In fact, within the same cell type such as human peripheral blood monocytes, subpopulations of monocytes possess different capacities to synthesize PGE_2 (67).

Furthermore, macrophages show quantitative differences in their capacity to synthesize AA metabolites depending on the source of free AA. For example, Scott et al. (68) showed that resting macrophages exposed to exogenous AA synthesized far more hydroxy-arachidonic acid than zymosan-activated macrophages, whereas the reverse is true in terms of PGE_2 synthesis. These observations may have some relevance in monocyte-lymphocyte interactions since it has also been shown that lymphocytes which do not synthesize significant amounts of AA metabolites can release free AA during mitogen stimulation (69,70). One may expect, therefore, that in in vivo situations where the two cell types exist in close proximity lymphocytes could provide the necessary substrate for synthesis of PGE_2 and other AA metabolites by the neighboring monocyte. This interaction could essentially provide a regulatory mechanism in cell-mediated immunity.

Recent discoveries of the leukotrienes have led to several studies involving macrophages. It now appears that macrophages are also capable of synthesizing LTC_4 and the mono-HETES in response to zymosan or A23187 (71-73). Interestingly, Humes et al. (74) have shown that LTC_4 formation is not tightly coupled to PGE_2 release. Using different stimuli, they showed that although zymosan phagocytosis stimulated both lipoxygenase and cyclooxygenase pathway, LPS and TPA selectively stimulated PGE_2 synthesis. Thus, despite the variety of factors capable of stimulating LTC_4 synthesis by macrophages, some specificity in the nature of the stimuli exists.

V. THE MODULATORY ROLE OF PGs IN THE IMMUNE RESPONSE

In 1971, Parker and co-workers (75) demonstrated that PG increased intracellular cAMP and depressed phytohemagglutinin (PHA)-induced lymphocyte transformation. The ability of PGs to modify cyclic nucleotide levels in lymphocytes has provided a basis for considering PGs as physiological modulators of immunity (76,77). However, the role of PGs and other AA metabolites in immunoregulation is complicated by many factors. The heterogeneous sets of cells involved in immune surveillance (T, B lymphocytes, monocytes-macrophages) appear capable of synthesizing and also responding to a number of these AA metabolites. Multifold interactions between these cells plus both positive and negative feedback signals complicate their involvement in cellular and humoral immune responses. It is, therefore, not surprising that both immunological enhancement and suppression have been reported for PGs. This is very much dependent on assay conditions. For example, species, age, sex, strain, biorhythm, nutritional status, environmental conditions, and concurrent infection of the animal used, as well as the dose, route, duration, and time of administration of the PG, will help determine the experimental outcome.

Diverse pharmacological activity and lability also add to difficulties in defining a specific role for these AA metabolites in regulating immune reactivity.

Before discussing the evidence that suggests a major regulatory role for PGs in the immune response it should be noted that, in addition, these substances may play a central role in initiation and regulation of those diseases classified as cancer (78). For example, a number of reactive AA metabolites and their intermediates (e.g., malondialdehyde) are capable of covalent attachment to DNA, an event that contributes to spontaneous carcinogenesis (79). These metabolites may oxidatively convert noncarcinogenic compounds such as benz(a)pyrene, benzanthracene, and benzidine to carcinogens (80-82). PGs are also thought to play an important role in tumor promotion without being tumor promoters per se (78). For example, the mechanism of tumor promotion by substances such as TPA, although well established, has been attributed to its ability to enhance PG levels in a variety of tissues (40).

A. Lymphocytes

Numerous studies have implicated a regulatory role for PGs on lymphocytes. PGE has been shown to be capable of modulating many functions of both the efferent and afferent limbs of the immune response.

The addition of PGE to thymocytes in vitro produces an increase in thymocyte cAMP levels which leads to thymocyte differentiation (83,84). Additionally, the induction of T-cell differentiation by PGE is also indicated in experiments where the expression of T-cell differentiation marker Thy 1 was examined. Under these conditions, it was shown that marker expression was enhanced (85).

One of the most commonly measured parameters for lymphocyte activation is the proliferative response to mitogen and antigen. Much of the earlier work that showed inhibition of T-cell proliferation by PGE employed pharmacological concentrations of PGs which were not normally found in the cellular environment (75,86,87). More recent work, however, suggests that lymphocyte proliferation can be inhibited at more physiological concentrations, although the degree of inhibition was very much dependent on the mitogen concentration (88-94). Inhibition of 0-75% has been reported in the presence of PGE, and it has been argued that such diverging results may be the consequence of variability in cell division, PG content of sera used in cultures, PG binding to protein, or the number of lymphocytes. Several studies have also shown that PGE inhibition of blast transformation is a time-dependent event. Addition of PGE to cultures at the same time as antigen or shortly thereafter resulted in maximal inhibition of cell-mediated immunity. The continued presence of PGE is required for inhibition since removal of PGE from the culture allowed the proliferative response to proceed.

Several mechanisms have been proposed to account for the inhibitory activity of PGE. Current understanding of the regulation of cell-mediated immunity involves the interactions of suppressor macrophages, T suppressor (T_s), and T helper (T_h) cells. Under certain conditions where it is known that macrophage-mediated suppression predominates, PGE is believed to be the macrophage product responsible for the suppression of lymphocyte activation (95-97). Consistent with this hypothesis is the observation that macrophages constitute the major cell type involved in PGE synthesis (see Sec. IV). Indeed, removal of a glass-adherent cell population from lymphocyte cultures enhances the mitogenic response with a concomitant decrease in PGE levels (97). What is not known, however, is whether macrophage-mediated suppression is a direct or indirect phenomenon. There appears to be a subpopulation of T_s cells that is sensitive to activation by PGE which may be derived from macrophages (98,99).

Although lymphocyte proliferation is universally used as an index of lymphocyte activation, certain aspects of lymphocyte activity may not be associated with the proliferative response. For example, lymphokine production by lymphocytes is independent of blast transformation. In these systems PGE caused significant inhibition of certain lymphokines but not others. Production of migration-inhibitory factor is inhibited (100, 101), but osteoclast-activating factor is unaffected (102).

There are a few reports implicating PGE in the role of cytotoxicity. PGE has been shown to inhibit the ability of cytotoxic T cells to specifically lyse tumor target cells (103). Addition of PGE at the time of the primary sensitization of spleen cells in culture results in inhibition of cellular cytotoxicity on day 4 of culture (104). Further investigations have revealed that primary cytotoxic T cells (generated during the proliferative response to antigen) are more sensitive to PGE than secondary cytotoxic T cells (105). Thus, it appears that PGE modulates the induction of a T-cell population more efficiently than the effector function of these cells. This hypothesis is supported by the work of Plaut (106) who showed that the lytic activity of effector cells generated in vitro was unaffected by PGE, whereas cytotoxic lymphocytes generated in vivo were inhibited.

A third population of T cells that is affected by PGE is natural killer (NK) cells (107). It is increasingly evident that these cells play an important role in immunosurveillance against neoplastic cells. Brunda et al. have recently shown that PGE caused marked suppression of NK activity (108). Both spontaneous and interferon (IFN)-induced NK activity was inhibited. However, Kendall and Targan (109) showed that, depending on the type of target cells, PGE at physiological concentrations can either inhibit or enhance NK activity. Furthermore, the time of PGE addition was once again critical such that addition of PGE during cellular induction resulted in inhibition of the lysis whereas addition after completion of full express of NK activity produced enhancement (110,111).

Several studies have demonstrated modulation of the humoral arm of immunity by PGE (112-114). First indications of the effects of PGE on antibody production came from the work of Webb and Nowowiejski in vivo (113). They showed that PGE levels produced by spleen cells correlated with the number of PFC cells from mice immunized with a T-dependent antigen [sheep red blood cells (SRBC)]. Antibody production is enhanced when PGE is administered early but inhibited when PGE is given during the late stages of antibody production (115). Taken together these observations would suggest that the final expression of humoral immunity (i.e., antibody production) is controlled and regulated at different steps which may not respond in a similar manner to PGE.

In vivo PGE_1 reduced adjuvant disease and hemagglutination titers to SRBCs without suppressing delayed hypersensitivity (DH) to purified protein derivative (PPD) in rats (116), suggesting PGE_1 might be immunosuppressive via B lymphocytes. Furthermore, PGE_1 did not affect homograft rejection in mice, yet depleted splenic B lymphocytes (112).

B. Macrophages

Macrophages play a pivotal role in regulating immune reactivity (117). In contrast to T cells or B cells, macrophages are neither clonally restricted nor antigen specific, but function as nonspecific accessory cells. They present antigen to lymphocytes and participate as accessory cells in both limbs of the immune response.

Since macrophages are known to secrete large amounts of PGE (see Sec. IV.B), several studies have been devoted to an investigation of the effects of PGE on macrophages from various sources. In most studies, PGE inhibited macrophage activities such as lysosomal enzyme release (118), phagocytosis (119,120), chemotaxis, spreading, and adherence (121). This may partially be attributed to a direct effect on macrophage membranes rather than through a rise in cAMP levels. Macrophage colony formation induced by colony-stimulating factors (CSF) is also inhibited by PGE, and it has been suggested that there is a bidirectional link between CSF and PGE production by macrophages (122-124). Apart from CSF, PGE may also serve as a feedback regulator of macrophage activity in response to other stimuli. For example, during zymosan stimulation, PGE inhibited zymosan induction of phagocytosis and chemiluminescence (125).

One area of macrophage activity which is receiving increasing attention is the role of macrophages in tumor cell killing. A large variety of agents have the ability to arm macrophages for tumoricidal activity. Schultz et al. (126) recently postulated that PGE may act as a negative feedback regulator of macrophage tumoricidal activity. When PGE was added simultaneously with IFN to resting macrophages, the IFN induction of tumoricidal macrophages was inhibited. Inhibition was achieved even when added after macrophage activation, suggesting that the modulation involved later events. This work has been confirmed and extended by Taffet and Russell (127) who showed that endogenously produced PGE can inhibit macrophage-mediated tumoricidal activity. It was further shown that PGE did not completely block the induction of cytolytic activity, and for PGE to be effective, mitogen preincubation was required. Interestingly, more recent work indicates that a lymphokine lowers the response threshold of macrophages (i.e., reducing the sensitivity of activated macrophages to PGE) (128).

C. PGs as Inhibitors of Tumor Growth

Although the evidence so far presented implicates PGs in the irritation and enhancement of tumor growth and further describes the largely beneficial effect of PG synthesis by cyclooxygenase inhibitors, there are also claims which suggest PGs limit tumor growth. Exogenous PGs and their synthetic analogs inhibit growth of animal and human tumors both in vivo and in vitro (129-131). Clinical evaluation of the PGs has not been encouraging; for example, administration of PGE_2, PGA_1, and PGA_2 was ineffective in patients with breast cancer and leukemia (131). Indeed, the suggestion has been made than an inhibitor of PG synthesis given in combination with a PG or analog might prove to be an optimal preparation for cancer chemotherapy. However, this has not been substantiated experimentally.

A similar paradox is apparent when one considers the role of PGs in inflammation. Both pro- and anti-inflammatory actions are exerted by the products of AA metabolism (132). PGs are mediators of the early stages of inflammation causing vasodilatation and increased capillary permeability. However, as the inflammation progresses to a chronic form, PGs may exert more of a protective function regulating lymphocyte activation and granuloma formation.

VI. EFFECTS OF CYCLOOXYGENASE INHIBITORS ON THE IMMUNE RESPONSE

From the above sections it is to be expected that cyclooxygenase inhibitors will reverse many of the numerous immunological effects of the PGs. However, as discussed earlier, these drugs possess activities other than inhibition of PG synthesis and consequently the effects resulting from their administration are not always those expected.

In general, indomethacin augments lymphocyte proliferation, although tremendous variation exists in the degree of enhancement (89,91,133). The effects of indomethacin on T-cell proliferation seem critically dependent on the dose of mitogen. For example, several investigators reported that indomethacin at 1 μg/ml enhanced blast transformation only when suboptimal concentrations of mitogen were used. Indeed, when T-cell responses from 18 people were compared, indomethacin either inhibited or enhanced the mitogenic response at a particular concentration of mitogen (91). Such diverging results may be explained in terms of indomethacin having more than just PG-inhibitory activity, although this is unlikely since aspirin and Ro 20-5720 (structurally unrelated cyclooxygenase inhibitors) also cause significant increased blast transformation at concentrations comparable with those affecting PG synthesis. The effects of indomethacin on lymphocytes isolated from patients suffering from Hodgkin's disease (134), sarcoidosis (135), rheumatoid arthritis (136), and aging people (137) have also been studied. The in vitro depressed cell-mediated immunity in these patients has been shown to be reversed in the presence of indomethacin.

Macrophages, as discussed earlier, constitute the major PG-producing cells among immune cells, and current concepts seem to indicate that pharmacological intervention by indomethacin in the immune response is targeted at cells of the monocytic lineage. Indeed, where macrophage suppressor activity is known to regulate lymphocyte proliferation, indomethacin is a potent inhibitor of the suppressive effect of macrophages (138). In contrast, T_s cell-mediated suppression is unaffected by indomethacin (i.e., the effector function of T_s cells is not inhibited). More recent evidence, however, suggests that the induction of T_s cells may also be affected by cyclooxygenase inhibitors. Orme and Shand (98) have found that concanavalin A (ConA)-induced suppressor T cells were sensitive to indomethacin and meclofenamic acid, but only when added concomitantly with ConA. Incubation of T cells and ConA for a few days gives rise to a suppressor cell population which is no longer sensitive to indomethacin or meclofenamic acid. This would suggest that, unlike macrophage-mediated suppression, T_s cell functions can only be altered by cyclooxygenase inhibitors during the early stages of a primary immune response when the T cells are relatively undifferentiated (99).

The effects of indomethacin on lymphokine production have also been investigated. The data indicate that both indomethacin and Ro 20-5720 inhibited the production of osteoclast-activating factor and vascular permeability factor (101,102). On the other hand, the synthesis of migration-inhibitory factor was enhanced in the presence of indomethacin. Thus, it appears that indomethacin has differential effects on lymphokine production.

Cyclooxygenase inhibitors have been examined in a number of models of delayed hypersensitivity with varying results depending on the antigen, species, and time of administration. For example, they have been shown to suppress methylated bovine serum albumin (MBSA) response in mice (139) and *Bordetella pertussis* responses in rats (140) and tuberculin-induced DH in guinea pigs (141); however, these effects were obtained using high doses and were often not dose related.

Both in vivo and in vitro data indicate that cyclooxygenase inhibitors can modulate B-cell reactivity (113,114,142). Both indomethacin and Ro 20-5720 produce an enhancement of the in vivo anti-SRBC IgM and IgG plaque-forming cell (PFC) response (143, 144). Since the effect was not observed early in the response, it has been suggested that drug treatment affected the later regulation of differentiation and proliferation. However, when the PFC response was induced by a soluble antigen such as chicken serum albumin in Freund's complete adjuvant (FCA), indomethacin treatment produced a long-lasting depression of antibody production. In contrast, when chicken serum albumin was administered in the absence of FCA, indomethacin and Ro-2920 enhanced the subsequent antibody response. Further, indomethacin treatment enhanced the PFC response to a chicken lysozyme-lipolysaccharide but did not greatly affect the PFC response to pneumococcal polysaccharide. These results suggest that cyclooxygenase inhibitors can both inhibit or enhance B reactivity. Such contrasting observations may be explained by the fact that the net antibody production is the result of T-cell, B-cell, and monocyte interactions, and the relative contribution of each cell leading to antibody production varies with the antigen. Cyclooxygenase inhibitors have also been demonstrated to inhibit the development of IFN-induced antiviral state (145); furthermore, IFN stimulates PG synthesis (146,147).

VII. EFFECTS OF CYCLOOXYGENASE INHIBITORS ON TUMORS

The provocative effects of PG cyclooxygenase inhibition on tumor growth has been the subject of a number of recent reviews. In view of the complex modulatory role of PGs described in Sec. V, and the ill-defined immune involvement in many different types of cancers, it would be astonishing to expect that these drugs should have a uniform effect. Nevertheless, the majority of studies performed in vivo have demonstrated that cyclooxygenase inhibitors inhibit tumor growth (Table 2). A number of studies show minor inhibition or no effect (148-152), and one study reported that development of tumors was hastened by indomethacin (152). Most studies measure only tumor size. This may be insufficient evidence of a beneficial effect of drug therapy since the drug may actually increase tumor cell proliferation without affecting tumor size or weight. A smaller tumor size after cyclooxygenase inhibitors may also simply be a reflection of a reduced inflammatory response and does not necessarily indicate a direct influence on tumor cell proliferation.

Metastatic spread and survival appears to be either inhibited or not influenced by cyclooxygenase inhibitors (Table 2).

The mechanism of anticancer activity of PG cyclooxygenase inhibitors is not known. The well-known anti-inflammatory actions of these agents with concomitant reduction in vascularity and disruption of energy supplies to the tumor site seem to play a minor role. Tumor-mediated suppression of cell-mediated and humoral immune responses is well established. It has been postulated that reducing tumor PG production should have a profound effect on tumor growth by reducing PG-induced inhibition of the immune response (158). Indeed, tumor-mediated suppression of cell-mediated and humor immune responses can be reversed by treatment of the host with cyclooxygenase inhibitors (158, 164). However, in one of the latter studies (164) no effect was observed on tumor growth.

Cyclooxygenase inhibitors prevent platelet aggregation, and it has been implied that metastatic spread is associated with platelet aggregability (see Sec. VIII). Finally, Bennett (170) has also suggested that, as in the gastric mucosa, tumor cell PGs possess a cytoprotective function and prevent attack by the host's immune response.

An intriguing form of tumor therapy is the combination of a cyclooxygenase inhibitor and conventional chemotherapy. Studies in animals and humans have shown that administration of cyclooxygenase inhibitors, when resistance to conventional chemotherapy has developed, is effective against tumors. Tumor sensitivity has been restored

Table 2 Effect of Cyclooxygenase Inhibitors on Experimental Tumors[a]

Species	Tumor	Drug	Effect on tumor size			Ref.
			1°	2°	Survival	
Rat	Walker carcinoma	Indo, Asp	↓	0	–	153
Mouse	MCA6 ascites sarcoma T 241 sarcoma Mammary carcinoma	Asp	–	↓	–	154
Mouse	Fibrosarcoma HSDM	Indo	↓	–	–	155
Mouse	Malony sarcoma	Indo	↓	–	–	156
Mouse	Malony sarcoma	Indo	↓	–	0	157
Mouse	MC16	Indo	↓	–	–	158
Mouse	P815 mast cell ascites	Asp,	↓	–	0	159
		Indo	↓	–	0	159
	Lewis lung carcinoma	Asp	↓	–	–	159
Rabbit	VX2 carcinoma	Indo	0	slight	0	160
Mouse	McC3-I	Indo	↓	–	↑	161
Mouse	NC mammary carcinoma	Indo	↓	0	↑	162
		Flur	↓	0	↑	162
Mouse	Lewis lung carcinoma	Flur	0	0	–	163
	B16 melanoma		–	0	–	163
	Sarcoma 180		slight	↓	–	163
Mouse	Lewis lung carcinoma	Indo	0	–	0	164
		Flur	0	–	0	164
		Fentiazac	0	–	0	164
Mouse	Sarcoma 180	Indo	0	–	–	148
Mouse	B16 melanoma	Indo	0[b]	–	–	151
Mouse	B16 melanoma	Indo	↓[b]	–	–	130
Mouse	NC mammary carcinoma	Indo	–	–	0	165
		Flur	–	–	0	165

[a]↓, reduction; ↑, enhancement; 0, no effect; Indo, indomethacin; Asp, aspirin, Flur; Flurbiprofen.
[b]Increase in nontumor cells observed.

when indomethacin or flurbiprofen was administered to rat tumors made resistant to chlorambucil (167,168). Similarly, melphalan and methotrexate were ineffective against tumor size or survival time following excision of NC carcinoma in mice, yet survival time was increased when flurbiprofen was administered with chemotherapy to animals with resected primary tumors (169,170). Flurbiprofen appeared to reduce the recurrence of tumor growth at the site of excision, whereas individual therapeutic regimens were ineffective (169). However, flurbiprofen did not protect against the toxic effects of chemotherapy (165), although indomethacin apparently reduced the toxicity of methotrexate on gut and bone in rats (167,168). These beneficial effects of cyclooxygenase inhibitors were not observed when flurbiprofen was administered to animals also receiving cyclophosphamide, suggesting that the form of chemotherapy may be important (171).

In contrast to these favorable effects of cyclooxygenase inhibitors administered in combination with chemotherapy, Hofer et al. (152) have reported that indomethacin had no additional beneficial effect after chemotherapy was administered to mice receiving B16 melanoma. These studies have been criticized on the grounds of experimental variation and questionable interpretation (166).

The above data using animals suggest that cyclooxygenase inhibitors may prove to be of value as adjuvants in cancer, but human trials, currently in progress for flurbiprofen, are sorely needed before this form of therapy can be recommended as safe and efficacious.

VIII. THE ROLE OF MISCELLANEOUS ARACHIDONIC ACID METABOLITES IN THE IMMUNE RESPONSE AND TUMOR GROWTH

Recent interest has been aroused concerning the role of TxA_2, PGI_2, HETEs, and leukotrienes in modulating the immune response. Several reports have described the effects of TxA_2 and PGI_2 synthesis inhibitors on the immune response (172-175). It has been proposed that PGI_2 is a negative regulator and TxA_2 a positive regulator of lymphocyte activation (173). A major concern of these studies is that several of the putative TxA_2 inhibitors may not be as specific as originally thought (174). They may affect the synthesis of other arachidonic acid metabolites as well as having non-PG effects at higher concentrations. For example, imidazole, which is frequently used as a TxA_2 inhibitor, also inhibits carbonic anhydrase (176), stimulates phosphodiesterase (177), and affects calcium-dependent processes (178). Thus, whereas Kelly et al. (172) found imidazole and L8027 to inhibit lymphocyte proliferation, other investigators using several TxA_2 inhibitors of varying specificity failed to correlate specificity of Tx inhibition with the inhibition of mitogen response (174). Similarly, the evidence supporting the notion PGI_2 is a negative regulator of the immune response is based solely on the observation that tranylcypromine, a putative PGI_2 inhibitor, augmented lymphocyte proliferation (173). Clearly, if these inhibitors are to be used to support the role of a particular PG, it is necessary to show that the modification is not in fact a result of increasing or decreasing the synthesis of other PGs potentially synthesized by the system under study.

The second group of arachidonic acid metabolites that may potentially influence the immune response are the products of the lipoxygenase pathway. Preliminary observations from various laboratories have already indicated that 15-HPETE, 15-HETE, LTD_4, and LTE_4 inhibit the lymphocyte response to PHA and lipopolysaccharide (LPS) (179-181). LTD_4 and LTE_4 were nearly 1000 times more potent than PGE_2 as inhibitors of proliferation. Although 15-HPETE and 15-HETE are not as potent, it is believed that the inhibition of lymphocyte proliferation by these agents is irreversible.

Paradoxically, inhibitors of the lipoxygenase pathway such as NDGA and ETYA also blocked lymphocyte activation (172). This conflicting result may once again be explained by the inadequate specificity of these agents. More recently, BW 755C, which inhibits both the cyclooxygenase and lipoxygenase pathways, has been shown to enhance and suppress lymphocyte activation of low and high doses, respectively (182). Since the concentrations of BW 755C used were lower than those reported to affect arachidonic acid metabolism, it was suggested that this property of BW 755C may be unrelated to arachidonic acid metabolism.

Honn et al. (186) have recently proposed that the balance between TxA_2/PGI_2 plays a critical role in tumor metastasis. Current concepts regarding these particular arachidonic acid metabolites suggest they are involved in the regulation of platelet homeostasis since TxA_2 has been shown to be a potent aggregating substance while PGI_2 when released from the endothelial cells prevents the aggregation of platelets. Several tumor cell types have been shown to have the capacity to aggregate platelets (185), and disseminated neoplasia is closely related to thromboembolic disease (185). Taken together, it is suggested that an imbalance favoring the formation of TxA_2 could lead to the spread of tumor malignancy. This hypothesis is supported by the observation that PGI_2 produces a dose-related reduction in experimental metastasis of the B16a melanoma (186). Metastases to the liver and spleen were also reduced, suggesting that the decrease in metastasis was not a result of tumor cell redistribution. The combination of theophylline and PGI_2 potentiated the antimetastatic activity of PGI_2 supporting the concept the cAMP regulates cell proliferation. The amelioration of tumor metastasis was also achieved when nafazatrom, a new antimetastatic agents, was administered to animals bearing B16 tumors. Subsequent work with this agent suggests that it could be acting through enhancement of PGI_2 synthesis (187) or through the inhibition of lipoxygenase (188). It is interesting to note that 15-HPETE exacerbates the metastatic process. Although it has been claimed that 15-HPETE acts through the inhibition of PGI_2 synthesis more recent evidence indicates that this arachidonic acid metabolite could also act through the inhibition of lipoxygenease activity (189).

Several TxA_2 synthesis inhibitors such as U51605, U54071, and U54874 were shown to be effective antimetastatic agents (183). These agents were effective in inhibiting 60% of the pulmonary metastasis from subcutaneous B16 melanoma and Lewis lung carcinoma tumors, and this suggests that endogenous TxA_2 production by the tumor cells is indeed a signal for proliferation.

IX. SUMMARY

Considerable multidisciplinary interest has been generated concerning the role of PGs in the initiation and growth of tumors in the last decade. The value of cyclooxygenase inhibitors as adjuvants in the treatment of cancer needs to be confirmed in order to extend some initial encouraging findings in animals. Clearly the therapeutic importance of manipulating PGs in cancer and immunity will be an area of considerable interest in the future. However, the next decade for prostaglandinologists is likely to be spent establishing the biological importance of the newly discovered leukotrienes. The immune reactivity of these arachidonic acid metabolites is not yet defined and their interaction with the PGs will no doubt further complicate the already highly complex series of events that makes up the immune response.

ACKNOWLEDGMENT

We would like to thank Mary Ludovici and Maritza Salicrup for their help during the preparation of this manuscript.

REFERENCES

1. J. R. Vane, *Nature* (*New Biol.*), *231*:232 (1971).
2. S. H. Ferreira, S. Moncada, and J. R. Vane, *Nature* (*New Biol.*), *231*:237 (1971).
3. J. B. Smith and A. L. Willis, *Nature* (*New Biol.*), *231*:235 (1971).
4. R. J. Flower, *Pharmacol. Rev.*, *26*:33 (1976).
5. P. J. Piper, *SRS-A and Leukotrienes*, Research Studies Press, Chichester, 1981.

6. R. Nickander, F. G. McMahon and A. S. Ridolfo, *Ann. Rev. Pharmacol. Toxicol.*, *19*:469 (1979).
7. J. R. Vane, R. J. Flower, and J. A. Salmon, in *Prostaglandins and Cancer: First International Conference* (T. J. Powles, R. S. Bockman, K. V. Honn, and P. Ramwell, eds.), A. R. Liss, New York, 1982, pp. 21-45.
8. D. M. Bailey and L. W. Chakrin, *Ann. Rep. Med. Chem.* (H. J. Hess, ed.), Academic Press, New York, 1981, pp. 213-228.
9. B. F. Sloane, S. Makin, J. R. Dunn, R. Lacoste, M. Theodorou, J. Battista, R. Alex, and. K. V. Honn, in *Prostaglandins and Cancer: First International Conference* (T. J. Powles, R. S. Bockman, K. V. Honn, and P. Ramwell, eds.), A. R. Liss, New York, 1982, pp. 789-792.
10. H. S. Hansen, *Prostaglandins*, *12*:647 (1976).
11. A. G. A. Flores and G. W. G. Sharp, *Am. J. Physiol.*, *223*:1392 (1972).
12. H. S. Kantor and M. Hampton, *Nature*, *276*:841 (1978).
13. G. A. Higgs, K. E. Eakins, K. G. Mugridge, S. Moncada,and J. R. Vane, *Eur. J. Pharmacol.*, *66*:81 (1980).
14. D. C. Atkinson, *Agents Actions*, *9*:480 (1979).
15. R. J. Flower and G. J. Blackwell, *Biochem. Pharmacol.*, *25*:285 (1976).
16. B. Haye, S. Champion, and C. Jacquemin. *FEBS Lett.*, *30*:253 (1973).
17. H. Kunze and W. Vogt, *Ann. N.Y. Acad. Sci.*, *180*:123 (1971).
18. G. J. Blackwell, W. G. Duncombe, R. J. Flower, R. J. Parsons, and J. R. Vane, *Br. J. Pharmacol.*, *59*:353 (1977).
19. T. K. Bills, J. B. Smith, and M. J. Silver, *Biochim. Biophys. Acta*, *424*:303 (1976).
20. F. Hirata, J. Axelrod, and F. T. Crews, *Proc. Natl. Acad. Sci. USA*, *76*:4813 (1979).
21. F. Hirata and J. Axelrod, *Science*, *209*:1082 (1980).
22. R. L. Bell, D. A. Kennerly, N. Stanford, and P. W. Majerus, *Proc. Natl. Acad. Sci. USA*, *76*:3238 (1979).
23. D. A. Kennerly, T. J. Sullivan, P. Sylvester, and C. W. Parker, *J. Exp. Med.*, *150*:1039 (1979).
24. S. Rittenhouse, *J. Biol. Chem.*, *255*:2259 (1980).
25. H. Nugteren, *Biochim. Biophys. Acta*, *380*:299 (1975).
26. P. Borgeat and B. Samuelsson, *Proc. Natl. Acad. Sci. USA*, *76*:2148 (1979).
27. B. A. Jakschik, A. Kulczycki, H. H. MacDonald, and C. W. Parker, *J. Immunol.*, *119*: 618 (1977).
28. E. J. Goetzl and F. F. Sun, *J. Exp. Med.*, *150*:406 (1979).
29. P. Borgeat and B. Samuelsson, *Proc. Natl. Acad. Sci. USA*, *76*:3213 (1979).
30. E. J. Corey, Y. Arai, and C. Mioskowski, *J. Am. Chem. Soc.*, *101*:6748 (1979).
31. P. Borgeat and B. Samuelsson, *J. Biol. Chem.*, *254*:2643 (1979).
32. O. Radmark, C. Malmsten, B. Samuelsson, D. A. Clark, G. Goto, A. Marfat, and E. J. Corey, *Biochem. Biophys. Res. Commun.*, *92*:954 (1980).
33. R. C. Murphy, S. Hammarstrom, and B. Samuelsson, *Proc. Natl. Acad. Sci. USA*, *76*:4275 (1979).
34. L. Orning, S. Hammarstrom, and B. Samuelsson, *Proc. Natl. Acad. Sci. USA*, *77*: 2014 (1980).
35. H. R. Morris, G. W. Taylor, P. J. Piper, and J. R. Tippins, *Nature*, *285*:104 (1980).
36. R. A. Lewis, K. F. Austen, J. M. Drazen, P. A. Clark, A. Marfat, and E. J. Corey, *Proc. Natl. Acad. Sci. USA*, *77*:3710 (1980).
37. S. L. Hong, C. M. Wheless, and L. Levine, *Prostaglandins, 13:271* (1977).
38. F. A. Fitzpatrick and D. A. Stringfellow, *Proc. Natl. Acad. Sci. USA*, *76*:1765 (1979).
39. V. A. Poggi, A. Dallolio, G. Balconi, G. De Gaetano, and M. B. Donati, *Thromb. Haemoest.*, *42*:339 (1979).

40. L. Levine, *Adv. Cancer Res.*, *35*:49 (1981).
41. A. Bennett, M. Del Tacca, I. F. Stamford, and T. Zebro, *Br. J. Cancer*, *35*:881 (1977).
42. A. Bennett, J. S. Simpson, A. M. McDonald, and I. F. Stamford, *Lancet*, *2*:1218 (1975).
43. A. Bennett, A. M. McDonald, I. F. Stamford, E. M. Charlier, J. S. Simpson, and T. Zebro, *Lancet*, *1*:624 (1977).
44. M. Sandler, S. M. M. Karim, and E. D. Williams, *Lancet*, *11*:1053 (1968).
45. E. D. Williams, S. M. M. Karim, and M. Sandler, *Lancet*, *1*:22 (1968).
46. E. L. Kaplan, G. W. Sizemore, G. W. Peskin, and B. M. Jaffe, *Surgery*, *74*:21 (1973).
47. R. M. Zusman, J. J. Snider, A. Cline, B. V. Caldwell, and L. Speroff, *N. Engl. J. Med.*, *290*:843 (1974).
48. A. Bennett, R. L. Carter, I. M. F. Stamford, and N. S. B. Tanner, *Br. J. Cancer*, *41*: 204 (1980).
49. W. E. Kibbey, D. G. Brown, and J. P. Minton, *Lancet*, *1*:101 (1978).
50. N. Feller, T. Malachi, and I. Halbrecht, *J. Cancer Res. Clin. Oncol.*, *93*:275 (1979).
51. D. C. Klein and L. G. Raisz, *Endocrinology*, *86*:1436 (1970).
52. G. R. Mundy, in *Prostaglandins and Cancer: First International Conference* (T. J. Powles, R. S. Bockman, K. V. Honn, and P. Ramwell, eds.), A. R. Liss, New York, 1981, pp. 501-511.
53. A. H. Tashjian, E. F. Voelkel, and L. Levine, in *Prostaglandins and Cancer: First International Conference* (T. J. Powles, R. S. Bockman, K. V. Honn, and P. Ramwell, eds.), A. R. Liss, New York, 1981, pp. 513-523.
54. T. J. Martin and N. C. Partridge, in *Prostaglandins and Cancer: First International Conference* (T. J. Powles, R. S. Bockman, K. V. Honn, and P. Ramwell, eds.), A. R. Liss, New York, 1981, pp. 525-540.
55. R. P. Robertson, D. J. Baylink, J. J. Marini, and H. W. Adkinson, *J. Clin. Endocrinol. Metab.*, *41*:164 (1975).
56. R. S. Bockman, W. P. L. Myers, S. C. Kempin, and D. Bajorunas, *Clin. Res.*, *25*:387A (1977).
57. H. W. Seyberth, G. V. Segre, J. L. Morgan, B. J. Sweetman, J. T. Potts, and J. A. Oates, *N. Engl. J. Med.*, *293*:1278 (1975).
58. S. M. M. Karim and B. Rao, in *Advances in Prostaglandin Research* (S. M. M. Karim, ed.), MTP Press, Lancaster, England, 1976, p. 303.
59. M. E. Goldyne and J. D. Stobo, *CRC Crit. Rev. Immunol.*, *2*:189 (1981).
60. R. J. Bonney, P. D. Wightman, P. Davies, S. Sadowski, F. A. Kuehl, Jr., and J. L. Humes, *Biochem. J.*, *176*:433 (1978).
61. K. Brune, M. Glatt, H. Kalin, and H. Peskar, *Nature*, *274*:261 (1978).
62. J. L. Humes, P. Davies, R. J. Bonney, and F. A. Kuehl, Jr., *Fed. Proc.*, *27*:1318 (1978).
63. J. Chang, F. M. Wigley, and D. S. Newcombe, *Proc. Natl. Acad. Sci. USA*, *77*:4736 (1980).
64. J. H. Passwell, J. M. Dayer, K. Gass, and P. J. Edelson, *J. Immunol.*, *125*:910 (1980).
65. L. M. Wahl, C. E. Olsen, S. M. Wahl, J. B. McCarthy, A. L. Sandberg, and S. E. Mergenhagen, *Ann. NY Acad. Sci.*, *332*:271 (1970).
66. J. L. Humes, S. Burger, M. Galavage, F. A. Kuehl, Jr., P. D. Wightman, M. E. Dahlgren, P. Davies, and R. J. Bonney, *J. Immunol.*, *124*:2110 (1980).
67. M. E. Goldyne, M. S. Kennedy, and J. D. Stobo, in *Adv. in PG and Thromboxane Res.*, Vol. 8, (B. Samuelsson, P. W. Ramwell, and R. Paoletti, eds.), 1980, p. 1655.
68. W. A. Scott, N. A. Pawlowski, M. Andreach, and Z. A. Cohn, *J. Exp. Med.*, *155*: 535 (1982).
69. C. W. Parker, J. P. Kelly, S. F. Falkenhein, and M. G. Haber, *J. Exp. Med.*, *149*:1487 (1979).
70. C. W. Parker, *J. Immunol.*, *128*:393 (1982).

71. C. A. Rouzer, W. A. Scott, Z. A. Cohn, P. Blackburn, and J. M. Manning, *Proc. Natl. Acad. Sci. USA*, *77*:4928 (1980).
72. N. A. Pawlowski, W. A. Scott, M. Andreach, and Z. A. Cohn, *J. Exp. Med.*, *155*: 1653 (1982).
73. D. Gemsa, M. Seitz, W. Kramer, W. Grimm, G. Till, and E. Rasch, *Exp. Cell. Res.*, *118*:55 (1979).
74. J. L. Humes, S. Sadowski, M. Galavage, M. Goldenberg, E. Subers, R. J. Bonney, and F. A. Kuehl, Jr., *J. Biol. Chem.*, *257*:1951 (1982).
75. J. W. Smith, A. L. Steiner, W. M. Newberry, and C. W. Parker, *J. Clin. Invest.*, *50*: 432 (1971).
76. L. M. Pelus and H. R. Strausser, *Life Sci.*, *20*:903 (1977).
77. J. S. Goodwin and D. R. Webb, *Clin. Immunol. Immunopathol.*, *15*:106 (1980).
78. K. V. Honn, R. S. Bockman, and L. J. Marnett, *Prostaglandins*, *21*:833 (1981).
79. L. J. Marnett, *Life Sci.*, *29*:531 (1981).
80. J. A. Miller and E. C. Miller, in *Prostaglandins and Cancer: First International Conference* (T. J. Powles, R. S. Bockman, K. V. Honn, and P. Ramwell, eds.), A. R. Liss, New York, 1981, pp. 81-96.
81. J. A. Miller and E. C. Miller, in *Prostaglandins and Cancer: First International Conference* (T. J. Powles, R. S. Bockman, K. V. Honn, and P. Ramwell, eds.), A. R. Liss, New York, 1981, pp. 123-141.
82. T. Eling, J. Boyd, and K. S. Sivarajah, in *Prostaglandins and Cancer: First Inter-National Conference* (T. J. Powles, R. S. Bockman, K. V. Honn, and P. Ramwell, eds.), A. R. Liss, New York, 1981, pp. 123-141.
83. R. Taetle and A. Koessler, *Cancer Res.*, *40*:1223 (1980).
84. R. S. Bockman and M. Rothschild, *J. Clin. Invest.*, *64*:812 (1979).
85. W. Singh and J. J. T. Woen, *Eur. J. Immunol.*, *5*:286 (1975).
86. J. W. Smith, A. L. Steiner, and C. W. Parker, *J. Clin. Invest.*, *50*:442 (1971).
87. T. B. Strom, C. B. Carpenter, M. R. Garavsky, K. F. Austen, J. P. Merrill, and M. Kaliner, *J. Exp. Med.*, *138*:387 (1973).
88. C. C. Muscoplat, D. J. Klausner, C. J. Brunner, E. D. Sloane, and D. W. Johnson, *Infect. Immun.*, *26*:311 (1979).
89. J. S. Goodwin, A. D. Bankhurst, and R. P. Messner, *J. Exp. Med.*, *146*:1719 (1977).
90. T. Sims, J. A. Clagett, and R. C. Page, *Clin. Immunol. Immunopathol.*, *12*:150 (1979).
91. K. M. K. Rao, S. A. Schwartz, and R. A. Good, *Cell. Immunol.*, *48*:155 (1979).
92. A. Novogrodsky, A. L. Rubin, and K. H. Stezzel, *J. Immunol.*, *122*:1 (1979).
93. T. Okazaki, M. Shimuzu, C. E. Arbesman, and E. Middleton, Jr., *Prostaglandins*, *15*:423 (1978).
94. S. Burchiel, *Prostaglandins Med.*, *3*:315 (1979).
95. D. R. Webb and A. T. Jamieson, *Cell. Immunol.*, *24*:45 (1976).
96. D. R. Webb and I. Nowowiejski, *Cell. Immunol.*, *41*:72 (1978).
97. D. R. Webb and I. Nowowiejski, *Cell. Immunol.*, *63*:321 (1981).
98. I. M. Orme and F. L. Shand, *Int. J. Immunopharmacol.*, *3*:15 (1981).
99. A. Fischer, A. Durandy, and C. Griscelli, *J. Immunol.*, *126*:1452 (1981).
100. D. Gordon, M. Bray, and J. Morley, *Nature*, *262*:401 (1976).
101. M. A. Bray, D. Gordon, and J. Morley, *Agents Actions*, *6*:171 (1976).
102. T. Yoneda and G. R. Mundy, *J. Exp. Med.*, *150*:338 (1979).
103. C. S. Henney, H. R. Bourne, and L. M. Lichtenstein, *J. Immunol.*, *108*:1526 (1972).
104. K. H. Leung and E. Mihich, *Int. J. Immunopharmacol.*, *4*:205 (1982).
105. T. L. Darrow and R. H. Tomar, *Cell. Immunol.*, *56*:172 (1980).
106. M. Plaut, *J. Immunol.*, *123*:692 (1977).
107. H. S. Koren, S. J. Anderson, D. G. Fischer, C. S. Copeland, and P. J. Jensen, *J. Immunol.*, *127*:2007 (1981).

108. M. J. Brunda, R. B. Herberman, and H. T. Holden, *J. Immunol.*, *124*:2682 (1980).
109. R. A. Kendall and S. Targan, *J. Immunol.*, *127*:1424 (1981).
110. A. Silva, B. Bonavida, and S. Targan, *J. Immunol.*, *125*:479 (1980).
111. S. R. Targan, *J. Immunol.*, *127*:1424 (1981).
112. F. Quagliata, V. J. W. Lawrence, and T. M. Phillips-Quagliata, *Cell. Immunol.*, *6*: 457 (1973).
113. D. R. Webb and I. Nowowiejski, *Cell. Immunol.*, *33*:1 (1977).
114. D. R. Webb and P. L. Osheroff, *Proc. Natl. Acad. Sci. USA*, *63*:1300 (1976).
115. R. Kishimoto and K. Ishizaka, *J. Immunol.*, *116*:534 (1976).
116. R. B. Zurier and F. Quagliata, *Nature*, *234*:304 (1971).
117. D. S. Nelson, *Immunobiology of the Macrophage*, Academic Press, New York, 1976.
118. J. Schnyder, B. Dewald, and M. Baggiolini, *Prostaglandins*, *22*:411 (1981).
119. E. Razin, S. Bauminger, and A. Globerson, *J. Reticuloendothel. Soc.*, *23*:237 (1977).
120. R. L. Oropeza-Rendon, V. Speth, G. Hiller, K. Weber, and H. Fischer, *Exp. Cell. Res.*, *119*:365 (1979).
121. W. D. Cantarow, H. T. Cheung, and G. Sundharadas, *Prostaglandins*, *16*:39 (1978).
122. J. I. Kurland, P. W. Kincade, and M. A. S. Moore, *J. Exp. Med.*, *146*:1420 (1977).
123. R. G. Cook, A. B. Stavistsky, and H. W. Harold, *Cell. Immunol.*, *40*:128 (1978).
124. L. M. Pelus, H. C. Broxmeyer, J. E. Kurland, and M. A. S. Moore, *J. Exp. Med.*, *150*:277 (1979).
125. M. J. Weidemann, B. A. Peskar, K. Wrogemann, E. T. Reitschel, H. Standinger, and H. Fischer, *FEBS Lett.*, *89*:136 (1978).
126. R. M. Schultz, N. A. Pavlidis, W. A. Stylos, and M. A. Chirigos, *Science*, *202*:320 (1978).
127. S. Taffet and S. W. Russell, *J. Immunol.*, *126*:424 (1981).
128. S. M. Taffet, J. L. Pace, and S. W. Russell, *J. Immunol.*, *127*:121 (1981).
129. M. G. Santoro, G. W. Philpott, and B. M. Jaffe, *Nature*, *263*:777 (1976).
130. P. J. M. Tutton and D. H. Barkla, *Br. J. Cancer*, *41*:47 (1980).
131. T. J. Powles, R. C. Coombes, M. Depledge, J. Muindi, and R. Powles, in *Prostaglandins and Cancer: First International Conference* (T. J. Powles, R. S. Bochman, K. V. Honn, and P. Ramwell, eds.), A. R. Liss, New York, 1981.
131a. M. Fukushima, T. Kato, R. Ueda, K. Ota, S. Narumiya, and D. Hayaishi, *Biochem. Biophys. Res. Commun.*, *105*:956 (1982).
132. I. L. Bonta and M. J. Parnham, *Biochem. Pharmacol.*, *27*:1611 (1978).
133. J. S. Goodwin, R. P. Messner, and G. T. Peake, *J. Clin. Invest.*, *62*:653 (1978).
134. J. S. Goodwin, R. P. Messner, A. D. Bankhurst, G. T. Peake, J. H. Saiki, and R. C. Williams, *N. Engl. J. Med.*, *297*:963 (1977).
135. J. S. Goodwin, R. Dehoratius, H. Israel, G. T. Peake, and R. P. Messner, *Ann. Int. Med.*, *90*:169 (1979).
136. J. Morley, *Prostaglandins*, *8*:315 (1974).
137. J. S. Goodwin and R. P. Messner, *J. Clin. Invest.*, *64*:434 (1979).
138. J. Kemp, D. Louie, J. Mattingly, J. Bennett, C. Higuchi, J. Preteu, M. Horowitz, and R. Gershon, *J. Immunopharmacol.*, *2*:471 (1980).
139. A. J. Lewis, J. Parker, J. Diluigi, L. J. Datko, and R. P. Carlson, *J. Immunopharmacol.* *3*:289 (1981).
140. P. A. Dieppe, D. A. Willoughby, E. C. Huskisson, and E. Arrigoni-Martelli, *Agents Actions*, *6*:618 (1976).
141. R. Wojnar, R. J. Brittain, and E. Dzelzkalns, *J. Pharm. Sci.*, *68*:12 (1979).
142. D. R. Webb and M. Zimecki, *J. Immunol.*, *117*:2158 (1976).
143. J. M. Rojo, I. Barasoain, and A. Lortoles, *Int. J. Clin. Pharmacol. Ther. Toxicol.*, *19*:250 (1981).
144. R. P. Schleimer and E. Benjamini, *Immunopharmacology*, *3*:205 (1981).

145. K. A. Chandrabose, R. Pottahil, E. C. Borden, R. Fox, and P. Cuatrecasas, in *Prostaglandins and Cancer: First International Conference* (T. J. Powles, R. S. Bockman, K. V. Honn, and P. Ramwell, eds.), A. R. Liss, New York, 1981, pp. 345-364.
146. M. Yaron, I. Yaron, D. Rotman Gurari, M. Revel, H. R. Lindner, And U. Zor, *Nature*, *267*:457 (1977).
147. F. A. Fitzpatrick and D. A. Stringfellow, *J. Immunol.*, *125*:431 (1980).
148. J. A. C. Sykes and I. S. Maddox, *Nature* (*New Biol.*), *237*:57 (1972).
149. I. Feher and J. Gidali, *Nature*, *247*:550 (1974).
150. M. Pollard, G. R. Burleson, and P. H. Luckert, in *Cancer Invasion add Metastasis: Biologic Mechanisms and Therapy* (S. B. Day, ed.), Raven Press, New York, 1977, pp. 357-72.
151. C. Favalli, E. Garaci, E. Etheridoe, M. G. Santoro, and B. M. Jaffe, *J. Immunol.*, *125*:897 (1980).
152. D. Hofer, A. M. Dubitsky, P. Reilly, M. G. Santoro, and B. M. Jaffe, *Prostaglandins*, *20*:1033 (1980).
153. T. J. Powles, S. A. Clark, D. M. Easty, G. C. Easty, and A. M. Neville, *Br. J. Cancer*, *28*:316 (1973).
154. G. J. Gasic, T. Gasic, and S. Murphy, *Proc. Am. Assoc. Cancer Res.*, *14*:87 (1973).
155. A. H. Tashjian, E. F. Voelkel, P. Goldhaber, and L. Levine, *Prostaglandins*, *3*:515 (1973).
156. J. L. Humes, J. J. Cupo, and H. R. Strausser, *Prostaglandins*, *6*:463 (1976).
157. H. R. Strausser and J. L. Humes, *Int. J. Cancer*, *15*:724 (1975).
158. O. J. Plescia, A. H. Smith, and K. Grinwich, *Proc. Natl. Acad. Sci. USA*, *72*:1868 (1975).
159. V. Hial, Z. Horakova, R. E. Shaff, and M. A. Beaven, *Eur. J. Pharmacol.*, *37*:367 (1976).
160. C. S. B. Galasko and A. Bennett, *Nature*, *263*:508 (1976).
161. N. R. Lynch, M. Castes, M. Astioin, and J. C. Salomon, *Br. J. Cancer*, *38*:503 (1978).
162. A. Bennett, J. Houghton, D. J. Leaper, and I. F. Stamford, *Prostaglandins*, *17*:179 (1979).
163. K. Hellman and B. A. Pym, in *Prostaglandins and Cancer: First International Conference* (T. J. Powles, R. S. Bockman, K. V. Honn, and P. Ramwell, eds.), A. R. Liss, New York, 1981, pp. 767-776.
164. A. J. Lewis, R. P. Carlson, and F. J. Gregory, *Proc. Am. Assoc. Cancer Res.*, *22*: 273 (1981).
165. A. Bennett, D. A. Berstock, and M. A. Carroll, *Br. J. Cancer*, *45*:762 (1982).
166. A. Bennett, in *Prostaglandins and Cancer: First International Conference* (T. J. Powles, R. S. Bockman, K. V. Honn, and P. Ramwell, eds.), A. R. Liss, New York, 1981, pp. 759-766.
167. T. J. Powles, P. Alexander, and J. L. Miller, *Biochem. Pharmacol.*, *27*:1389 (1978).
168. T. J. Powles and J. L. Millar, *Cancer Treat. Res.* (Suppl.), *6*:63 (1979).
169. D. A. Berstock, J. Houghton, and A. Bennett, *Cancer Treat. Res.* (Suppl.), *6*:69 (1979).
170. A. Bennett, D. A. Berstock, and M. A. Carroll, *Br. J. Pharmacol.*, *71*:2084 (1981).
171. S. E. Heckford, S. A. Eccles, T. J. Powles, and P. Alexander, in *Prostaglandins and Cancer: First International Conference* (T. J. Powles, R. S. Bockman, K. V. Honn, and P. Ramwell, eds.), A. R. Liss, New York, 1981, pp. 815-817.
172. J. P. Kelly, M. C. Johnson, and C. W. Parker, *J. Immunol.*, *122*:1563 (1979).
173. K. H. Leung and E. Mihich, *Nature*, *288*:597 (1980).
174. D. Gordon, A. M. E. Nouri, and R. U. Thomas, *Br. J. Pharmacol.*, *74*:469 (1981).
175. E. Pick, Y. Keisari, A. Jakubowski, Y. Bromberg, and M. Freund, in *Lymphokines and Thymic Hormones: Their Potential Utilization in Cancer Therapeutics*

(A. L. Goldstein and M. A. Chirigos, eds.), Raven Press, New York, 1981, pp. 177-185.
176. H. Wolphert, C. Shader, and R. G. Khalifab, *Biochemistry, 16*:5717 (1977).
177. R. Butcher and E. Sutherland, *J. Biol. Chem., 237*:1244 (1962).
178. K. Nilsson, L. Djarv, and R. Anderson, *Acta Physiol. Scand., 98*:407 (1976).
179. M. G. Goodman and W. O. Weigle, *J. Immunol., 125*:593 (1980).
180. J. M. Bailey, R. W. Bryant, C. E. Low, M. B. Pupillo, and J. Y. Vanderhock, *Cell. Immunol., 67*:112 (1982).
181. D. R. Webb, I. Nowowiejski, C. Healy, and T. J. Rogers, *Biochem. Biophys. Res. Commun., 104*:1617 (1982).
182. A. T. M. Mobarok Ali and J. Morley, *Br. J. Pharmacol., 75*:1628 (1982).
183. G. J. Gasic, T. B. Gasic, N. Galanti, T. Johnson, and S. Murphy, *Int. J. Cancer, 11*:704 (1973).
184. G. H. Sack, Jr., J. Levin, and W. R. Bell, *Medicine, 56*:1 (1977).
185. D. Menter, G. Neagos, J. Dunn, R. Palazzo, T. T. Tchen, J. D. Taylor, and K. V. Honn, in *Prostaglandins and Cancer: First International Conference* (T. J. Powles, R. S. Bockman, K. V. Honn, and P. Ramwell, eds.), A. R. Liss, New York, 1981, pp. 809-813.
186. K. V. Honn, B. Cicone, and A. Skoff, *Science, 212*:1270 (1981).
187. J. Vermylen, D. A. Chamone, and M. Verstraete, *Lancet, i*:518 (1979).
188. K. V. Honn and J. R. Dunn, *FEBS Letts., 139*:65 (1982).
189. J. Y. Vanderhoeck, R. W. Bryant, and J. M. Bailey, *J. Biol. Chem., 255*:5996 (1980)

Index